An Introduction to Neuropathology

For Churchill Livingstone

Publisher Geoff Nuttall
Project Editor Lowri Daniels
Editor Jennifer Bew
Production Controller Mark Sanderson
Promotion Executive Duncan Jones

An Introduction to Neuropathology

J. Hume Adams

DSc MD PhD FRCPath FRCP (Glas.) FRSE

Emeritus Professor of Neuropathology,
University Department of Neuropathology,
Institute of Neurological Sciences,
Southern General Hospital, Glasgow

D.I. Graham

MB BCh PhD FRCPath FRCP (Glas.) FRSE

Professor of Neuropathology,
University Department of Neuropathology,
Institute of Neurological Sciences,
Southern General Hospital, Glasgow

with special chapters by

Janice R. Anderson

MA MBBS FRCPath

Consultant Neuropathologist,
Addenbrooke's Hospital,
Cambridge

Rosalind H.M. King

PhD

Senior Lecturer in Neurological Sciences,
Royal Free Hospital,
London

I. Bone

MB ChB FRCP (Lon. & Glas.)

Consultant Neurologist,
Institute of Neurological Sciences,
Glasgow

W.R. Lee

MD FRCPath FCOph FRSE

Professor of Ophthalmic Pathology,
University of Glasgow,
Glasgow

Foreword by

Roderick N.M. MacSween

BSc MD FRCP (Glas/Edin) FRCPath FIBiol FRSE

Professor of Pathology, University of
Glasgow; Honorary Consultant Pathologist,
Western Infirmary, Glasgow

CHURCHILL LIVINGSTONE
EDINBURGH LONDON MADRID MELBOURNE NEW YORK AND TOKYO 1994

CHURCHILL LIVINGSTONE
Medical Division of Longman Group Limited

Distributed in the United States of America by Churchill
Livingstone Inc., 650 Avenue of the Americas, New York,
N.Y. 10011, and by associated companies, branches and
representatives throughout the world.

First edition 1988
Second edition 1994
  Reprinted 1995

ISBN 0 443 04495 3

British Library Cataloguing in Publication Data
A catalogue record for this book is available from the British
Library.

Library of Congress Cataloging in Publication Data
Adams, J. Hume.
  An Introduction to neuropathology / J. Hume Adams and
  D. I. Graham with special chapters by Janice R. Anderson
  ... [et al.]. — 2nd ed.
    p.   cm.
  Includes bibliographical references and index.
  ISBN 0-443-04495-3
  1. Nervous system—Diseases. I. Graham, David I.R.
  II. Anderson, Janice R, III. Title.
  [DNLM: 1. Nervous System Diseases—pathology. WL 100
  A2141 1993]
  RC347.A28 1993
  616.8′047—dc20
  DNLM / DLC
  for Library of Congress   93-4546

The
publisher's
policy is to use
**paper manufactured
from sustainable forests**

Produced by Longman Singapore Publishers Pte Ltd

Printed in Singapore

Contents

NPEL BASIC REACTIONS (Google)
Introduction to neuropathology

Foreword   vii

Preface   ix

Acknowledgements   x

1. Introduction   1

2. Functional neuroanatomy   13
   I. Bone

3. The central nervous system and its reactions to disease   29

4. Intracranial expanding lesions, cerebral oedema and hydrocephalus   49

5. Vascular and hypoxic disorders   63

6. Bacterial infections   91

7. Virus and other infections   103

8. Trauma   133

9. Demyelinating diseases   157

10. Metabolic disorders   169

11. Deficiency disorders and intoxications   191

12. System disorders   211

13. Developmental and perinatal disorders   223

14. Ageing and the dementias   251

15. Tumours   269

16. Diseases of the orbit   309
    W. R. Lee

17. Diseases of muscle   337
    Janice R. Anderson

18. Diseases of peripheral nerves   373
    R. H. M. King

Index   405

Foreword

I am delighted and honoured to write the foreword for the second edition of this book, an edition which appears just 5 years after the first – an indication that the book has made a considerable impact and has been identified as an outstanding monograph. The justification for both editions, however, lies primarily in the excellence and experience of its contributors who have devoted many years to the study of the morphology of diseases of the central nervous system.

The role of pathology in the study of diseases of the central nervous system is a changing one and continues to expand. In the first edition of *Muir's Textbook of Pathology* in 1924 less than two pages were devoted to tumours of the nervous system (gliomas being considered under the generic title histiomata) and, with the exception of general paralysis of the insane (dealt with under syphilis), there was no account of the morphological changes associated with ageing and the dementias nor of the morphology of metabolic disorders and the demyelinating diseases. The section on tumours in the current text runs to 38 pages and this chapter has had to be updated in view of the new WHO classification. The advances in our knowledge of the neuropathology of ageing and dementia and of the metabolic and demyelinating diseases are concisely and clearly summarized, in some areas embracing advances which have been made at the ultrastructural and molecular level. All the chapters appearing in the first edition have been extensively revised, and in addition, two new chapters appear, one on functional neuroanatomy and one on diseases of the orbit.

In their preface Professors Adams and Graham indicate that the book is not meant to compete with large reference textbooks such as *Greenfield's Neuropathology* (the 5th edition of which was co-edited by Professor Adams). The book is precisely what its title states – an introduction, but it also represents a scholarly review of the state of the art. It clearly meets the needs of the trainee histopathologist but, in addition, it has been identified as a most valuable introductory bench book by the practising histopathologist and as a most useful source of information by clinicians and research workers in the neurosciences. At a time when disciplinary demarcation and borders are no longer sharply defined, the role of pathology continues to be one of providing reliable guidelines to recognise disease. Neuropathology may be carried out by histopathologists, clinicians and research scientists but, irrespective of this, it will retain a key role in diagnosis, in establishing prognostic criteria and in leading to a better understanding of pathogenetic mechanisms.

In these days of 'core and options' in medical education *An Introduction to Neuropathology* might be seen as the core and the larger texts as optional. The concept of 'core and options' in continuing medical education is perhaps not entirely a satisfactory one. In another connotation the core is something which is relatively indigestible and which is disposed of. However, these cores also contain the seeds and the need to preserve and conserve them is not optional. In warmly commending this text I have no doubt but that it will simultaneously be the core and seed for trainee and practising histopathologists, and for all neuroscientists, thus contributing to both basic and continuing education in the discipline of neuropathology.

Glasgow, 1994   R.N.M. MacS.

Preface

The first edition of this book was published in 1988 and reviews have been generally complimentary. We have also been encouraged by the many personal observations that the book had achieved precisely what we had aimed for. It certainly seems to be used in many countries of the world by trainees in pathology and in the neurosciences. It has already been reprinted with some improvements, but the time has now come for a second edition incorporating some wholesale revisions and reflecting recent developments.

As in pathology in general, many basic concepts and common processes in neuropathology, e.g. infarction, infection and tumours, remain relatively unchanged over decades; nevertheless, we have updated all of the original chapters. The chapter on tumours has been entirely rewritten to conform to the recent new nomenclature recommended by the World Health Organization, and there are two entirely new chapters: one on Functional Neuroanatomy by Dr I. Bone of the Institute of Neurological Sciences, Glasgow, and one on Diseases of the Orbit by Professor W. R. Lee of the University of Glasgow. Furthermore, two chapters have been completely rewritten by internationally recognized authorities in their fields – the chapter on Diseases of Muscle by Dr Janice R. Anderson of Addenbrooke's Hospital, Cambridge, and the chapter on Diseases of Peripheral Nerves by Dr Rosalind H. M. King of the Royal Free Hospital, London. We are most grateful to all of these contributors. We are also grateful to Dr William L. Maxwell, Lecturer in Anatomy in the University of Glasgow, for advising us on points of anatomical detail and for providing several new illustrations.

As with the first edition, we would urge general pathologists to submit autopsy and biopsy material to Departments of Neuropathology for specialist study. If this is not possible, however, we hope that this book will help the pathologist to examine a brain intelligently and methodically. Once again, it has not been our intention to compete with major reference works on neuropathology that provide much more detailed information on structural abnormalities, immunohistochemistry and electron microscopy. For this reason we have decided not to include many specific references, but only to recommend particularly relevant publications at the end of each chapter.

We would again like to acknowledge with sincere thanks the help we have received from our secretaries, Mrs J. Rubython and Mrs A. Whyte; the loyal help over many years of Mr L. M. Miller, Senior Chief MLSO in this Department, and his staff; and the assistance of Mr A. McIlroy, Head of the Department of Medical Illustration in the Southern General Hospital and his staff – in particular Miss Linda Scott, Medical Photographer and Mr Charles Orr, Medical Artist.

J.H.A.
D.I.G.

Glasgow 1994

Acknowledgements

We are indebted to the following publishers for permitting us to reproduce illustrations we have used in the past: Cambridge University Press for Figures 1.1 to 1.12 which first appeared in *An Atlas of Post-Mortem Techniques* (Adams J.H. and Murray M. F., 1982); Edward Arnold (Publishers) Ltd, London for Figures 5.2, 5.10, 5.14, 5.15 a & b, 6.11, 9.4, 9.7, 9.11b and 9.18 which appeared in *Greenfield's Neuropathology*, 4th edition (Eds. Adams, J. H., Corsellis, J.A.N. and Duchen, L.W., 1984), and for Figures 13.7, 13.14 and 13.24 which appeared in *Muir's Textbook of Pathology*, 12th edition (Ed. Anderson, J.R., 1985); and Blackwell Scientific Publications, Oxford, for Figures 15.6, 15.11, 15.33, 15.34 and 15.40 which were published in *Applied Surgical Pathology* (Eds. Stuart, A.E., Smith, A.N. and Samuel, E., 1975).

We are also indebted to Lloyd-Luke (Medical Books), London for allowing us to modify Figures 22 and 23 taken from *Pathology of the Spinal Cord*, 2nd edn. by J. Trevor Hughes in the design of Figure 5.4; and also to Churchill Livingstone, Edinburgh, for the use of Figure 7.15a from *Systemic Pathology*, 3rd edn (Ed. Weller, R.O., 1990) and figures 17.11, 17.12, 17.23, 17.32 and 17.40 from *Atlas of Skeletal Muscle Pathology* (Anderson, Janice R., 1985); MTP Press Ltd, Lancaster.

1. Introduction

The central nervous system (CNS) is complex, and its proper study requires special investigations, including the use of various staining techniques and the application of modern methods such as electron microscopy and immunohistochemistry. Nevertheless, many of the principles of general pathology are relevant, so that a training in general pathology is a prerequisite to a proper appreciation of neuropathology.

Disease of the CNS is often manifest by the signs and symptoms of focal neurological deficit. It is for this reason that some knowledge of its structure, function and metabolism is important. The ability to localize and better characterize lesions *in vivo* has improved enormously in the last decade with high resolution computed tomographic scanning (CT), magnetic resonance imaging (MRI), single photon emission computed tomography (SPECT) and proton emission tomography (PET). In spite of these advances, however, there remains a need for traditional methods such as the examination of cerebrospinal fluid (CSF), the microscopical examination of biopsy specimens, and autopsies in order to achieve accurate clinicopathological correlations. These mainstays of clinical neuropathology are now run, however, in parallel with techniques that include tissue culture and sampling of specimens for neurochemical analysis. As the fundamental nature of disease becomes better understood, so the importance of genetics and molecular pathology become increasingly apparent. This might suggest that the role of the neuropathologist is limited, but on the contrary he is in a singular position to make full use of the material at his disposal and to help realize its full potential.

In this introductory chapter we would like to comment briefly on certain technical points, some of which have been dealt with in greater detail elsewhere (see guides to further reading at the end of the chapter).

TECHNIQUES IN NEUROPATHOLOGY

The pathologist should see the clinical records so that the type of neurological illness can be determined and, if necessary, further advice sought from a neuropathologist. It can then be decided in advance if some brain tissue has to be retained unfixed for microbiological or neurochemical studies, if the spinal cord and posterior root ganglia require to be removed, and what, if any, muscles and peripheral nerves have to be taken for histological examination. The pathologist will also be alerted to any potential hazards, e.g. serum positivity for HBsAg or HIV or the possibility that the patient is suffering from Creutzfeldt–Jakob disease or AIDS. Local codes of practice can then be put into effect and the Code of Practice for the Prevention of Infection in Clinical Laboratories and Post-mortem Rooms consulted.

REMOVAL OF THE BRAIN AND SPINAL CORD

Pathologists should remove the brain themselves – or at least witness the procedure – so that they can ascertain the tightness of the dura, and the presence and volume of blood in either the extradural or subdural spaces.

The saw cut through the calvaria should be made immediately above the supraorbital ridge and continued horizontally round the skull to the

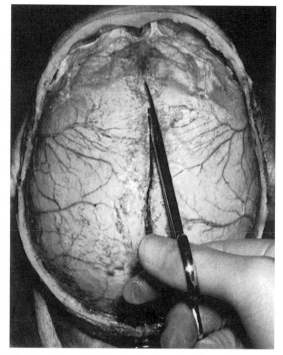

Fig. 1.1   Removal of the brain. Opening the superior sagittal sinus.

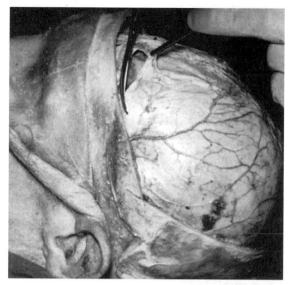

Fig. 1.2   Removal of the brain. Opening the dura along the line of the saw cut.

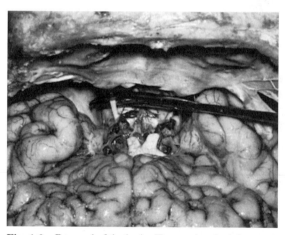

Fig. 1.3   Removal of the brain. Transecting the left oculomotor nerve.

occiput. The dura should not be breached, although this may be difficult when it is tightly adherent to the skull as is common in infants and in the elderly. The skull cap can be prised loose by twisting a T-shaped chisel along the saw cut and, if necessary, this can be tapped gently with a mallet if the skull has not been completely cut through. Force, however, must be avoided as this may produce damage to the bone that might be misinterpreted as a fracture. If the dura is tightly adherent to the skull, a malleable retractor is a useful means of separating the two. The superior sagittal sinus is now opened and inspected to establish whether or not it contains thrombus (Fig. 1.1). The dura is then incised along the line of the saw cut, preferably with curved scissors (Fig. 1.2), taking care not to damage the underlying cortex. The tenseness of the dura is established at this stage. The falx is freed from the cribriform plate and the dura retracted to allow inspection of the bridging veins draining into the sagittal sinus. The frontal poles are then retracted gently and the rostral cranial nerves, the pituitary stalk and the internal carotid arteries cut

(Fig. 1.3). The attachment of the tentorium cerebelli to the skull is then incised to expose the structures in the posterior fossa (Fig. 1.4). The next stage is to divide the remaining cranial nerves and the vertebral arteries (Fig. 1.5) as they enter the skull. The upper end of the spinal cord is transected and the brain gently removed from the skull taking care not to damage the brain stem.

If an abnormality in the lower brain stem or upper cervical cord is suspected, a central wedge

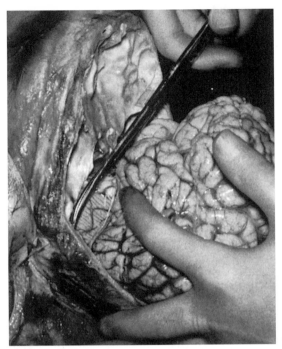

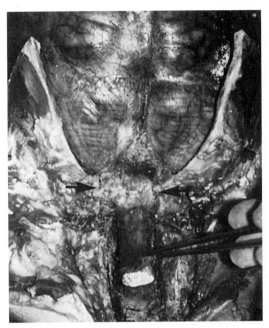

Fig. 1.4   Removal of the brain. Incising the lateral edge of the tentorium cerebelli.

Fig. 1.6   Removal of the brain. Elevating the transected cervical spinal cord after removing part of the occipital bone and the arches of the upper cervical vertebrae, and exposing the foramen magnum (arrows).

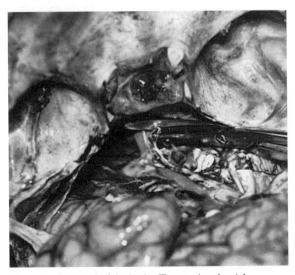

Fig. 1.5   Removal of the brain. Transecting the right vertebral artery.

of occipital bone should be removed along with the spines and laminae of the upper cervical vertebrae, so that the brain and the upper segments of the spinal cord can be removed in one block (Fig. 1.6).

The spinal cord may be removed by either an anterior or posterior approach. Advantages of the anterior approach are that the autopsy can be carried out through a single midline ventral incision, and that dorsal root ganglia and the vertebral arteries in the transverse processes of the cervical vertebrae are more easily identifiable. After the cord has been fully exposed, it should be removed within its dural sheath. Angulation of the cord during its removal must be avoided since this can cause remarkable distortion of its intrinsic architecture (the so-called 'toothpaste effect'). In some situations it is desirable to remove the vertebral column *en bloc* and to fix the cord *in situ*.

Some observations on removing infants' brains are made in Chapter 13.

EXAMINATION OF RELATED STRUCTURES

In cases of cerebrovascular disease the major extracranial cerebral arteries in the neck have to be examined. These should be dissected in one block rather than opened *in situ*. This is most easily done by exposing the arch of the aorta after opening the pericardium and then dissecting along its major branches. The block that is finally removed therefore consists of the arch of the aorta, the innominate artery, the common carotid arteries, the proximal parts of the external carotid arteries, the internal carotid arteries up to the base of the skull, the proximal parts of the subclavian arteries and the proximal parts of the vertebral arteries to the point where they enter the foramina of the 6th cervical vertebrae (Fig. 1.7). After fixation the presence or absence of atheromatous stenosis and/or occlusion can be assessed by serial transverse sections. The cavernous portions of the carotid arteries should also be examined.

Examination of the base of the skull depends on the type of lesion that is being sought. The dura, however, has to be stripped from the bone to identify fractures and to allow examination of the various air and venous sinuses and the middle

ears. It may be necessary in certain cases to explore the contents of the orbit through the floor of the anterior cranial fossa. Finally, the pituitary gland should be examined in all cases; the first step is to make a transerve cut along the posterior margin of the diaphragma sellae before removing the posterior clinoid processes. (Fig. 1.8). If this is not done, part of the posterior lobe tends to be removed with the bone.

FIXATION

It is rarely possible to obtain precise information about the distribution of any lesion in the brain if it is cut in the unfixed state. Furthermore, some lesions, such as small plaques of demyelination or a recent infarct, may not be identifiable in the unfixed brain, even by an experienced neuropathologist. Portions of the unfixed brain may of course have to be removed for virological studies or neurochemical analysis. In cases of massive subarachnoid haemorrhage, it is advisable to dissect the arteries at the base of the brain prior to fixation and to wash away the blood clot with normal saline in an attempt to define any aneurysm or other vascular malformation.

After preliminary observations have been made, the brain should be fixed intact as soon as possible after removal from the skull. If it is allowed to lie on the dissecting table, even for a

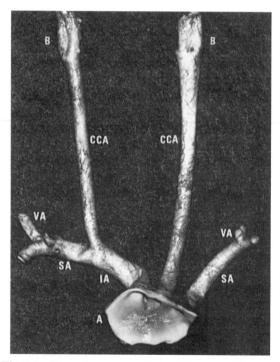

Fig. 1.7 The major arteries in the neck. A = aorta; IA = innominate artery; SA = subclavian artery; VA = origin of vertebral artery; CCA = common carotid artery; B = bifurcation of common carotid artery.

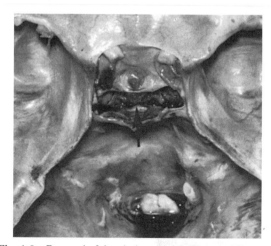

Fig. 1.8 Removal of the pituitary gland. The posterior part of the diaphragma sellae has been incised and the clinoid processes retracted to expose the posterior lobe of the pituitary gland (arrow).

short time, it will become permanently deformed. The brain should be placed in a 2 gallon polythene bucket containing neutral 4% formaldehyde in normal saline. Once the brain has been immersed, a paperclip attached to a piece of string tied across the top of the bucket can be slipped under the basilar artery (Fig. 1.9) and the brain allowed to hang freely, care being taken to ensure that no surface of the brain is in contact with the bottom or sides of the bucket. The fixative should be changed after 3 days and then at weekly intervals. The spinal cord still within the dura is best fixed vertically in a large measuring cylinder.

DISSECTION

The brain should be fixed for 3–4 weeks and then washed in running water for an hour or so prior to dissection. The plane in which the dissection is carried out depends to some extent on how best to correlate the morbid anatomy with the neuroradiological findings. In general, however, our standard procedure is to cut the cerebral hemispheres in the coronal plane, since we find this to be the most informative technique.

Prior to dissection the intact brain is examined for external abnormalities such as flattening of the convolutions, selective or generalized atrophy, thickening or other abnormalities of the meninges, vascular malformations, and tentorial or tonsillar herniation. Any focal abnormalities, such as areas of 'softening' are noted. Our initial procedure is to detach the hindbrain from the cerebrum by transecting the upper pons. A further transverse cut is made through the cerebral peduncles, to obtain a block of the midbrain including the aqueduct (Fig. 1.10). A coronal cut is then made through the cerebral hemispheres at the level of the mamillary bodies, and the hemispheres cut into slices 1 cm thick with the aid of two angles made of metal (Fig. 1.11). The brain knife should be pulled smoothly across the brain. Sometimes a lesion in the cerebellum can best be displayed by a transverse cut, but it is usually more informative to separate the cerebellum from the brain stem by cutting through the cerebellar peduncles on each side. The hemispheres can then be cut at right angles to the folia and slightly nearer the vermis than the lateral border: this is the best method for demonstrating the folial pattern and the dentate nuclei. A further 1 cm thick slice of the lateral part of each hemisphere is then obtained by using the angles referred to above. A further cut is then made through the

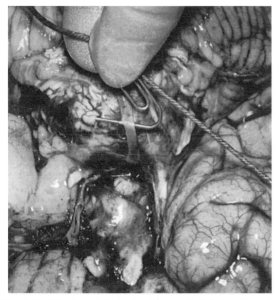

Fig. 1.9 Fixation of the brain. A paperclip is being slipped under the basiliar artery by which it will be suspended in formol saline.

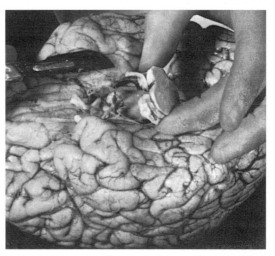

Fig. 1.10 Dissection of the brain. Transecting the midbrain after having detached the hindbrain at the level of the upper pons.

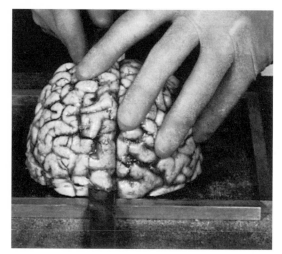

Fig. 1.11 Dissection of the brain. Making a coronal slice through the brain with the aid of 1 cm thick metal cutting angles.

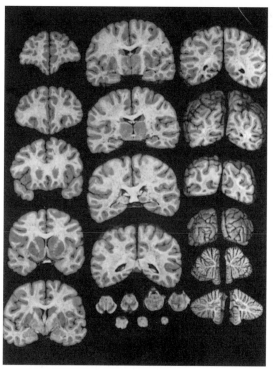

Fig. 1.12 Dissection of the brain. The brain laid out ready for inspection.

vermis. A series of transverse cuts is made through the pons and medulla. The slices are laid out in a standard fashion so that any abnormalities, the size and shape of the ventricles, and the presence of any distortion and/or displacement of the midline structures can be identified easily (Fig. 1.12).

The first step in examining the spinal cord is to open the dura in the midline along its dorsal and ventral aspects. Any external abnormalities are noted, including atrophy of nerve roots. A series of transverse cuts through the full thickness of the cord is then made and any intrinsic abnormalities noted. The ventral surface of the cord is easily identified by the single anterior spinal artery. Even if the cord has been damaged *post mortem*, it is usually possible to identify the segments approximately by identifying the lowest large ventral nerve root of the cervical plexus: this is usually T1.

There are occasions when the brain should be cut in the midline sagittal plane to demonstrate the third ventricle, the aqueduct and the pineal region and, increasingly, there is a need to cut the cerebral hemispheres in the horizontal plane in order to correlate the appearances with CT scanning and magnetic resonance imaging.

The sides from which blocks have been taken for microscopical examination should be recorded. It is often helpful to adopt some standard method of identifying from which side of the brain the block has been taken, for example by making a small hole or nick in all blocks taken from one or other hemisphere.

HISTOLOGICAL TECHNIQUES

The principal histological techniques used by neuropathologists are listed in Table 1.1, from which it can be seen that much information can be gained from a limited number of techniques that are often used routinely in departments of pathology. Thus many abnormalities in cells and myelin can be identified in sections stained with haematoxylin and eosin (H & E), provided fairly thick sections (7–8 μm) are examined. It is easy to recognize the difference between grey and white matter and to appreciate that the architectural arrangements of the cerebral cortex differ from those of the basal ganglia, the hippocampus, the cerebellum and the brain stem. Indeed, it is often possible to identify from which subcortical area of the brain a section has been taken by noting

Table 1.1   Histological techniques in neuropathology

Type of preparation	Stain	Colour reaction and application
Smears	Polychrome methylene blue; Toluidine blue	Blue: rapid diagnosis
	Haematoxylin and eosin	Pink and blue
Paraffin	Haematoxylin and eosin	Pink and blue: general purpose
	van Gieson	Red: collagen
		Yellow: other tissues
	Reticulin stain	Black: reticulin
	Cresyl violet (may be used with Luxol fast blue or Palmgren)	Violet: Nissl substance of neurons
	Palmgren	Black: axons and neurons
	Bodian	
	Glees and Marsland	
	Loyez	Black: myelin
	Luxol fast blue	Deep blue: myelin
	Holzer	Blue purple: glial fibres and astrocytes
	Phosphotungstic acid haematoxylin	
	Nauomenko and Feigin	Black: microglia
	Perls' stain	Blue: ferric iron
	Masson Fontana	Black: melanin
	Periodic acid–Schiff	Magenta: glycogen and mucopolysaccharide
Frozen	von Braunmuhl King's amyloid	Black or brown-black: neurons and axons, senile plaques and neurofibrillary tangles
	Cajal	Black: astrocytes
	Hortega silver carbonate	Black: astrocytes
	Penfield's modification of Hortega silver carbonate	Black: oligodendrocytes
	Marchi	Black: degenerating myelin
	Oil red O	Red: degenerating myelin
	Acidified cresyl violet	Purple-brown: metachromatic leukodystrophy
Celloidin	Cresyl violet	Violet: neurons
	Woelke's modification of Heidenhain's method	Black: myelin
	Bielschowsky's method	Black: axons
CSF	Leishman	Blue/pink: cytology
	May-Grunwald-Giemsa	
	Southgate's mucicarmine	Pink: mucin

the size, shape and pigmentation of neurons: unfortunately, this is rarely possible in the cerebral cortex. The use of haematoxylin/van Gieson (H/VG) helps to distinguish between collagen and glial fibrils. Phosphotungstic acid haematoxylin (PTAH) is also often used as a general stain as it identifies myelin and collagen as well as glial fibres. A particularly useful general stain is the combined cresyl violet and Luxol fast blue technique. The cresyl violet stains neurons and their Nissl granules, whereas the Luxol fast blue stains myelin a rich blue colour.

Specialized techniques are, however, essential for the identification of specific structural abnormalities such as those affecting axons and myelin. Commonly used techniques for axons are the silver impregnation methods of Palmgren, Bodian, and Glees and Marsland. The basic principles of how to identify abnormalities in myelin are somewhat confusing, but in essence there are two principal types of staining reaction. First, loss of myelin can be identified by negative staining; the demyelinated areas are pale when stained with Luxol fast blue, haematoxylin lakes or H & E, or H/VG; secondly, the breakdown products of myelin can be stained positively by either the Sudan stains (Oil red O) or by the Marchi technique. Both of these are applicable to frozen sections, but material that has been impregnated by the Marchi method can be embedded in paraffin wax.

There is often a need to identify both normal

and fibre-forming astrocytes. Although PTAH frequently gives good results in postmortem material that has been fixed for a number of weeks, it is rarely satisfactory with surgical specimens. Immunohistochemical methods are therefore being used increasingly to overcome some of the difficulties (see below). Silver techniques are available for the selective impregnation of *astrocytes, oligodendrocytes* and *microglia.* As with all silver techniques, sections have to be stained individually, thus ensuring that they are properly differentiated. Even with experience, it is still likely that various types of cell will be impregnated, with the result that cellular morphology has to be taken into account in the interpretation of the sections.

There are many occasions when pigment requires to be identified. In most instances this can be resolved by the use of Perl's stain which demonstrates iron, and the Masson Fontana technique which identifies melanin.

In patients with diffuse brain damage due, for example to cardiac arrest, hypoglycaemia or some other generalized disease process, large sections of brain have to be examined so that the precise anatomical distribution of the brain damage can be defined. Some laboratories prefer large celloidin-embedded sections to paraffin sections; the former can then be stained by cresyl violet for the study of neurons, by Woelke's modification of Heidenhain's method for myelin and by the Bielschowsky silver impregnation method for axons.

Brain biopsy is a standard procedure in most neurosurgical units. Two principal techniques are available when a rapid diagnosis is required – smears or frozen sections. Our preference is the smear technique, which is simple and rapid. After fixation in alcohol the smears can be stained with 1% toluidine blue, polychrome methylene blue, H & E etc. If the biopsy is too tough to smear, frozen sections are indicated.

Cytology of cerebrospinal fluid (CSF)

Cytological examination of CSF has become of increasing value in recent years because of the development of improved techniques such as membrane filter, cytospin, and sedimentation techniques. The most important prerequisites for good cytology are fresh specimens correctly handled and prepared. Considerable experience, however, is required to differentiate reactive from tumour cells, but in any patient where the CSF cell count is raised cytological examination should be undertaken, with the aim of identifying precisely the nature of the nucleated cells. Cytospin specimens are usually stained routinely by the Leishman or May–Grunwald's Giemsa methods, but various other techniques can be used, such as Southgate's mucicarmine for the identification of mucin-secreting metastatic carcinoma and the periodic acid–Schiff technique. Various antibodies are being used increasingly to help in the identification of nucleated cells, particularly when tumour cells are present in the CSF. In meningeal leukaemia, there are many leukaemic cells in the CSF.

What blocks to examine?

General pathologists often require some guidance as to what regions of the brain they should examine. If a specific diagnosis is suspected clinically, reference to the appropriate chapter in this book should be of assistance. Not infrequently, however, in a patient thought clinically to have some generalized but poorly defined disorder of the CNS, the brain may appear normal macroscopically. In such cases our approach is to examine the following blocks: the dorsal angle of each cerebral hemisphere in the posterior frontal and parietal regions, each insula, each thalamus, each hippocampus, the hypothalamus including the mamillary bodies, each cerebellar hemisphere and representative levels of the brain stem stained by H & E and by Luxol fast blue-cresyl violet. The remainder of the brain is retained lest other regions require to be examined, or other techniques applied.

IMMUNOHISTOCHEMISTRY

As in other systems in the body, particular functions have been ascribed to various cells in the nervous system. These specific functions are to a large extent mediated by proteins, many of which may be unique to the CNS (Table 1.2). Immunohistochemical techniques have, therefore,

Table 1.2 Immunohistochemistry in neuropathology

Antigen	Types of cell identified
S-100 protein	Glia and cells derived from neural crest
Neuron-specific enolase	γγ Dimer specific for neurons and neuroendocrine cells in other parts of the body Isomer present in astrocytes
Glial fibrillary acidic protein Glutamine synthetase	Astrocytes
Galactocerebroside Myelin basic protein Myelin-associated glycoprotein Anti-*Leu 7*	Oligodendroglia and myelin
Fibronectin	Fibroblasts
Factor VIII-related antigen Angiotensin-converting enzyme	Endothelial cells
Fc receptor Activated complement C3b Class II major histo-compatibility antigen Ricin agglutinin	Macrophages and microglia
Prolactin Growth hormone ACTH Follicle-stimulating hormone Luteinizing hormone Thyroid-stimulating hormone	In anterior pituitary
Monoamines Acetylcholine γ-aminobutyric acid (GABA) Neuropeptides	Neurotransmitter substances
Neurofilaments Synaptophysin	Neurons, axons and synapses
Cytokeratin Epithelial membrane antigen	Cells of epithelial tissues
Vimentin	Cells of mesenchymal and glial origin
Desmin Myosin	Cells of myogenic origin
Chorionic gonadotrophin α_1-Fetoprotein	Cells of trophoblastic origin
Carbonic anhydrase C	Choroid plexus
Leucocyte common antigen T and B cells	Lymphocytes

been used to characterize the proteins of various cells within the CNS that are probably involved in these functions. Morphological information obtained from these studies, combined with biochemical data, continues to be an extremely valuable means of studying the development, structure and the functional components of the CNS.

S-100 protein is found in substantial amounts in glial cells and cells derived from the neural crest. Its value in tumour diagnosis, however, is limited because it also occurs in small amounts in other cell types. The S-100 protein is, therefore, not brain-specific but is a useful general marker indicating an origin from the embryonic neural crest. Another marker is *neuron-specific enolase*, which exists as a number of subunits designated α, β, and γ, tissue extracts containing both homodimers and heterodimers of the isoenzymes. It has been shown by immunoperoxidase staining that most neurons, and neuroendocrine cells in other parts of the body, stain for γ-enolase, whereas glial cells, particularly astrocytes, stain strongly for α-enolase. There is considerable variation in the intensity of the staining for enolase between various types of neuron, Purkinje cells in particular giving a very weak reaction. Neurons do not stain for α-enolase. Antibodies raised to *neurofilaments* are also useful in the identification of neurons and their axons, and antibodies raised to *synaptophysin* have been used as a marker of synaptic vesicles in neurons. Synaptic vesicles contain *neurotransmitter substances* such as monoamines (noradrenalin, dopamine and serotonin), acetylcholine and amino acids (glutamate and γ-aminobutyric acid (GABA)). Furthermore, certain *neuropeptides* such as substance P, encephalin, vasoactive intestinal peptide and somastostatin and many others behave as either neurotransmitters or neuromodulators, which modify the action of neurotransmitters. The immunohistochemical identification and localization of these substances is increasingly being used to determine the mechanisms of a number of neurological diseases, such as parkinsonism and Alzheimer's disease.

Glial fibrillary acidic protein (GFAP) is a major component of astrocytic fibres and was first isolated from 'burnt-out' plaques of multiple sclerosis. It is apparently the subunit of the 8–9 nm intermediate filament of astrocytes, and with antisera to the protein there is intense immunohistochemical staining of the cell bodies and their processes. To all intents and purposes, GFAP is confined to astrocytes in normal mature brain and is a very useful marker for identifying normal, reactive and tumour astrocytes. Although GFAP is now most widely used to identify astrocytes, glutamine synthetase, which is confined to astrocytes in the CNS, is an alternative marker. Astrocytes can also be identified using antibodies raised to α-enolase.

Since both oligodendrocytes and myelin are unusually rich in the glycolipid *galactocerebroside*, antisera raised against this component have been applied extensively to the investigation of white matter. Because of the particular importance of oligodendrocytes in demyelinating diseases, antibodies to *myelin basic protein* and *myelin-associated glycoprotein* have been used extensively in the study of myelinogenesis and demyelination. Myelin basic protein is the most extensively studied brain-specific membrane protein, and has been localized in myelin with fluorescent-labelled antibodies and, more specifically, to the major dense line by electron microscopy. In contrast, myelin-associated glycoprotein appears to be localized to the cell bodies of oligodendrocytes. It is against myelin-associated glycoprotein that the antibody *Leu 7* is now thought to react. Increasing use is being made of antibodies raised against several enzymes which are either specific for the myelin membrane, e.g. carbonic anhydrase (isoenzyme 2 or C) and the soma of the oligodendrocyte (glycerol phosphate dehydrogenase).

The *lympho-reticular system* in the CNS has been studied traditionally by its metallophil staining reactions, a feature that suggests a relationship between microglia and macrophages. These staining reactions, however, are variable and so the increasing availability of antibodies for identifying lymphocytic and phagocytic cells has provided useful information about these cell types in normal, reactive and neoplastic conditions. Although antibodies to α_1-antichymotrypsin can be used as a relatively specific cell marker for macrophages in the CNS in paraffin sections, use is increasingly being made of recently introduced monoclonal antibodies, e.g. EBM 11, which react with both macrophages and normal microglia in cryostat sections. Macrophages also react for the *Fc receptor, class II major histocompatibility complex (MHC)* antigens and with *ricin agglutinin*. The markers *fibronectin* for fibroblasts and *factor VIII-related antigen* and *angiotensin-converting enzyme* for endothelial cells are also available. In the study of tumours the ability to identify *vimentin filaments*, *desmin* and *myosin* in cells of mesenchymal origin may be helpful.

The application of various conventional stains to the cells of the anterior lobe of the pituitary gland is not a satisfactory means of correlating morphological features with secretory activity. The introduction of immunohistochemistry has allowed the specific localization of various *pituitary hormones*, e.g. prolactin, growth hormone and ACTH (adrenocorticotrophic hormone), in tissue that has been fixed in formalin and embedded in paraffin wax. Surgical biopsies are often small, and it is sometimes difficult to distinguish between metastatic carcinoma and some types of malignant neuroepithelial tumour. Antibodies for identifying metastatic carcinoma, such as *cytokeratin* and *epithelial membrane antigen*, may aid in establishing the diagnosis. Likewise, the presence of *chorionic gonadotrophin* and α_1-*fetoprotein* are important in the identification of cells of trophoblastic origin in germ-cell tumours arising in the region of either the hypothalamus or the pineal gland.

It is probably true to say that at present there are no specific immunocytochemical markers for ependyma, although antibodies to *carbonic anhydrase C* may be used to identify choroid plexus.

A small number of lymphocytes are commonly present in the CSF of normal subjects, and in many disease processes the numbers of lymphocytes and monocytes increase and in certain circumstances there is infiltration by plasma cells. All leucocytes react with antibodies to *leucocyte common antigen*, and further classification can be obtained by using antibodies specific for T and B lymphocytes. Where lymphoid tumours are suspected, myelomas and B-cell lymphomas can be further classified using antibodies to κ and λ light chains and immunoglobulin heavy chains.

FURTHER READING

Adams J H, Murray M F (1982) *Atlas of Post-Mortem Techniques in Neuropathology.* Cambridge: Cambridge University Press.

Adams J H, Graham D I & Doyle D (1981) *Brain Biopsy: The Smear Technique for Neurosurgical Biopsies.* London: Chapman & Hall.

Advisory Committee on Dangerous Pathogens (1990) *HIV: The Causative Agent of AIDS and Related Conditions.* 2nd Revision of Guidelines. London: HMSO.

Bullock G R, Petrusz P (eds.) (1982) *Techniques in Immunocytochemistry*, Vols 1, 2, 3, 4. London: Academic Press.

Health and Safety Commission's Health Services Advisory Committee (1991) *Safe Working and the Prevention of Infection in Clinical Laboratories.* London: HMSO.

Health and Safety Commission's Health Services Advisory Committee (1991) *Safe Working and the Prevention of Infection in the Mortuary and Post-Mortem Room.* London: HMSO.

Health and Safety Commission's Health Services Advisory Committee. (1991) *Safe Working and the Prevention of Infection in Clinical Laboratories – Model Rules for Staff and Visitors.* London: HMSO.

Polak J M, McGee J.O'D (eds.) (1990) *In situ Hybridization: Principles and Practice.* Oxford: Oxford University Press.

Polak J M, & Van Noorden S, (eds.) (1986) *Immunocytochemistry: Modern Methods and Applications*, 2nd edn. Bristol: John Wright.

Sternberger L A, (1979) *Immunocytochemistry*, 2nd edn. New York: John Wiley.

2. Functional neuroanatomy

I. Bone

The purpose of this section is to introduce the pathologist to the basic essentials of functional neuroanatomy, so that the relationship of the nervous system to clinical symptoms and signs can be more fully understood. A knowledge of functional anatomy also ensures that the pathologist, when carrying out an examination, concentrates attention on clinically relevant regions of the central and/or peripheral nervous systems. Precise anatomical localization of symptoms and signs has been dependent upon clinicopathological correlations carried out by previous generations of neurologists and neuropathologists. The development of structural imaging such as computed tomography (CT) and magnetic resonance imaging (MRI), as well as the more recent development of functional imaging, positron emission tomography (PET) and single photon emission computed tomography (SPECT), has, over the last two decades, taught clinicians that old dogmas and concepts of localisation were not always correct. This is especially pertinent to the function of the cerebral cortex. Whereas previously specific areas had been associated with particular tasks, it is now realized that there is a complex integration of function that renders precise clinical localization an outmoded goal. Also, the face of clinical psychiatry has changed greatly in recent years, from the analytical to the organic or neurobehavioural, and pathologists may expect in the future to be asked to explore the anatomical substrate of disorders such as schizophrenia. In the peripheral nervous system the knowledge of nerve and muscle disease has been greatly advanced by the development of new electrophysiological techniques, which may, for instance, demonstrate early or presymptomatic disease before the development of abnormal neurological signs. In summary, the advances in diagnostic technology have greatly enhanced our concepts of functional neuroanatomy. In this section we shall deal predominantly with signs and symptoms of disease of the central nervous system (CNS), so that common terms such as apraxia or dystonia will come to have a meaning in terms of the possible site of origin of such symptomatology.

THE CEREBRAL CORTEX

The cerebral cortex was, until the mid-19th century, regarded as being functionally homogeneous – the seat of the soul and mind. Pierre Broca first demonstrated localized dysfunction when describing impaired language (dysphasia) in a patient with a lesion in the posterior third of the left third frontal convolution. Subsequent observations in patients with cerebrovascular disease, brain tumours or focal epilepsy led to the awareness that different regions of the cortex had specific functions. It was next realized in the 1960s that subcortical disease could 'disconnect' one area of cortical function from the next. The appreciation of these *disconnection syndromes* led to the acceptance that, whereas certain skills were localized to specific sites within the cerebral cortex, connection between these sites is essential for normal integrated cortical function.

The cerebral hemisphere may be divided into frontal, parietal, temporal and occipital lobes (Fig. 2.1). The *frontal lobe* extends from the frontal pole backwards to the central sulcus (fissure of Rolando), and downwards on the lateral surface of the hemisphere to the lateral fissure.

13

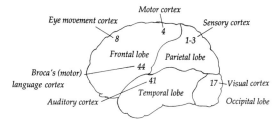

Fig. 2.1   Lateral aspect of a cerebral hemisphere with the principal Brodmann's areas labelled.

The *parietal lobe* extends from the central sulcus to the parieto-occipital fissure, and again laterally to the lateral cerebral fissure. The *temporal lobe* lies inferior to the lateral cerebral (Sylvian) fissure and extends back to the parieto-occipital fissure. The *occipital lobe* has a pyramid-like configuration and lies behind the parieto-occipital fissure. Each of these lobes can be divided into specific subdivisions. Within the lateral fissure lies an important buried island or *insula* of cerebral cortex. A further deeply situated constituent of the cerebral hemispheres is the *rhinencephalon*, a phylogenetically old portion of the cerebral hemisphere comprising the olfactory bulb and tract, the anterior perforated substance and the pyriform area, this region being associated with the perception of olfactory sensation. Further deeper structures such as the *fornix* and *hippocampal formation* play an important role in modifying behaviour responses and memory processing.

Histologically, the cerebral cortex appears to be made up of six definable layers (Fig. 2.2).

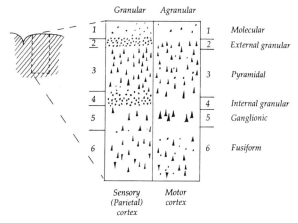

Fig. 2.2   The structure of the cerebral neocortex with diagrammatic representation of neurons.

These layers are not of homogeneous thickness throughout the cerebral cortex, but show considerable regional variation; for example, in that part of the neocortex that receives major sensory projections the granular layers are more prominent than the pyramidal layer (*granular cortex*), the opposite being the case in areas from which major motor projections emanate (the *agranular* or *pyramidal cortex*). Based on these subtle differences in cytoarchitecture, Von Economo and Brodmann divided the cerebral cortex into specific regions, implying that each discrete area had a specific and unique function. Brodmann's classification is most commonly used and the areas defined by him have been used as a reference base for the localization of physiological and pathological processes. Ablation or stimulation of these regions, electrically and with chemicals in experimental animals, has confirmed their functional importance. Important Brodmann areas are illustrated in Figure 2.1. For example, Area 4 is a principal motor cortex, whereas Area 8 is concerned with the control of eye movements and pupillary responses, and Area 17 is the striate or principal visual cortex surrounded by Areas 18 and 19, the visual association cortex.

Studies in patients with lateralized hemisphere disease suggest that there is a *major* or *dominant* cerebral hemisphere which is functionally distinct from the opposite or *minor* hemisphere. In all right-handed and approximately 95% of left-handed persons, the left hemisphere appears dominant in that in it reside the verbal, linguistic, calculating and analytical functions, whereas the non-dominant or minor hemisphere is concerned with visual, spatial and perceptual skills. Hemisphere dominance appears to be established within the first 3–5 years of life, although in trauma and disease dominance can switch in later childhood. Such *plasticity* does not occur in adolescence or adult life. Anatomical differences are evident in the structure and symmetry of the dominant and minor hemispheres. This is most evident in the upper surface of the temporal lobe, where Heschl's gyrus (Brodmann Area 41) is found to be larger in the left cerebral hemisphere in the majority of brains examined.

The degree of disability and symptomatology that a patient may manifest in cortical disease is variable, being influenced by the tempo of the illness as well as the nature of the disease process and the capacity of the cerebral hemispheres to show plasticity. This means that functional recovery following a lesion may occur as a consequence of cortical neuronal reorganisation, possibly through secondary or supplementary areas within the cerebral cortex that can 'take over' function in the face of focal disease. It therefore follows that the size and site of lesion do not always produce a predictable deficit.

SYMPTOMS OF FRONTAL LOBE DISEASE

In normal health the frontal lobes are responsible for contralateral movement in the face, arms, legs and trunk. The dominant hemisphere contains the centre for the expression of language (Broca's area). The frontal lobes also control contralateral head and eye turning, inhibition of bladder and bowel voiding, and play an important part in the maintenance of personality and initiative. The *motor cortex* (Fig. 2.3) lies anterior to the central sulcus, with the areas subserving movement in the face, arms and trunk on the lateral surface and those subserving movement in the legs on the medial surface. It can be seen from Figure 2.3 that certain functions, such as hand or lip movements, have a greater area of cortex responsible for refined and particular movement, whereas movement at a large joint has only a small area of cortical initiation.

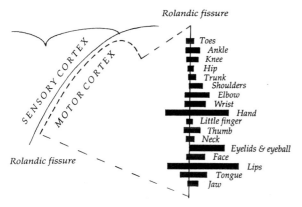

Fig. 2.3   The motor and sensory homunculus (proportional representation). (After Penfield and Rasmussen.)

Damage to the motor cortex results in contralateral *hemiplegia*. If the medial cortex is affected primarily, as in occlusion of the anterior cerebral artery or by compression from a parasagittal meningioma, paralysis is evident in the leg, with sparing of the trunk, upper limb and face. If the lateral surface only is affected, as in occlusion of the middle cerebral artery, then paralysis is present in the face, arm and trunk, with relative sparing of the leg. In destructive disease there is also a tendency for functions with greater cortical representation to be more severely affected. For instance, a patient recovering from occlusion of a middle cerebral artery may regain movement at the shoulder, elbow and wrist but no useful fine hand movement.

When *Broca's area* (Brodmann Area 44, Fig. 2.1) is diseased in the dominant hemisphere there is a loss of expressive language, the patient being able to comprehend and carry out commands, but not to produce meaningful language. This form of disturbance is referred to as *expressive dysphasia*, and sometimes, because of its hesistant nature, non-fluent dysphasia. Damage to the *paracentral lobule* on the medial surface of the frontal lobe results in 'frontal incontinence'. Here, the normal cortical inhibition of a full bladder or bowel is lost, resulting in loss of sphincter control.

Involvement of the *prefrontal areas* (the vast part of the frontal lobes anterior to the motor cortex, as well as the undersurface/orbital surface of the frontal lobes) produces predominantly disturbances in behaviour. When the *orbitofrontal cortex* is affected, disinhibition, inappropriate jocularity, emotional lability and distractability occur. When the *lateral surfaces of both frontal lobes* are affected, apathy, indifference and perseveration (the repetition of motor or language tasks) is evident. When the *medial surface* of the prefrontal cortex is affected the patient may become akinetic, lacking spontaneous movements and gestures and with sparse verbal output; this state is often referred to as *akinetic mutism*, and is associated with frontal incontinence.

Frontal lobe dysfunction may be associated with the presence of *primitive reflexes*. These reflexes are normally apparent in very early infancy and then diminish. They take the form of a *grasp reflex*, in which the patient may clutch the examiner's hand and tighten upon it, or a *snout reflex* when, if the mouth is tapped with a tendon hammer, pouting movements of the lips are made. Finally, in frontal lobe disease that affects the *corpus callosum* a disconnection between the initiation and execution of gait may occur. This results in an *apraxia* of gait, the patient appearing to have normal power in the limbs but being unable to initiate movement of them when attempting to walk.

Unilateral disease of the frontal lobe may be caused by cerebrovascular disease or infection, such as brain abscess and tumour. Bilateral frontal lobe disease may be caused by large subfrontal tumours (Fig. 2.4), tumours of the corpus callosum, hydrocephalus, degenerative disease such as Pick's dementia, and haematoma or vasospasm in association with anterior communicating artery aneurysm.

SYMPTOMS OF PARIETAL LOBE DISEASE

The *main sensory cortex* lies behind the central sulcus (Fig. 2.3) and shows topography and representation similar to the motor cortex. The dominant hemisphere contains part of the receptive language area (*Wernicke's area*) as well as being implicated in other language-related skills. The fibres of the *optic radiation* responsible for perception of vision in the lower homonymous visual fields pass deep through the parietal lobe. In disease affecting the sensory cortex there is *contralateral loss of discriminatory sensation*, with impaired awareness of touch, shape and form. Disease of the dominant hemisphere results in an inability to appreciate or understand spoken language. This is referred to as a *receptive dysphasia*, or sometimes, because spoken language is rapid and nonsensical, *fluent dysphasia*. There is also impaired calculation (*acalculia*), impaired handwriting (*dysgraphia*) and disturbed reading ability (*dyslexia*). In the non-dominant hemisphere loss of body image and spatial orientation occur, with neglect of environment and inability to follow simple drawing constructional tasks (*constructional apraxia*) and to dress (*dressing apraxia*). Visual field loss will occur if the *optic radiation* is affected.

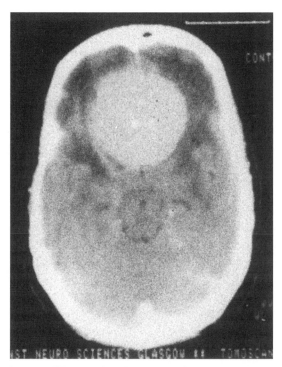

Fig. 2.4   CT scan. There is a large subfrontal meningioma with surrounding oedema. The patient presented with loss of sense of smell (anosmia) and dementia, and symptoms of increased intracranial pressure.

Bilateral parietal lobe disease is uncommon, although it may occur as a consequence of a hypotensive episode with ischaemic damage in arterial boundary zones (see p. 79). Unilateral disease is most commonly the consequence of cerebrovascular disease, and may form part of a complete middle cerebral artery occlusion syndrome or else may be the consequence of occlusion of the parietal branches of that vessel. Haematomas may also occur in the parietal lobe, as may suppurative infection and tumours.

SYMPTOMS OF TEMPORAL LOBE DISEASE

The temporal lobe is made up of its lateral cortex, buried insular cortex and the deep limbic lobe, which includes part of the rhinencephalon, hippocampus and associated structures. The *lateral cortex* serves some memory function and posteriorly it is involved in the reception of language. The *auditory cortex* lies buried in the insula. *Limbic structures* are important in the perception of smell and taste, emotion and affect and memory processing. The *optic radiation* from the upper contralateral homonymous fields again passes deep through the temporal lobes. Disease of the dominant temporal lobe will result again in a *receptive* or *fluent dysphasia*, with impaired verbal memory. Disease of the minor temporal lobe will result in impaired visual memory. Unilateral damage to the auditory cortex will not result in hearing loss, as hearing has bilateral cortical representation. Bilateral lesions are rare but may result in *cortical deafness*. Disease of the limbic system may result in aggressive or anti-social behaviour, and may be associated with the inability to establish new memories. Damage to the optic radiation will result in an upper homonymous quadrantanopia.

Unilateral temporal lobe disease may occur as a consequence of vascular or neoplastic processes, and abscesses may occur as a consequence of extension of localized infection from the middle ear or mastoid. Bilateral temporal lobe disease may occur in herpes-simplex virus encephalitis, vascular disease or in Wernicke's encephalopathy, where limbic structures are affected. The most common disease affecting temporal lobe function is *epilepsy*. This usually gives rise to positive phenomena, such as memory disturbance, déja vu or jamais vu, transient hallucinations of smell and taste and formed visual hallucinations. Psychomotor seizures are associated with primitive limb or truncal movements. In persons with temporal lobe epilepsy between seizures, certain features are noted which are felt to have their origin within the temporal lobe. *Hypergraphia* (rapidity of handwriting), paranoid ideas, hyposexuality and excessive religiosity are frequently encountered.

DISEASES OF THE OCCIPITAL LOBE

The occipital lobe is concerned with the perception of vision (the *visual cortex*) and the interpretation of this (the *parastriate* or association visual cortex). A unilateral cortical lesion will produce loss of vision in the homonymous fields. The macula or central vision is represented at the occipital pole. Diseases that extend to this will result in a loss of macular or central vision. *Cortical blindness* occurs with an extensive bilateral cortical lesion affecting the striate cortex (Fig. 2.5). In this situation the pupillary light reflex is retained despite the absence of any conscious perception of light. This situation may occur in a patient who has already had an occipital infarct from posterior cerebral artery occlusion who then develops a similar event on the opposite side. Simultaneous occipital infarction may be the consequence of distal basilar artery occlusion, transtentorial herniation with compression of the posterior cerebral arteries, or may occur as a result of a hypoxic ischaemic event, such as status epilepticus. *Anton's syndrome* is a situation where extension to the association visual cortex results in the patient being unaware of his or her blind-

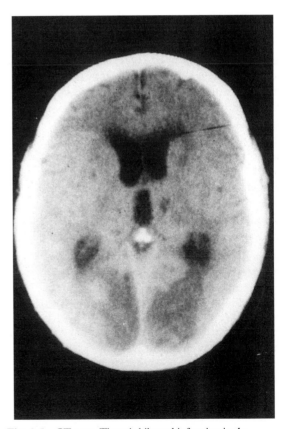

Fig. 2.5 CT scan. There is bilateral infarction in the occipital lobes. The patient presented with cortical blindness with denial of visual loss (Anton's syndrome).

ness and insisting, despite obvious visual loss, that they can see normally.

Visual hallucinations of an unformed nature, with stripes or lines before the eyes, are common in migraine and have either a retinal or an occipital cortical origin. Subtle degrees of occipital dysfunction may also be noted in disease where a patient may have difficulty in interpreting an object presented to them – *visual agnosia* – or difficulty putting a name to a familiar face – *prosopagnosia*.

THE DISCONNECTION SYNDROMES

When the large subcortical fibre connections between one area of the cortex and the next are damaged, a disconnection syndrome develops. There are several forms of these, e.g. the isolation of the hearing from the language cortex may result in *pure word deafness*. Here the patient can hear sounds but is unable to interpret the meaning of words. Another type of disconnection syndrome has already been described where the anterior corpus callosum is diseased, for instance by tumour (Fig. 2.6). This results in an *apraxia* of movement, the patient having normal power in the limbs but being unable to initiate movement, for instance being unable to walk and therefore confined to a chair. Another form of disconnection is where the sensory language cortex, Wernicke's area, is disconnected from the motor language cortex, Broca's area. This results in a form of language disturbance termed *conduction aphasia*, a characteristic of which is impaired repetition.

THE THALAMUS

These paired masses of grey matter are egg-shaped and lie in relation to the lateral wall of the third ventricle. Anatomically and functionally four regions can be identified: anterior, posterior, medial and lateral. Efferent connections from the thalamus (Fig. 2.7) project to the frontal lobes, the hypothalamus, the cingulate gyrus, the mesial parietal cortex and the orbitofrontal cortex. Afferent connections are received from the mamillary bodies, the hippocampus, the frontal lobes, the amygdala, the hypothalamus, other basal ganglia

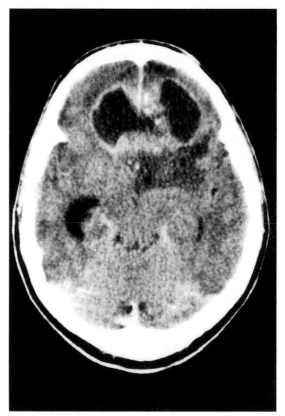

Fig. 2.6 CT scan. There is a bifrontal enhancing tumour. The patient presented with change in personality, seizures, apraxia of gait and the features of raised intracranial pressure.

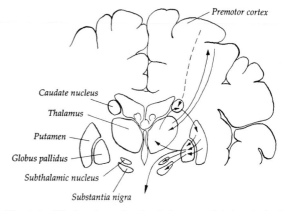

Fig. 2.7 The basal ganglia, the thalamus and their principal connections.

Premotor cortex

Caudate nucleus
Thalamus
Putamen
Globus pallidus
Subthalamic nucleus
Substantia nigra

structures and the sensory afferent pathways. These complex connections result in a plethora of symptoms and signs in disease. Four syndromes can be recognized, depending on the site of the lesion. Disease of the *anterior thalamic region* in the dominant hemisphere may cause dysphasia, inattention and memory impairment. Extension of disease into the *subthalamic region* may cause a movement disorder which takes the form of wild involuntary movements of the contralateral limbs (*hemiballismus*). Disease of the *medial thalamic region* results in impairment of recent memory, apathy, agitation, impaired attention and, occasionally, coma. Extension of the lesion into the midbrain region may result in impairment of ocular movements. *Ventrolateral thalamic* lesions result in sensory loss on the contralateral side of the body, often associated with paroxysmal sensory discomfort or pain. Finally, involvement of a *posterior thalamic* region results in hemianaesthesia or sensory loss on the contralateral side of the body, often with visual field impairment and, again with pain.

Thalamic pain is a very specific symptom. It is unpleasant, often excruciating in quality and generally appears when the sensory loss following a thalamic lesion is recovering. The pain feels superficial and is exacerbated by touching the skin. When impairment of sensation is associated with this pain, the term *anaesthesia dolorosa* is used. Thalamic pain and thalamic syndromes are rare, and although they occur with tumours they are usually more indicative of cerebrovascular disease, in particular disease affecting the small perforating blood vessels.

THE HYPOTHALAMUS AND PITUITARY GLAND

The hypothalamus also lies in the lateral wall of the third ventricle, being separated from the thalamus by a short sulcus. The hypothalamus can be divided into four regions (Fig. 2.8): anterior, posterior, medial and lateral, with specific nuclei lying in each. There are connections to the midbrain and to the reticular formation, these being responsible for alertness. There are also connections to the limbic system, important in behaviour and memory; and, finally, connections to the sympathetic and parasympathetic nuclei of the brain stem and spinal cord, controlling autonomic function. The precise localization of function to specific areas of the hypothalamus

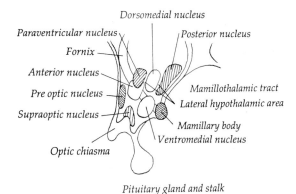

Fig. 2.8 The hypothalamic nuclei and their relationship to surrounding structures.

remains uncertain, and is compounded by the identification of multiple neuropeptides associated with this region and active in the control of body temperature, cardiac and respiratory function, fluid balance, behaviour, reproductive function and circadian rhythm. The hypothalamic control of vegetative function is to a greater extent mediated through the pituitary gland, the control of hormonal secretions from the anterior pituitary being regulated by hypothalamic releasing factors. Bilateral hypothalamic disease is a prerequisite for the development of symptoms. Involvement of the *anterior hypothalamus* will result in cachexia, diabetes insipidus and hypothermia. *Posterior hypothalamic* involvement will produce hypothermia, coma and apathy. Involvement of the *medial hypothalamic* structures results in excessive water intake, inappropriate secretion of antidiuretic hormone (ADH), obesity, memory impairment and aggression. Involvement of the *lateral hypothalamus* results in reduced water intake, dehydration, emaciation and apathy. The identification of specific neuropeptides that control body temperature, food intake and emotion has greatly enhanced understanding of these disorders. Hypothalamic peptides also play an important role in controlling the release of anterior pituitary hormones. The hypothalamus may be damaged by trauma, vascular disease or, rarely, by neoplasia.

Lesions that affect the pituitary gland may present hormonally with either decreased or increased pituitary hormone production. Increased production is associated with *pituitary adenomas*.

Excess *growth hormone* causes gigantism in children and acromegaly in adults. Increased *prolactin* causes delayed puberty in children and, in adult females, amenorrhea, galactorrhea and infertility. In males it may be associated with impotence, infertility and, rarely, galactorrhea. Increased *thyrotropin* results in hyperthyroidism, and increased *luteinizing hormone* and *follicle-stimulating hormone* will produce precocious puberty in children and, in adults, infertility, hypogonadism and the polycystic ovary syndrome. An expanding lesion in the pituitary gland will often give rise to headache as a consequence of stretching the diaphragma sella. Due to the proximity to the optic chiasm, visual field defects are commonly associated with large pituitary tumours, the usual presentation being that of a *bitemporal hemianopia*.

THE BASAL GANGLIA

Deep subcortical paired masses of grey matter are referred to collectively as the basal ganglia (see Fig. 2.7) and include the *corpus striatum*, consisting of the putamen and caudate nucleus, the *substantia nigra*, the *globus pallidus* and the *subthalamic nuclei*. The basal ganglia are responsible for the control and modulation of movements and the maintenance of posture. The anatomical connections are complex and circuitous, there being multiple interconnections as well as afferent and efferent projections from all parts of the cerebral cortex. The majority of striatal efferents project to the globus pallidus, the rest to the substantia nigra. The globus pallidus projects to the hypothalamus and to the subthalamic nuclei.

The observation that certain drugs can produce symptoms identical to those found in disease of the basal ganglia has clarified to an extent the neurochemical basis of many movement disorders, and has delineated the central role of certain specific neurotransmitters. The major two within the basal ganglia are *acetylcholine*, synthesized in striatal cells, and *dopamine*, synthesized by cells of the substantia nigra. In disease of the basal ganglia two types of symptom are noted: *negative symptoms*, in which there may be a loss or slowness of movement or impairment of posture, and *positive symptoms*, which take the form of involuntary movements. Specific types of such movement disorder are associated with distinct anatomical substrates.

CHOREA

Choreiform movements are brief, sudden involuntary movements of an irregular nature, appearing like jerks or fidgeting. These movements are classically encountered in Huntington's and Sydenham's choreas, although they may occur in a host of metabolic, degenerative and drug-induced disorders. Pathological studies suggest that choreiform movements are associated with disease of the caudate nucleus and putamen.

ATHETOSIS

These slow writhing movements are encountered in Wilson's disease, kernicterus and perinatal hypoxia. Damage to the cerebral cortex, globus pallidus and substantia nigra have been identified.

DYSTONIA

These can be defined as sustained muscle contractions, often with a twisting and repetitive quality. Dystonia may be encountered in multiple disorders, and may be focal or generalized. An example of the former is spasmodic torticollis; of the latter, dystonium musculoram deformans. Dystonia has been associated with lesions affecting the contralateral basal ganglia.

HEMIBALLISMUS

These wide-amplitude violent flinging or flailing movements appear to affect proximal limb muscles. They are rarely bilateral and can result in self-injury. Such movements are associated with lesions in the contralateral subthalamic nucleus and may be encountered in tumours, demyelination or cerebrovascular disease.

TREMOR

Tremor is not necessarily a symptom of the basal ganglia. It can occur physiologically as well as in certain metabolic and cerebellar disorders. It can also occur in peripheral neuropathy. Tremor, however, is a consistent finding in parkinsonism, whether idiopathic or drug-induced. Parkinson's disease is a consequence of striatal dopamine deficiency and results in degeneration of the pigmented neurons in the pars compacta of the substantia nigra. The tremor characteristically occurs at rest, is coarse in quality and is associated with rigidity and paucity of movement (bradykinesia).

THE BRAIN STEM

The relationship of the brain stem to the cerebral hemispheres and cerebellum is shown in Fig. 2.9. The brain stem is classically divided into midbrain, pons and medulla. Each of these regions contains cranial nerve nuclei as well as ascending and descending pathways. A knowledge of the anatomy of the brain stem is essential in clinical neurology, not only in order to localize disease to a specific level, but also to help distinguish intrinsic brain-stem disease from an extrinsic compressive process.

THE MIDBRAIN

The midbrain lies between the pons and the cerebral hemispheres (Fig. 2.10), the dorsal aspect being made up of the paired *superior* and *inferior colliculi*. The *cerebral peduncles* converge upon one another, entering the pons at its upper surface. The *IIIrd* and *IVth cranial nerve nuclei* and their emergent nerves, as well as part of the interconnecting *medial longitudinal fasciculus* that

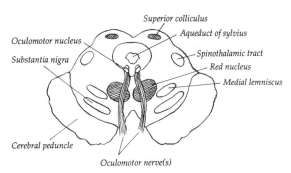

Fig. 2.10 Section through the midbrain.

coordinates ocular movements, lie within the midbrain associated with the ascending sensory and descending motor pathways. Symptoms of midbrain disease take the form of contralateral spastic hemiplegia if a cerebral peduncle is diseased, *diplopia* if destruction of the IIIrd and/or IVth cranial nerve nuclei occurs, and impairment of vertical eye movements and convergence if the superior colliculus is damaged. There are three specific midbrain syndromes: *Weber's syndrome* takes the form of an ipsilateral complete IIIrd nerve palsy associated with contralateral hemiplegia; *Benedikt's syndrome* results from damage to the red nucleus and the IIIrd nerve fasciculus, giving tremor and cerebellar signs contralateral with an ipsilateral IIIrd nerve palsy; *Parinaud's syndrome* results from damage to the superior colliculus, with impaired upward gaze and convergence. This syndrome may be seen with posterior third ventricular tumours, pineal region tumours and hydrocephalus.

THE PONS

As well as containing descending motor and ascending sensory pathways, the pons (Fig. 2.11) is linked to the cerebellum by the *anterior* and *middle cerebellar peduncles*. It contains the *Vth to the VIIIth cranial nerve nuclei* and their emergent nerves, as well as the continuation of the pathway linking the nuclei involved in coordinated ocular movements in the *medial longitudinal fasciculus*. The vestibular and cochlear nuclei of the VIIIth nerve lie at about the pontomedullary junction. Three pontine syndromes are recognized, usually associated with vascular disease. In *dorsolateral*

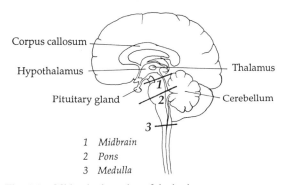

Fig. 2.9 Midsagittal section of the brain.

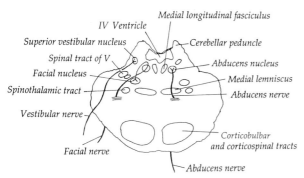

Fig. 2.11   Section through the pons.

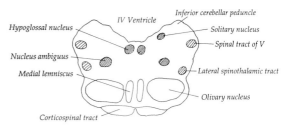

Fig. 2.12   Section through the medulla.

infarction an ipsilateral Horner's syndrome is associated with contralateral loss of pain and temperature from limbs and body, usually with sparing of the face. Ipsilateral cerebellar ataxia is also present, and impaired lateral ocular gaze to the side of the lesion is common. Other associated features, such as deafness and nystagmus, may occur if these specific cranial nerve nuclei are affected. The corticobulbar and corticospinal tracts are spared. *Paramedian infarction* may affect the VIth nerve and the associated VIIth nerve fibres as they sweep around the VIth nerve nucleus. The medial lemniscus may also be affected, with loss of touch and proprioception on the opposite side of the body. Finally, *basilar infarction*, if unilateral, will result in a contralateral hemiplegia associated with VIth and VIIth nerve palses (Millard–Gubler syndrome). Bilateral basilar infarction will result in quadriplegia.

MEDULLA OBLONGATA

The medulla oblongata is a pyramid-shaped section of the brain stem connecting the pons with the spinal cord (Fig. 2.12). The lower part contains the floor and body of the *fourth ventricle*. As well as ascending sensory and descending motor pathways, the medulla oblongata contains the *IXth to the XIIth cranial nerve nuclei* and their emerging nerves. It also contains specific centres for vital function involved in respiration and cardiac control. Two vascular syndromes are recognized: *dorsolateral infarction* (Wallenberg's syndrome or lateral medullary syndrome) is usually the consequence of occlusion of the posterior inferior cerebellar artery. It results in an ipsi-

lateral Horner's syndrome with contralateral loss of pain and temperature perception. Ipsilateral facial sensation is usually affected. Vertigo and vomiting are common, ipsilateral ataxia is usually present, and the IXth and Xth cranial nerves are occasionally affected. *Paramedian* or *basilar infarction* usually occurs as a consequence of basilar artery occlusion. Here, bilateral damage to the medulla results in the patient being mute and quadriplegic, often with impaired sensation in the medial lemnisci and relatively spared lateral spinothalamic pathways. This results in the so-called 'locked-in syndrome', in which the patient is quadriplegic and unable to communicate, although fully conscious.

Throughout the brain stem runs the *reticular formation*, consisting of scattered groups of neurons responsible for activation of the thalamus and cortex. The reticular formation plays a major role in the maintenance of consciousness and its integrity is essential for arousal from sleep, wakefulness and attention. Impaired function results in comatose states. The reticular formation may be damaged by vascular disease, but is also influenced by drugs and anaesthetic agents.

The brain stem is susceptible to compression at any point in its course. This may occur as a consequence of a fusiform aneurysm in the posterior fossa or the cerebellopontine angle, or an ectatic basilar artery, as well as tumours lying in the posterior cranial fossa. These tumours usually present initially with cranial nerve dysfunction, such as loss of sensation in the face in the case of a trigeminal schwannoma, or impaired hearing in the case of an acoustic schwannoma (neuroma), long before secondary brain-stem compression occurs with resultant central brain-stem symptomatology. Advances in imaging have made such separation on clinical grounds alone unnecessary. The clinician should, however, always be aware that the development of subtle unilateral hearing loss or disturbed facial sensation may be the initial presentation of an extrinsic tumour which may eventually cause complex brain-stem symptomatology.

THE CEREBELLUM

The cerebellum is located in the posterior cranial fossa behind the pons and medulla (see Fig. 2.9) and is connected to these structures by *three paired peduncles*. The cerebellum is composed of a small unpaired median portion referred to as the *vermis* and the two large paired *cerebellar hemispheres*. Deep within the cerebellum are located groups of nuclei – the *dentate*, *emboliform*, *globus* and *fastigial* nuclei. The function of the cerebellum is to modulate motor activity, controlling and smoothing out movements and maintaining stance, posture and gait. The major symptom of cerebellar disease is *ataxia*. This implies a disturbance in the smooth performance of voluntary motor acts. This results in movement that is no longer smooth but becomes broken up into small jerky components, with abnormal excessive excursions. There is difficulty in performing rapid alternating tasks with the limbs, unsteadiness of the feet while walking, and the necessity to walk and turn with the feet placed widely apart. Slurring of speech occurs as a consequence of poor motor control of articulatory movement (*dysarthria*). Tremor is present, as is disturbance of smooth eye movement, and nystagmus (jerks of eye movement) is commonly encountered. Certain specific cerebellar syndromes are recognised: *anterior cerebellar lobe* involvement results in the patient walking with a broadened gait but with no evidence of limb incoordination, disturbance of speech or ocular movements. Such cerebellar dysfunction is often found as a consequence of nutritional or alcohol indiscretion. It may also result from long-term drug treatments.

Posterior cerebellar vermis syndrome takes the form of a more profoundly disturbed gait, with an inability to stand without swaying. Again there is no evidence of limb ataxia and no disturbance of ocular movement. This syndrome may also be associated with alcohol and drug abuse, but is also encountered in cerebrovascular disease.

Finally a *cerebellar hemisphere syndrome* occurs with unilateral cerebellar disease. This results in marked incoordination of the ipsilateral limbs, unsteadiness of gait with a tendency to lurch to the diseased side, slurring or dysarthria of speech, and nystagmus with fast beats to the affected side. This hemisphere syndrome may be encountered with cerebellar tumours, infarction or haematoma (Fig. 2.13).

A further syndrome is recognized in which all features of cerebellar function are involved. In this so-called *pan-cerebellar syndrome* there is marked disturbance of gait and balance, ataxia in all four limbs, disturbed ocular movements and dysarthria. A pan-cerebellar syndrome is encountered in certain degenerative disorders and may also occur as a non-metastatic manifestation

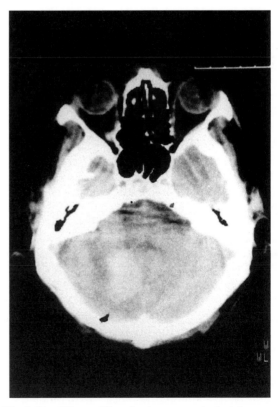

Fig. 2.13   CT scan. There is a haematoma in the left cerebellar hemisphere. The patient presented with sudden headache, unsteadiness and incoordination of the ipsilateral limbs.

of occult malignancy. Cerebellar disease may be the consequence of developmental disorders such as cerebellar hypoplasia, vascular disease (either ischaemic or haemorrhagic) and tumours arising from midline structures such as medulloblastoma, or in a hemisphere such as glioma, haemangioblastoma or metastases. There is also a large group of degenerative, hereditary and metabolic disorders such as sporadic acquired cerebellar degeneration, the familial spinocerebellar degenerations and certain inborn areas of metabolism. Infective disorders, in particular viral infection in childhood, may give rise to a short-lived self-limiting 'cerebellitis'.

Finally, cerebellar symptoms and signs, as well as brain stem dysfunction, are commonly encountered in demyelinating disease, either in the form of acute disseminated encephalomyelitis or, more commonly, in multiple sclerosis.

RAISED INTRACRANIAL PRESSURE

The skull is a rigid structure and its contents – blood, brain and cerebrospinal fluid – are incompressible. An increase in one constituent or an expanding mass within the skull will result in *increased intracranial pressure*. The primary causes of raised intracranial pressure are many, and are compounded by the development of brain oedema, which may arise around an intrinsic lesion within brain tissue or in relation to traumatic ischaemic or toxic brain damage. The clinical effects of raised intracranial pressure are the development of headache, vomiting and papilloedema as well as the shift of structures within intracranial compartments. The pathologist should be aware of the clinical features of *brain shift syndromes* (see Fig. 4.1). Four specific types of herniation syndrome are recognized. *Subfalcine* midline shift occurs with unilateral space-occupying lesions and seldom produces any clinical effects, although compression of the ipsilateral anterior cerebral artery with infarction of the medial aspect of the frontal lobe has been documented. *Transtentorial herniation* (lateral) with a unilateral expanding lesion causes tentorial or uncal herniation, with the medial part of the temporal lobe passing through the tentorial hiatus. This results in compression of the IIIrd cranial nerve in its intra-cranial course, and manifests clinically as an ipsilateral dilated pupil unreactive to light, associated with ptosis and downward and outward deviation of the eye. Lateral shift at the tentorial hiatus may result in compression of the ipsilateral cerebral peduncle (*Kernohan's notch*). Clinically this will result in hemiparesis ipsilateral to the mass lesion causing herniation, and is consequently regarded as 'a false localizing sign'.

Tentorial herniation (central) results in buckling of the midbrain, with distortion and stretching of the perforating blood vessels. This leads to deterioration of conscious level, and initially small pupils which then become intermediate in size and unreactive to light and to accommodation. Compression on the upper midbrain may result in impairment of upward gaze (*Parinaud's syndrome*), and downward compression on the pituitary stalk and hypothalamus may result in diabetes insipidus. *Tonsillar herniation* caused by an infratentorial expanding mass will cause the cerebellar tonsils to prolapse or herniate through the foramen magnum. This will result in neck stiffness, often with a head tilt, depression of consciousness and disturbance of vital respiratory and cardiac function.

THE SPINAL CORD

The spinal cord extends from the level of the cranial border of the atlas, where it is continuous with the medulla, to the first lumbar vertebra. In fetal life the spinal cord extends beyond this to the end of the sacrum, but as elongation of the vertebral column occurs during life the spinal cord retreats, although still remaining connected to the sacrococcygeal region by the *filum terminale*. The cross-sectional anatomy of the spinal cord is shown in Fig. 2.14. There is variability in the size of fibre tracts at specific levels and, therefore, the cross-sectional appearance of the spinal cord is variable, depending on whether this be at cervical, thoracic or lumbar levels. Also, the *intermediolateral grey column* giving rise to preganglionic sympathetic autonomic fibres extends only from T1 to L2. A laminar cytoarchitecture of nine layers within the central grey matter of the spinal cord is recognized. This comprises sensory neurons dorsally and motor neurons ventrally. *The*

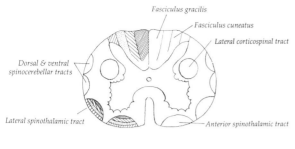

Fasciculus gracilis

Fasciculus cuneatus

Lateral corticospinal tract

Dorsal & ventral spinocerebellar tracts

Lateral spinothalamic tract

Anterior spinothalamic tract

Lamination of tracts (fibre distribution)

Cervical /// Thoracic ·   Lumbar \\\ Sacral ▨

Fig. 2.14 Schematic section through the spinal cord.

major ascending tracts carry sensation to the thalamus and cerebral cortex, finely myelinated or unmyelinated sensory fibres passing through the dorsal root, terminating in neurons in the dorsal horns and then crossing over the next few segments to form the *lateral* and *anterior spinothalamic tracts*, conveying the sensations of pain, temperature and light touch to consciousness. The more heavily myelinated fibres in the dorsal roots pass into the dorsal horns and then ascend in the *posterior columns*, ending in the nucleus gracilis and nucleus cuneatus on the dorsal surface of the medulla, then decussating within the medulla to form the medial lemnisci and passing up to the ventral nucleus of the thalamus and on to the primary sensory cortex. These fibres carry discriminatory sensations (vibration, weight, proprioception, pressure). Other ascending pathways include the dorsal and ventral spinocerebellar tracts, which convey unconscious proprioceptive information from the trunk and lower half of the body to the cerebellum.

The *descending pathways* all exert their influence on α and γ motor neurons lying in the ventral layers of the central grey matter of the anterior horns of the spinal cord. The major pathway is the corticospinal tract, arising predominantly from the primary motor cortex, passing down through the internal capsule into the cerebral peduncle of the midbrain and the basis of the pons, with projections to motor cranial nerve nuclei (corticobulbar fibres) before descending to the pyramidal decussation in the lower part of the medulla, arm fibres decussating before lower limb fibres. It follows from this that any disorder of the spinal cord will result in a combination of motor, sensory and autonomic dysfunction. Also important in the understanding of diseases of the spinal cord is an awareness of its complex blood supply. Paired *posterior spinal arteries* arise from the posterior inferior cerebellar artery and pass on the dorsal aspect of the spinal cord, where they form a plexus which is joined in its course down the spinal cord by approximately 12 unpaired radicular feeding arteries. This rich circulation protects the posterior part of the spinal cord from vascular disease. The *anterior spinal artery* is a single vessel formed by two branches of the vertebral artery running together. The anterior spinal artery lies in the median fissure of the spinal cord and receives approximately 7–10 unpaired radicular branches during its course, these arising in the cervical region as well as from intercostal blood vessels. The anterior spinal artery is at its narrowest in the lower dorsal region, and its largest radicular vessel, the *artery of Adamkiewicz*, enters between T10 and T12. This blood supply can be easily compromised, most often at a mid-dorsal level, which is the watershed area and thus vulnerable to damage by prolonged hypotension.

DISORDERS OF THE SPINAL CORD

Localization to a specific level of the spinal cord is dependent upon a knowledge of the segmental innervation of limb reflexes, the level of decussation of the spinothalamic fibres and the assessment of motor and sensory levels. By careful clinical examination, it is possible to delineate certain specific spinal cord syndromes synonymous with particular disease processes. The history and clinical examination may help distinguish extrinsic or *extramedullary* lesions from intrinsic or *intramedullary* pathology. In the former, *root pain* is a common initial symptom and cord compression, when it occurs, appears selective, compromising motor before sensory pathways. Also, disturbance of bladder and bowel function is a late feature. In intramedullary spinal cord disease there is often a sparing of lower lumbar or sacral sensory modalities (*sacral sparing*), which reflects the lamination of fibres within the spinothalamic pathways, in that sacral and lumbar segments lie to the outside whereas thoracic and cervical segments lie to the inside and are thus more susceptible to intrinsic pathology. In intramedullary lesions bladder and bowel dysfunction commonly occur early, and motor and sensory upsets tend to occur in conjunction.

The spinal cord syndromes (Fig. 2.15)

Complete transection

Complete transection of the spinal cord will result in loss of power below the level of transection. If this is in the cervical region, quadriplegia ensues; if in the thoracic region, paraplegia. Below the level of transection all sensory function to pain and temperature as well as discriminatory sensation is lost, and a clear level of sensory loss can be documented on the trunk. Bladder and bowel function is also lost, the bladder becoming automatic, unable to be emptied at will but emptied by means of manual compression. Disturbances of blood pressure and temperature control are common. Complete cord transection is usually the consequence of trauma, but may occur following inflammation in transverse myelitis, or be the end result of an untreated compressive lesion.

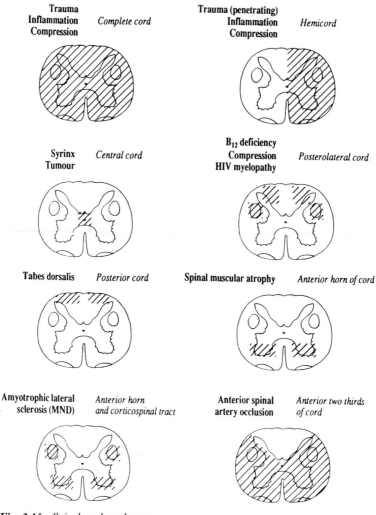

Fig. 2.15   Spinal cord syndromes.

Hemicord or Brown–Séquard syndrome

Here, one side of the spinal cord is diseased but the other is spared. Reflex, motor and sensory dysfunction is evident. There is loss of discriminatory sensation on the same side of the body, and limb paresis with loss of spinothalamic (i.e. temperature and pain perception) on the contralateral side. This syndrome is encountered with penetrating injuries to the spinal cord as well as inflammatory and compressive lesions.

Central syndrome

Lesions within the centre of the spinal cord first affect the decussating fibres of the spinothalamic pathways conveying pain and temperature. This results in a loss of those modalities of sensation, with retention of discriminatory or dorsal column sensation. This is referred to as *dissociated sensory loss*, and often takes the form of a cape-like distribution affecting the arm, shoulder and trunk, with sparing of the face, abdomen and lower limbs. This means that an upper and lower segmental level can be defined. As the central cord lesion progresses, anterior horn-cell involvement ensues, with wasting and paralysis and loss of reflexes. Extension into the dorsal columns will eventually result in the loss of discriminatory sensation, and extension into the corticospinal tracts will result in spasticity and upper motor neuron paresis of limbs distal to the lesion. This syndrome is classically encountered in *syringomyelia*, but it may occur with any intramedullary tumour and has been reported following severe hyperextension neck injuries.

Selective involvement of specific ascending and descending pathways

Tabes dorsalis predominantly affects the dorsal columns and posterior root entry regions. This results in a loss of discriminatory sensation as well as pain and temperature perception in the absence of paralysis. *Posterolateral degeneration* (subacute combined degeneration of the spinal cord) is classically the result of vitamin B_{12} deficiency. Here the dorsal columns conveying discriminatory sensation are involved, but also

the corticospinal pathways, resulting in spasticity. Peripheral nerve involvement is also encountered, accounting for loss of limb reflexes.

The anterior horn region of a spinal cord may be specifically involved. This classically occurs in poliomyelitis, where wasting and loss of reflexes occur in a segmental distribution with no impairment of sensory function. A similar, although more chronic, and generally symmetrical picture is encountered in the progressive muscular atrophy form of motor neuron disease, as well as in other rarer forms of motor neuron diseases (spinal muscular atrophies). *Combined anterior horn cell* and *corticospinal tract dysfunction* is seen in amyotrophic lateral sclerosis (classic motor neuron disease). Here, segmental wasting and weakness is associated with hyperreflexia.

Finally, *vascular syndromes* of the spinal cord are commonly encountered, in particular the *syndrome of infarction in the anterior spinal artery* territory. Here, the anterior two-thirds of the spinal cord are affected, with preservation of posterior function, paralysis being associated with loss of spinothalamic sensation but retention of dorsal column sensation.

The causes of spinal cord disease are multiple. Compression may be secondary to degenerative disease of the cervical or thoracic spine, or may be the consequence of lesions such as neurofibroma, meningioma and metastatic carcinoma. It may also result from direct trauma to the spinal cord, or inflammatory processes such as transverse myelitis or multiple sclerosis. The spinal cord may be affected in a variety of nutritional and metabolic disorders, as well as by infection such as tuberculous spinal compression, HIV myelopathy or spinal abscess. The spinal cord is also susceptible to radiation injury, such as after radiotherapy, and other physical insults including hypothermia and electrocution.

DISORDERS OF PERIPHERAL NERVES

The function of the peripheral nervous system is to convey information to and from the central nervous system with regard to motor, sensory and autonomic activities. The *axon* is an elongation of the neuron, either lying within the central nervous system, in the α and γ neurons of the spinal anterior horn, or else in an outlying ganglion such as the dorsal root ganglion, whose peripheral and central axons are responsible for conveying sensory information to the spinal cord. Peripheral nerves can be divided into those insulated by a myelin sheath and those that are unmyelinated. Diseases of the peripheral nervous system are selective, in that they may affect either motor, sensory or autonomic fibres or else they preferentially affect myelinated or unmyelinated fibres, sparing others. The clinical features of *peripheral neuropathy*, the commonest disorder of the peripheral nervous system, are those of distal motor weakness and/or distal sensory loss accompanied by a loss of deep tendon reflexes. In some of the hereditary neuropathies, peripheral nerves are palpable and skeletal abnormalities such as pes cavus occur in association. The commonest causes of peripheral nerve damage seen in clinical practice in western Europe and the USA are diabetes mellitus, alcohol abuse and nutritional disturbance. Neuropathy may also occur as a non-metastatic syndrome, in association with collagen vascular disease and as the consequence of a host of drugs and toxins.

There are specific circumstances when *nerve biopsy* is essential to direct appropriate management. This is particularly the case in the chronic, inflammatory demyelinating neuropathies and in neuropathy due to vasculitic disease. A nerve biopsy is not routinely performed in the evaluation of peripheral nerve disease, but only in highly specific circumstances where a combination of clinical presentation, electrophysiological investigations and ancillary laboratory tests suggest it is appropriate.

DISEASES OF MUSCLE

Disease of skeletal muscle may present with obvious wasting and/or weakness, or give rise to more subtle symptomatology, taking the form of aches and pains in muscles induced by exercise in the context of normal muscle bulk and strength on formal examination. There is an increasing recognition of *mitochondrial disorders*, which may present without muscle symptomatology and yet muscle histology may prove to be diagnostic. The *muscular dystrophies* are genetically determined myopathies in which progressive degeneration, wasting and weakness occur; the pathogenesis is unknown. Muscular dystrophies may have sex-linked, autosomal dominant or autosomal recessive inheritance and are diagnosed clinically on the topography of weakness, age of onset and the presence or absence of associated features such as contractures, muscle hypertrophy, cardiomyopathy, etc. Inflammatory myopathies often present in childhood as *dermatomyositis*, or in adult life as *polymyositis*. These conditions are usually acute or subacute in onset, predominantly affecting proximal muscle groups often associated with weakness of neck flexion and, often, difficulties in swallowing. Skin and joint features may be characteristic. Muscle enzymes (creatinine kinase) are profoundly elevated and the diagnosis can be confirmed by muscle biopsy, which is essential in view of the complexity of treatment in patients resistant to conventional treatment.

Metabolic myopathies are often easily diagnosed clinically in view of the associated features, e.g. thyrotoxicosis, acromegaly, hypoparathyroidism, etc. Other more subtle metabolic myopathies such as those of phosphorylase (McArdle's disease) and acid maltase deficiency require biopsy for confirmation. Finally, the mitochondrial disorders may present with a variable phenotype of neurological features, including myoclonic epilepsy, stroke-like syndromes and a relatively non-progressive polymyopathy. In these conditions a muscle biopsy is essential for diagnosis.

FURTHER READING

Bradley W G, Daroff R B, Fenichel G & Marsden C D (eds) (1991) *Neurology in Clinical Practice*. Oxford: Butterworth-Heinemann.
Brodal A (1981) *Neurological Anatomy in Relation to Clinical Medicine*, 3rd edn. Oxford: Oxford University Press.
Chusid J G (1982) *Correlative Neuroanatomy and Functional Neurology*, 18th edn. Los Altos, CA: Lange Medical Publications.
Lindsay K, Bone I & Callendar R (1991) *Neurology and Neurosurgery Illustrated*, 2nd edn. Edinburgh Churchill Livingstone.

3. The central nervous system and its reactions to disease

MICROSCOPY OF THE NORMAL NERVOUS SYSTEM

THE NEURON

A neuron consists of a cell body (perikaryon) and its processes. Neurons vary considerably in shape and size, ranging from the small granule cells of the cerebellum that measure about 5 μm in diameter to the large motor cells in the ventral horns of the spinal cord that measure up to 120 μm in diameter. Each possesses a single axon that also varies considerably in length, ranging from a few millimetres to up to 90 cm. The number of its dendrites varies from one to as many as 80, according to the type of neuron. Whatever their size or function, neurons share certain features: they have a high metabolic rate, they are vulnerable to lack of oxygen and/or glucose, and in postnatal life they lose the ability to multiply.

Large neurons have vesicular nuclei, prominent nucleoli and a coarsely granular cytoplasm (Fig. 3.1). These basophilic granular masses (Nissl substance) are composed of RNA-rich stacks of rough endoplasmic reticulum and intervening groups of polyribosomes (Fig. 3.2a and b). Mitochondria are numerous and the Golgi apparatus is usually highly developed. Neurofibrils are present in all neurons and are of two principal types, 20–30 nm microtubules, and 6–10 nm neurofilaments, both of which resemble similar structures in axons and dendrites. There are organised mechanisms that transport material within axons both away from (*anterograde*, which has fast and slow components) and towards (*retrograde*) the perikaryon. Fast anterograde flow (up to 1000/mm per day) transports mitochondria and neurosecretory vesicles: the slow component

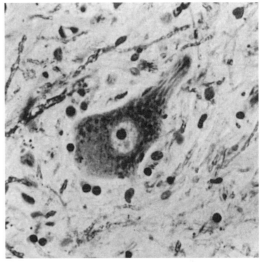

Fig. 3.1 Normal neuron. Ventral horn cell from lumbar spinal cord. The nucleus is round and centrally placed, and contains a prominent nucleolus: the cytoplasm contains large numbers of Nissl bodies that extend into dendrites. (Cresyl violet.)

(up to 5 mm per day) conveys components of the cytoskeleton. Retrograde flow (about 200 mm per day) transports lysosomes and a heterogeneous collection of small vesicles that are either disposed of or recycled in the perikaryon.

Neurotransmitters are transported to the *boutons terminaux* which form *synapses* on the dendrites and perikarya of other neurons. The cytoplasm of synapses contains mitochondria and neurofibrils similar to and continuous with those in the perikaryon, but the characteristic organelle of the bouton is the *synaptic vesicle* (Fig. 3.3) in which the neurotransmitter is stored. In catecholaminergic excitatory fibres the synaptic vesicles usually have a dense osmiophilic core, but in

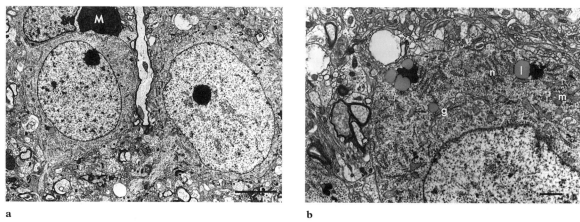

a   b

Fig. 3.2   Large neuron in human cerebral cortex. (a) The pale cytoplasm contains membranous organelles and Nissl substance. An electron-dense perineuronal microglial cell (M) lies in close relation to one neuron. (b) The pale central nucleus is surrounded by cytoplasm containing mitochondria (m), Golgi apparatus (g), Nissl substance (n) and lipofuscin granules (l). (Transmission electron micrographs. Bar (a) 5 μm; (b) 1 μm.)

inhibitory neurons the vesicles are clear and agranular. Larger vesicles are seen in some neurons, and in the hypothalamus take the form of neurosecretory granules associated with peptide hormones and their carriers. Although neuro- transmitters exhibit great diversity in many of their properties, all are stored in vesicles in nerve terminals and are released to the extracellular space. In some terminals more than one type of transmitter substance is released.

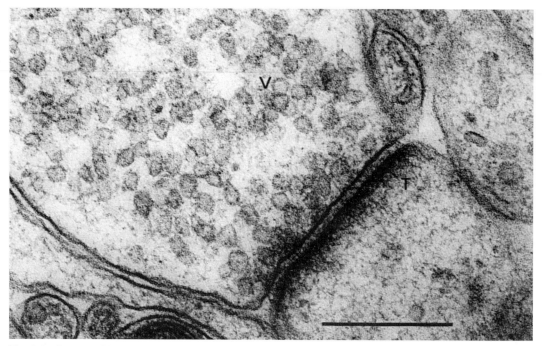

Fig. 3.3   Synapse. Clear round synaptic vesicles (V) predominate in the presynaptic element and there is prominent post-membranous thickening (T) in the postsynaptic element. Bar = 0.5 μm.

Lipofuscin is a cytoplasmic organelle which measures about 1 μm diameter (Fig. 3.2b) and is a type of lysosome (residual body) in which non-metabolisable substances accumulate: it stains bright red with Sudan dyes and is PAS-positive. It is membrane-bound and usually has an electron-dense and an electron-light component, which is presumably responsible for its light yellow colour. It is a normal organelle that is particularly conspicuous in certain neurons, such as those in the olivary nuclei and the ventral horns of the spinal cord, but it increases with age, and an increased number of lipofuscin granules is seen in certain pathological conditions, such as ageing and dementia. It is also found in many somatic cells, e.g. skeletal and cardiac muscle, and liver. In certain sites, e.g. the substantia nigra and locus ceruleus, granules of *neuromelanin* are normal cytoplasmic consituents.

THE NEUROGLIA

Astrocytes

Two types of astrocytes are recognized, *protoplasmic* and *fibrillary* (fibrous). Only their round or ovoid 8–10 μm nuclei can be recognized in routinely stained sections, and special techniques (e.g. PTAH, Holzer and immunoperoxidase) are required to stain their processes which, by electron microscopy, contain glycogen and large amounts of 9 nm intermediate filaments. *Fibrillary astrocytes* are widely distributed throughout the white matter of the CNS, and their numbers increase with age. They occur in the white matter of the CNS as a thick layer beneath the pia (Fig. 3.4a). A similar layer is seen beneath the ependyma (Fig. 3.4b). Between these two surfaces, fibrillary astrocytes are intimately associated with neurons and myelinated fibres, and there is a close association with the microvasculature, the basement membrane of all capillaries being enveloped by the foot processes of astrocytes. *Protoplasmic astrocytes* are largely confined to grey matter (cortex and basal ganglia),

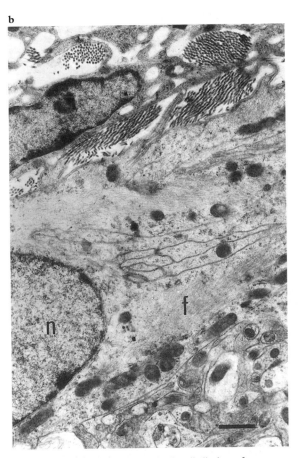

Fig. 3.4 (a)   Subpial astrocytic fibres from spinal cord of elderly subject. H&E. (b)   An astrocyte in the glia limitans from human cerebral cortex. The nucleus (n) has a characteristic electron-dense rim. Bundles of intermediate filaments (f) occur in the cytoplasm among other organelles. (Transmission electron micrograph. Bar - 1 μm.) (Courtesy of Dr W. L. Maxwell, Department of Anatomy, University of Glasgow.)

where they closely invest neurons and their processes except at synapses. The processes of protoplasmic astrocytes are short and stout and they branch more often than the long, fine processes of the fibrillary astrocytes. The Bergmann cells found in the granule layer of the cerebellum near the Purkinje cells are a variant of astrocytes.

Multiple functions have been ascribed to astrocytes, in addition to that of a structurally supportive role. Thus, during fetal development the radial glia guide migrating neurons to their permanent positions in the cerebral and cerebellar cortex. There is also an increasing awareness of the metabolic functions of astrocytes because of the close functional relationships that exist between them and neurons: these include regulation of the ionic composition of the extracellular fluid and their influence on calcium and neurotransmitter metabolism. Another major role is healing and repair after damage to the CNS.

Corpora amylacea are 10–15 µm diameter rounded, laminate bodies (Fig. 3.5) that are often present in the periventricular and subpial white matter, and in the spinal cord, particularly of elderly subjects. They stain grey or greyish-blue in H & E preparations and are PAS-positive. They are thought to represent end-stage degeneration of astrocytes.

Oligodendroglia

There are two main types of oligodendroglia. In grey matter they are closely related to neurons, when they are referred to as *perineuronal satellite cells*: in white matter they are lined up between myelinated fibres as the *interfascicular glia*. The cytoplasm of normal oligodendrocytes is more electron-dense than that of astrocytes (Fig. 3.6).

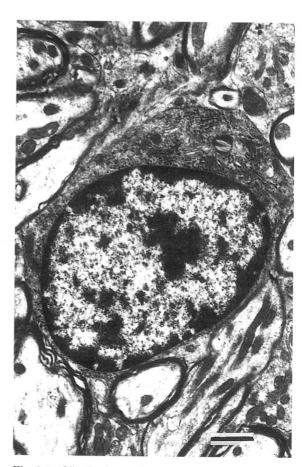

Fig. 3.6   Oligodendrocyte from the white matter in man. Punctate heterochromatin occurs within the nucleus. The cell cytoplasm forms a thin, electron-dense perinuclear sheath. (Transmission electron micrograph. Bar = 1 µm.) (Courtesy of Dr W. L. Maxwell, Department of Anatomy, University of Glasgow.)

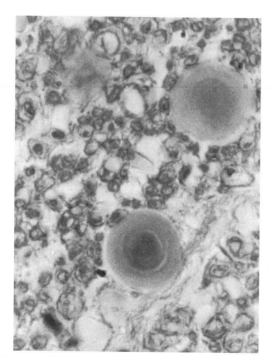

Fig. 3.5   Corpora amylacea in subpial white matter. (H & E.)

They contain the usual organelles apart from cytoplasmic filaments, e.g. glial fibrillary acidic protein.

Myelin in the CNS is formed and maintained by oligodendrocytes. It consists of the compaction of the oligodendrocyte cell membrane, the resulting laminated structure of many successive layers of protein and lipid wrapped around the axon, having a characteristic ultrastructural appearance with a regular periodicity in which the major dense period line is formed where the cytoplasmic components of the cell membranes fuse, and the interperiod line from the fusion of the outer surfaces of the oligodendroglial membrane. Schwann cells subserve the same function in peripheral nerves (Fig. 3.7). A unique feature of the oligodendrocyte is that it myelinates a single internode of up to 10–15 axons: this contrasts with the Schwann cell (see Ch. 18), which can only form a single internode of myelin. There is some relationship both in the CNS and PNS between the thickness of the myelin sheaths formed by oligodendrocytes and Schwann cells respectively, and the diameter of the axon and the length of the internode. Thus, in general, large-diameter axons have thick myelin sheaths and small-diameter axons thin myelin sheaths, whereas the internodes on large-diameter axons are longer than those on small diameter axons. The constituents of myelin include cholesterol, phospholipids and cerebroside in a ratio of 2:2:1, and there are large amounts of *Folch–Lees phospholipid* and *myelin basic protein*. Myelin acts as an insulating material and prevents excitation of the axolemma other than at the *nodes of Ranvier*. At the nodes, the myelin sheaths at either side form end loops of cytoplasm and attachment zones between the sheath and axon. These form the glial–axonal junction (Fig. 3.8a and b). Conduction of a nerve impulse is mediated through polarization and repolarization at the nodes of Ranvier, the impulse passing in a *saltatory fashion*.

Ependyma

The ventricles and the central canal of the spinal

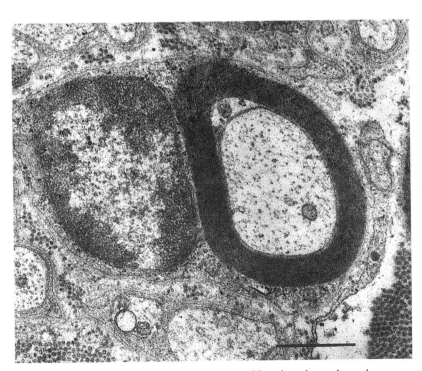

Fig. 3.7 Myelinated fibre from a peripheral nerve. Note the pale axoplasm, the myelin sheath and the associated Schwann–cell nucleus. (Transmission electron micrograph. Bar = 1 μm.) (Courtesy of Dr W. L. Maxwell, Department of Anatomy, University of Glasgow.)

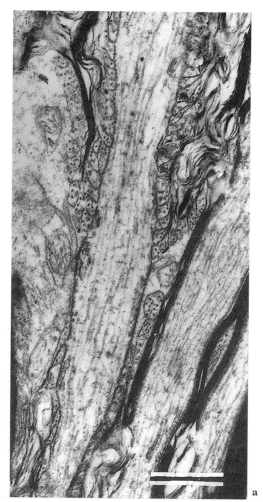 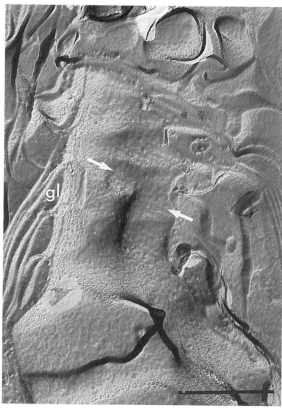

Fig. 3.8   (a) This is a longitudinal section of a central myelinated nerve fibre to illustrate the structural features of the nodal and paranodal regions. (Transmission electron micrograph. Bar = 1 μm.) (b) Central myelinated nerve fibre of a non-human primate. The glial end loops (gl) closely abut the axolemma. Helical particulate arrays (arrows) occur on the axolemma at the sites of the glial–axonal junctions. (Freeze-fracture replica. Bar = 1 μm.) (Courtesy of Dr W. L. Maxwell, Department of Anatomy, University of Glasgow.)

cord are lined by ciliated cuboidal or columnar cells known as ependymal cells (Fig. 3.9). At the base of the cilia of the ependymal cells are small bodies known as *blepharoplasts*. The blepharoplast stains with PTAH and corresponds to the basal corpuscle seen with the electron microscope. The ependyma is normally a continuous layer, although both tight and gap junctions exist between the cells, but with increasing age it becomes discontinuous and there is thickening of the subependymal layer of astrocytes. It seems highly likely that a primary function of the ependymal cells is related to circulation of the CSF.

CHOROID PLEXUS

There are vascular structures (Fig. 3.10) in the lateral, third and fourth ventricles. They are covered by non-ciliated cuboidal cells and are the major source of CSF, the circulation of which is dealt with in Chapter 4.

A small quantity of CSF is formed by exudation through the ependyma.

MICROGLIA

These are thought to be the equivalent of the lymphoreticular system in the CNS, and reach

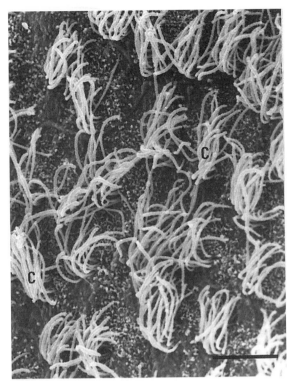

Fig. 3.9 Ependyma from a lateral ventricle. There are numerous cilia. (Scanning electron micrograph. Bar = 10 μm.) (Courtesy of Dr W. L. Maxwell, Department of Anatomy, University of Glasgow.)

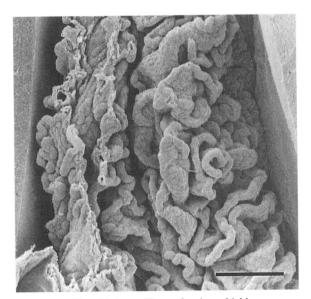

Fig. 3.10 Choroid plexus. The surface has a highly convoluted appearance. (Scanning electron micrograph. Bar = 5 mm.) (Courtesy of Dr W. L. Maxwell, Department of Anatomy, University of Glasgow.)

the brain during embryonic development through the 'fountains of Hortega', which are subpial collections of amoeboid cells situated in the tela choroidea of the lateral and fourth ventricles and beneath the pia covering the cerebral peduncles. They have elongated nuclei that are similar to the endothelium of capillaries. Their cytoplasm is scanty and silver impregnation techniques show that their processes are fewer than those of astrocytes. Resting microglia are normally found in grey matter near small blood vessels.

THE NEUROPIL

This term is used to designate the intercellular matrix in the CNS. In H & E stained sections it appears as 'ground substance', whereas electron microscopy has established that it consists of a dense complex of glial and neuronal processes together with some myelin. Between the membranes of adjacent cells there is a potential extracellular space, which is estimated by electron microscopy to be 20 nm wide, and it is in this space that ionic movements are believed to occur.

BLOOD VESSELS OF THE BRAIN AND THE BLOOD–BRAIN BARRIER

The blood supply to the brain is derived from vessels lying in the subarachnoid space that ultimately perforate its surface (see Ch. 5). The traditional view was that the *Virchow–Robin space* seen around the larger blood vessels as they enter the brain represents an extension of the subarachnoid space, but recent observations have demonstrated that there is a structural barrier between the subarachnoid and Virchow–Robin spaces. There is no space around capillaries, where the basement membranes of the endothelial cells, perivascular astrocytes and pericytes fuse to form the basement membrane of the capillaries. A potential space, however, remains at arteriolar level because, in cases of pyogenic or carcinomatous meningitis, cells may accumulate and separate the perivascular astrocytes from the endothelial cells.

In contrast with several other tissues of the body, the rate at which various substances pass from the bloodstream into the CNS is usually slow, reflecting the activity of membrane pumps. This selective permeability is referred to as the *blood–brain barrier* and numerous dyes such as trypan blue, have been used to study it. Current views attribute the blood–brain barrier to the relative impermeability of the specialized endothelium of the capillaries. Capillaries in the brain, unlike those in the remainder of the body, have circumferential tight junctions (zonula occludens) which prevent or retard the passage of large and small molecules from the blood to the intraventricular (blood–CSF barrier) or interstitial space. Some substances do, however, pass through the endothelium in pinocytotic vesicles, the number of which increases considerably under certain conditions.

There are sites where the blood–brain barrier is deficient–the area postrema on the floor of the fourth ventricle, the pineal gland, the choroid plexus and the ganglia of the dorsal spinal nerve roots. It may be that toxins and some neurotropic viruses gain access to the CNS at these apparently more permeable sites.

ARTEFACTS

Pathologists must be aware of these so that they are not interpreted as evidence of structural damage to the brain. Provided refrigeration has been adequate, *post-mortem autolysis* is not usually too advanced to preclude reasonable light microscopy. An exception to this is when the patient has been maintained on a life support system. Once a patient is clinically 'brain-stem dead', the brain undergoes *in vivo* autolysis since there is no cerebral blood flow. At *post mortem* the brain, the so-called 'respirator brain', may be increased in weight; it becomes semifluid in consistency and hardens poorly or not at all in formalin. The tissue is usually discoloured and there is loss of definition between grey and white matter and disintegration of tissue, particularly in the deep grey matter, in the corpus callosum and in the cerebellum. Fragments of the latter may be found around the spinal cord. Histologically, the neurons have large, pale nuclei

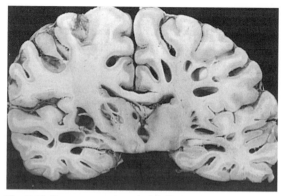

Fig. 3.11 Post-mortem 'autolysis'. 'Swiss cheese change'.

with indistinct nucleoli and their cytoplasm is frequently vacuolated, an appearance that is referred to as *hydropic cell change*. These changes are particularly severe in the granule cells of the cerebellum: in contrast, Purkinje cells are relatively well preserved.

Another artefact is '*Swiss cheese change*' when smooth-walled cysts occur in the deep white matter of the brain (Fig. 3.11). These cysts are formed by gas-producing organisms that continue to proliferate after death and before adequate refrigeration. Organisms can be identified histologically in the cysts in the absence of any inflammatory reaction.

Histological artefact is seen in most surgical specimens that are placed in 10 per cent formalin immediately after removal. The neurons near the surface of the specimen are shrunken, their nuclei stain deeply with basic dyes and their axons and dendrites are twisted in a corkscrew fashion. This is referred to as *dark cell* change, which can easily be confused with the *ischaemic cell process* (see below), an important vital reaction. This artefact can be prevented, or at least reduced, by minimising handling of fresh and unfixed brain tissue. In experimental animals it can be obviated by perfusion fixation and leaving the brain in the skull for several hours before its removal. Other common artefacts include swollen hydropic cells and '*perineuronal* and *perivascular spaces*', which are probably due to shrinkage occurring during tissue processing. They are commonly seen in paraffin sections, particularly of paediatric material, and can be reduced only by prolonging the duration of each stage of dehydration, clearing and impregnation with paraffin wax. They are rarely obvious in tissue embedded in celloidin. Another artefact is the formation of *mucocytes*, which appear as metachromatic bodies in the white matter of frozen sections, although they may also be seen in both paraffin- and celloidin-embedded tissue.

REACTIONS OF THE NERVOUS SYSTEM TO DISEASE

NEURONS

Structural changes resulting from hypoxia

Neurons are more vulnerable to a lack of oxygen than the neuroglia, whereas microglia and capillaries are least vulnerable. Neurons are particularly susceptible to hypoxia since they have an obligative aerobic glycolytic metabolism. The respiratory quotient of the brain is almost unity and glucose is the principal source of energy by oxygenation.

The identification of alterations in neurons attributable to hypoxia may be difficult in the human brain because of the frequent occurrence of histological artefacts (see above). They are due partly to post-mortem handling and to the slow penetration of fixative. Although these artefacts will obscure the earliest stages of hypoxic neuronal changes, the later stages of the same process after a survival of days or weeks are easily recognizable as loss of neurons and a glial reaction. The use of perfusion-fixed material in experimental animals, and selected human material, has shown that there is an identifiable sequence of events, namely the *ischaemic cell process*, which is the neuropathological common denominator in all types of hypoxia (*see* Ch. 5).

The earliest histological feature of hypoxic damage to neurons is *microvacuolation* when the perikaryon of an essentially otherwise normal neuron becomes vacuolated. Most of the vacuoles are swollen mitochondria, although some may be due to dilatation of endoplasmic reticulum. This rather subtle change is difficult to identify in human material but has been recognized in experimental animals after only 5–15 minutes of hypoxia. If the neuron is irreversibly damaged, there is a gradual transition from the stage of microvacuolation to that of *ischaemic cell change* in which the cell body and nucleus become shrunken and triangular in shape (Fig. 3.12a). The cytoplasm stains intensely with eosin and from bright blue to dark mauve with the combined Luxol fast blue and cresyl violet technique; the nucleus stains intensely with basic aniline dyes. The next stage of ischaemic cell change is the development of small dense granules lying on or close to the surface of the neuron known as *incrustations*. (Fig. 3.12b) These are electron-dense profiles of the neuronal cytoplasm (Fig. 3.12c) which are formed into projections from the cell surface, which is indented and distorted by clear, swollen astrocytic processes. Such appearances have been seen between 30 and 90 minutes after an episode of hypoxia in experimental animals, and they may persist for 48 hours. Finally, the neuron undergoes *homogenizing cell change* when the cytoplasm becomes progressively paler and homogeneous and the nucleus smaller. This type of change is most commonly seen in the Purkinje cells of the cerebellum (Fig. 3.13), where it may be seen a few hours after hypoxia and persist for 10 days or longer. The end stage of hypoxic cell damage (*ghost cell change*) is a shrunken, pyknotic and fragmented nucleus without recognizable cytoplasm.

The time course of ischaemic cell change is relatively constant for neurons according to their size and site, so that the interval between a hypoxic episode and death, if between 2 and 24 hours, can be assessed with reasonable accuracy. The ischaemic cell process is energy-dependent, and occurs only if the patient has been resuscitated for a sufficient length of time after the period of critical hypoxia. It therefore does not occur after brain-stem death. In such circumstances any evidence of ischaemic cell change must be interpreted as having preceded the onset of brain-stem death.

Changes in the neuroglia and blood vessels resulting from hypoxic brain damage are proportional to the severity of neuronal destruction. Thus, if selective neuronal necrosis is mild, so also is the *reaction*; if, however, it is severe, then

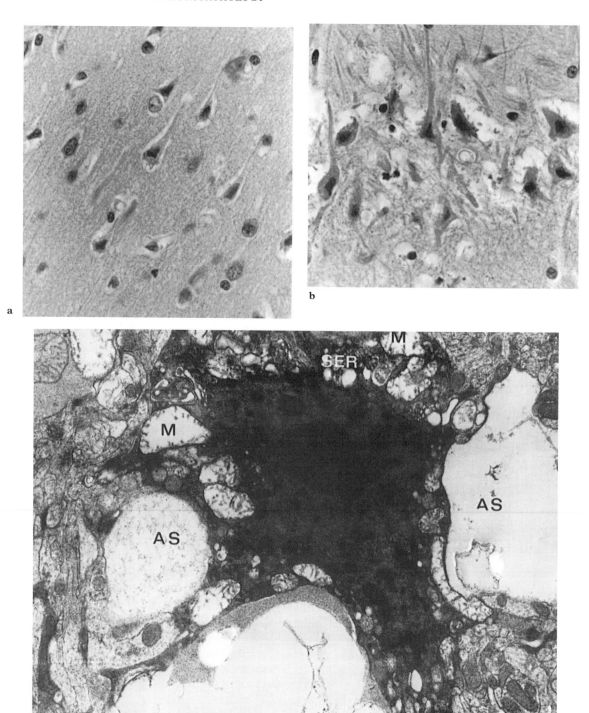

Fig. 3.12 Ischaemic cell process. (a) Ischaemic cell change in cortical neurons. The cell bodies are shrunken and the nuclei triangular. The cytoplasm was intensely eosinophilic. (b) Ischaemic cell change with incrustations in hippocampal neurons. The small dense incrustations project from the surface of the neurons. (c) Electron micrograph of a neuron showing ischaemic cell change with incrustations. The incrustations are electron-dense portions of the perikaryon and dendrites distorted by swollen astrocytic profiles (AS). Numerous vacuoles are seen in the perikaryon and appear as mitochondria with disrupted cristae (M) and profiles of smooth endoplasmic reticulum (SER). ((a) and (b) H & E; (c) bar = 1 μm).

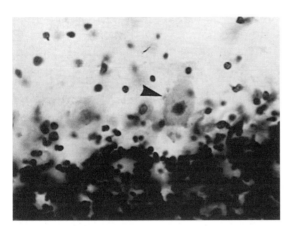

Fig. 3.13 Ischaemic cell process. Homogenizing cell change (arrow head) in a Purkinje cell in the cerebellum. (Celloidin; cresyl violet.)

the reaction is intense and the tissue comes ultimately to be represented by a firm, shrunken scar.

Neuronophagia

In this process macrophages engulf, and eventually digest, irreversibly damaged neurons (Fig. 3.14). The macrophages, which appear to be both microglial and monocytic in origin, are stimulated to react in this way when neurons undergo rapid death as, for example, in viral infections and in hypoxic brain damage. The clustering of the macrophages indicates the position of the dead neuron, which may still be recognizable by its outline. Neuronophagia is less evident in conditions in which necrosis is less acute.

Transneuronal degeneration

This process takes place when a neuron becomes *deafferentated*, from which can be inferred that the normal appearance of a neuron is the product of a number of factors, one of which is its synaptic input. The rate at which neurons undergo transneuronal degeneration is dependent upon age, it being slower with advancing years, and the degree of deafferentation. Affected neurons undergo one of two processes. Most commonly, they become atro-

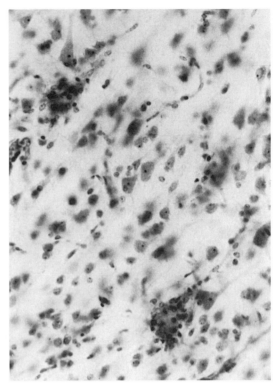

Fig. 3.14 Neuronophagia. Macrophages surround necrotic neurons. (Celloidin; cresyl violet.)

phied, eventually dying and being replaced by gliosis. This type of degeneration is seen at a number of sites, viz, in the lateral geniculate body after the loss of an eye or lesions of the optic nerve, and in the gracile and cuneate nuclei after loss of sensory fibres in the posterior columns of the spinal cord. A second, and less common, type of transneuronal degeneration is seen in the cells of the inferior olivary nucleus, which undergo an initial phase of enlargement associated with vacuolation of the cytoplasm and a fibrillary gliosis. If many neurons are affected, the olives undergo hypertrophy, a finding that is particularly common after lesions of the central tegmental tract.

Reactions to axonal transection

These include both the central somal response of central *chromatolysis* and the peripheral axonal response of *Wallerian degeneration*. The two processes are often discussed separately, but they constitute basic reactions to the same injury.

Central chromatolysis

This term describes a process that is characterized by swelling of the cell body (soma), displacement of the nucleus to the periphery of the cell, folding of the nuclear membrane and enlargement of the nucleolus (Fig. 3.15). At the same time there is dispersion of the Nissl substance (chromatolysis), a change that is particularly marked in the centre of the cell body. Electron microscopy has shown that the chromatolytic change is due to fragmentation and dispersion of the granular endoplasmic reticulum and the ribosomal rosettes. Other ultrastructural changes include an increase in the amount of neurofilamentous material and lysosomal bodies.

The chromatolytic reaction occurs in both central and peripheral neurons, and may be followed by recovery of the neuron with or without axonal regeneration, or may proceed to degeneration and ultimate death of the neuron. The changes tend to develop more rapidly and

to a greater degree if the axonal damage is close to the cell body. Chromatolysis may be identifiable within a day or so of injury, and the changes may persist for some weeks or months. They are particularly obvious in the perikarya of neurons whose axons project out of the CNS into cranial or peripheral nerves, e.g. the motor neurons of the brain stem and spinal cord. Whereas such neurons may recover, neurons whose projections lie entirely within the CNS tend eventually to degenerate and die.

There is considerable biochemical evidence that chromatolysis is accompanied by a net increase in the amount of RNA and protein synthesis, features which are very strongly suggestive of a *regenerative process* rather than a degenerative one. In general, however, although the severity of chromatolysis appears to be a measure of the initial cell injury, its significance in terms of cell function is not clear.

Axonal degeneration (Wallerian degeneration)

After an axon is disrupted, the severed ends of both the proximal and distal stumps swell to form *axonal bulbs*. These swellings, which are due to the accumulation of neurofilaments, microtubules, mitochondria and dense bodies, are attributed to anterograde and retrograde axoplasmic flow, which continues in spite of the axonal damage. Axonal bulbs can be seen by electron microscopy in experimental preparations within hours of injury, but usually they are not identifiable by light microscopy much before 8 hours, and in routine human material until some 18–24 hours after injury. They are most frequently seen adjacent to infarcts, or in certain types of head injury, as homogeneous eosinophilic bodies: they are much more readily apparent in sections stained for axons by silver impregnation (see Fig. 8.11). The proximal bulbs may reach a size in excess of 50 μm in diameter, and it is from such swellings that regeneration of fibres occurs in the peripheral nervous system. In contrast, the distal portion of the transected axon undergoes progressive degeneration and by 3–4 days the whole length of the axon is irregularly fusiform. Later,

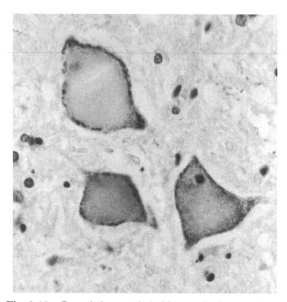

Fig. 3.15 Central chromatolysis. Neurons in the ventral horn of the spinal cord have become rounded. The nuclei are eccentric and there is loss of Nissl bodies from the central part of the perikaryon. (Luxol fast blue/cresy violet.)

fragmentation occurs, a feature that can be best seen in silver impregnation preparations. Most of the axonal debris has been removed by phagocytosis within about one month of injury. Commensurate with axonal bulb formation are degenerative changes within the terminal innervation fields of the affected axons. Again, these are best seen in silver impregnation preparations, which show the characteristic argyrophilic terminals of degenerating *boutons termineaux*. The degenerating terminals are removed rapidly by phagocytosis, and consequent neurogenic atrophy in muscle (see Ch. 17) are important sequelae of axonal transection.

As the distal part of the axon degenerates, so also does the myelin: this is referred to as *Wallerian degeneration*, during which myelin breaks down into ovoid bodies. Within the peripheral nervous system most of the breakdown products of myelin are removed by macrophages within weeks. In contrast, the process within the CNS is very much slower, demonstrable macrophages remaining within the affected tissue for many months or even years. Once myelin debris has been phagocytosed its staining properties change, largely due to the *production of cholesterol esters*, which stain red with Sudan dyes and black with osmium in the Marchi technique (Figs 3.16a and b). Loss of myelin can also be demonstrated by the Heidenhain method, which stains normal myelin black. Zones where myelin has been lost do not stain (see Figs 8.24 and 8.25).

Regeneration and recovery of function

If the optic nerve or spinal cord in man is severed, irreversible blindness and paraplegia ensue respectively. Not so in the frog or fish, for within weeks the frog's vision will be restored. For many years it has been taught that, although axons in the CNS of adult mammals are capable of regeneration, growth ceases by 2 weeks, thereby apparently confirming the early work of Cajal. Recent evidence has accrued to the contrary, namely that under certain experimental circumstances, in both the adult and fetal mammalian brain, axons can regenerate to form synapses and recover some function. The capacity for generation depends on age, being much less in old than in young animals, and on the nature of the system damaged, being greater in noradrenergic fibres and dopaminergic and cholinergic neurons than in serotonergic and GABAergic neurons. Apart from these special circumstances, regeneration is thought to be abortive, either because of the concomitant development of a glial or collagen scar at the site of injury which acts as an impenetrable barrier to the passage of regenerating axons, or because trophic or growth factors are absent from the adult CNS.

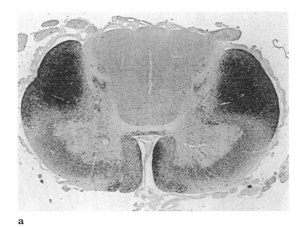 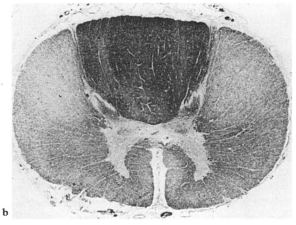

a   b

Fig. 3.16   Wallerian degeneration. (a) Descending degeneration below level of lesion. There is degenerating myelin (dark area) in the lateral and anterior white columns. (b) Ascending degeneration above lesion. There is degenerating myelin in the posterior white columns.) (Marchi preparations.)

There has been considerable interest in the last few years in the capacity of transplants to survive and form connections when grafted to adult central or peripheral nervous systems. At the present time only embryonic or early post-natal donor tissue from the CNS can survive, and there is no evidence of immunological rejection of the CNS tissue transplanted into brain. If hippocampal primordia is transplanted into the hippocampal region of adult rat hosts, the grafts differentiate and send mossy fibres to the host brain and receive mossy fibres from it. Dopamine deficiency in animal models of Parkinson's disease has been reversed by the transplantation of fetal substantia nigra or fetal adrenal medulla into the lateral ventricle adjacent to the dopamine-deprived caudate nucleus. These encouraging experiments give some credence to the belief and hope that transplantation in the future may be a form of therapy for paraplegia and degenerative disorders such as parkinsonism.

It is well recognized that some recovery of function may continue to appear in neurologically damaged patients for some time after the initial injury. Because actual regeneration of the originally damaged axons is unlikely to have occurred, the functional improvement has been attributed to *plasticity*. This is attributed to an adaptation whereby a deafferented neuron becomes reinnervated.

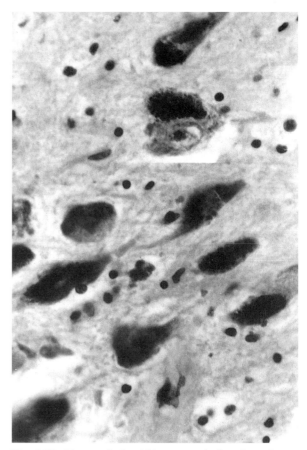

Fig. 3.17   Neuromelanin within neurons in the substantia nigra. (H & E.)

Pigment in the nervous system

Variable amounts of *melanin* are found in the meninges. Although some of the melanin-containing cells are probably melanophores, others appear to be melanoblasts and are thought to be the origin of the rare examples of primary melanoma of the meninges.

Neuromelanin is found in some nuclei of the brain stem, e.g. the locus ceruleus, the substantia nigra (Fig. 3.17) and the dorsal motor nucleus of the vagus. Whereas the melanin in the locus ceruleus appears at an early stage in fetal development, pigmentation of the substantia nigra is delayed until about the age of 2 years.

Neurons in the vicinity of old infarcts often become encrusted with iron and calcium (ferrugination) (Fig. 3.18).

Other alterations in neurons

A variety of structural abnormalities occur within neurons, and some are characteristic of specific diseases. Although many of these will be described in greater detail in ensuing chapters, brief descriptions of the more common types will be incorporated in this chapter.

Alzheimer's neurofibrillary degeneration

This type of degeneration is easily identifiable by light microscopy in frozen or paraffin sections stained by silver impregnation techniques as a skein (tangle) of thick neurofibrils in the

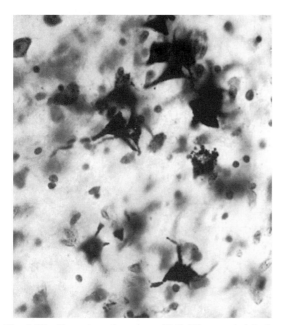

Fig. 3.18   Ferruginated neurons. (Celloidin; cresyl violet.)

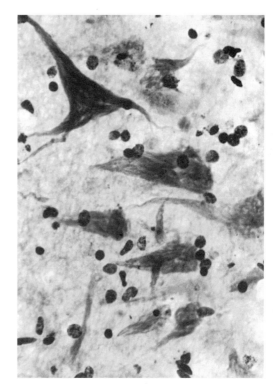

Fig. 3.19   Neurofibrillary tangles. (King's amyloid.)

perikaryon of affected neurons (Fig. 3.19). Ultrastructurally, the tangles consist of paired helical filaments with a characteristic periodicity. Occasional tangles may be seen in the cerebral cortex in normal old age, but they are abundant and widely distributed in Alzheimer's disease (see Ch. 14) and in cases of Down's syndrome surviving into adulthood: they also occur in the brain stem in postencephalitic parkinsonism and in the parkinsonism–dementia complex of Guam.

Granulovacuolar degeneration

This refers to one or more 3–4 μm diameter vacuoles in the cytoplasm of neurons, particularly in the pyramidal cells of the hippocampus (Fig. 3.20). Within each vacuole there is a centrally placed 0.5–1.5 μm diameter haematoxyphilic and argyrophilic inclusion. This degenerative change is rare before the age of 65 years, but thereafter it increases in frequency even in non-demented elderly people. It is particularly apparent in Alzheimer's disease (see Ch. 14), and its occurrence has also been described in certain nuclei of the brain stem in progressive supranuclear palsy.

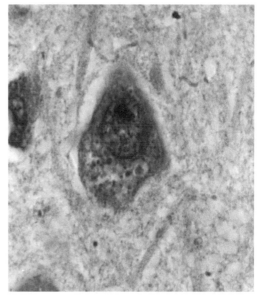

Fig. 3.20   Granulovacuolar degeneration. Darkly stained cytoplasmic granules are surrounded by clear spaces. (H & E.)

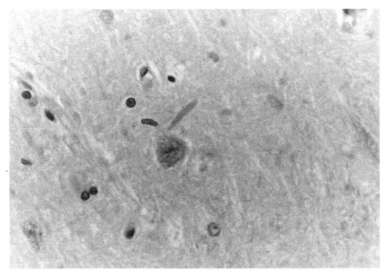

Fig. 3.21 There is an elongated eosinophilic body beside a neuron in the hippocampus. (H & E.)

Hirano bodies

In sections stained with H & E, these bodies are elongated eosinophilic structures that measure from 10–30μm in length and between 8 and 15 μm in diameter (Fig. 3.21). Ultrastructurally they consist of filamentous aggregates and can be found at all ages and in various conditions. They are seen frequently, however, in Alzheimer's disease.

Cytoplasmic inclusions in Pick's disease

The Pick body, which is said to be characteristic of Pick's disease (see Fig. 14.6), consists of a hyaline eosinophilic mass of material that distends the cytoplasm of affected neurons and displaces the nucleus to the periphery. It is argyrophilic and on electron microscopy is a mass of neurofilaments and microtubules.

Lewy bodies

These are hyaline, eosinophilic concentrically laminated inclusions, often with a central core, with surrounding pale peripheral rims (Fig. 3.22). They may be single or multiple, and occur characteristically in the substantia nigra and locus ceruleus in patients with idiopathic parkinsonism.

Lysosomal enzyme disorders

In several metabolic disorders that affect the nervous system there is an increased number of normal cytoplasmic organelles within neurons, or abnormal cytoplasmic bodies (cytosomes) within which non-metabolizable substrates

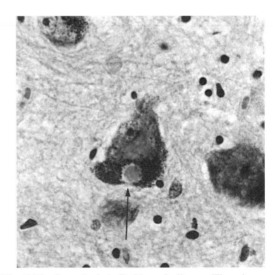

Fig. 3.22 Lewy body in Parkinson's disease. There is a rounded concentric hyaline inclusion (arrow) in the perikaryon of a pigmented neuron of the substantia nigra. (H & E.)

accumulate, thus leading to greatly swollen neurons often referred to as 'ballooned' (see Fig. 10.1); the cytoplasmic bodies may be the primary site of the cellular defect or they may represent secondary adaptive changes. The metabolic defect in many of these cellular disorders has not been clearly defined, although are thought to be lysosomal in origin. The better-recognized inclusion bodies of this type are the *membranous cytoplasmic body* of Tay–Sachs' disease and the *zebra body* of gargoylism (see Fig. 10.6). In many of these conditions the affected neurons also contain large amounts of lipofuscin.

Viral inclusions

These are, in general, visible by light microscopy as homogeneous pink, round or oval, intranuclear or intracytoplasmic bodies that displace the normal components of the cell and are usually surrounded by a thin clear rim. They may be sparse or numerous, and are most often seen in herpes simplex encephalitis (see Fig. 7.5) and in subacute sclerosing panencephalitis.

ASTROCYTES

Damage to the CNS, whatever its cause, is invariably accompanied by hypertrophy and hyperplasia of astrocytes (Figs 3.23a, b, c and and Fig. 7.17), processes that are referred to as *astrocytosis*. The stimulus to this process is probably soluble factors derived from neurons, axons and myelin. Within 48 hours of tissue damage, both fibrillary and protoplasmic astrocytes begin to divide, this response being associated with the production of large amounts of glial fibrillary acidic protein (GFAP). As the proliferation continues, astrocytic nuclei become clustered in pairs or groups of four or more. Neuronal loss is invariably accompanied by astrocytosis and hyperplasia of microglia (*gliosis*). The term gliosis is, however, used loosely to mean astrocytosis.

Characteristically, gliotic tissue is firmer than normal and tends to appear grey and translucent, as in plaques of multiple sclerosis, in relation to cystic infarcts and in the walls of syringomyelic cavities. Usually the glial fibres are laid down in an irregular manner, but occasionally they assume a regular and parallel arrangement (*isomorphic gliosis*), as is seen not uncommonly, for example, in the molecular layer of the cerebellum when there has been loss of Purkinje cells. In areas of long-standing gliosis, in some gliomas and in certain types of leukodystrophy, *Rosenthal fibres (granular bodies)* may be seen. These are eosinophilic structures which may be round, oval or elongated, ranging in size from 10 to 40 µm in length. The nature of the centre of these structures is uncertain even with electron microscopy, but their periphery consists of glial fibres which are GFAP-positive by light microscopy.

Another type of astrocytic response is seen in oedematous white matter, when the cell body enlarges, becomes rounded and acquires an eosinophilic homogeneous cytoplasm, and the nucleus becomes eccentric. These cells are known as *gemistocytic astrocytes* (Fig. 3.23c) and have been found in the white matter within as little as 6 hours after the onset of acute oedema. They are seen also in relation to tumours and infarcts. If the lesion resolves, they become fibrillary astrocytes and lay down glial fibres. Giant astrocytes containing many small nuclei are occasionally encountered, particularly in relation to necrotic tumours and abscesses.

Gliosis is the principal response of the CNS to injury but in certain circumstances, when there has been tissue necrosis, there is often a mixed glial and fibroblastic response referred to as a *gliomesodermal reaction*. This is most frequently seen as a capsule around subacute and chronic abscesses.

Neurons are more vulnerable to hypoxia than astrocytes. In a cerebral infarct, however, astrocytes undergo a sequence of changes that culminates in death, i.e. *cloudy swelling*, in which the cell and its processes swell, followed by pyknosis and disappearance of the nucleus and fragmentation of cell processes.

Alzheimer type 2 astrocytes occur principally in hepatocerebral degeneration (Wilson's disease), and in hepatic encephalopathy, particularly when associated with portocaval shunts (see Ch. 10). They have swollen vesicular nuclei, a

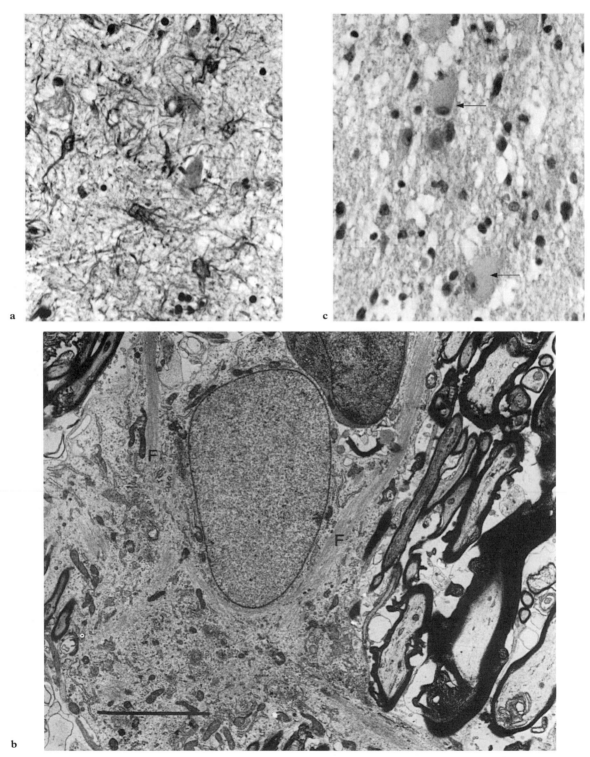

Fig. 3.23   Reactive astrocytes. (a) Hypertrophy and hyperplasia of fibre-forming astrocytes. (b) Electron micrograph of fibre-forming astrocyte. The nucleus contains evenly dispersed chromatin and there are large numbers of glial filaments (F) in the perikaryon. (c) Gemistocytic astrocytes in oedematous white matter (arrows). ((a) PTAH; (b) bar = 5 μm; (c) H & E.)

distinct nuclear membrane and one or more prominent nucleoli (see Fig. 10.10). They seem to be peculiar to man and may indeed be artefactual, since they have not been seen in similar experimental situations.

OLIGODENDROCYTES

An increased number of oligodendrocytes around a neuron is called *satellitosis*: this is a non-specific response seen in a variety of degenerative conditions and as a normal occurrence with ageing. There are, however, many conditions in which oligodendrocytes undergo *acute swelling*, but this too may be a non-specific phenomenon related to delayed fixation.

Damage to oligodendrocytes may be due to infecting lytic viruses, immunological mechanisms, specific antimetabolites, and as a bystander effect in inflammatory reactions. The resulting demyelination follows a stereotyped pattern, with only minor differences in morphology which can be related either to the mode of action of the damaging agent and/or the speed and scale of the subsequent demyelination (see Ch. 9). Although somewhat controversial, it is generally accepted that oligodendrocytes are not phagocytic and therefore do not play any part in the removal of effete myelin. The process of *Wallerian degeneration* has already been described (see p. 40).

MICROGLIA

The microglia respond rapidly to any noxious process, but it is not yet clear what proportion

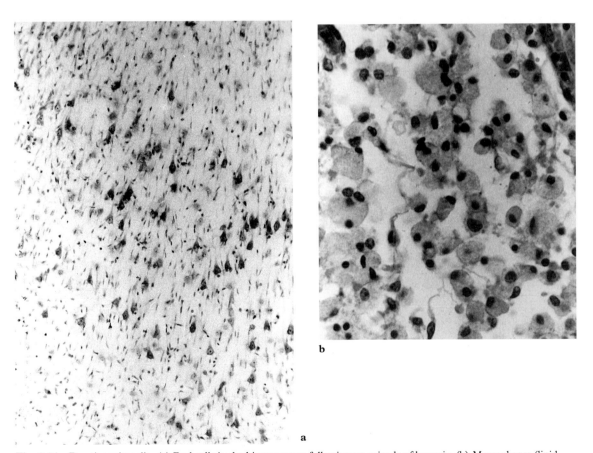

Fig. 3.24   Reactive microglia. (a) Rod cells in the hippocampus following an episode of hypoxia. (b) Macrophages (lipid phagocytes) (H & E.)

of reactive microglia are derived from microglia already present in the CNS, and what proportion from circulating monocytes. *Neuronophagia* has already been described (see p. 39). In the presence of any irritative process, e.g. subacute encephalitis or selective neuronal necrosis, microglia become elongated and their processes more apparent but confined mainly to the extremity of the cells: these cells are referred to as *rod cells* (Fig. 3.24a). When brain tissue is destroyed, the microglia act as phagocytes: the cell becomes enlarged and rounded, the nucleus eccentric, and the cytoplasm filled with ingested material–usually the breakdown products of myelin: these cells–*lipid phagocytes* (Fig. 3.24b) –are sudanophilic and react strongly for acid phosphatase. They are most commonly seen in cerebral infarcts and in recent plaques of demyelination. Microglia also ingest the breakdown products of haemoglobin, when they are referred to as *siderophages* and stain positively with Perls' Prussian blue reaction. The ultimate fate of these macrophages remains unclear, but many appear to migrate into the perivascular spaces and then either into blood vessels or into the subarachnoid space to be absorbed through the arachnoidal villi.

Small clusters of reactive microglia are frequently seen throughout the CNS in patients with a bacteraemia, and in the white matter in patients who have sustained diffuse axonal injury as a result of a head injury (see Ch. 8).

EPENDYMAL CELLS

Ependymal cells have relatively little capacity to react to pathological conditions or to regenerate. The most commonly seen pathological change is *granular ependymitis*, which is a response to some irritant process and is seen in neurosyphilis, chronic ventriculitis and, often, in association with hydrocephalus. The small granules seen on the ependyma, however, do not consist of proliferating ependymal cells but of small collections of reactive subependymal astrocytes, usually covered by ependyma.

FURTHER READING

Brown A W (1977) Structural abnormalities in neurons. *Journal of Clinical Pathology* **30**, Supplement (Royal College of Pathologists) 155–169.

Esiri M M & Oppenheimer D R (1989) *Diagnostic Neuropathology*. London: Blackwell Scientific.

Lantos P L (1990) Cytology of the normal central nervous system. In: *Systemic Pathology, Nervous System, Muscle and Eyes*, 3rd edn, Vol. 4. Edited by R O Weller. Edinburgh: Churchill Livingstone, pp. 3–35.

Lantos P L (1990) Histological and cytological reactions. In: *Systemic Pathology, Nervous System, Muscle and Eyes*, 3rd edn, Vol. 4. edited by R O Weller. Edinburgh: Churchill Livingstone, pp. 36–63.

Reier P J, Bunge R P & Seil F J (eds) (1988) *Current Issues in Neural Regeneration Research. Neurology and Neurobiology*, Vol. 48. New York: Alan R Liss Inc.

Sears T A (ed) (1982) *Neuronal–Glial Cell Interrelationships*. Berlin: Springer.

Weller R O (1984) *Colour Atlas of Neuropathology*. London: Harvey Miller.

4. Intracranial expanding lesions, cerebral oedema and hydrocephalus

These three topics are dealt with together because they have in common the propensity to increase *intracranial pressure* (*ICP*). The basic principle is that, once the fontanelles have closed, the intracranial contents – consisting of the brain (about 70% of the intracranial volume), cerebrospinal fluid (CSF, about 15%) and blood (about 15%) – are enclosed in a rigid bony container. Any increase in the volume of one of these components will, unless compensated for by a corresponding reduction in the volume of the other components, lead to an increase in ICP.

In both clinical and experimental studies, four stages have been defined in the genesis of an increased ICP. In stage 1, the period of *spatial compensation*, any increase in one of the components is accommodated by a compensatory decrease in the other components. In stage 2, once this compensatory mechanism has become exhausted, ICP rises slowly; for a time the systemic arterial blood pressure (SAP) may increase as ICP increases (the Cushing response) in an attempt to maintain *cerebral perfusion pressure*, i.e. the difference between ICP and SAP (see p. 66), with the result that SAP may become very high. This response, however, is usually only transient if ICP reaches high levels. In stage 3, ICP rises rapidly and the cerebral perfusion pressure may fall to a critical level; and in stage 4, which rapidly follows stage 3 unless the process can be arrested, there is *cerebral vasomotor paralysis*, when intrinsic vasomotor tone is lost in the cerebral arterioles. When this occurs, ICP equals SAP, the cerebral circulation ceases, and brain-stem death occurs (see p. 36).

The widespread introduction of continuous monitoring of ICP during life has shed considerable light on various pathophysiological concepts in patients with intracranial expanding lesions. In particular, it has been established that various types of *pressure wave*, i.e. transient increases of ICP, are common in patients who are decompensated (stages 2 and 3) and that *pressure gradients* between intracranial compartments and the spinal subarachnoid space (see below) are of great importance. The skull is divided into three compartments – two supratentorial and one infratentorial (often referred to as the posterior fossa) – by the dura mater (Fig. 4.1). The *falx cerebri* projects downwards between the cerebral hemispheres: there is a space between its lower border and the anterior part of the corpus callosum, but posteriorly, where the falx fuses with the tentorium, it is closely related to the splenium of the corpus callosum. The *tentorium cerebelli* separates the cerebral hemispheres from the cerebellum and centrally embraces the midbrain – the *tentorial incisura*. In normal circumstances, the supratentorial spaces, the infratentorial space and the spinal subarachnoid space are in continuity via the tentorial incisura and the foramen magnum respectively. The normal upper limit of ICP is about 2.7 kPa (20 mmHg). A moderately elevated ICP is between 2.7 kPa and 5.4 kPa (20–40 mmHg), whereas a level above 5.4 kPa (40 mmHg) must be considered high.

The commonest cause of a raised ICP in clinical practice is an intracranial expanding lesion and, as a result of distortion and herniation of the brain (see below), this leads frequently to impaction of brain tissue in the tentorial incisura or in the foramen magnum (Fig. 4.1): this results in a *pressure gradient* between the supratentorial and infratentorial compartments of the skull, or between the intracranial and spinal subarachnoid

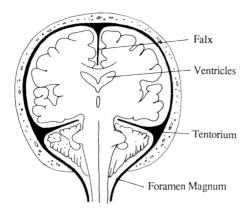

a

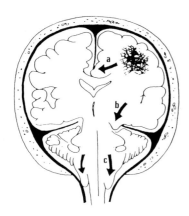

b

Fig. 4.1 (a) The intracranial compartments. (b) The effects of an intracranial expanding lesion. a = supracallosal hernia; b = tentorial hernia; c = tonsillar hernia.

spaces. Such a gradient leads to rapid deterioration of the patient's clinical state (the patient is often said to have 'coned'), and may be produced by ill-considered lumbar puncture in a patient with an intracranial expanding lesion. Removal of CSF from the lumbar subarachnoid space 'opens' a 'closed' space, thus allowing caudal movement of the cerebral hemispheres and/or the cerebellum. There is no such thing as a 'careful' lumbar puncture in a patient with a high ICP because CSF continues to leak through the defect in the dura into the spinal epidural space. If the subarachnoid space is already obliterated at the tentorial incisura or at the foramen magnum, the high ICP is not transmitted to the spinal subarachnoid space, and CSF pressure at lumbar

puncture may be normal. In contrast, when there is free communication between the supratentorial, infratentorial and spinal subarachnoid spaces, as in benign intracranial hypertension (see p. 61), remarkably high ICPs may be well tolerated by the patient.

The account that follows is based on the closed skull. The situation is different in infants, when any increase in the volume of the intracranial contents results in bulging of the fontanelles and starting of the sutures, leading to enlargement of the skull.

INTRACRANIAL EXPANDING LESIONS

A wide variety of pathological processes may present as intracranial expanding (space-occupying) lesions. The lesion may be a malignant tumour, such as a glioma or metastatic carcinoma; a simple tumour, such as a meningioma or a schwannoma; or a non-neoplastic process, such as a haematoma, an abscess, a swollen infarct or a granuloma. It may affect the brain in one or more of three ways: local distortion of the brain, producing localizing neurological signs; displacement and herniation of the brain; and, ultimately, an increase in ICP, the clinical features of which are headache, vomiting, a depressed conscious level and papilloedema. Herniation of the brain and increased ICP are often of greater immediate significance with regard to the survival and the clinical state of the patient than the nature of the expanding lesion itself.

RAISED INTRACRANIAL PRESSURE (ICP)

Distortion and displacement of the brain usually precede any clinically significant increase in ICP, because of the intrinsic compensatory mechanisms by which the total volume of the intracranial contents does not necessarily increase as soon as an expanding lesion develops. Were it not for this spatial compensation, the addition of a very small extra volume of fluid or tissue to the cranial cavity would produce an abrupt and rapidly fatal increase in ICP.

Spatial compensation

In the presence of an intracranial expanding lesion the volume of CSF is reduced. The ventricles become small and the subarachnoid space is partly or totally obliterated. The volume of blood within the cranial cavity can be reduced by compression of the major venous sinuses, and in certain circumstances – the best example is a slowly growing non-infiltrating tumour such as a meningioma – there may be local loss of brain tissue.

The concept of spatial compensation is most easily understood by referring to the *pressure volume curve* (Fig. 4.2), which expresses the relationship between ICP and the volume of the intracranial contents. Initially, the addition of a small volume to the intracranial contents produces little change in ICP because of a corresponding reduction in the volume of CSF, but once the ICP begins to rise smaller increments of volume produce larger increases in ICP because the compensatory mechanisms are becoming exhausted. A critical stage occurs at the steepest part of the curve, when a very small increase in the volume of the intracranial contents produces an abrupt and considerable increase in ICP. This is one reason why the clinical state of a patient with an intracranial expanding lesion of some duration may suddenly deteriorate. The most labile of the intracranial contents is the volume of circulating blood, because of the rapidity with which cerebral arterioles dilate in response to hypercapnia. An individual with normal intracranial contents can tolerate these states without experiencing a significant increase in ICP, but a patient on the steep part of the pressure–volume curve cannot, and any respiratory problems producing hypercapnia can precipitate a sudden dramatic deterioration in the clinical state: conversely, rapid correction of the blood gases can have an equally dramatic beneficial effect. Volatile anaesthetic agents may also produce cerebral vasodilatation, and general anaesthesia for any cause in a patient with an intracranial expanding lesion may increase the ICP.

Other factors affect the rate of increase of ICP. Probably the most important is the rate of expansion of the lesion. Thus, when it expands rapidly, compensatory mechanisms are exhausted rapidly and the ICP soon increases. Patients with acute intracranial haematomas rarely survive for long unless the haematoma is small or amenable to surgical evacuation. On the other hand, a slowly growing non-invasive tumour like a meningioma may attain a remarkably large size before there is any clinically significant increase in ICP. Furthermore, in older age groups, when there is some pre-existing cerebral atrophy and therefore an increased volume of CSF in the ventricles and subarachnoid space, the potential for spatial compensation is greater than in a younger individual.

ALTERATIONS PRODUCED IN THE BRAIN

Focal neurological signs may occur as a result of local distortion of the brain produced by an expanding lesion. The affected part of the brain may function abnormally, leading to epilepsy, or it may fail to function, resulting in paralysis, hemianopia, dysphasia etc. Generalized distortion of the brain with the production of brain shift and herniation as the expanding lesion becomes larger are, however, of greater importance. Shift and herniation are more severe when the lesion expands slowly, since with rapidly fatal expanding lesions there is less time for such structural changes to occur.

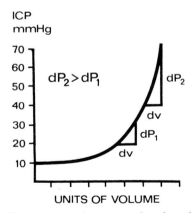

Fig. 4.2 The pressure–volume curve. As volume increases and ICP rises, uniform increments of volume (d/v) produce progressively larger increase in ICP (dP$_1$) and dP$_2$). Increases or decreases in volume cause correspondingly greater changes in ICP on the steep part of the curve.

Supratentorial expanding lesions

A common type of expanding lesion is one within a cerebral hemisphere. Although the various changes will be dealt with separately, they occur progressively and synchronously, and during the period of spatial compensation there may be considerable distortion of the brain without the ICP becoming high.

As the lesion expands so also does the hemisphere: the surface of the brain is pressed against the unyielding dura, gyri are flattened, sulci are narrowed and, as CSF is displaced from the subarachnoid space, the surface of the brain becomes dry. The ventricle on the side of the lesion becomes reduced in size and there is a lateral shift of the midline structures, namely, the pericallosal arteries, the interventricular septum and the third ventricle, away from the lesion (Fig. 4.3). There is frequently enlargement of the contralateral ventricle (see Fig. 4.8) because of obliteration of the interventricular foramen. There may be deformities on the surface of the brain where it has come into contact with bony protuberances on the base of the skull, e.g. the body and the lesser wings of the sphenoid bone. If the expanding lesion has been present for some time, cerebral cortex may actually push through the dura to form small nodules on its outer surface.

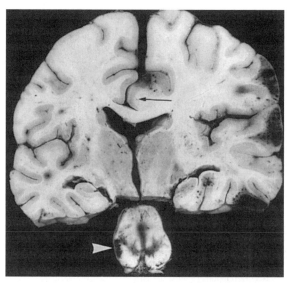

Fig. 4.4 Expanding lesion in right cerebral hemisphere. There is a conspicous supracallosal hernia (arrow). There is also secondary haemorrhage in the midline of the brain stem and a contralateral penduncular lesion (arrow head).

The next stage is the appearance of *internal herniae*, i.e. displacement of brain tissue from one intracranial compartment to another (see Fig. 4.1).

A *supracallosal hernia* (subfalcine or cingulate hernia) occurs when the ipsilateral cingulate gyrus herniates under the free edge of the falx. The pericallosal arteries are selectively displaced from the midline (Fig. 4.4). Because of the relationship of the falx to the corpus callosum (see p. 49), an anterior supracallosal hernia can occur without downward displacement of the roof of the ipsilateral ventricle. As the hernia enlarges, however, the roof of the lateral ventricle is displaced downwards, and posteriorly a supracallosal hernia cannot occur until the roof of the lateral ventricle is so displaced. A small wedge of pressure necrosis may occur in the cortex of the cingulate gyrus where it is in contact with the falx and, occasionally, when the circulation through the pericallosal arteries is severely impaired because of their displacement, widespread infarction may occur in the territories they supply.

A *tentorial hernia* (uncal or lateral transtentorial hernia), i.e. herniation of the uncus and the medial part of the ipsilateral parahippocampal gyrus through the tentorial incisura (Figs 4.1 and 4.5)

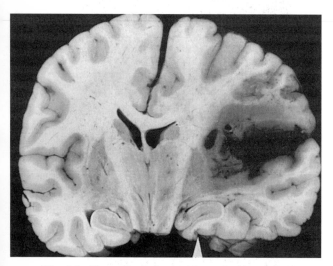

Fig. 4.3 Expanding lesion in right cerebral hemisphere. There is a shift of the midline structures to the left and haemorrhagic pressure necrosis along the line of a tentorial hernia (arrow).

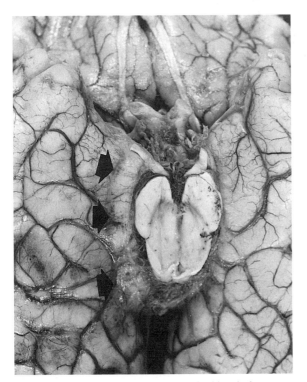

Fig. 4.5 Expanding lesion in right cerebral hemisphere. There is a conspicuous tentorial hernia (arrow heads). There is also compression of the right oculomotor nerve and a contralateral peduncular lesion.

Dilatation of the ipsilateral pupil is the earliest consistent sign of a tentorial hernia and may occur before there is any impairment of consciousness. As the hernia enlarges it produces a groove on the upper surface of the adjacent cerebellar hemisphere. As with a supracallosal hernia, a wedge of pressure necrosis, often accompanied by haemorrhage, may occur along the line of the groove in the parahippocampal gyrus (Fig. 4.3). If there is no haemorrhage, the wedge of pressure necrosis may only be identifiable microscopically. Clinicopathological studies on patients in whom the ICP has been continuously monitored during life have established that when the increase in ICP has been produced by a supratentorial expanding lesion, there is always pressure necrosis in the parahippocampal gyrus when the ICP exceeds 5.4 kPa (40 mmHg). Thus the pathologist can conclude that the ICP has been high even when it has not been monitored during life.

A tentorial hernia also produces selective compression of the posterior cerebral artery, and a common secondary effect is infarction of the cortex on the medial and inferior surfaces of the ipsilateral occipital lobe (Fig. 4.6), which are supplied by the posterior cerebral artery. In some cases infarction is more extensive and extends

is of great clinical significance because of its consequential effects on other structures. Tentorial herniation is characteristically most marked when the expanding lesion is in the temporal lobe, but it can occur in association with any supratentorial expanding lesion. As the medial part of the temporal lobe pushes towards the midline and over the free edge of the tentorium, the midbrain is narrowed in its transverse axis, the aqueduct is compressed, and the contralateral cerebral peduncle is pushed against the opposite free edge of the tentorium. This may be sufficiently severe to cause infarction (the Kernohan lesion – Figs 4.4 and 4.5) in the peduncle, leading to the potentially misleading clinical sign of a hemiparesis ipsilateral to the expanding lesion. The ipsilateral oculomotor nerve becomes compressed between the free edge of the tentorium and the posterior cerebral artery. The nerve then becomes angled over the artery and, if herniation is severe, there may be haemorrhage into it (Fig. 4.5).

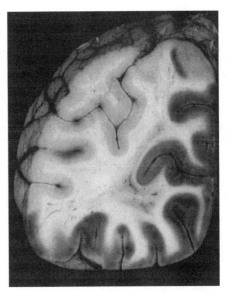

Fig. 4.6 Raised ICP. There is haemorrhagic infarction in the cortex of the medial and inferior surfaces of the occipital lobe.

anteriorly along the inferomedial angle of the temporal lobe involving the cortex, the subjacent white matter and the hippocampus. This type of infarction is often haemorrhagic, when it is easily seen macroscopically, but on other occasions the infarction is pale and, if of short duration, can only be identified microscopically. The infarction may be bilateral, and occasionally it may be contralateral to the expanding lesion, the mechanism here being similar to that of the contralateral peduncular damage referred to above. Other arteries may also be so compressed that infarction, again usually haemorrhagic, occurs in the territories they supply, e.g. compression of the anterior choroidal arteries may cause infarction in and adjacent to the globus pallidus (Fig. 4.7), and compression of the perforating arteries arising from the posterior communicating artery may result in unilateral or bilateral infarction in the thalamus (Fig. 4.8) and in the splenium of the corpus callosum, whereas compression of the superior cerebellar arteries may cause infarction in the cerebellum.

As well as lateral shift there is *caudal movement* of the brain, leading to displacement of the mamillary bodies backwards and downwards, and stretching and compression of the pituitary stalk. Infarction may therefore occur in the anterior lobe of the pituitary gland due to impairment of

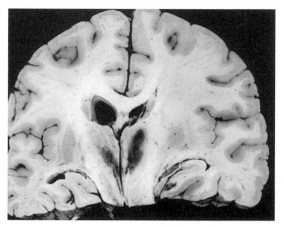

Fig. 4.8   Raised ICP. There is bilateral haemorrhagic infarction in each thalamus. There is also a shift of the midline structures to the left and enlargement of the left (contralateral) ventricle.

blood flow through the hypothalamo-hypophyseal portal vessels.

Haemorrhage and infarction in the midbrain and pons also occur as a result of lateral and caudal displacement of the brain stem (see Fig. 4.4). Emphasis is usually placed on haemorrhage, since this is obvious macroscopically, but microscopical examination often shows that infarction is more widespread than frank haemorrhage. Both types of lesion occur mainly adjacent to the midline in the tegmentum of the midbrain and in the tegmental and basal parts of the rostral pons. Their pathogenesis is controversial. They may be attributable partly to venous obstruction, to the increase in blood pressure often associated with a high ICP (the Cushing response), or to shear strains on the perforating arteries leading to spasm, infarction and/or haemorrhage.

A *tonsillar hernia* (cerebellar cone), i.e. downward displacement of the cerebellar tonsils through the foramen magnum, can occur in association with a supratentorial expanding lesion because of transmission of a high ICP from the supratentorial to the infratentorial compartment. The tentorium cerebelli is displaced downwards, the upper surface of each cerebellar hemisphere becomes concave, the volume of the posterior cranial fossa is reduced and a tonsillar hernia develops. The hernia compresses the medulla and apnoea frequently results. Normal cerebellar tonsils vary considerably in size and shape, and

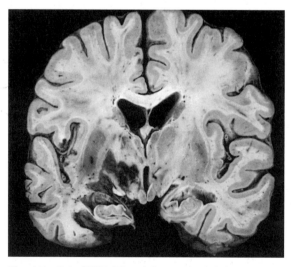

Fig. 4.7   Raised ICP. There is haemorrhagic infarction in the territory supplied by the left anterior choroidal artery.

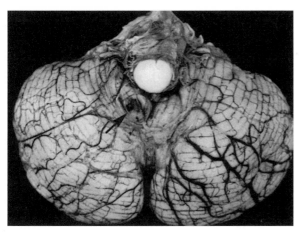

Fig. 4.9   Raised ICP. The tonsils are displaced downwards and there is focal haemorrhagic necrosis affecting the right tonsil (arrow) – a tonsillar hernia.

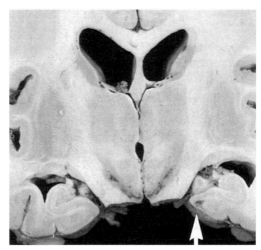

Fig. 4.10   Previous episode of raised ICP. There is an old scar (arrow) in the right parahippocampal gyrus (cf. Fig. 4.3).

herniation can only be said to be present if there is impaction of the tonsils in the foramen magnum, producing a depression on the ventral surface of the medulla where it has been compressed against the foramen magnum, or if there is necrosis of the tips of the tonsils (Fig. 4.9).

Supratentorial extracerebral expanding lesions such as extradural or subdural haematoma produce a sequence of events similar to intracerebral lesions. One difference observed is that convolutional flattening associated with a subdural haematoma is restricted to the contralateral hemisphere, the blood in the ipsilateral subdural space preventing flattening of the convolutions.

When brain swelling is diffuse and bilateral, as in *diffuse cerebral oedema*, the ventricles become small and symmetrical and there is no lateral shift of the midline structures. Tentorial herniae may occur but they are usually relatively small and often bilateral, their size depending on the rate of brain swelling and the size of the tentorial incisura. Caudal displacement of the diencephalon and the brain stem will be more severe than with a unilateral expanding lesion.

If shift and herniation of the brain regress as the result of treatment of a high ICP (> 5.4 Kpa), evidence of the previous high ICP remains in the form of wedge-shaped scars in the cingulate and parahippocampal gyri (Fig. 4.10). There may also be evidence of previous infarction in the medial occipital cortex (Fig. 4.11), in the terri-

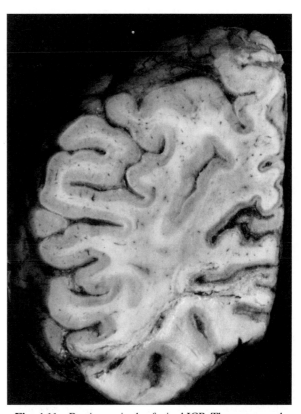

Fig. 4.11   Previous episode of raised ICP. The cortex on the medial and inferior surfaces of the occipital lobe is narrowed and granular (cf. Fig. 4.6).

tory supplied by the anterior choroidal artery, and in the brain stem. Patients who have sustained damage to the brain stem secondary to an intracranial expanding lesion rarely survive for more than a few weeks, even if the primary lesion has been treated.

Infratentorial expanding lesions

Increase in the size of the lateral ventricles (hydrocephalus) is the commonest abnormality associated with an expanding lesion in the posterior fossa. This leads in turn to enlargement of the cerebral hemispheres, and convolutional flattening. When the lesion is not in the midline, the aqueduct and fourth ventricle are compressed and displaced to the other side. Tonsillar herniation is more severe than with supratentorial expanding lesions. When there is a severe tonsillar hernia, the posterior inferior cerebellar arteries may be so compressed that infarction occurs in the inferior part of one or both cerebellar hemispheres.

Herniation of the cerebellum may also occur in an upward direction through the tentorial incisura – the so-called *reversed tentorial hernia*, and if the lesion is expanding very slowly, upward herniation of the superior vermis can produce considerable distortion of the parahippocampal gyri.

OTHER EFFECTS OF EXPANDING LESIONS

Erosion of bone is a characteristic feature of a long-sustained moderate increase in ICP. In adults the pituitary fossa is the first structure to be affected. At first there is loss of detail of the cortex anteriorly at the lower part of the fossa. In infants and children up to about 10 years old, the first sign of raised intracranial pressure is often separation of the sutures of the vault. Enlargement of the skull, thinning of the bones of the vault and prominence of the convolutional impressions may also occur in children. If the evolution of the expanding lesion has been particularly slow, the floor of the pituitary fossa may be thinned, this being attributed to downward pressure on the diaphragma sellae. Certainly a deeply cupped diaphragma sellae is often

seen *post mortem* in patients with slowly expanding lesions. Occasionally there may also be erosion of the lesser wings of the sphenoid bone and of the orbital roof.

Systemic changes that may occur in association with a high ICP and distortion and herniation of the brain include subendocardial haemorrhage in the outflow tract of the left ventricle, foci of necrosis in the myocardium and haemorrhagic congestion and ulceration of the mucosa of the stomach, duodenum and urinary bladder. These changes are related in some way to sympathetic overactivity.

OEDEMA AND SWELLING OF THE BRAIN

These remain controversial and poorly understood conditions. The term *cerebral oedema* means that there is an increase in the water content of the brain tissue, leading to an increase in the volume of all or part of the brain. The normal water content of grey matter is 80 per cent of the wet weight, and of white matter 68 per cent of wet weight. The content in cerebral oedema would be some 81–82 per cent and 76–79 per cent respectively. Swelling may also be brought about by *congestive brain swelling* as a result of an increase in the cerebral blood volume. In either case there is ultimately an increase in the volume of one of the intracranial constituents, leading to the sequence of events described in the previous section.

In many types of intracranial expanding lesion, e.g. simple and malignant tumours and traumatic haematomas, the effective size of the lesion may be considerably increased by associated vasodilatation or oedema (Fig. 4.12): these can often be controlled by hyperventilation or by the administration of steroids, respectively. In other types of expanding lesion, e.g. infarcts and haematomas, such treatment is ineffective. The principal aim of treatment therefore is to remove, or at least reduce, the volume of the expanding lesion. If no definitive treatment is possible, any attempt to reduce ICP by removing part of the vault of the skull is contraindicated since the brain simply extrudes through the defect in the skull. This is referred to as an *external hernia cerebri*.

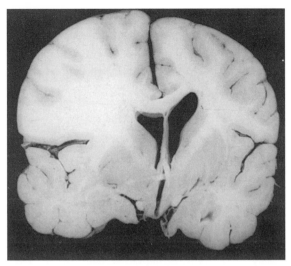

Fig. 4.12 Cerebral oedema. The left cerebral hemisphere is markedly expanded, and there is a shift of the midline to the right and a supracallosal hernia. There was a small deposit of metastatic carcinoma in an adjacent brain slice.

CEREBRAL OEDEMA

There are several types of cerebral oedema, and the increased water content may be *extracellular* or *intracellular*.

Vasogenic oedema

In this type of oedema the blood–brain barrier is defective, and water, sodium and protein molecules are extravasated into the extracellular space.

The oedema occurs particularly in white matter and, when severe, the affected white matter may have a pale green colour. On microscopical examination there is pallor of myelin staining and the myelin sheaths appear rather vacuolated and beaded. Gemistocytic astrocytes are conspicuous. If the oedema persists for some time there is some destruction of myelin, as shown by the appearance of lipid phagocytes. The causes of the breakdown of the blood–brain barrier in this type of oedema include physical disruption due to trauma, and necrosis of vessel walls in tumours and infarcts. In some instances where the anatomical barrier appears to be intact, dysfunction is thought to be due to an increase in pinocytotic activity.

Cytotoxic oedema

The commonest cause of this type of oedema is ischaemic damage to the brain, and it is essentially an intracellular type of oedema. It occurs as a result of energy failure within neurons and is therefore more prominent in grey than in white matter. Vasogenic oedema may, however, develop adjacent to an infarct (see Ch. 5).

Cytotoxic oedema can be produced experimentally by certain toxins, such as triethyltin and hexachlorophane.

Hydrostatic oedema

A sudden increase in intravascular pressure can overcome the cerebrovascular resistance, leading to flooding of the capillary bed within the brain, followed rapidly by extravasation of protein-poor fluid into the extracellular space. This type of oedema is seen in hypertensive encephalopathy and may occur when neurosurgical procedures are undertaken on patients with a very high intracranial pressure. The oedema increases when an intracranial tumour is removed, a large external hernia cerebri may develop when a bone flap is turned in a patient with pre-existing high intracranial pressure.

Interstitial oedema

The water content of the periventricular tissue increases in acute obstructive hydrocephalus (see below). Fluid under high pressure is forced into the periventricular white matter through damaged ependyma.

Hypo-osmotic oedema

This type of oedema may develop when the serum osmolality is severely reduced, and may explain the cerebral oedema that sometimes occurs in the treatment of diabetic coma, when there may be a relative reduction of serum osmolality compared with brain tissue where the glucose level is still high.

Effects and resolution of cerebral oedema

There is no evidence to suggest that any increase in brain water content directly interferes with a patient's neurological state. It exerts its effects only when it is sufficiently severe to produce an increase in ICP. This is clearly demonstrable when steroids are administered to a patient with vasogenic oedema around a cerebral tumour, who is becoming decompensated (see p. 51). The precise effect of steroids in this condition is not known but even a slight reduction in the oedema can result in a dramatic improvement in the patient's clinical state because they are on the steep part of the pressure–volume curve (see Fig. 4.2). Unfortunately, steroids do not exert a similar effect on the other types of cerebral oedema.

It has been shown experimentally that, in vasogenic oedema related to focal brain damage (e.g. a lesion produced by intense cold), most of the oedema fluid is produced within or immediately adjacent to the lesion. Some of this fluid then traverses the white matter to enter the ventricular system. This has been referred to as 'the oedema front', but it is now clear that there are many other sites of reabsorption of oedema fluid into blood vessels.

CONGESTIVE BRAIN SWELLING

This can occur remarkably rapidly, particularly in children who have sustained a head injury and in patients with an acute subdural haematoma (see Ch. 8). The precise pathogenesis is not known, but arterioles dilate without there being hypercapnia or hypoxaemia and the capillary bed is flooded with stagnant blood. There would therefore appear to be some element of vasomotor paralysis, possibly attributable to trauma.

Congestive brain swelling tends to be diffuse, affecting one or both cerebral hemispheres, and leads to rapid expansion of the affected brain, particularly when arterial blood pressure is high. This, in turn, will induce dysfunction of the blood–brain barrier with the result that ICP may increase rapidly, leading to the sequelae described above.

HYDROCEPHALUS

The formation and circulation of cerebrospinal fluid (CSF) is summarized diagrammatically in Figure 4.13. The volume of the CSF is about 120 ml, and it is changed some 3–5 times per day. The term hydrocephalus means an *increased volume of CSF* within the cranial cavity.

TYPES OF HYDROCEPHALUS

In *internal* hydrocephalus the increased volume of CSF is within the ventricular system and, in general, the term hydrocephalus is used to denote this type of hydrocephalus. In *external* hydrocephalus the excess CSF is in the subarachnoid space. The hydrocephalus is said to be *communicating* if CSF can flow freely from the ventricular system to the subarachnoid space; if it cannot, it is *non-communicating*. In *active* hydrocephalus there is progressive enlargement of the ventricular system and an increased intraventricular pressure. Hydrocephalus is said to be *arrested* when ventricular enlargement ceases and intraventricular pressure is normal. *Compensatory* hydrocephalus (sometimes referred to as *ex vacuo*) occurs when the increased volume of CSF is compensatory to loss of brain tissue.

Pathogenesis of hydrocephalus

The commonest cause of hydrocephalus is ventricular enlargement secondary to cerebral atrophy (see Ch. 14): in these circumstances intracranial pressure is not increased. Hydrocephalus of acute onset with an increased intracranial pressure is most often due to *obstruction* to the free flow of CSF. The ventricles enlarge and there is a reduction in the bulk of the white matter in the cerebral hemispheres, despite the fact that CSF flows into the adjacent white matter causing interstitial oedema. As a result of this there is a reduced density of the periventricular white matter in CT scans (Fig. 4.14). In experimental studies it has been shown that there is disruption of the ependyma as the ventricles enlarge, but after some weeks hydrocephalus usually becomes arrested, presumably because the amount of CSF absorbed is in equilibrium with the volume of

Superior sagittal sinus

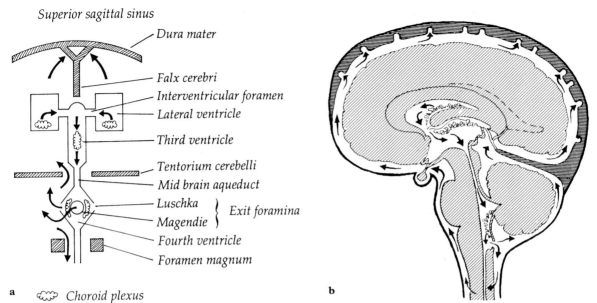

a   ꙮ *Choroid plexus*   b

Dura mater
Falx cerebri
Interventricular foramen
Lateral ventricle
Third ventricle
Tentorium cerebelli
Mid brain aqueduct
Luschka } *Exit foramina*
Magendie }
Fourth ventricle
Foramen magnum

Fig. 4.13 (a & b) The formation and circulation of CSF. The bulk of the CSF is produced in the choroid plexuses of the lateral, third and fourth ventricles. The direction of intraventricular flow is shown by the arrows. CSF leaves the lateral ventricles via interventricular foramina, and the fourth ventricle via the exit formanima in the fourth ventricle (Luschka and Magendie) to enter the subarachnoid space. Some descends through the foramen magnum into the spinal subarachnoid space where it is absorbed in the prolongations of the subarachnoid space along spinal nerve roots. Most circulates through the posterior fossa and then reaches the supratentorial space through the tentorial incisura. It then flows over the cerebral hemispheres to be absorbed in the superior sagittal sinus.

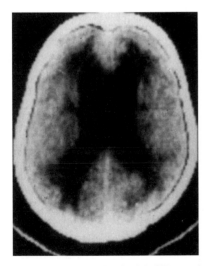

Fig. 4.14 Acute hydrocephalus. In this CT scan the ventricles are enlarged and the periventricular white matter is of reduced density (interstitial oedema). (Courtesy of Dr Peter Macpherson, Department of Neuroradiology, Institute of Neurological Sciences, Glasgow.)

CSF produced. A similar arrest of hydrocephalus may occur in man, but death can occur with remarkable rapidity, e.g. when a colloid cyst in the third ventricle (see Ch. 15) blocks the interventricular foramina. In patients with acute hydrocephalus, however, there is usually time to establish ventricular drainage to remove CSF. The ventricles then rapidly reduce in size and the cerebral mantle returns to its normal width (Fig. 4.15), but the mechanism which allows this restoration remains unexplained.

In obstructive hydrocephalus in man it is the site of the lesion rather than its nature which is of importance. Thus, a small lesion in a sensitive site adjacent to an interventricular foramen or the aqueduct in the midbrain is of much greater significance than a large expanding lesion in a frontal or occipital lobe. The abnormality, however, need not be adjacent to the ventricular system, since any process such as previous

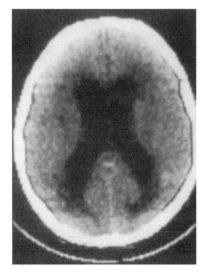 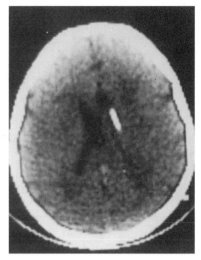

a   b

Fig. 4.15 Hydrocephalus. CT scans (a) before and (b) after ventricular drainage. Note the difference in the width of the cerebral mantle. The tip of the catheter is seen in the right lateral ventricle. (Courtesy of Dr Peter Macpherson, Department of Neuroradiology Institute of Neurological Sciences, Glasgow.)

meningitis or subarachnoid haemorrhage that results in obliteration of the subarachnoid space – particularly at the level of the tentorial incisura (see Fig. 4.13) – will obstruct the free flow of CSF. It is also clear from Fig. 4.13 that hydrocephalus will be produced rapidly by a lesion in the infratentorial compartment of the skull. This may be a conventional expanding lesion, but rarer causes include ectasia and tortuosity of the basilar artery, and abnormalities of the base of the skull, e.g. Paget's disease, achondroplasia etc. Several of the obstructive lesions causing hydrocephalus are congenital, e.g. the Chiari malformations and the Dandy–Walker syndrome (see Ch. 13). A rare cause of hydrocephalus is *gliosis of the aqueduct* in late adolescent or young adult life. This appears to be produced by a proliferation of periaqueductal astrocytes, leading to progressive stenosis of the aqueduct.

In essence, the ventricular system proximal to the obstruction enlarges. If the obstruction is at an interventricular foramen (Monro), one lateral ventricle enlarges; if it is in the third ventricle or the aqueduct, both lateral ventricles enlarge; if it is at the exit foramina of the fourth ventricle due to some previous inflammatory process, the entire ventricular system enlarges; if the obstruction is in the subarachnoid space at the level of

the tentorium, again the entire ventricular system enlarges but on this occasion the hydrocephalus is communicating in type.

Other theoretical causes of hydrocephalus are *increased production* of CSF, or *decreased absorption*. Increased production of CSF may occur in patients with a papilloma of the choroid plexus (see Ch. 15), but there may also be an obstructive element since shedding of tumour cells or haemorrhage from the tumour may have an irritant effect leading to obliteration of the subarachnoid space. It has been suggested that decreased absorption of CSF may be a sequel to subarachnoid haemorrhage, the arachnoidal granulations being partly obliterated by macrophages containing haemosiderin.

Clinical features of hydrocephalus

In acute hydrocephalus the clinical features are basically those of a high ICP. It would appear, however, that unless there is a total intraventricular obstruction to the free flow of CSF in man, active hydrocephalus often becomes arrested.

When hydrocephalus develops before the sutures of the skull have closed, the head enlarges and may become enormous, and the ventricles become extremely large. It is remarkable how, on occasion, intellect is surprisingly well maintained despite the fact that the cerebral mantle is extremely thin.

Normal pressure hydrocephalus

This syndrome has attracted considerable attention in recent years and is characterized by ventricular enlargement and a clinical syndrome consisting of progressive dementia, disturbance of gait and urinary incontinence or urgency. Routine measurement of the CSF pressure may show it to be normal, but if patients with this type of hydrocephalus are subjected to continuous monitoring of ICP, episodes of moderate intracranial hypertension can often be demonstrated, particularly during sleep. For this reason it has been suggested that a more appropriate descriptive term would be *intermittent hydrocephalus*. The importance of this type of hydrocephalus is that the patient's condition may be improved by surgical measures to reduce hydrocephalus, such as a ventriculoperitoneal shunt.

This is a particularly frustrating syndrome for pathologists, who often find some ventricular enlargent in elderly patients who have had some degree of dementia. It is, however, impossible *post mortem* to distinguish compensatory hydrocephalus brought about by cerebral atrophy from normal pressure hydrocephalus.

BENIGN INTRACRANIAL HYPERTENSION

This is another controversial subject and it is not yet clear whether it represents a single entity or is merely one of several different disease processes which cause raised ICP. The patients – women more frequently than men – have a high ICP, papilloedema and headache, but neuroradiological studies show that the ventricular system is not enlarged. Because the high ICP is evenly distributed throughout the craniospinal axis, there are no intracranial pressure gradients, and no shift or herniation of the brain.

FURTHER READING

Adams J H & Graham D I (1976) The relationship between ventricular fluid pressure and the neuropathology of raised intracranial pressure. *Neuropathology and Applied Neurobiology* **2**, 323–332.

Betz A L & Crockard A (1992) Brain edema and the blood–brain barrier. In: *Neurosurgery: the Scientific Basis of Clinical Practice*. Edited by A Crockard, R Hayward & J T Hoff. Oxford: Blackwell Scientific Publications, pp. 353–372.

Graham D I (1990) The pathophysiology of raised intracranial pressure. In: *Systemic Pathology, Nervous System, Muscle and Eyes*, 3rd edn, Vol. 4. Edited by R O Weller. Edinburgh: Churchill Livingstone, pp. 64–77.

Klatzo I (1967) Neuropathological aspects of brain oedema. *Journal of Neuropathology and Experimental Neurology* **26**, 1–14.

Langfitt T W (1969) Increased intracranial pressure. *Clinical Neurosurgery* **16**, 436–471.

Miller J D & Piper I A (1992) Raised intracranial pressure and its effect on brain function. In: *Neurosurgery: the Scientific Basis of Clinical Practice*. Edited by A Crockard, R Hayward & J T Hoff. Oxford: Blackwell Scientific Publications, pp. 373–390.

Reulen H-J, Baethmann A, Fenstermacher J, Marmarou, A & Spatz, M (eds) (1990) *Brain Edema VIII. Acta Neurochirurgica Supplementum 51*. Wien: Springer Verlag.

5. Vascular and hypoxic disorders

'Strokes' or 'cerebrovascular accidents' are clinical terms that describe the rapid onset of a focal disturbance of cerebral function of presumed vascular origin and of more than 24 hours' duration. The commonest causes are *cerebral infarction* and *spontaneous intracranial haemorrhage*. Although it may be difficult to make the correct diagnosis clinically, modern neuroimaging techniques such as CT and MRI have greatly facilitated a precise diagnosis. Despite the difficulties of comparing clinical and pathological material, prospective epidemiological studies such as that at Framingham, Massachusetts, USA, have provided much useful information about the morbidity, mortality and pathogenesis of cerebrovascular disease. In the UK, as in other westernized countries, cerebrovascular disease constitutes a major health problem accounting for some 10 per cent of all deaths, and is surpassed only by heart disease and cancer. In those patients who survive a 'stroke' that persists for 24 hours, about 50 per cent are permanently disabled and only 10 per cent return to normal activity. Although commonest in the elderly, strokes occur in all age groups.

Estimates of the incidence of the various types of 'stroke' vary depending on the source of the information. However, data from prospective epidemiological studies suggests that some 84 per cent are due to *infarction* (53 per cent thrombotic, 31 per cent embolic), leaving some 16 per cent due to *haemorrhage* (10 per cent with spontaneous intracerebral haemorrhage, 6 per cent with subarachnoid haemorrhage from a ruptured aneurysm).

There is general agreement that any significant reduction in death and disability from cerebro-vascular disease will come about by prevention rather than by more effective medical or surgical treatment. Hence considerable resources have been used in an attempt to identify factors that increase the risk of 'stroke', i.e. *risk factors*. With respect to cerebral infarction, atheroma and hypertension have been shown to play dominant roles, but other important factors include abnormalities in serum lipids, diabetes mellitus, coronary artery disease, cardiac failure and atrial fibrillation. Less important factors include a raised haematocrit, open surgery on the heart and the great vessels of the neck, and certain medications such as oral contraceptives. Various environmental factors have also been incriminated and include cigarette smoking, diet, obesity, whether the drinking water is hard or soft, coffee drinking, alcohol consumption, stress, physical activity and climate. On the other hand, factors that predispose to spontaneous intracranial haemorrhage are hypertension, congenital anomalies, vascular malformations, arteritis and bleeding diatheses.

A sharp distinction is usually made on clinical grounds between *transient ischaemic attacks (TIAs)* – a fully reversible neurological deficit often lasting for no more than a few minutes but occasionally for up to 24 hours, in which it is assumed that no structural brain damage has occurred – and a *'stroke'*, where permanent brain damage has occurred even if the patient makes a good clinical recovery. Some 30 per cent of cases have only a single TIA, but most have between two and 10. About 80 per cent of TIAs occur in the carotid arterial territories. Some occur in the vertebrobasilar territory.

The pathogenesis of TIAs closely resembles that of cerebral infarction. Estimates of the risk of a subsequent permanent stroke within 4 years of the first TIA range from about 10 to 35 per cent. Most, however, develop their permanent stroke within 6 months, indicating that there is an urgent need to recognize and treat TIAs.

BLOOD SUPPLY OF THE CENTRAL NERVOUS SYSTEM

The cerebral hemispheres

The *arterial supply* to the cerebral hemispheres is derived from branches of the *circle of Willis* at the base of the brain, which is essentially an anastomosis between the *vertebrobasilar* and the *internal carotid systems*. The configuration of the circle of Willis is subject to considerable variation, but the 'normal' circle is illustrated in Figure 5.1. The *posterior cerebral arteries* are the end branches of the basilar artery and supply the cortex of the occipital lobes, including the visual cortex, and the medial and inferior surfaces of the temporal lobes excluding the temporal poles (Fig. 5.2). The *middle cerebral artery* supplies the lateral surface of the cerebral hemisphere, except for strips along the upper border (anterior cerebral artery) and the lower border (posterior cerebral

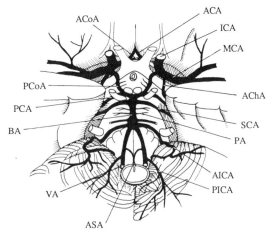

Fig. 5.1   Diagram of the circle of Willis.
ACA = anterior cerebral artery; ICA = internal carotid artery; MCA = middle cerebral artery; AChA = anterior choroidal artery; SCA = superior cerebellar artery; PA = pontine artery; AICA = anterior inferior cerebellar artery; PICA = posterior inferior cerebellar artery; ASA = anterior spinal artery; VA = vertebral artery; BA = basilar artery; PCA = posterior cerebral artery; PCoA = posterior communicating artery; ACoA = anterior communicating artery.

artery) (Fig. 5.2). Included in this area is the auditory cortex and the insular cortex deep to the Sylvian fissure. The *anterior cerebral artery* supplies the medial surface of the hemisphere as far back

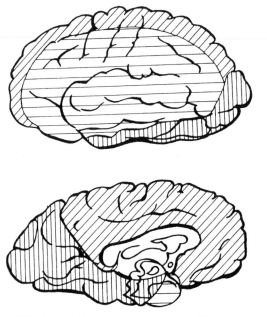

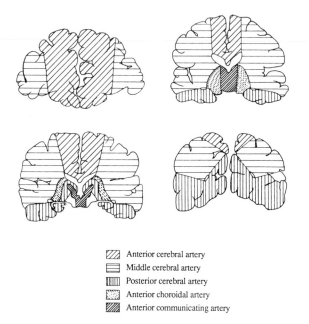

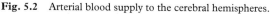

Anterior cerebral artery
Middle cerebral artery
Posterior cerebral artery
Anterior choroidal artery
Anterior communicating artery

Fig. 5.2   Arterial blood supply to the cerebral hemispheres.

as the parieto-occipital sulcus, plus the superior rim of the lateral surface not supplied by the middle cerebral artery (Fig. 5.2). There are anastomoses between these arteries on the surface of the brain. The deep grey and white matter are supplied by *striate arteries* which arise from the circle of Willis and the proximal parts of the cerebral arteries as perforating branches. These are essentially end arteries.

There are three main groups of *external cerebral veins* which drain the surfaces of the hemispheres. These are the superior, the superficial middle and the inferior veins, all linked by two anastomotic veins: the superior (between the superior and the superficial middle) and the inferior (between the superficial middle and the inferior). There are about a dozen *superior cerebral veins* which drain via the bridging veins into the *superior sagittal sinus*. The posterior veins are oblique and enter the sinus against the direction of blood flow. The *superficial middle cerebral vein* runs forwards in the Sylvian fissure and drains into the *cavernous sinus* on either side of the pituitary fossa. The *inferior veins* are inconspicuous and drain into the nearest venous sinus. The *paired internal cerebral veins* form when the thalamostriate and choroidal veins run backwards in the roof of the third ventricle; they then unite to make the *great cerebral vein of Galen*, which empties into the *straight sinus*. The great cerebral vein receives many tributaries from the deeper structures of the cerebral hemispheres.

The hindbrain

The blood supply of the hindbrain is derived chiefly from the vertebrobasilar system (Fig. 5.3). The peripheral branches of this system are not end arteries and their territories overlap. The upper surface and dorsal angle of a cerebellar hemisphere is supplied by the *superior cerebellar artery*: the artery curves around the brain stem in the pontomesencephalic groove and is separated from the posterior cerebral artery by the oculomotor nerves proximally and by the tentorium cerebelli distally. The deep parts of the cerebellum are supplied by the *anterior inferior cerebellar artery*, which is usually the smallest of the three cerebellar arteries. The *posterior inferior cerebellar artery* arises from the vertebral artery usually

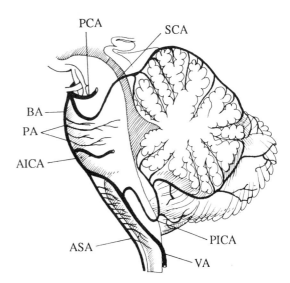

Fig. 5.3   Arterial blood supply to the hindbrain. Abbreviations as in Fig. 5.1.

some 2 cm below the pontomedullary junction and supplies the dorsolateral quadrant of the medulla, the inferior surface of the cerebellar hemisphere, the roof of the fourth ventricle and its choroid plexus. The brain stem derives its blood supply from the paramedian and short circumferential branches of the vertebrobasilar system.

The venous drainage of the brain stem is chiefly a rostral continuation of the spinal veins, and the cerebellum drains mainly into the great cerebral vein of Galen and the straight venous sinus.

The circle of Willis, the anastomotic channels between the major cerebral arteries on the surface of the cerebral hemispheres and the cerebellum, and the potential anastomosis via the ophthalmic artery between the external and internal carotid arterial systems are of the greatest importance if the blood flow through the internal carotid or vertebral arteries is compromised in any way. Thus, there is an increased incidence of cerebral infarction if these potential anastomoses are deficient as a result of some anomaly in the circle of Willis, or acquired arterial disease such as atheromatous stenosis.

Spinal cord

The *blood supply* of the cord is derived from the

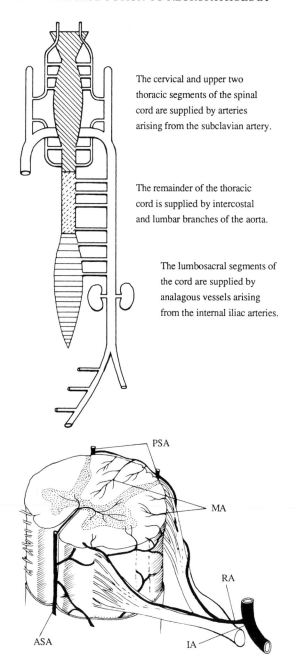

The cervical and upper two thoracic segments of the spinal cord are supplied by arteries arising from the subclavian artery.

The remainder of the thoracic cord is supplied by intercostal and lumbar branches of the aorta.

The lumbosacral segments of the cord are supplied by analagous vessels arising from the internal iliac arteries.

Fig. 5.4 Arterial blood supply to the spinal cord. PSA = posterior spinal artery; MA = branches of meningeal arteries; RA = radicular artery; IA = intercostal artery; ASA = anterior spinal artery.

spinal branches of the vertebral, deep cervical, intercostal and lumbar arteries which arise from the aorta in a segmental manner (Fig. 5.4). Each spinal artery divides into an *anterior and posterior*

radicular artery which run along the ventral and dorsal nerve roots respectively. The initial arrangement provides each segment of the cord with its own blood supply, but the pattern has undergone considerable phylogenetic change and in man most of the anterior radicular arteries are small and never reach the cord. Between four and nine anterior radicular arteries, of which one, the *artery of Adamkiewicz* (which usually lies between T8 and L1 on the left) is considerably larger than the others, reach the anterior sulcus of the cord and contribute to the longitudinal anastomoses of the *anterior spinal artery*. Variations in the anatomy of the anterior radicular arteries are of considerable surgical importance. The anterior spinal artery in the ventral median fissure gives rise to central branches which supply the ventral grey and white matter of the cord. The posterior radicular arteries are much more variable in number and size, and there are more of them than anterior radicular arteries. They contribute to the freely anastomosing *posterior spinal arteries*, the central branches of which supply the dorsal third of the cord. The territories overlap but no anastomoses have been reported within the cord.

The venous drainage of the cord is via six tortuous plexiform longitudinal vessels, one along each median sulcus and the others on either side of it.

MAINTENANCE OF CEREBRAL BLOOD FLOW AND OXYGEN SUPPLY

The brain is very susceptible to oxygen deprivation. The supply of oxygen depends on the *cerebral blood flow* (CBF) and the oxygen content of the blood. Cerebral blood flow, in turn, depends on the *cerebral perfusion pressure* (CPP), which is the difference between the *mean systemic arterial pressure* and the *intracranial pressure*. Since the most important factor in maintaining an adequate supply of oxygen to the brain is the CBF, there are protective mechanisms to preserve it.

Preservation of CBF, when systemic arterial pressure is low, is brought about by *autoregulation*, which can be defined as the maintenance of a relatively constant blood flow in the face of changes in CPP. As the systemic arterial pressure falls, the cerebrovascular resistance also falls because of autoregulatory dilatation of cerebral arterioles, with the result that CBF remains within normal limits over a wide range of systemic arterial pressure. When cerebral vasodilatation is maximal, however, cerebrovascular resistance cannot fall further (the lower limit of auto-regulation): the critical level of systemic arterial pressure at which autoregulation fails is about 50 mmHg (Fig. 5.5). Thus, when systemic arterial pressure falls below this level, CBF also falls. There is also an upper limit of auto-regulation beyond which the autoregulatory vaso-constriction of the cerebral arterioles is inadequate (about 160 mmHg); CBF then increases and dysfunction of the blood–brain barrier develops (hypertensive encephalopathy).

Cerebral arterioles also respond to alterations in the blood gases when systemic arterial pressure is within normal limits: an increase of $Pa\text{CO}_2$ or a decrease of $Pa\text{O}_2$ produces arteriolar vasodilatation and hence a fall in cerebrovascular resistance and an increase in CBF. Thus, if arteriolar vasodila-tation resulting from hypoxia or, in particular, hypercapnia, exists prior to any reduction in systemic arterial pressure, maximal vasodilatation will occur at a higher systemic arterial pressure

than in the normocapnic normoxic state. Hence CBF will become linearly related to systemic arterial pressure at a relatively high systemic arterial pressure. Patients with pre-existing arteriolar vasodilatation are particularly vulner-able to a fall in systemic arterial pressure because the potential autoregulatory preservation of CBF is impaired. Autoregulation may also be deficient if a patient is hypoxaemic, for example in the postanaesthetic period, and appears to be lost, or at least severely impaired, in a wide range of acute conditions producing brain damage, e.g. acute head injury, haemorrhagic and ischaemic strokes or a brief episode of hypoxia. Such patients are particularly susceptible to any episode of acute cardiorespiratory failure and especially a fall in systemic arterial pressure. In patients with chronic hypertension, there is a shift of the auto-regulatory curve to the right, with the result that CBF commences to fall at a higher systemic arterial pressure than in normotensive individuals (Fig. 5.5).

Energy is produced in the brain almost entirely from the oxidative metabolism of glucose. The amount of glucose consumed is very high (60 mgl per min), reflecting the inability of the brain to make use of other substrates. Oxidative metabolism of glucose yields energy in the form of high-energy phosphate compounds, the most important of which is adenosine triphosphate (ATP).

Experimental work in the last decade has, however, suggested that both the nature of the neuronal change and its distribution in the brain are different in hypoglycaemia and following ischaemia.

In many medical emergencies, for example cardiorespiratory arrest, a severe episode of hypotension, status epilepticus, carbon monoxide or barbiturate intoxication or hypoglycaemic coma, the vital factor with regard to the ultimate clinical outcome is whether or not satisfactory resuscitation can be achieved before irreversible brain damage has occurred.

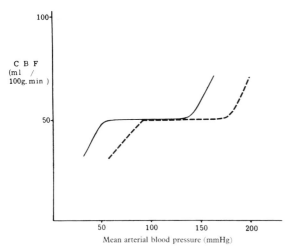

Fig. 5.5 Autoregulation of cerebral blood flow. Diagrammatic representation of the relationship between cerebral blood flow (CBF) and mean arterial blood pressure in normotensive and hypertensive subjects. Note the 'shift to the right' of the autoregulatory curve in the hypertensive subjects. —— normotensive subjects; - - - - hypertensive subject.

'SELECTIVE VULNERABILITY'

The differing susceptibility of brain cells to hypoxia has been known for many years: in general, neurons are the most sensitive, followed by oligo-dendroglia and astrocytes, whereas the microglia and blood vessels are the least 'vulnerable'. Two major hypotheses have been advanced to explain the characteristic distribution of hypoxic brain damage. The 'vascular theory' invokes anatomical factors, such as the length and tortuous course of a particular artery, as well as physiological factors, whereas the concept of 'pathoclisis' postulates particular physicochemical properties of the individual cells. Recent work suggests that local metabolic rather than vascular factors determine selective vulnerability. The former has received a considerable boost in the last 10 years from the development of the concept of excitotoxicity, which established a strong correlation between the excitatory properties of glutamate and related amino acids and their ability to induce neuronal damage, mediated through various glutamate receptor subtypes, principal among which are three named after their selective agonists – *N*-methyl-D-aspartate (NMDA), quisqualate and kainate. These receptors play an important role in the selective neuronal loss that occurs after cardiac arrest, although the pattern of damage does not correlate precisely with the density of NMDA receptors. More likely, the pattern of selective vulnerability is determined by the localization of calcium-binding proteins and their vulnerability to the action of excitotoxic amino acids.

The pattern of 'selective vulnerability' in its classic form is best seen after an episode of cardiac arrest, when evidence of neuronal necrosis may be limited to certain layers of the cortex, parts of the hippocampus, and the Purkinje cells of the cerebellum (see p. 76).

STRUCTURAL CHANGES RESULTING FROM HYPOXIA

Structural damage resulting from hypoxia ranges from *selective neuronal necrosis*, i.e. limited to neurons, to frank *infarction*, i.e. additional involvement of glia and blood vessels. *Partial infarction* describes the situation when there is involvement of glia but not blood vessels.

Selective neuronal necrosis

Studies in experimental animals and selected human material have shown that there is an identifiable sequence of changes, the *ischaemic cell process*, which is the neuropathological common denominator in all types of hypoxia and has been described in detail in Chapter 3. The identification of neuronal changes that are attributable unequivocally to hypoxia may be difficult in the human brain because of histological artefact. This results partly from autolysis, partly from slow penetration of fixative, and partly from shortcomings in the processing of tissue, leading to artefacts such as *dark cells*, *hydropic cells*, *perineuronal* and *perivascular spaces* and the features of the *respirator brain* (see Ch. 3). In any histological assessment of the brain, it is of the utmost importance that the pathologist recognizes the ischaemic cell process and can distinguish it from these artefacts. The artefacts do not coincide with areas of selective vulnerability, they are more numerous on the surface of the brain, and are not related to the duration of survival after an episode of hypoxia. Thus any evidence of the ischaemic cell process or of a vital reaction in a 'respirator brain' (see Ch. 3) must be interpreted as having preceded the onset of clinical brain-stem death.

Neuronal damage induced by excitatory amino acids

Two main types have been recognized. First, there may be glutamate-induced *acute swelling* of the dendrites and spinous processes of susceptible neurons, followed by acute degenerative changes in intracellular organelles and the clumping of nuclear chromatin, which progresses rapidly to nuclear pyknosis. Because axons passing through or terminating in the damaged area remain normal in appearance, the lesion has been termed a 'dendrosomatotoxic' but 'axon-sparing' type of histological reaction. Secondly, via non-NMDA receptor-mediated mechanisms the changes of *delayed neuronal death* may occur, in which affected neurons become contracted and darkly staining some 72 hours after the hypoxic insult.

Infarction

Cerebral infarction, i.e. necrosis of neurons, neuroglia and blood vessels, is due to a local arrest or reduction in the cerebral blood flow. It is usually centred on a particular arterial territory within the cerebral hemispheres, the cerebellum or the brain stem. It can affect an entire arterial territory or, if there is some collateral circulation from adjacent arterial territories, the infarct may be restricted to the central part of the arterial territory (Fig. 5.6).

There are basically three stages in the development of an infarct, depending on its age. Recent infarcts are slightly soft and distinctly swollen: indeed a large infarct may swell to the extent of acting as an intracranial expanding lesion to produce distortion and herniation of the brain and an increase in intracranial pressure (Fig. 5.7). It may be *anaemic* or *haemorrhagic*, depending on whether or not some blood flow has been restored through the infarct and on whether or not necrosis of vessel walls has occurred, thus allowing extravasation of blood into the necrotic tissue. An intensely haemor-

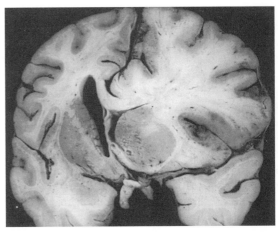

Fig. 5.7   Cerebral infarction. There is a large swollen infarct in the territories supplied by the right anterior and middle cerebral arteries. Note the shift of the midline structures to the left and the supracallosal hernia. There was a tentorial hernia and secondary haemorrhage into the brain stem.

rhagic infarct may superfically resemble a haematoma but the distinctive feature of a haemorrhagic infarct (see previous text) is the preservation of intrinsic brain architecture within it. In brain

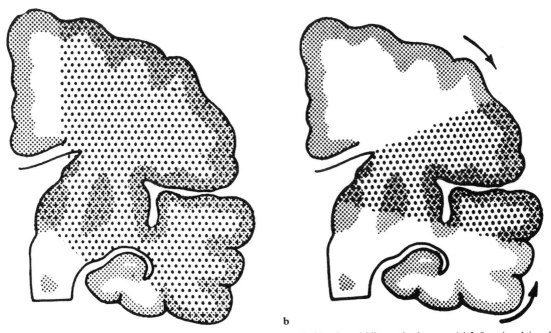

a   b

Fig. 5.6   Diagrammatic representation of infarcts in the territory supplied by the middle cerebral artery. (a) Infarct involving the entire territory. (b) Infarct restricted to the central territory. Arrows in (b) indicate collateral inflow from the anterior and posterior cerebral arteries.

that has undergone recent infarction, the histological appearances are those of *coagulation necrosis*. Within grey matter the outlines of dead neurons are recognizable, their cytoplasm is intensely eosinophilic and the nucleus stains poorly with haematoxylin. This picture, which is recognizable within the first 4–6 hours, is followed by patchy decreasing stainability (Fig. 5.8a). Incrustations are not seen in the central region of a large infarct but occur frequently at its edges. Within 12–15 hours an infarct has a sharply demarcated edge (Fig. 5.8b) due to a spongy appearance of the neurophil caused by a combination of the swelling of astrocytic processes and of axons, and loss of staining of myelin. Neutrophil polymorphs may be conspicuous in relation to the necrotic walls of small vessels. Within about 24 hours early reactive changes, as shown by proliferation of microglia, astrocytes and capillaries, occur in the normal tissue adjacent to the infarct: reactive microglia also appear early around any surviving vessels within the infarct. Within 1–2 weeks the infarct becomes extremely soft and the swelling resolves. Affected grey matter may already be slightly shrunken and granular. At this stage, in addition to the reactive changes mentioned above, there are sheets of lipid-containing macrophages throughout the infarct (see Fig. 3.24b). If the patient survives for several months or more, the dead tissue is removed and the infarct ultimately comes to be represented by a shrunken cystic lesion (Fig. 5.9). The cysts are often traversed by small vessels and glial fibrils, and some lipid-containing macrophages usually persist. If the infarct is in a cerebral hemisphere, shrinkage of the infarct is usually accompanied by enlargement of the adjacent lateral ventricle. Wallerian-type degeneration will occur in any nerve fibres that have been destroyed. Thus, if the infarct involves the internal capsule, there is progressive degeneration and shrinkage of the corresponding pyramidal tract in the brain stem and in the spinal cord (see Fig. 5.23).

PATHOGENESIS OF CEREBRAL INFARCTION

Embolism

According to the Framingham Study, some 31 per cent of ischaemic strokes are due to

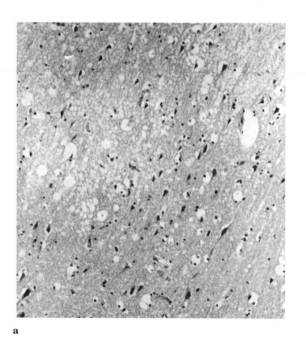
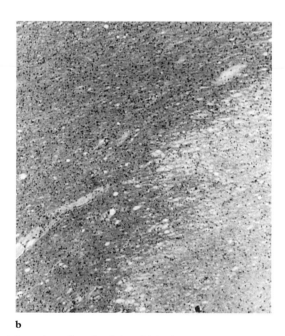

a   b

Fig. 5.8   Recent infarction: (a) in the cerebral cortex, where there is irregular pallor of staining; (b) in the white matter, where there is a sharply defined border between the abnormal (pale) and normal white matter. (a) and (b) H & E.

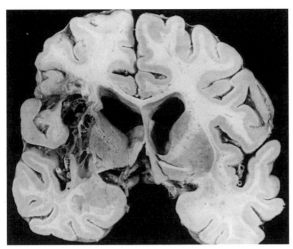

Fig. 5.9 Old infarction. The original infarct is represented by shrunken cystic tissue.

embolism, but other studies have estimated that between 50 and 60 per cent are of embolic origin.

About 75 per cent of patients who have had a 'stroke' have cardiac failure, atrial fibrillation or an enlarged heart, and there is a two to fivefold increased incidence of 'stroke' in patients with ischaemic heart disease. The embolus may arise from thrombus formed on endocardium overlying an infarct: in two-thirds of cases this complication develops within the first 3 weeks after acute myocardial infarction. Sometimes, however, cerebral infarction appears to occur at the same time as myocardial infarction as a result of hypotension and a failure of cerebral perfusion pressure. Other causes of embolism include infective endocarditis, calcific aortic stenosis, prolapsed mitral valve, myxoma of the left atrium, non-bacterial thrombotic endocarditis in association with the cachexia of advanced chronic disease, cardiomyopathy and arrhythmias. Rarely, a thrombotic embolus reaching the heart from the systemic veins may pass through a patent foramen ovale to enter the systemic arterial circulation (*paradoxical embolism*). Brain damage due to embolism may also complicate cardiac surgery and, more recently, open heart surgery with cardiopulmonary bypass has created new sources of cerebral embolism that include air, fat, particles of silicone and platelet/fibrin emboli from the pump oxygenator.

If the intimal covering of an atheromatous plaque breaks down, excavation of the lesion by the bloodstream may dislodge fatty and crystalline debris. Thrombus on ulcerated atheromatous lesions in the aorta and in the cervical arteries to the brain is also a common source of embolism.

Atheroma (atherosclerosis)

This is the most common and important arterial disease in adults in developed countries. Although it may occur to some extent in young adults, it is much more severe and extensive in the middle-aged and elderly. As the plaques gradually enlarge they become confluent and encroach upon the lumen of the vessel and may be complicated by calcification and ulceration. The process may progress to complete occlusion of the vessel, due either to intramural bleeding in the base of the plaque or, more often, to the formation of thrombus.

The vessels most commonly affected are the internal carotid and vertebral arteries, followed by the basilar and middle cerebral arteries and then by the posterior inferior cerebellar arteries. Atheroma of the cerebral arteries is usually associated with atheroma in other parts of the body, including the arteries of the limbs. Correlation between the occurrence of coronary atheroma and that of cerebral atheroma is usually close, although coronary atheroma tends to be more severe. Occasionally, however, a person with marked atheroma in the aorta and coronary arteries may have little or no disease in the cerebral arteries; the reverse may also occur.

Extensive atheroma does not necessarily lead to cerebral infarction because at normal blood pressure the internal cross-sectional area of an artery must be reduced by up to 90 per cent before blood flow is impaired. If, however, there is an episode of hypotension (see below), the flow may be reduced sufficiently to cause ischaemic damage.

Stenosis and occlusion of the extracranial cervical arteries

Atheroma of the *internal carotid arteries* in the neck and of the *cervical vertebral arteries* is of considerable importance in the pathogenesis of cerebral infarction. Atheroma is particularly common at the lower end of the internal carotid artery, which may become severely stenosed and, ultimately, occluded by thrombus, but many individuals with thrombosis of one or even both internal carotid arteries do not necessarily develop a cerebral infarct because of the collateral circulation. Other causes of carotid artery occlusion include embolism, dissecting aneurysm, trauma, blood dyscrasias, the aortic arch syndrome and inflammation at the base of the skull. When an internal carotid artery is occluded, reverse flow through the ophthalmic artery connecting the external carotid artery with the upper end of the internal carotid artery is an important source of a collateral circulation.

Occlusion of an internal carotid artery may be without symptoms or signs, may reveal itself by episodic attacks of transient motor or sensory impairment, or present as a gradual or sudden onset of permanent hemiplegia. If infarction occurs, it may take several forms: massive infarction within the entire territory supplied by the middle cerebral artery (Fig. 5.6) and sometimes involving the anterior cerebral arterial territory as well; infarction of the cortex around the Sylvian fissure with or without involvement of the basal ganglia and the internal capsule; infarction restricted to the internal capsule (so-called capsular infarct); small infarcts distributed throughout the white matter; and infarction within the boundary zone between the territories supplied by the anterior and middle cerebral arteries.

Stenosis or occlusion of the vertebral arteries affects the vertebrobasilar territory and, if the collateral circulation is inadequate, there is infarction in the brain stem, in the cerebellum or in the posterior cerebral arterial territories. Indeed, in patients with the clinical syndrome of infarction in the territory of one posterior inferior cerebellar artery, the occlusive arterial disease is often in the vertebral artery and not in the posterior inferior cerebellar artery itself.

Thus, the haemodynamic disturbance leading to cerebral infarction is complex and it is often difficult to ascribe an infarct to a particular arterial lesion and, particularly in the presence of arterial stenosis, cerebral infarction is often the result of a combination of systemic circulatory insufficiency and atheroma of extracranial or intracranial cerebral arteries, or of both.

Obstruction of the *subclavian and brachiocephalic (innominate) arteries* is rarely a cause of cerebral infarction but is of some clinical importance as a causative factor in the *subclavian steal syndrome*. In this condition, clinical evidence of cerebral ischaemia may be precipitated by exercise of the upper limbs, thus 'stealing' blood from the basilar artery and the circle of Willis to the subclavian artery distal to the occlusion.

Occlusion of intracranial arteries

The anatomical distribution of arteries in the brain is remarkably constant and the neurological deficit that results from occlusion of individual vessels may be so well defined that clinicians can often say with confidence which artery, or branch of an artery, in the carotid and/or vertebrobasilar system is involved.

Common causes of occlusion of these vessels are embolism (mainly from the heart or internal carotid arteries), thrombosis (formed locally on atheroma or propagated from extracranial cervical arteries), vasospasm in patients with rupture of a saccular aneurysm, arteritis (micro-organisms, collagen diseases etc.), and mechanical deformation in patients with mass lesions that are producing midline shift and internal herniation The *middle cerebral artery* is more often occluded than any other cerebral artery, and it is often secondary to embolism or the cephalad extension of thrombus from the internal carotid artery. Infarction within the distribution of the *posterior cerebral artery* is a common incidental finding post mortem in the elderly.

Autopsy studies have established that occlusion of one *vertebral artery* may be asymptomatic. Whereas thrombus forming on atheroma is the most common cause of vertebral artery occlusion, these vessels may also be distorted by osteoarthritis of the cervical spine which, together with atheroma, may be sufficient to cause obstruction as a result of certain temporary movements of the neck, namely hyperextension, intubation for general anaesthesia, osteopathic manipulation etc. Other causes of occlusion include subluxation of the atlanto-occipital joint in rheumatoid arthritis, and as a birth injury following assisted cephalic breech presentation. Occlusion of the *basilar artery* is usually due to atheroma. Most of the clinical syndromes associated with vertebrobasilar disease represent ischaemia either of the hindbrain or of the medial portions of the occipital lobes. In some patients there is extensive infarction of the brain stem and the patient dies, whereas others develop the 'locked-in' syndrome in which a conscious mute patient is completely paralysed apart from eye movements.

Occlusion of the spinal arteries

Occlusion of the *anterior spinal artery* causes infarction of the ventral two-thirds of the cord and is more common than occlusion of the *posterior spinal artery*. Occlusion is usually due to thrombosis secondary to trauma, subluxation of the spine, cervical spondylosis, syphilis (now rare) or embolism. Occlusion of the spinal arteries is a common complication of a dissecting aneurysm of the aorta, the pattern of damage being determined by the location of the dissection. Mid and lower thoracic regions of the cord are the most vulnerable due to interference of blood flow through the intercostal arteries. Sometimes the entire cord is involved, but on other occasions the damage is limited to the central grey matter. Infarction in either or both of these vascular territories may occur without arterial occlusion, when it is precipitated by changes in spinal blood flow, as may occur after prolonged hypotension, disease of the aortic ostia of the intercostal or lumbar arteries, embolism following surgery, and in association with coarctation of the aorta.

Hypertension

There is considerable evidence that *atheroma* of the larger cerebral vessels is aggravated by hypertension. In chronic severe hypertension, atheroma can in addition be found in the penetrating arteries of the internal capsule, basal ganglia and pons. Hypertension also produces changes in the walls of arteries and arterioles, the latter undergoing *hyaline arteriolosclerosis*. *Lacunes* are small cavities in the basal ganglia (Fig. 5.10) and in the

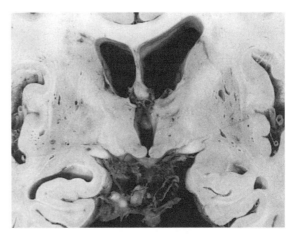

Fig. 5.10   Lacunes. There are small cysts in the basal ganglia.

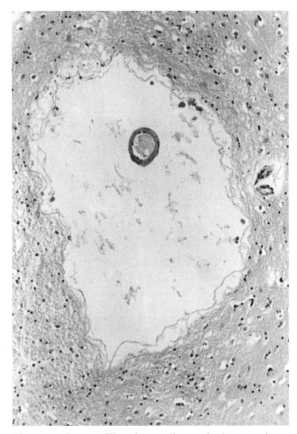

Fig. 5.11   Lacune. There is a small artery in the space that its spiralled course now occupies. (H & E.)

pons in elderly subjects, some 90 per cent of which are associated with hypertension. Some appear as expanded perivascular spaces (Fig. 5.11), others as small infarcts or resolving haemorrhages. When numerous in grey and white matter, the terms *état lacunaire* and *état criblé* respectively are used. There is also an association between hypertension and *multi-infarct dementia* (see Ch. 14).

Rarely, *hypertensive encephalopathy* may complicate acute glomerulonephritis, toxaemia of pregnancy and malignant-phase hypertension. Although severe hypertension is accepted as the underlying cause of hypertensive encephalopathy, the exact pathogenesis remains uncertain. It has been attributed to spasm of the cerebral vessels and to excessive vasodilatation, damage to the blood–brain barrier and cerebral hyperaemia. There is also an association between a slowly developing dementia (*subcortical arteriosclerotic encephalopathy: Binswanger's disease*) and hypertension.

There is a close association between hypertension and spontaneous *intracranial haemorrhage* (see below).

Cerebral arteritis

There are many types of vasculitis that cause cerebral infarction including arteritis due to micro-organisms, collagen diseases and a miscellaneous group of disorders.

Arteritis due to micro-organisms

In the preantibiotic era acute carotid arteritis sometimes developed in children and young adults with tonsillitis and retropharyngeal inflammation. In some cases of acute purulent meningitis, particularly due to *pneumococci* or *meningococci*, there is often histological evidence of acute arteritis of the pial blood vessels, where they are surrounded by inflammatory exudate. In subacute or chronic meningitis, as in *tuberculous meningitis* and in *meningovascular syphilis*, the blood vessels become thickened and narrowed due to endarteritis obliterans (Fig. 5.12). Arteritis may also be caused by various fungal and parasitic diseases, such as *aspergillosis, mucormycosis* and *cryptococcosis*.

Collagen diseases

Polyarteritis nodosa affects the CNS in 20 per cent

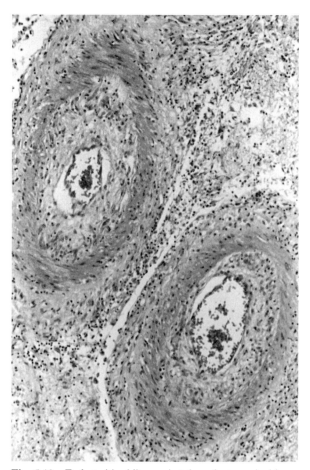

Fig. 5.12 Endarteritis obliterans in tuberculous meningitis. The adventitia is thickened and infiltrated by chronic inflammatory cells. The media is normal and there is marked concentric thickening of the intima. (H & E.)

of cases, when the intracranial arteries may have a beaded appearance due to multiple aneurysms. Rupture of these aneurysms is, however, uncommon, subarachnoid haemorrhage rarely being a presenting feature. Many of the patients are severely hypertensive, so some of the terminal features may be due to hypertensive encephalopathy. Clinical evidence of CNS involvement in *systemic lupus erythematosus* is said to occur in some 50 per cent of patients. In *giant-cell arteritis (temporal arteritis)* there is a pangranulomatous reaction as shown by the presence of lymphocytes, plasma cells and occasional neutrophil polymorphs in the walls of arteries of all sizes. Giant cells of either Langhans' or foreign-body type are almost invariably present (Fig 5.13a), either in

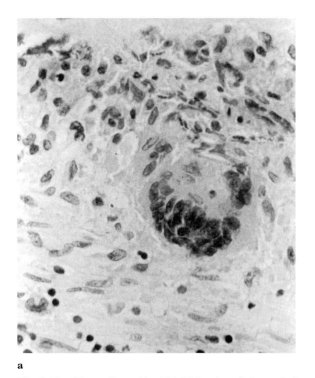

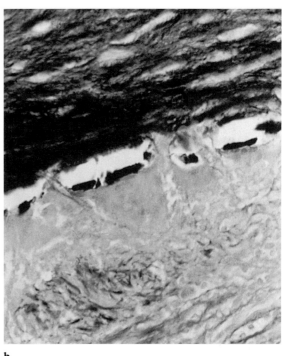

a   b

Fig. 5.13   Giant-cell arteritis. (a) Multinucleated giant cell close to junction between intima and media. There is infiltration of the intima and media by monocytes and some lymphocytes. (b) Irregularly damaged internal elastic lamina in relation to multinuclear cells. (a) H & E; (b) Van Gieson/elastica.

the media close to the damaged internal elastic lamina (Fig. 5.13b) or in the adjacent intima. Involvement of the ophthalmic arteries, including the ciliary arteries and the central artery of the retina, is particularly important. The disease process often involves the superficial temporal arteries, which become swollen, tortuous and nodular. Because of its accessibility, the temporal artery is the most popular choice for biopsy. Other varieties of vasculitis classified as collagen disorders include *Behçet's disease, rheumatic fever* and *thrombotic thrombocytopenic purpura*.

Miscellaneous causes of cerebral infarction

These include the *aortic arch syndrome* (pulseless disease or Takayasu's arteritis), which is the name given to a constellation of clinical signs and symptoms that arise following a progressive reduction of blood flow in the territories of the brachiocephalic (innominate), left common carotid and left subclavian arteries. There are many causes of this condition, but when it occurs in young patients there is often evidence of more generalized disease with the features of a 'collagenosis'. The early cases were described in young Japanese women, but it is now appreciated that it occurs in older women and men throughout the world.

Moya Moya disease is seen predominantly in children in whom cerebral angiography shows an unusual netlike appearance of small blood vessels (resembling a 'puff of smoke') at the base of the brain. There is a preponderance in the Japanese race. Pathologically there is stenosis or occlusion of the terminal portions of the internal carotid arteries and the proximal portions of the anterior and middle cerebral arteries, and numerous dilated small arteries branching from the circle of Willis. The aetiology is unclear, but two main hypotheses have been advanced. The first is that it is a true congenital vascular malformation, and the second that the abnormal angiographic appearances represent a collateral circulation.

The brain and spinal cord may be damaged by *X-irradiation*. The immediate response may be an acute inflammatory vasculitis, but more characteristically there is a delayed response in which small vessels undergo marked proliferative changes, with hyaline degeneration in their walls and necrosis of surrounding brain tissue.

Radiological evidence of *vasospasm* of the cerebral arteries is seen commonly in association with subarachnoid haemorrhage due to rupture of a saccular aneurysm (see below) and after severe head injury. In both situations it is an important factor in the genesis of ischaemic brain damage.

Vascular complications are common in patients who develop brain shift and internal herniation as a result of *raised intracranial pressure* (see Ch. 4).

Failure of cerebral perfusion as a result of cardiac arrest or an episode of hypotension (see below) may also cause cerebral infarction.

There is an association between cerebrovascular disease and various blood disorders. For example, transient ischaemic attacks, cerebral infarction and cerebral haemorrhage are all recognized complications of *polycythaemia rubra vera*. The nervous system is also involved in some 25 per cent of patients with *sickle-cell disease* and in other types of *haemoglobinopathy*. Neurological complications are also common in patients with *macroglobulinaemia*.

It is now appreciated that there is a six to ninefold increase of cerebral infarction due to thromboembolic occlusion of the internal carotid artery or a major branch of an intracranial artery in women taking *oral contraceptives*. The thrombotic tendency seems to be related to the oestrogen content of the preparation, which in turn produces a hypercoagulable state and an increase in platelet adhesiveness. There is also a positive association between cerebral infarction and *pregnancy* and the *puerperium*. Until recently this was regarded as being usually due to cerebral venous thrombosis, but it is now clear that the majority of cases are due to arterial thrombosis.

Occlusive vascular disease has also been recorded in cases of addiction to *heroin* and *LSD*, as a complication of *inflammatory bowel disease*, in association with *migraine* and in patients with inherited disorders of *connective tissue*.

BRAIN DAMAGE DUE TO CARDIAC ARREST

Brain damage brought about by cardiac arrest is characterized by *widespread selective neuronal necrosis* in the cerebral cortex that tends to increase in severity from the frontal and temporal poles to the occipital poles. The necrosis may be total or it maybe restricted to layers III, V and VI (see Ch. 2) (Fig. 5.14). It is more severe within sulci than on the crests of gyri. The hippocampi are particularly vulnerable, especially the Sommer sector (CA1; Fig. 5.15). Neuronal necrosis is also common in the amygdaloid nuclei. The pattern of damage in the basal nuclei is less constant, but tends to be most common and severe in the caudate nucleus and in the adjacent part of the putamen. In the thalamus,

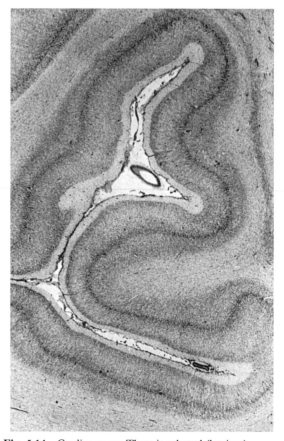

Fig. 5.14 Cardiac arrest. There is subtotal (laminar) necrosis of the III, V and VI cortical layers with selective sparing of the II and IV layers (darker staining). Celloidin; cresyl violet.

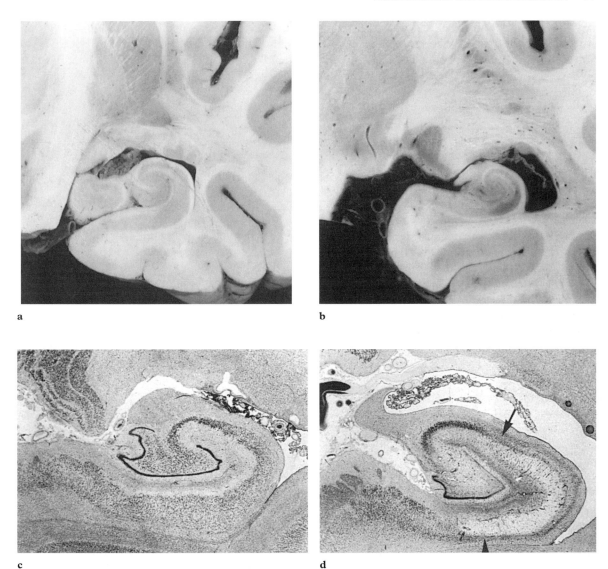

Fig. 5.15   Hippocampus. (a) Normal. (b) There is necrosis of the CA1 sector. (c) Normal. (d) There is neuronal necrosis of the CA1 sector (between arrows). (c) and (d) Celloidin; cresyl violet.

the anterior, dorsomedial and ventrolateral nuclei are the most susceptible. In the cerebellum there is characteristically diffuse necrosis of Purkinje cells. Damage to nuclei in the brain stem is relatively uncommon in the adult but it may be widespread and severe in young children.

Patients may die soon after an episode of cardiac arrest, when there will be no abnormalities identifiable in the brain. If the individual lives for about 12 hours, the brain may again appear

entirely normal macroscopically even when it has been properly fixed prior to dissection, but a microscopic analysis will show widespread neuronal necrosis in the sites referred to above. In this context little significance should be attached to pallor of nuclear staining, swelling or vacuolation of cytoplasm or loss of Nissl granules, since these can be brought about by autolysis of the brain. Furthermore, many of the patients may have been maintained on artificial ventilation for some hours and during this period autolytic change may proceed in the brain (see Ch. 3). What the pathologist must identify is incontrovertible evidence of classic ischaemic cell change with or without incrustations (see Ch. 3). If the patient survives for more than 24–36 hours, the pathologist's task is made easier because of more established abnormalities in neurons, and the appearance of early reactive changes in astrocytes, microglia and endothelial cells. With the passage of a few days many of the dead neurons disappear and reactive changes become more intense, including the formation of lipid phagocytes. At this stage it may also be possible to identify macroscopically selective damage in the hippocampus (Fig. 5.15b) and in the cerebral cortex within sulci, particularly in the occipital lobes. A particularly conspicuous histological abnormality is the proliferation of microglia in the form of rod cells in the cerebellar cortex in

relation to the disintegrating dendrites of the Purkinje cells. This is often referred to as 'microglial shrubwork' (Fig. 5.16), and is clear evidence that some Purkinje cells have been destroyed. Indeed, a pathologist should hesitate to state that there is loss of neurons in any part of the brain unless there are corresponding reactive changes. Occasionally, patients who have sustained severe hypoxic brain damage remain alive in a vegetative state for long periods. When this occurs the affected grey matter becomes shrunken and often cystic. Because the axons of the neurons that have been destroyed undergo Wallerian-type degeneration, there is also a loss of bulk of the white matter throughout the brain, leading to symmetrical enlargement of the ventricular system (compensatory hydrocephalus) (Fig. 5.17).

There is very little accurate information available about the shortest period of cardiac arrest that is likely to produce brain damage in man, but in the context of true circulatory arrest at normal body temperature, complete clinical recovery is unlikely if the period of arrest is more than about 10 minutes. It is important to realize, however, that adequate cerebral perfusion does not necessarily recommence as soon as the heart rate and arterial pressure become recordable, and that a poor prearrest or postarrest circulatory state may be as important as the duration of complete arrest in the pathogenesis of brain damage.

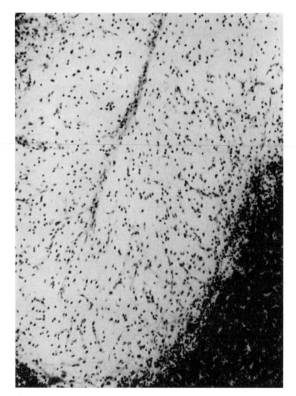

Fig. 5.16 Hypoxic damage in the cerebellum. The Purkinje cells have undergone necrosis and as a result there is a reactive astrocytosis and proliferation of microglia in the molecular layer. Celloidin; cresyl violent.

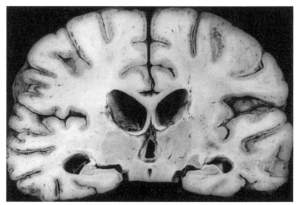

Fig. 5.17 Cardiac arrest. The cortex is greatly narrowed and there is enlargement of the ventricles. The hippocampi and the thalami are small.

BRAIN DAMAGE DUE TO HYPOTENSION

Brain damage due to a generalized reduction in CBF occurs characteristically in association with an episode of severe systemic hypotension. Brain damage may take several forms, but in the commonest type ischaemic damage is concentrated in the boundary zones between the main cerebral and cerebellar arterial territories (Fig. 5.18). If the patient survives only a short time, the brain will appear normal macroscopically. After a few days, however, it is usually possible to see wedge-shaped, often haemorrhagic, infarcts in the arterial boundary zones (Fig. 5.19). They may, however, be small, when they take the form of sharply defined irregular foci of necrosis, mainly in the cortex but sometimes also in the adjacent white matter. The infarcts tend to be largest in the parieto-occipital regions, where the territories of the anterior, middle and posterior cerebral arteries meet. There is variable involvement of the basal nuclei, particularly of the head of the caudate nucleus and in the upper third of the putamen. The hippocampi, despite their extreme vulnerability to hypoxia, are usually not involved.

This type of brain damage appears to be caused by a major and abrupt episode of hypotension followed by a rapid return to normal arterial pressure. Because of the precipitate decrease in arterial pressure, autoregulation fails in the regions most remote from the parent arterial stems, i.e. the boundary zones, which are thus subjected to the greatest reduction in cerebral blood flow. Many examples of this pattern of brain damage have been described, but in the great majority there has been a known episode of hypotension or good clinical grounds for suspecting that the patient had experienced at least a transient episode of hypotension, such as brain damage occurring in the course of a major operation under general anaesthesia or in association with a myocardial infarct. If the brain damage is particularly severe the hippocampi may be involved, but if the hypotension is less severe and of longer duration, damage to neurons is more widespread, is usually accentuated in the arterial boundary zones and there is again relative sparing of the hippocampi. Structural damage due to a generalized reduction in cerebral perfusion pressure is characteristically bilateral and may occur in the absence of any occlusive arterial disease. One hemisphere may be more severely affected than the other, and this is readily explicable because of the frequency with which there are anatomical variations in the circle of Willis.

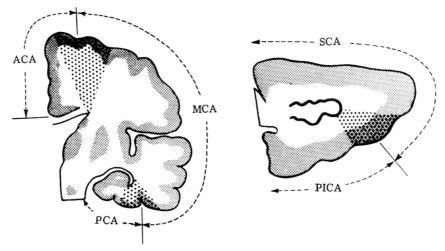

Fig. 5.18   Arterial boundary zones (heavy stippling) in the cerebral and cerebellar hemispheres. They lie between the ACA/MCA, MCA/PCA and SCA/PICA territories. ACA = anterior cerebral artery; MCA = middle cerebral artery; PCA = posterior cerebral artery; SCA = superior cerebellar artery; PICA = posterior inferior cerebellar artery.

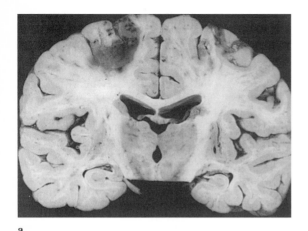

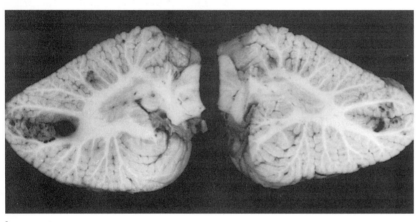

a

b

Fig. 5.19 Infarction in arterial boundary zones. (a) There is asymmetrical haemorrhagic infarction of the sides and depths of the superior frontal sulci in the boundary zones between the anterior and middle cerebral arteries. (b) There is haemorrhagic infarction in the boundary zones between the superior cerebellar and posterior inferior cerebellar arteries.

Since hypotension can produce severe brain damage in the absence of any occlusive arterial disease, the significance of any reduction in cardiac output in a patient with pre-existing atheromatous stenosis in the pathogenesis of hypoxic brain damage should now be clear. It seems likely that such a combination of circumstances more often accounts for the coexistence of cerebral and myocardial infarction than the widely held view that cerebral infarcts in patients with recent myocardial infarcts are usually embolic in type.

BRAIN DAMAGE DUE TO CARBON MONOXIDE POISONING

Carbon monoxide may give rise to structural brain damage because its affinity for haemoglobin is about 250 times that for oxygen The remaining normal haemoglobin has a normal oxygen saturation and blood oxygen tension is normal but the oxygen content is reduced. Furthermore, the dissociation curve of oxyhaemoglobin is shifted to the left, so that less oxygen is available to the tissues at a particular oxygen tension.

Although there is a particular predilection for selectively severe structural damage in the globus pallidus, there is also widespread neuronal necrosis in other vulnerable areas, such as the hippocampi and the cerebellar cortex. In some cases of carbon monoxide poisoning abnormalities are more conspicuous in white matter than in grey. The reasons for this are not understood, especially since this type of damage tends to occur particularly in patients who develop delayed signs of intoxication after a period of relative normality following acute poisoning. The histological features are those of a marked astrocytosis in the affected regions accompanied by various degrees of periaxial demyelination (see Ch. 9).

EPILEPSY

Epilepsy is an episodic disorder of the CNS due to the synchronous and sustained electrical activity of a group of neurons. The clinical features of an epileptic attack can range from a transient arrest of movement, an episode of disordered thought or an 'absence', to sustained generalized clonic and tonic movements. The aetiology of epilepsy is poorly understood, but from the point of view of the neuropathologist it is useful to distinguish between *primary or idiopathic epilepsy* (cryptogenic epilepsy) for which there is no obvious cause, and *secondary or symptomatic epilepsy* in which the underlying cause of the seizures may, for example, be trauma, tumour or an infection. With the increasing use and sophistication of neuroimaging techniques, the accuracy of the clinical diagnosis of symptomatic epilepsy has greatly improved.

Idiopathic epilepsy

Abnormalities are few, but thorough histological examination may reveal changes which could be responsible for the seizures. Three main types of lesion have been identified, namely, minor dysgenetic lesions in which there are disturbances of the normal cytoarchitecture of the cerebellum, the hippocampus and the neocortex; consequences of trauma that include healed contusions; and neuronal loss and gliosis. The latter changes are common, the hippocampus being damaged in some 50–60 per cent of patients, the cerebellum in 45 per cent and the thalamus, amygdala and neocortex each in 25 per cent. The common abnormality in the hippocampus is atrophy of the medial part of the temporal lobe due to gliosis of the CA1 sector (Sommer sector) known as Ammons horn sclerosis (Fig. 5.20). Changes in the cerebellum consist of loss of Purkinje cells, some loss of granule cells and an associated astrocytosis.

The aetiology of the neuronal loss and gliosis is not clear. The question as to whether these abnormalities are the cause or the result of

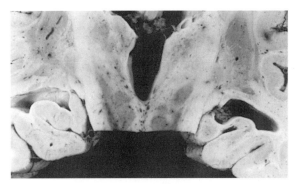

Fig. 5.20 Unilateral sclerosis of the right hippocampus. There is associated enlargement of the temporal horn.

epilepsy remains controversial. Thus it has been suggested that they may be secondary to hypoxia occurring during birth, when the circulation through the posterior cerebral arteries may be compromised. However, lesions may be found in structures supplied by other arteries, raising the possibility that the lesions may be secondary to the epilepsy and not the cause of it.

Symptomatic epilepsy

This may be caused by a wide variety of systemic and cerebral diseases. The incidence of the underlying causes varies according to the age of the patient. For example, in the neonatal period about a quarter are due to metabolic disease (hypocalcaemia, hypoglycaemia, etc.), about a quarter to intracranial haemorrhage, birth injury and infection, some 10 per cent to malformations, and a further 10 per cent to perinatal hypoxia. In children about 50 per cent are due to vascular accidents, head injury, acute infections, malformations and tumour, some 20 per cent are of uncertain cause and in the remaining 30 per cent there is no evidence of brain disease. This is in contrast to adults, in whom trauma and tumours are the most important identified factors, and in the elderly the underlying causes are most likely to be cerebrovascular disease or degenerative disorders. Alcoholism may also play a part in adults.

Epilepsy occurs in some 50 per cent of patients with intracranial tumours, seizures being more common if the tumour lies in the frontal or parietal lobe near the central sulcus, and if it is slow growing and relatively benign, e.g. oligo-dendroglioma, rather than a rapidly growing glioblastoma.

A penetrating head injury is more likely than a closed head injury to be complicated by epilepsy. After a penetrating injury to the skull perhaps as many as 40 per cent of patients during a 5-year period develop seizures: this is in contrast to some 15 per cent of patients who develop late epilepsy following closed head injury, the number increasing if there is a depressed fracture of the skull, sepsis or focal signs.

Many different types of infection of the nervous system may result in epilepsy. These include acute viral encephalitis, toxoplasmosis and cysticercosis.

Temporal lobe epilepsy

As the lesions causing this type of epilepsy may be small it is very important that each specimen, either a surgically resected temporal lobe or a brain, is cut into thin slices and examined systematically. Recent studies have distinguished eight types of lesion:

1. Ammon's horn sclerosis, which was by far the commonest abnormality.
2. Hamartomas made up of glia, mixed neuronal glia and vascular lesions in the temporal lobe.
3. Lesions made up of astrocytes and/or oligodendrocytes that are probably neoplastic.
4. Lesions composed of glial and neuronal tissue, which may appear either as hamartomas or gangliogliomas.
5. Vascular lesions which are angiomatous malformations.
6. Inflammatory lesions.
7. A sequel of head injury.
8. Developmental abnormalities consisting of cysts and cortical malformations such as polymicrogyria.

In spite of this catalogue of abnormalities, it is necessary to remember that one out of four temporal lobes appears to be normal, or shows only minor non-diagnostic changes.

Febrile convulsions and status epilepticus

About 29 per 1000 of children under 5 years of age experience one or more febrile convulsions, about 10 per cent of whom subsequently experience afebrile seizures. Conversely, of patients with epilepsy, about 10 per cent have experienced febrile convulsions in childhood. Febrile convulsions therefore carry the risk of permanent brain damage, which may include Ammon's horn sclerosis, cerebral hemiatrophy and generalized damage in those areas most vulnerable to hypoxia.

Status epilepticus is a convulsive episode lasting over an hour without an intervening period of consciousness. It poses a threat at any age, but particularly in young children. In many cases it is symptomatic of underlying brain disease, although pre-existing cryptogenic epilepsy may also be a risk factor. In fatal cases naked eye abnormalities may be limited to swelling, although subsequent microscopy will probably – if survival has been long enough (see Ch. 5) – show widespread irreversible hypoxic damage in vulnerable areas. Experimental studies have shown that in both acutely induced and chronic epilepsies neuronal damage is probably due to the influx of calcium as a direct consequence of the epileptic activity.

HYPOGLYCAEMIC BRAIN DAMAGE

Hypoglycaemia in man may lead to permanent brain damage in such diverse situations as an excess of insulin given for the treatment of diabetes mellitus or psychosis, in the rare instances of islet-cell tumours of the pancreas, and in examples of hypoglycaemia in infants.

In cases of short survival, the brain may appear normal macroscopically. If survival is for more than a few weeks, there may be atrophy of the cortex and hippocampi, and enlargement of the ventricular system. Microscopy shows that the brain damage is very similar in type and distribution to that seen after cardiac arrest, except that there is often relative sparing of the Purkinje cells in the cerebellum.

Experimental work has shown that the blood glucose must fall to about 1 mmol/l before brain damage is produced, although a higher level of blood sugar may produce similar damage if complicated by hypotension, hypoxaemia or epileptic activity.

THROMBOSIS OF THE VEINS AND VENOUS SINUSES

There are two principal types, namely *primary* (non-infectious) and *secondary* (due to pyogenic infection). Primary thrombosis of the cortical veins and superior sagittal sinus may complicate pregnancy and the puerprium, various haematological disorders and the use of oral contraceptives as well as extreme dehydration in children (*marasmus*). If several cortical veins or the sagittal sinus are occluded by thrombus, the interference with venous drainage leads to venous infarction (Fig. 5.21).

Secondary thrombosis is most often found as a complication of pyogenic infection. For example, the superior sagittal sinus may become thrombosed if infection spreads from the frontal sinuses or a compound fracture of the skull. Likewise, the lateral and cavernous sinuses may become occluded if infection spreads from either the middle ear or the central part of the face respectively. If the thrombus fragments and is carried into the bloodstream, pyaemia and systemic abscesses may develop.

SPONTANEOUS INTRACRANIAL HAEMORRHAGE

Figures from the Framingham study suggest that some 16 per cent of 'strokes' are due to haemorrhage, of which 10 per cent are due to *intracerebral haemorrhage* and 6 per cent to subarachnoid haemorrhage from rupture of an *intracranial (saccular) aneurysm*. There are other, less common, causes of spontaneous intracranial haemorrhage. Traumatic haemorrhage is considered in Chapter 8. The commonest types occur in late middle-aged individuals with hypertension. They were attributed by Charcot in the middle of the 19th century to haemorrhage from miliary aneurysms on the small perforating cerebral arteries, and this view has been confirmed by *post-mortem* micro-angiographic studies which have demonstrated the existence of microaneurysms on these arteries. They are usually multiple, tend to occur on arteries less than $25\,\mu m$ in diameter, and may attain a diameter of $2\,mm$. They occur mainly in hypertensive subjects over the age of 50. In contrast, microaneurysms are rare in normotensive individuals, although a few can be demonstrated in people over the age of 65 years, and are considered to be the origin of spontaneous intracranial haematomas in elderly normotensive individuals.

In four-fifths of cases the haematoma is in the region of the basal ganglia – the so-called 'capsular haemorrhage' (Fig. 5.22). Since the haemorrhage is arterial in origin, the haematoma usually enlarges rapidly and causes considerable destruction of brain tissue. Because of the rapidly expanding lesion and distortion and herniation of the brain, death often occurs within 24–48 hours as a result

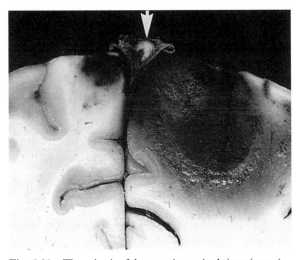

Fig. 5.21 Thrombosis of the superior sagittal sinus (arrow). There is haemorrhagic necrosis of the dorsal angles of the cerebral hemispheres.

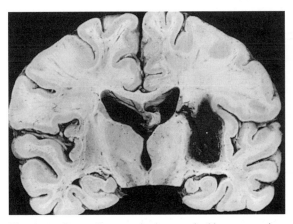

Fig. 5.22 Recent hypertensive intracerebral haematoma in the basal ganglia.

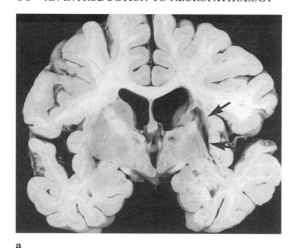

a

Fig. 5.23   Old hypertensive haematoma. (a) There is an 'apoplectic cyst (arrows) in the basal ganglia, the walls of which were orange/brown in colour. Compare location with Fig. 5.22. (b) In the brain stem of the same patient there is unilateral descending degeneration in the corticospinal tract.

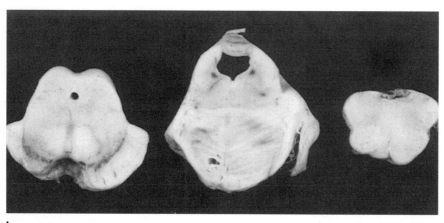

b

of raised ICP. The haematoma often ruptures into the ventricles or through the surface of the brain directly into the subarachnoid space. A few patients may survive the acute episode, presumably because the haematoma is relatively small or because it has developed slowly, thus leaving more time for spatial compensation (see Ch. 4). The haematoma becomes brown in colour and reactive changes in astrocytes, microglia and small vessels appear around it. If the patient survives, the clot is ultimately completely absorbed and replaced by xanthochromic fluid, thus forming a so-called *apoplectic cyst* (Fig. 5.23).

In the remaining one-fifth of cases the haematoma occurs in the hindbrain, either in the pons or in the cerebellum (Figs 5.24, 5.25). Primary pontine haemorrhage has to be distinguished from haemorrhage secondary to raised ICP and

internal herniae (see Ch. 4). This is usually not difficult, although a large primary supratentorial haematoma may track downwards into the upper brain stem.

Less common causes of haemorrhage are *vasculitis*, particularly in patients with collagen diseases, and rupture of a *mycotic aneurysm*, a *saccular aneurysm* or a *vascular malformation* (see below). In some instances, however, the cause cannot be determined in spite of careful examination of the brain. In such circumstances the haematoma is probably due to rupture of a small hidden angioma. Haemorrhage may occasionally occur in either primary or secondary *brain tumours*. The former is most likely to occur in patients with anaplastic astrocytoma, glioblastoma and oligodendroglioma. Bleeding into metastatic tumour may be severe, and occurs most often

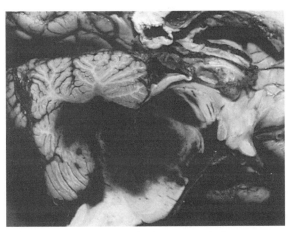

Fig. 5.24 Recent hypertensive haematoma in the pons.

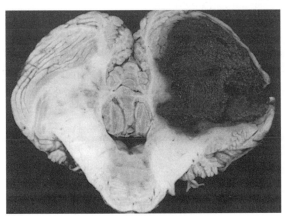

Fig. 5.25 Recent hypertensive haematoma in the cerebellum.

into deposits from primary carcinoma of the bronchus, cutaneous malignant melanoma and choriocarcinoma.

There has been an increasing awareness of *cerebral amyloid angiopathy* as a cause of intracerebral haemorrhage in an aytpical site in normotensive individuals. The amyloid infiltrates the media and adventitia of the blood vessels, often giving a 'double-barrel' appearance. Rupture may follow the formation of microaneurysms. This type of amyloid (βA4) is not related to systemic amyloidosis, but it does appear to have an association with Alzheimer-type dementia (see Ch. 14).

Multiple haemorrhages are often seen in the white matter in patients with *thrombocytopenia*.

Such patients fall into two main categories: those with and those without leukaemia. Thrombocytopenia is also probably the most important factor in the bleeding tendency sometimes seen in alcoholics and in patients with aplastic anaemia or disseminated intravascular coagulation. Patients on anticoagulant therapy or those with various factor deficiencies, such as haemophilia, more often bleed into the subdural space than into the brain parenchyma.

HAEMORRHAGE INTO THE SPINAL CORD

Bleeding into the spinal cord (*haematomyelia*) is common after trauma and often occurs without any evidence of fracture or subluxation. Spontaneous bleeding is rare, although it may occur in patients with thrombocytopenia or a spinal vascular malformation.

SUBARACHNOID HAEMORRHAGE

There are several causes of blood in the subarachnoid space, the commonest of which is probably acute head injury. The term subarachnoid haemorrhage, however, tends to be used in the clinical sense for spontaneous rupture of a saccular aneurysm. Intracerebral haematomas may also rupture into the ventricular system or directly into the subarachnoid space.

Thus, in about 65 per cent of patients presenting clinically with spontaneous (non-traumatic) subarachnoid haemorrhage, it is due to rupture of a saccular aneurysm on one of the major cerebral arteries. In another 5 per cent it is due to rupture of an arteriovenous malformation and in a further 5 per cent it is due to some other disease, such as a blood dyscrasia or the extension of an intracerebral haematoma into the subarachnoid space. In up to 10 per cent of patients no cause is found even after complete cerebral angiography.

Saccular aneurysms

These occur on the arteries at the base of the brain in about 1–2 per cent of the adult population (Fig. 5.26a). They are found more commonly in women than in men and are a not

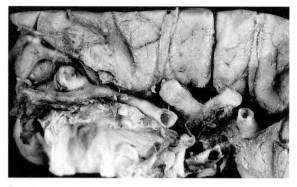

a

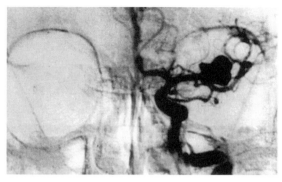

b

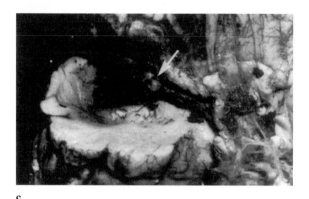

c

Fig. 5.26 Saccular aneurysm. (a) An intact aneurysm arising from middle cerebral artery. (b) Angiographic demonstration of aneurysm arising at the bifurcation of a middle cerebral artery. (c) Subarachnoid and intracerebral haemorrhage due to rupture of an aneurysm (arrow) arising from middle cerebral artery. (Fig. 5.26b courtesy of Dr Peter Macpherson, Department of Neuroradiology, Institute of Neurological Sciences, Glasgow.)

uncommon incidental finding at autopsy. They are often referred to as congenital aneurysms, but the developmental abnormality is not the aneurysm itself but a defect in the medial coat of the artery at one of the bifurcations of the larger cerebral arteries within the subarachnoid space. Subsequent degeneration of the internal elastic lamina, probably brought about by early atheroma and hypertension, may be a prerequisite for the development of the aneurysm. The arterial wall at the bifurcation then commences to bulge, and it has been established from serial angiographic studies that the sac may enlarge progressively. Support for the role of haemodynamic stress in the formation of saccular aneurysms is provided by the coincidence of their occurrence on vessels supplying arteriovenous malformations. The contribution of elevated blood pressure to the development of an aneurysm is unclear, as the relative importance of these factors varies at different ages.

The great majority of aneurysms are thin-walled: they range in size from small aneurysmal blisters measuring some 1–2 mm in diameter to large sacs measuring several centimetres across. The latter are usually thick walled, often contain laminated thrombus and rarely rupture, but may cause focal neurological signs from local pressure on the brain or cranial nerves (Fig. 5.27). Most aneurysms that rupture measure 5–10 mm in diameter.

About 40 per cent of aneurysms are located at the junction between the internal carotid and the posterior communicating arteries, about 30 per cent at the junction between the anterior communicating and anterior cerebral arteries within the interhemispheric fissure, and about 20 per cent at the bi- or trifurcation of the middle cerebral artery within a Sylvian fissure. The commonest sites of the remaining 10 per cent are on the pericallosal artery as it winds around the anterior part of the corpus callosum, at the junction between the internal carotid and middle cerebral arteries, at the upper end of the basilar artery, at the junction between the vertebral and posterior inferior cerebellar arteries, and at the

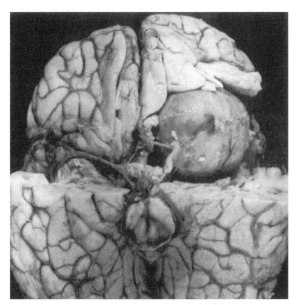

Fig. 5.27 Giant aneurysm. There is a large unruptured saccular aneurysm on the left middle cerebral artery.

junction between the internal carotid and ophthalmic arteries immediately beyond the cavernous sinus. Rupture occurs when the wall is no longer strong enough to withstand the stress, and generally occurs at the fundus. Multiple aneurysms are found in 10–15 per cent of patients with subarachnoid haemorrhage: in such patients there are usually two or three but sometimes five or more. There is said to be an association between multiple aneurysms and coarctation of the aorta, adult type III polycystic disease of the kidney and renal artery stenosis, the possible common denominator being hypertension. However, patients with these conditions are not invariably hypertensive and in at least some instances it is thought that there may be a developmental abnormality in the form of a collagen type 3 deficiency.

Early intracranial complications

Some 10 per cent of patients die during the first bleed and a further 30 per cent from its after-effects within the next few days. A further 35 per cent rebleed and die within the first year, most of these within the first two weeks. The causes include severe recurrent haemorrhage, intra-

cerebral haematoma, subdural haematoma and a caroticocavernous fistula.

Subarachnoid haemorrhage

When an aneurysm ruptures there is usually subarachnoid haemorrhage. This may be limited to the immediate vicinity of the aneurysm, but frequently there is extensive haemorrhage throughout the subarachnoid space. Recurrent haemorrhage is common and many patients who sustain severe subarachnoid haemorrhage have a recent clinical history of some headache and neck stiffness which was not recognized at the time as a minor subarachnoid haemorrhage. In fatal cases the basal cisterns and much of the subarachnoid space over the surfaces of the cerebral hemispheres and the cerebellum are filled with recent blood clot. When undertaking a post-mortem examination on such a case it is important to try to define the aneurysm prior to fixing the brain, since fixed blood clot is very difficult to remove without destroying the aneurysm. Blood also tracks along the spinal cord, most of it localizing in the subarachnoid space of the posterior surface of the cord. Sometimes quite a large haematoma may develop in the subarachnoid space, usually within the Sylvian fissure in association with an aneurysm on the middle cerebral artery, or between the medial surfaces of the frontal lobe in association with an aneurysm on the anterior communicating artery.

Intracerebral haematoma

This is also a common occurrence when an aneurysm ruptures. There is usually some subarachnoid haemorrhage in addition, but sometimes the fundus of the aneurysm is so deeply embedded in the brain, this possibly having been brought about by previous small leaks from the aneurysm, that the aneurysm ruptures directly into the brain without there being any obvious subarachnoid haemorrhage. The haematomas lie adjacent to the aneurysms and occur in the inferomedial part of the frontal lobe(s) in association with anterior communicating artery aneurysms (Fig. 5.28), and in the temporal lobe in association with an aneurysm on a middle

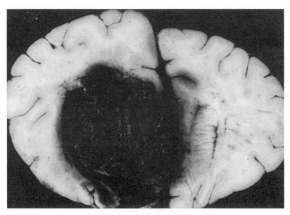

Fig. 5.28 Intracerebral haematoma. There is a haematoma in the inferomedial quadrant of the left frontal lobe due to rupture of an aneurysm arising from the anterior communicating artery.

cerebral artery or on a posterior communicating artery. The haematomas so formed may rupture into the ventricular system, particularly an aneurysm on the anterior communicating artery or at the bifurcation of the basilar artery. Rupture of an aneurysm on the middle cerebral artery may occasionally produce an *acute subdural haematoma*: this is particularly important in medicolegal cases where trauma is suspected. Also, an aneurysm on the internal carotid artery may rupture into the cavernous sinus, causing a *caroticocavernous fistula*.

Late intracranial complications.

These include cerebral infarction, hydrocephalus and haemosiderosis.

Cerebral infarction

Infarction occurs most commonly in the region of the brain supplied by the artery on which the aneurysm is situated, but it is not infrequently more widespread. The infarct is probably partly attributable to arterial spasm, which is frequently seen on cerebral angiograms of patients with recently ruptured aneurysms. The situation, however, is complex and the infarct is often due to a combination of factors including vasospasm, the mass effects of an intracerebral haematoma and raised ICP.

Hydrocephalus

There are two types: an acute variety within the first few days and a chronic type at about the second week. Both types are probably due to obstruction to the flow of CSF by blood in the subarachnoid space (see Ch. 4).

Haemosiderosis

If the subarachnoid haemorrhage is not massive and the patient survives, the blood is gradually absorbed and the pia-arachnoid becomes permanently stained brownish/yellow because of residual haemosiderin pigment within macrophages. If there are recurrent episodes of subarachnoid haemorrhage, the outer cortical layers become more deeply pigmented because of the presence of subpial haemosiderin-containing macrophages. This condition is known as *subpial haemosiderosis*, and is seen more commonly in association with vascular malformations than aneurysms.

Other types of aneurysm

Atheroma may be the cause of *fusiform enlargement* of a major cerebral artery, but such aneurysms rarely rupture. A rare but not unimportant entity is widespread *ectasia* of the major cerebral arteries (Fig. 5.29). This may be partly attributable to atheroma, but it seems more likely that there is some more generalized inherent defect of the vessel walls. When ectasia is severe, the tortuous basilar artery may produce considerable distortion of the ventral surface of the brain stem. It has also been suggested that ectasia of the basilar artery and its increased pulsation in the posterior fossa may be an occasional cause of hydrocephalus. *Mycotic aneurysms* produced by infected emboli may also occur on the cerebral arteries. They are found more commonly in adults than in children, and are said to be multiple in 20 per cent of cases. The aneurysms are most commonly due to *streptococci* and *staphylococci*, and the organisms spread rapidly from the impacted embolus to the vessel wall, which then undergoes acute inflammatory changes, necrosis and aneurysmal dilatation. Mycotic aneurysms are

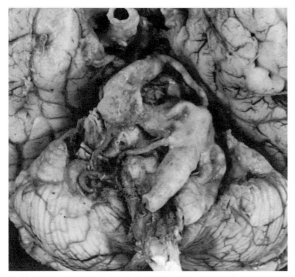

Fig. 5.29 Arterial ectasia. The basilar and left vertebral arteries are dilated and tortuous.

said to occur in between 3 and 10 per cent of patients with infective endocarditis. Fungal mycotic aneurysms are also encountered, most often in patients with aspergillosis or candidosis. They tend to be larger than aneurysms caused by bacteria and are found most commonly on the major arteries at the base of the brain. They are often multiple and the nasal sinuses or heart are frequent sources of infection.

Dissecting aneurysm of the aorta is the result of extensive haemorrhage into the media weakened by hypertension and idiopathic cystic medionecrosis. The haemorrhage usually commences as a tear in the ascending aorta and extends into the abdominal aorta. The dissection may extend into the extracranial cervical arteries, narrowing their lumina and impairing blood flow to the brain. Dissecting aneurysms of the carotid arteries in the neck and their major intracranial branches may be due to extension from the aorta, develop spontaneously, or be due to neck injury or follow carotid puncture for angiography. Dissecting aneurysms of the intracranial arteries are rare, and usually occur in children and young adults: the causes include head injury, migraine, arteritis, fibromuscular dysplasia, inflammation and homocystinuria. Following dissection, the aneurysm may rupture and cause subarachnoid haemorrhage or produce thrombotic occlusion of the vessel, with infarction of the tissue supplied by the affected artery.

VASCULAR MALFORMATIONS OF THE BRAIN AND SPINAL CORD

These may range in size from small capillary angiomas to massive lesions composed of a plexus of large, rather thick-walled vascular channels (Fig. 5.30). They occur most commonly in young adults and are usually on the surface of the brain or the spinal cord, but they are sometimes restricted to the deeper structures of the brain and do not reach the surface.

Rupture of a vascular malformation may produce a massive intracranial haematoma which is rapidly fatal, but a more frequent result is repeated episodes of mild subarachnoid haemorrhage leading to subpial haemosiderosis. Many vascular malformations are compatible with long survival.

Rupture of a spinal malformation may lead to subarachnoid or intramedullary haemorrhage. The latter is associated with the rapid onset of severe neurological symptoms, depending on the level of the malformation. In a condition known as subacute necrotic myelitis, or Foix–Alajouanine disease, which most often occurs in elderly males, small blood vessels within the lumbosacral parts of the spinal cord and in the adjacent sub-

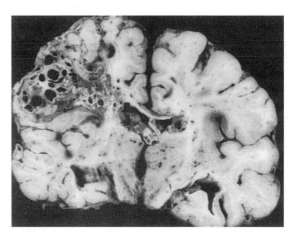

Fig. 5.30 Arteriovenous malformation.

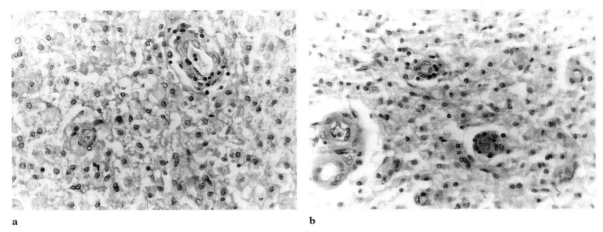

a   b

Fig. 5.31   Subacute necrotic myelitis of the spinal cord (Foix–Alajouanine disease). In the severely affected segments there are (a) numerous lipid-containing macrophages, and (b) striking vascular changes. ((a) and (b) H&E.)

arachnoid space have markedly thickened walls and may be cuffed by lymphocytes (Fig. 5.31). The structural changes that occur are those of small, often multiple, infarcts within the spinal cord, leading to various and often progressive degrees of paraparesis.

PURPURIC CONDITIONS AFFECTING THE BRAIN

This is a non-specific descriptive term applicable to any condition of the brain characterized by the occurrence of petechial haemorrhages. The petechiae vary considerably in number, but are usually confined to the white matter. There are many causes. They occur in some types of *head injury* (see Ch. 8), where they may be a manifestation either of severe primary injury or a secondary complication such as *fat embolism*. Petechial haemorrhages are also seen in cases of *cerebral malaria*, and in cases of *viral meningoencephalitis*, particularly if there is an associated vasculitis, as in acute necrotizing encephalitis due to herpes simplex. They are also seen in cases of *septicaemia* and *endotoxic shock*. Other causes include *acute haemorrhagic leukoencephalopathy, thrombotic thrombocytopenic purpura, disseminated intravascular coagulation* and *consumptive coagulopathy*. Other causes include *hypertensive encephalopathy* and as an *allergic sensitivity to drugs*, penicillin being the best known to have such an effect.

FURTHER READING

Allen C M C, Harrison M J E & Wade D T (1988) *The Management of Acute Stroke.* Colchester: Castle House Publications Ltd.

Barnett H J M, Mohr J P, Stein B M & Yatsu F M (eds) (1986) *Stroke: Pathophysiology, Diagnosis and Management, Vols 1 & 2.* Edinburgh: Churchill Livingstone.

Graham D I (1990) Vascular disease and hypoxic brain damage. In: *Nervous System, Muscle and Eyes, Systemic Pathology,* 3rd edn. Vol. 4. Edited by R O Weller. Edinburgh: Churchill Livingstone, pp. 89–124.

Russell R W R (ed) (1983) *Vascular Disease of the Central Nervous System.* Edinburgh: Churchill Livingstone.

6. Bacterial infections

Although it is convenient to deal separately with the principal types of infection of the CNS – bacterial, viral, fungal etc. – there are certain features that are common to all. The brain and spinal cord are relatively well protected by bone and by the dura from infective agents and, as a result of this, haematogenous infections are commoner than the direct spread of infection. The latter, however, may come about through a fracture of the skull or as a result of spread of infection from local sources, such as osteitis in the skull or vertebrae. The infective agent occasionally spreads along nerves. On the other hand, once infection is established local defensive mechanisms seem to be deficient, since many micro-organisms that are of low virulence in other sites can produce serious and often fatal infections of the CNS. Furthermore, once micro-organisms gain access to the CSF they can disseminate rapidly throughout the subarachnoid space and the ventricles, and opportunistic infections of the nervous system are a frequent terminal event in immunocompromised individuals. In any suspected infection of the CNS, *it is imperative that the pathologist takes appropriate specimens post mortem for microbiological examination.*

SITES OF INFECTION

There are six potential sites, singly or in combination (Fig. 6.1). The infection may be in *bone* in the form of osteitis in relation, for example, to a chronic suppurative otitis media or mastoiditis. Where tuberculosis is common, the vertebral column is often affected. The remaining sites are the *extradural space*, the *subdural space*, the *subarachnoid space*, *intracerebral* or *intraventricular*.

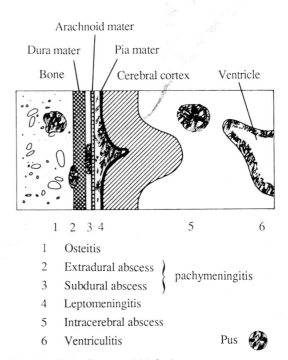

Fig. 6.1 Sites of intracranial infection.

Infections in the extradural or subdural space are examples of *pachymeningitis*, whereas infection of the subarachnoid space, properly known as *leptomeningitis*, is usually referred to simply as *meningitis*. The dura, the arachnoid and the pia appear to be fairly efficient barriers to the spread of micro-organisms because the infection often remains restricted to one particular compartment for a considerable period of time. Bacterial infections of the nervous system predominantly affect the meninges (*meningitis*) or brain tissue (*encephalitis*), but on histological examination there is usually evidence of meningitis and encephalitis, i.e. meningoencephalitis.

The cerebrospinal fluid (CSF) is almost invariably abnormal in infections of the CNS, although micro-organisms are unlikely to be cultured if the infection is restricted to the extradural or subdural spaces, or is intracerebral. Lumbar puncture is a prerequisite for the diagnosis of meningitis, since it is the only means whereby the causative organism can be identified and its sensitivity to antibiotics established. On occasion, lumbar puncture may have to be deferred until the coincident presence of a cerebral abscess has been eliminated by a CT scan. The clinical features of subarachnoid haemorrhage may be very similar to those of bacterial meningitis and, if a lumbar puncture has to be undertaken to distinguish between the two, this should also preferably be deferred until the presence of an intracranial haematoma has been excluded by a CT scan. Yet every pathologist must, on occasion, have encountered acute purulent meningitis *post mortem* in a patient thought to be a case of subarachnoid haemorrhage due to rupture of a saccular aneurysm (see Ch. 5).

In patients with meningitis, the CSF pressure on lumbar puncture is usually increased except in more chronic infections, e.g. tuberculous meningitis, where the exudate may have caused a 'spinal block'. In acute purulent meningitis the cell count is high because of the presence of many neutrophil polymorphs, there is some increase in protein content, and glucose is low or absent. In subacute bacterial meningitis the cell count is less increased, lymphocytes and plasma cells outnumber neutrophil polymorphs, the protein content is higher, and there is only a moderate reduction in the glucose content. Similar changes are seen in patients with diffuse meningeal tumour (see Ch. 15). In viral infections there is a moderate increase in protein and nucleated cells – mainly lymphocytes and monocytes, but neutrophil polymorphs may be present in the early stages of the disease – and the glucose remains normal. It is important to assess the blood glucose level when a lumbar puncture is undertaken, since CSF glucose closely follows the blood glucose level.

Bacterial infections of the nervous system may be *pyogenic* or *non-pyogenic*.

PYOGENIC INFECTIONS

PACHYMENINGITIS

This is most commonly caused by spread of infection from a focus of chronic osteitis in the skull, such as chronic suppurative otitis media, mastoiditis or frontal sinusitis. The first stage is the formation of an *extradural abscess*: such abscesses tend to be small because the dura is firmly attached to the skull. When the inflammatory process spreads through the dura into the subdural space to form a *subdural abscess*, the infection is again often localized because adhesions may develop in the subdural space in the region of an extradural abscess. If, however, the infection has proceeded rapidly and such adhesions have not developed, the inflammatory process spreads diffusely throughout the subdural space, which becomes filled with pus (*subdural empyema*). Quite large collections of pus may develop, not only on the surface of a cerebral hemisphere but also in the interhemispheric fissure and between the inferior surface of the cerebral hemispheres and the tentorium cerebelli. Pus in the subdural space wipes off the surface of the brain, in contrast to pus in the subarachnoid space which is retained in position by the arachnoid. Pachymeningitis may also be a sequel to a depressed fracture of the skull, whereas in infants and young children with a florid and acute leptomeningitis the infection may spread through the arachnoid into the subdural space, to produce a subdural empyema.

Within the vertebral canal extradural infections are commoner than subdural infections. One of the commoner lesions is an acute infection due either to staphylococci or coliform bacilli. On histological examination there is an active inflammatory process within which there is pus formation. Not infrequently, the inflammation is subacute, the result being a granulomatous mass within which there are loculi of pus. A chronic granulomatous mass in the extradural spinal space may be the presenting feature of brucellosis.

LEPTOMENINGITIS

In the account that follows the term *meningitis* will

be used for leptomeningitis. It is caused by the spread of pyogenic bacteria throughout the subarachnoid space, where they provoke an inflammatory reaction as a result of which purulent exudate is produced. It is almost invariably a medical emergency, and rapid clinical and laboratory diagnosis is necessary not only to save life but also to prevent permanent disability. Acute bacterial meningitis occurs most commonly at the extremes of life, i.e. in neonates and infants, and in the elderly.

Causes

Virtually any pyogenic bacteria can gain access to the subarachnoid space, but the causative micro-organisms vary with the age of the patient (see Tables 6.1 and 6.2). In the neonatal period the commonest organisms are *Escherichia coli* and *group B streptococci*. In other age groups the organisms most commonly identified are *Neisseria meningitidis*, *Haemophilus influenzae* and *Streptococcus pneumoniae*. The second of these is particularly common in children, and the last in the elderly. Less commonly encountered micro-organisms are listed in Tables 6.1 and 6.2.

Table 6.1 Bacterial meningitis

	Neonates	All other age groups
Escherichia coli	307	293
Group B streptococci	271	157
Listeria monocytogenes	62	203
Other streptococci (excluding *S. pneumoniae*)	32	157
Pseudomonas spp	30	269
Streptococcus pneumoniae	30	2512
Proteus spp	25	60
Staphylococcus aureus	25	331
Klebsiella spp	23	95
Neisseria meningitidis	22	3969
Haemophilus influenzae	19	3221
Citrobacter spp	19	10
Enterobacter spp	17	20
Serratia	10	15
Mycobacteria	0	277
Other organisms	28	679

(Causes of bacterial meningitis: 1975–83. *From:* Communicable Disease Surveillance Centre, London (1985) *Lancet* **290**, 778–779.)

Table 6.2 Bacterial meningitis

Neisseria meningitidis	265
Haemophilus influenzae	193
Streptococcus pneumoniae	67
Other streptococci	12
Staphylococci	5
Escherichia coli	27
Coliforms	4
Salmonella spp	5
Klebsiella spp	2
Proteus spp	2
Listeria monocytogenes	4
Other species	5
Organism not identified	147

Causes of acute bacterial meningitis in childhood (under 10 years of age). An analysis of 738 cases in the North-West Metropolitan Region, England. *From:* Goldacre, M.J. (1976) *Lancet* **i**, 28–31.

Routes of infection

There are four principal routes of infection.

Haematogenous

Most cases of acute pyogenic meningitis are caused by the haematogenous dissemination of bacteria. There is therefore always a bacteraemia and sometimes a septicaemia. The latter is particularly common in epidemics of meningococcal meningitis. The meningococci are spread by droplet infection from carriers who harbour the bacteria in the nasopharynx. Spread is favoured by poor hygienic conditions. In the course of an epidemic, patients may die as a result of the septicaemia before there is any clinical evidence of meningitis. A feature of meningococcal septicaemia is a haemorrhagic rash, and a common terminal event in rapidly fatal cases is haemorrhage into the adrenal glands (Waterhouse–Friderichsen syndrome). Pneumococcal meningitis is a relatively common occurrence in the elderly: its progress is so rapid that it is often thought that the patient has sustained a stroke. It is likely that septicaemia contributes to the rapid progress of this disease, the organisms originating in the respiratory tree or lungs.

Spread from the skull

Chronic osteitis has been referred to above. In

pyogenic infections of any of the sinuses in the skull, infection may occasionally spread to the subarachnoid space.

Compound fracture of the skull

This is another potential source of intracranial infection. Most fractures of the base of the skull also provide a means of entry of bacteria from air sinuses to the subarachnoid space (see Ch. 8), as do penetrating head injuries. Recurrent meningitis is a not uncommon occurrence in patients with a basal fracture, but a second well recognized cause is a congenital fistula between the skin and an intracranial or vertebral dermoid or epidermoid cyst.

Iatrogenic

This occasionally occurs as a result of the accidental introduction of bacteria in the course of lumbar or ventricular puncture or other invasive surgical or radiological procedures. Since the infecting agents are introduced directly into the CSF, a generalized meningitis ensues rapidly.

Structural changes

If the patient dies early in the course of the disease, abnormalities may be restricted to intense congestion of small vessels on the surface of the brain. Usually, however, there is a purulent exudate in the subarachnoid space, particularly where the subarachnoid space is widest, i.e. in the basal cisterns and within sulci. The spinal cord is usually also covered with pus, and there may also be purulent exudate within the ventricles. In rapidly fatal cases of acute pneumococcal meningitis, however, pus – which often has a distinctive green hue – may be restricted to the parasagittal regions of the brain at the vertex (Fig. 6.2). This should not be confused with the thickening and opalescence of the meninges which is commonly seen at the vertex in elderly people. It may therefore be necessary to confirm the diagnosis of meningitis histologically. In acutely fatal cases of streptococcal meningitis in neonates, the exudate is often haemorrhagic.

If the patient has survived for some days, there may already be moderate hydrocephalus since the purulent exudate rapidly interferes with the

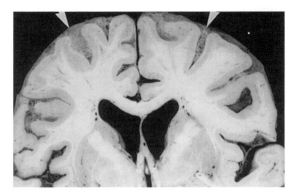

Fig. 6.2   Acute meningitis. There is a thick layer of pus in the subarachnoid space (arrows).

circulation of CSF. Occasionally, particularly in children, there may be necrosis of the superficial layers of the cerebral cortex and spread of the infection to the subdural space, within which there is a thin layer of pus. Again, mainly in children, the infection may occasionally spread to produce a suppurative encephalitis. Other complications include haemorrhagic infarction in the cerebral cortex, cortical thrombophlebitis and diffuse brain swelling.

On *histological examination* the exudate consists principally of neutrophil polymorphs, but even when the exudate appears frankly purulent macroscopically, there are many lymphocytes, plasma cells and cells of monocytic type within it (Fig. 6.3). It is remarkable how little the inflammatory process extends into perivascular spaces in the adjacent cortex. There is often an active vasculitis within the subarachnoid space, as shown by the presence of polymorphs in the intima, and occasionally necrosis of vessel walls (Fig. 6.4).

Since many patients make a complete recovery from acute pyogenic meningitis, it must be assumed that the exudate may resolve completely. If it does not, and this may be contributed to by a delay in initiating treatment, adhesions will inevitably develop in the subarachnoid space. This is sometimes particularly conspicuous in the posterior fossa, where it has in the past been referred to as *'posterior basal meningitis'*. Any obstruction to the free flow of CSF will produce varying degrees of obstructive hydrocephalus. Cranial nerve palsies and mental retardation are also complications of this type of meningitis.

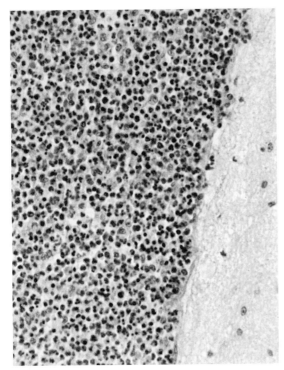

Fig. 6.3 Acute meningitis. The subarachnoid space is filled with inflammatory cells. (H & E).

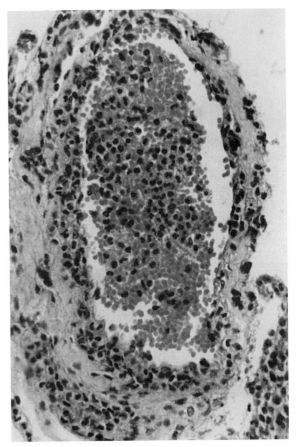

Fig. 6.4 Acute meningitis. The wall of this small blood vessel is infiltrated by inflammatory cells. (H & E.)

BRAIN ABSCESS

Causes

Because of the relatively poor resistance of the brain to infection, many organisms thought to be of low pathogenicity can produce a brain abscess (Table 6.3). Mixed infections are common and include anaerobic micro-organisms such as bacteroides and anaerobic streptococci. The pus, however, is often sterile as a result of prior antibiotic therapy.

Routes of infection

These are similar to those described above for pyogenic meningitis, but whereas haematogenous dissemination of micro-organisms is the commonest cause of meningitis, the most frequent cause of brain abscess in many countries is spread of infection from a *chronic suppurative otitis media* or a *chronic mastoiditis*. Indeed, brain abscess is an uncommon occurrence in countries where chronic infections of the ear are rare or well controlled.

Other causes of brain abscess are haematogenous dissemination of infection, penetrating head injuries and penetrating injuries of the orbit that enter the intracranial cavity through the orbital fissures.

Cerebral abscess secondary to osteitis

The bone adjacent to a chronic infection of the skull, usually chronic suppurative otitis media or chronic mastoiditis but occasionally chronic infections of other sinuses, becomes the seat of chronic osteitis and becomes eroded (Fig. 6.5). Infection extends to the extradural and subdural spaces. Precisely how the infection spreads across the subdural and subarachnoid spaces without producing a subdural empyema or a diffuse purulent meningitis is not clear, but it may be because the long-standing infection has produced local oblit-

Table 6.3   Brain abscess

Streptococci
   Strep. millen★
   Other viridans and non-haemolytic streptococci
   Enterococci
      β-haemolytic streptococci
   Peptostreptococci

Bacteroides group

Enterobacteriaceae
   Proteus sp.
   Escherichia coli
   Klebsiella sp.
Staphylococcus aureus†

★Most frequent organism isolated from intracranial pus
†Associated with post-traumatic and spinal lesions

(Bacteria commonly isolated from intracranial and intraspinal abscesses. *From* de Louvois, J. (1980) *J. Clin. Path.* **33**, 66–71.)

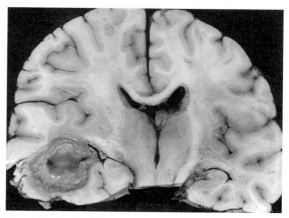

Fig. 6.6   Cerebral abscess. There is an encapsulated abscess in the left temporal lobe secondary to chronic suppurative otitis media.

eration of these spaces. Micro-organisms, however, gain access to the adjacent brain – the temporal lobe from a chronic suppurative otitis media, the cerebellum from a chronic mastoiditis, and the frontal lobe from a chronic frontal sinusitis. It has to be assumed that there is then an acute suppurative encephalitis, but this stage is rarely, if ever, seen by a neurosurgeon or pathologist since by the time most cerebral abscesses are diagnosed they are subacute or chronic. A chronic abscess has a grey and rather translucent capsule some 2 – 3 mm thick (Fig. 6.6): it may be unilocular or multilocular. The effective size of the abscess is often increased by oedema adjacent to it. An abscess

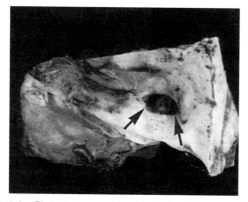

Fig. 6.5   Chronic suppurative otitis media. There is an oval defect in the roof of the middle ear (arrows).

therefore acts as an intracranial expanding lesion, producing local derangement of function and an increase in intracranial pressure (see Ch. 4). If the diagnosis is delayed, the abscess may rupture through the capsule to produce a progressive suppurative encephalitis. Further complications are rupture of the abscess into the ventricular system to produce an acute purulent ventriculitis, or rupture into the subarachnoid space to produce an acute purulent meningitis.

Structural changes

Three layers are recognizable in a chronic abscess. First, an inner zone comprising necrotic debris, neutrophil polymorphs and bacteria. This is surrounded by a capsule made up of collagen and glial fibres, among which there are numerous plasma cells, lymphocytes, lipid-containing macrophages and, occasionally, foreign-body giant cells. The outer zone consists of brain tissue in which there are reactive astrocytes, varying degrees of oedema, and blood vessels cuffed by plasma cells and lymphocytes. In a subacute abscess there is no clearly defined capsule but there is an active gliomesodermal reaction around it. If infection spreads through the capsule, there is necrosis of brain tissue and diffuse infiltration by polymorphs.

The *treatment* of brain abscess consists of aspiration of the pus and the administration of appropriate antibiotics. Practical points to remember are that in patients with chronic suppurative otitis media and mastoiditis there may be abscesses in both the temporal lobe and the cerebellum, and if the ear infection is not treated at the same time as the intracranial abscess the latter may recur very quickly. There may also be thrombosis of the sigmoid sinus, and a complication of this may be the haematogenous dissemination of bland or infected emboli to the lungs. Some of these features may be missed at autopsy unless the venous sinuses are opened and the dura stripped from the base of the skull.

Haematogenous brain abscess

These are similar in appearance to abscesses secondary to the direct spread of infection. There was in the past an association between suppurative bronchiectasis, pneumonia and empyema and haematogenous brain abscess, but these infections can now be controlled by antibiotics. Acute infective endocarditis is another common source of metastatic abscesses in the brain. In subacute infective endocarditis, however, the typical feature in the brain is the presence of numerous small foci of necrosis surrounded by hypertrophied microglia as a result of the dissemination of multiple small emboli. In many patients with haematogenous brain abscess, however, the source of the infection remains undetected, when it must be ascribed to transient bacteraemia, such as may occur after an apparently trivial procedure such as the extraction of a tooth. There is, however, an increased incidence of haematogenous brain abscess in individuals with congenital heart disease, particularly of cyanotic type, and abscesses caused, for example, by fungi are a not uncommon terminal event in patients with immunodeficiency or immunosuppression (transplantation, steroids etc.).

Haematogenous abscesses are often multiple (Fig. 6.7) and, although they can occur in any part of the brain, the superior parts of the cerebral hemispheres in the posterior frontal or parietal regions and the cerebellum are particularly frequently affected.

Lumbar puncture may be contraindicated in a patient suspected of having a cerebral abscess, but the classic feature is the presence of polymorphs in the CSF from which micro-organisms cannot be cultured.

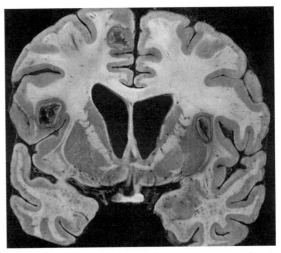

Fig. 6.7 Haematogenous brain abscess. Three separate abscesses are present.

NON-PYOGENIC INFECTIONS

TUBERCULOSIS

Infection of the CNS by *Mycobacterium tuberculosis* is always secondary to disease elsewhere in the body. Its frequency is therefore related to the incidence of tuberculosis in a given population. Where tuberculosis is widespread, tuberculous infection of the nervous system is most frequently encountered in young children; where the disease is well controlled, infection of the CNS may occur at any age. In countries where tuberculosis is uncommon, clinicians tend to forget that it may affect the CNS: thus, any patient with clinical evidence of a subacute infection of the CNS should be thought to be, and probably also treated as, a case of tuberculous meningitis until the correct diagnosis is established.

Tuberculous infection of the CNS takes two principal forms – tuberculous meningitis and tuberculomas.

Tuberculous meningitis

This is almost always caused by the haematogenous dissemination of tubercle bacilli, but it occasionally occurs as a result of spread of infection from a tuberculous lesion in the vertebral column. It may simply be one manifestation of miliary tuberculosis, but more often it appears to be due to the fortuitous deposition of bacilli in the CNS, the meningitis probably being secondary to the rupture of a small tuberculous focus in the choroid plexus or on the surface of the brain into the subarachnoid space.

Tuberculous meningitis is a subacute meningitis. The exudate is gelatinous or caseous and most abundant in the basal cisterns (Fig. 6.8), within sulci and around the spinal cord. Where exudate is minimal, small tubercles measuring 1–2 mm in diameter may be seen in the pia-arachnoid, usually adjacent to cortical blood vessels. The exudate obstructs the flow of CSF, with the result that there is almost invariably some degree of hydrocephalus in patients with tuberculous meningitis.

On *histological examination* the exudate is fibrinocaseous in type, diffusely permeated by lymphocytes, plasma cells and macrophages (Fig. 6.9). Langhans'-type giant cells are much less commonly seen than in tuberculous lesions elsewhere in the body, and classic tubercles are rarely seen. If the meningitis has persisted for some time there is considerable organization of the exudate, particularly around the spinal cord, which becomes ensheathed in a thick layer of tough exudate. Another feature is obliterative endarteritis, resulting in a great reduction in the lumina of affected arteries (see Fig. 5.12). As a result of this there are often superficial infarcts in the adjacent brain tissue, this being an important factor contributing to the frequent occurrence of focal neurological signs in patients with tuberculous meningitis.

In countries where tuberculosis is common, tuberculous meningitis can occasionally run an acute and fulminating course. This is particularly common in children, due to the spread of infection from a primary tuberculous focus, and is presumably a hypersensitivity phenomenon. Polymorphs are prominent in the exudate in the subarachnoid space, and in the adjacent brain there is a fulminating necrotizing encephalitis. This condition is referred to as *acute tuberculous encephalopathy*.

The *diagnosis* of tuberculous meningitis depends on examination of the CSF. Since it takes so long to culture *M. tuberculosis* and since the bacilli disappear rapidly from the CSF once treatment has been instituted, it is of the utmost importance in a suspected case to examine the first few specimens of CSF exhaustively in an effort to identify the bacilli, since this is the only means of establishing the diagnosis in the early stages of the disease. Clinicians must relay any suspicion of tuberculous meningitis to the bacteriologist so that an exhaustive search (as opposed to a less demanding routine approach) is undertaken. Some

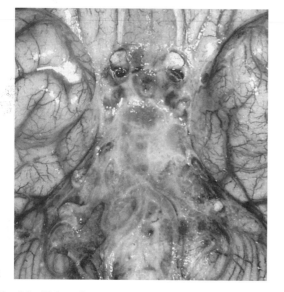

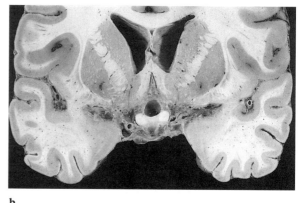

a   b

Fig. 6.8   Tuberculous meningitis. There is thick gelatinous exudate within the basal cisterns (a), and around the optic chiasma (b).

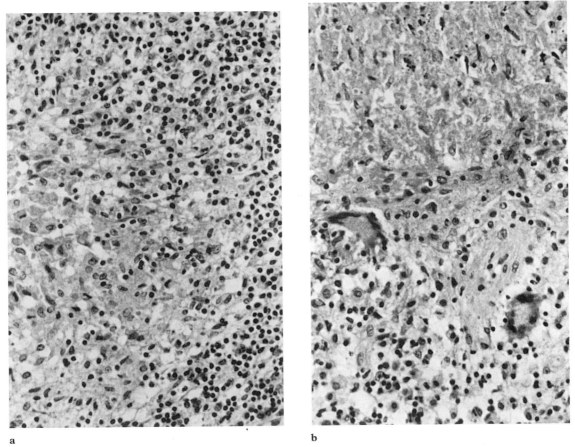

a   b

Fig. 6.9 Tuberculous meningitis. (a) The exudate consists mainly of lymphocytes, plasma cells and epitheliod cells. (b) There may also be caseation and occasional multinucleate giant cells. (H & E.)

studies have suggested that acid-fast bacilli can be identified in the centrifuged deposit in only about 20 per cent of cases, but in others a success rate of almost 90 per cent has been achieved.

Tuberculoma

These take the form of an encapsulated caseous mass in the brain (Fig. 6.10), and in countries where tuberculosis is rife they are a common cause of intracranial expanding lesions. In adults they usually occur in the cerebral hemispheres, but in children they have a particular predilection for the cerebellum. If they have been present for some

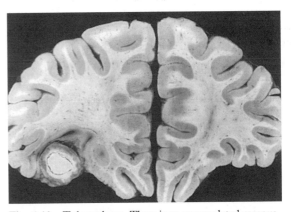

Fig. 6.10 Tuberculoma. There is an encapsulated caseous mass in the left frontal lobe.

time, they are frequently calcified. On histological examination they are composed of a core of caseous material surrounded by a broad band within which conventional tubercles and Langhans' cells are conspicuous.

SYPHILIS

Neurosyphilis is now so rare that there must be many experienced neuropathologists who have not encountered a case. The spirochaete *Treponema pallidum* gains access to the nervous system early in the secondary stage of the disease, as shown by some increase in cells and protein in the CSF, but only rarely does the patient exhibit the clinical features of a transient meningoencephalitis. Neurosyphilis presents in two principal forms – tertiary neurosyphilis and parenchymatous neurosyphilis.

Tertiary neurosyphilis

This may present as meningovascular syphilis or as a gumma. *Meningovascular syphilis* takes the form of a subacute meningitis, there being lymphocytes and plasma cells in the subarachnoid space and a periarteritis. Spread of the inflammatory process into cranial and spinal nerves and the periarteritis may cause focal neurological signs such as optic atrophy or pareses of cranial nerves.

Gummas occur in the meninges, particularly over the convexity of the cerebral hemispheres or over the cerebellum. They are usually attached to both the dura mater and to the brain, in which they become embedded, but occasionally they are confined to the dura mater. Within the abnormal tissue there is necrosis, a periarteritis, and infiltration by lymphocytes and plasma cells.

Pachymeningitis cervicalis hypertrophica is characterized by inflammatory thickening of the dura mater and the pia-arachnoid in the cervical region. First described as being syphilitic in origin, there may be other as yet undefined causes. The histological appearances are similar to a gumma and the obliterative endarteritis may ultimately produce ischaemic damage in the related segments of the spinal cord.

Parenchymatous neurosyphilis

This takes two forms, *general paralysis of the insane* (paretic dementia) and *tabes dorsalis*. Both forms sometimes coexist: *tabo-paresis*. The aetiology of these types of syphilis remains unknown, but their onset may be delayed for as long as 20 years after the primary infection – considerably longer than the interval between primary and tertiary syphilis.

General paralysis of the insane

This is a subacute encephalitis, the principal structural abnormalities being perivascular cuffing of vessels within the CNS by lymphocytes and plasma cells, and a similar inflammatory response in the subarachnoid space. If untreated there is progressive cerebral atrophy, as shown by the presence of small rounded gyri and widened sulci. Other structural abnormalities are the presence of large numbers of rod cells (hypertrophied microglia) in the cerebral cortex, many of which stain positively for iron with Perl's stain, and an intense astrocytosis in grey matter. The ventricles are enlarged and there is a granular ependymitis.

Tabes dorsalis

The basis of this disease is selective degeneration of posterior spinal nerve roots immediately proximal to the posterior root ganglia, but the pathogenesis of the degeneration is not known. The posterior nerve roots become grey and shrunken and the spinal cord also becomes reduced in size, particularly in its anteroposterior diameter, because of demyelination and shrinkage of the posterior columns as a result of Wallerian degeneration (Fig. 6.11). Tabes most frequently affects the lumbosacral nerve roots, but occasionally cervical nerve roots are the most severely affected; this is referred to as cervical tabes.

OTHER CAUSES OF NON-PYOGENIC MENINGITIS

These are many and varied, and only a proportion are due to bacteria such as leptospirosis and brucellosis. Other causes are viruses, amoebae and fungi, and these will be dealt with in Chapter 7.

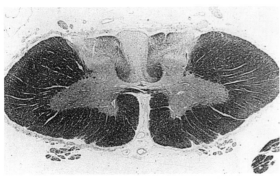

Fig. 6.11 Tabes dorsalis. There is shrinkage and loss of myelin in the posterior columns. (Luxol fast blue/cresyl violet.)

Sarcoidosis may affect the meninges, particularly in the hypothalamic region, involving the optic nerves and the infundibulum, and in the posterior fossa. The sarcoid granulomas are similar to those that occur elsewhere in the body and there may be perivascular cuffing by lymphocytes and plasma cells in the adjacent brain. Extension of the inflammatory process into cranial nerves may result in multiple pareses of cranial nerves.

Diffuse involvement of the subarachnoid space by tumour – *carcinomatosis, gliomatosis* or *meningeal leukaemia* – may present many of the clinical features of a subacute meningitis. It is for this reason that examination of the CSF for malignant cells is an essential investigation in patients with subacute meningitis.

Various irritant substances in the subarachnoid space may also mimic many of the clinical features of meningitis. The commonest is blood, but similar features may be produced by the intrathecal administration of drugs and contrast media in neuroradiological studies. The cell count in the CSF may be very high for a few days after air encephalography or myelography. In *chronic arachnoiditis* the spinal meninges become opaque and thickened, the subarachnoid space becomes obliterated, loculi containing CSF develop, and there is entrapment of nerve roots. The lumbar region is most often affected. Although commonly idiopathic, the arachnoiditis may be secondary to repeated trauma, neuroradiological procedures using contrast media, and previous surgery.

FURTHER READING

Kennedy D H & Fallon R J (1979) Tuberculous meningitis. *Journal of the American Medical Association* **241**, 264–268.

Kroll J S & Moxon E R (1987) Acute bacterial meningitis. In: *Infections of the Nervous System*. Edited by P G E Kennedy & R T Johnston. London: Butterworths, pp. 3–22.

Legg N J (1979) Intracerebral abscess. *British Journal of Hospital Medicine* **22**, 608–614.

Quagliarello V J & Scheld W M (1986) Review: recent advances in the pathogenesis and pathophysiology of bacterial meningitis. *American Journal of the Medical Sciences* **292**, 306–309.

Strong A J & Ingham H R (1983) Brain abscess. *British Journal of Hospital Medicine* **30**, 396–403.

7. Virus and other infections

VIRUS INFECTIONS

Although many of the systemic viral illnesses of man are caused by viruses with the capacity of infecting the nervous system, clinically evident virus infections of the CNS are uncommon. Yet it has been clearly established by serological surveys that many individuals possess circulating antibodies to such viruses, e.g. the enteroviruses, without them having had symptoms of an infection of the CNS. It is only in a small proportion of individuals infected with such viruses that the body's intrinsic defence mechanisms are unable to prevent disease of the CNS.

Because of the absence of specific treatment, much early interest in virus diseases of the CNS was inevitably rather academic and experimental. The diagnosis was often established on serological evidence after the acute infection had subsided, or even after the patient had died. The development of antiviral agents against DNA viruses, however, is now bringing viral infections of the nervous system into the category of potentially treatable diseases: there is therefore an ever-increasing awareness of these diseases and of the need – as with bacterial infections – to make the diagnosis as early as possible in the course of the disease. The pathologist can contribute by examining brain biopsies, but the precise diagnosis remains in the realm of the virologist. If there is any clinical evidence suggestive of a virus infection of the CNS, fresh tissue must always be taken at biopsy or autopsy for virological studies, together with specimens of serum and CSF.

Many viruses may affect the nervous system and in diverse ways. The two principal reasons for the diversity of pathological lesions are (i) different cell populations within the CNS vary in susceptibility to viruses, and (ii) viruses can have a variety of effects on cells, e.g. lysis, latency, transformation, fusion with neighbouring cells or simply to modify the antigen composition of the infected cell. A further essential factor is that, to be susceptible to infection by a particular virus, the host cell must have specific receptors on its plasma membrane. For a current classification of viruses the reader is referred to an appropriate reference work, but the requirement for specific receptors largely explains the selective vulnerability of different cell populations within the CNS to virus infection. Some viruses, such as herpes simplex virus, may infect all cell types in the CNS, albeit in selective regions within the brain (see below). Other viruses, such as polio, have a selective effect on motor neurons in the spinal cord and in the brain stem. Varicella zoster virus principally affects neurons in sensory ganglia, and other viruses, such as certain papovaviruses, may selectively affect oligodendrocytes, leading to subsequent demyelination.

Routes of infection

Most viruses gain entry to the body through the mucous membranes of the respiratory or gastro-intestinal tracts. Infection through the skin also occurs but usually via a bite or an abrasion or, accidentally, via a needle. Current evidence suggests that most viruses that affect the CNS replicate at some extraneural site, such as submucosal lymphoid tissue in the intestine, or muscle and subcutaneous tissue where viruses enter through the skin. During this incubation period the development of an effective immune response in the form of circulating antibodies frequently prevents the virus reaching the CNS. For example, in susceptible individuals infected with poliovirus, symptoms of involvement of the CNS develop in only about 1 per cent.

There are various routes by which virus may travel to the CNS but by far the commonest follows a viraemia, when virus passes through the blood–CSF barrier into the subarachnoid space or through the blood–brain barrier to neural tissue. Many viruses can be shown experimentally to travel along nerves, but this probably only occurs naturally with rabies virus, herpes simplex virus and varicella zoster virus. It has also been postulated that viruses may gain access to the CNS via the olfactory bulbs and tracts. Precisely how virus spreads within neural tissue, however, is not clear. It may be by cell to cell spread or along axons.

Types of infection

Viruses induce several types of disease in the nervous system. This may take the form of an *acute infection*, such as aseptic meningitis, acute infective encephalitis or encephalomyelitis. Other viruses cause *subacute infections*, such as subacute sclerosing panencephalitis, which is a persistent infection caused by the measles virus. Yet other agents, referred to as *slow viruses (prions)*, cause the spongiform encephalopathies, such as kuru and Creutzfeldt–Jakob disease.

Viruses that cause acute infections of the CNS have been referred to as *neurotropic* but, as indicated above, it does not follow that any individual infected with such a virus will necessarily develop an overt clinical neurological illness. As with most virus infections in man, many potentially neurotropic viruses produce a mild febrile illness, and immunity to reinfection is acquired without any serious illness at the time of the primary infection. There are, however, exceptions to this rule, since infection with rabies virus will regularly produce infection of the nervous system unless appropriate prophylactic measures are instituted.

As with bacterial infections, viruses usually cause inflammation of the brain and the meninges, i.e. there is a *meningoencephalitis*. Meningitis – usually referred to as aseptic meningitis – or encephalitis usually predominates. Patients with encephalitis, however, usually display some of the clinical features of meningitis. The term *encephalomyelitis* is used when the spinal cord is also involved, and *polioencephalitis* when the infection predominantly affects grey matter.

Abnormalities in the CSF

These tend to be consistent in acute viral infections of the CNS. The pressure may be slightly raised and the CSF usually appears normal macroscopically. The cell count varies from some 50 to 500 nucleated cells/mm^3. In the very early stages, particularly in acute poliomyelitis, some of the nucleated cells are neutrophil polymorphs but more frequently the cells are lymphocytes and monocytes, with a varying proportion of plasma cells. Lymphoplasmacytic cells with a rather primitive appearance are often seen in patients with acute herpes simplex encephalitis, and occasional mitotic figures are often identifiable. The protein is slightly raised. Glucose and chloride are characteristically normal.

ASEPTIC MENINGITIS

This is usually not a severe illness but it is a common acute infection of the CNS, particularly in children. It is most frequently caused by one of the many enteroviruses, including poliovirus, Coxsackie viruses and Echo viruses. Such infections are most commonly seen in early summer. The second common cause is mumps virus, particularly early in the year.

Since aseptic meningitis is rarely fatal, little is known about its pathology. There are no specific macroscopic abnormalities, and histological findings are restricted to infiltration of the subarachnoid space by lymphocytes, plasma cells and macrophages. There may be mild cuffing of blood vessels by similar cells in the superficial layers of the cortex.

ACUTE VIRUS ENCEPHALITIS

In a patient who dies in the acute phase of a viral encephalitis, the brain and spinal cord may appear normal since any localized brain swelling or early necrosis may be very difficult to recognize, even if the brain has been properly fixed prior to dissection. If the patient survives for some time, however, any areas of necrosis will become apparent as the tissue disintegrates and is removed by phagocytic activity.

There are, however, several characteristic and rather stereotyped histological abnormalities, since the inflammatory reaction of the brain tends to be similar in all types of virus encephalitis. The intensity and distribution of these abnormalities, however, as will be seen in the accounts that follow, vary with the type of virus causing the encephalitis and the pathologist may, on occasion be able to shed some light on the nature of the causal agent.

The general features of virus encephalitis

Infiltration by inflammatory cells

This is usually the most obvious histological abnormality, lymphocytes, plasma cells and cells

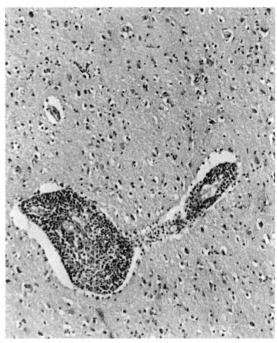

Fig. 7.2 Virus encephalitis. Blood vessels in the brain are cuffed by inflammatory cells. (H & E.)

of monocytic type characteristically occurring in the perivascular spaces ('perivascular cuffing') and in the subarachnoid space (Figs 7.1 and 7.2). There may also be a few neutrophil polymorphs in the early stages. Lymphocytes and plasma cells may, however, extend from perivascular spaces into brain tissue, particularly in regions where necrosis has occurred (Fig. 7.3).

Hyperplasia and proliferation of microglia

This is an almost constant feature throughout the grey matter and takes two forms: diffuse hyperplasia of microglia with the formation of rod cells (Fig. 7.4), and small clusters of microglia. Where necrosis has occurred, there are numerous lipid-containing macrophages.

Reactive changes in astrocytes

In the acute stage of the disease, changes in astrocytes are usually restricted to areas of tissue destruction, where reactive astrocytes become conspicuous. If the patient survives the acute

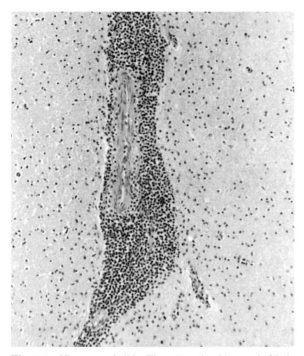

Fig. 7.1 Virus encephalitis. The subarachnoid space is filled with inflammatory cells. (H & E.)

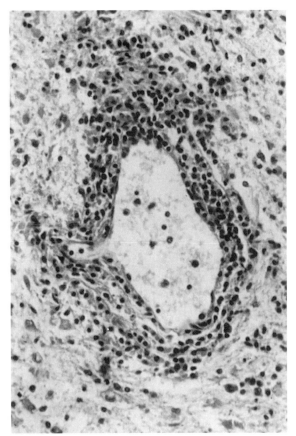

Fig. 7.3 Virus encephalitis. Lymphocytes and plasma cells are extending out from a perivascular space into the adjacent brain tissue. (H & E.)

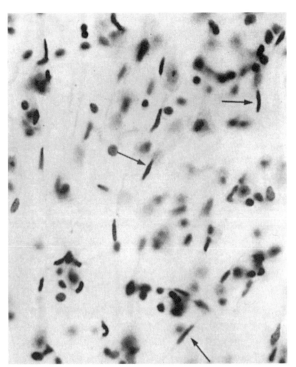

Fig. 7.4 Virus encephalitis. There are numerous rod cells (arrows). (Cresyl violet.)

stage, there is then a progressive fibrillary gliosis in the affected regions. In subacute encephalitis, hyperplasia of astrocytes and microglia leads to a widespread gliosis.

Abnormalities in neurons

Central chromatolysis, necrosis and neuronophagia (see Fig. 3.14) are frequently present. Various non-specific changes, such as some loss of Nissl granules, swelling of the perikaryon and pallor of staining of the cytoplasm, have been described in the past, but such changes must be interpreted with caution because of the possibility that they are not directly related to the viral infection but to terminal disturbances in the cerebral circulation or to autolysis.

Inclusion bodies

Various forms of inclusion body may be found in neurons, astrocytes and oligodendroglia. In light microscopic preparations they appear as round or oval, usually eosinophilic, bodies (Fig. 7.5). The larger type A inclusions are seen in several types of encephalitis, including those due to herpes simplex virus, B virus and cytomegalovirus, and in subacute sclerosing panencephalitis. The smaller type B intranuclear inclusion bodies may be seen in poliomyelitis. They are, however, not always present. Probably the only inclusion body that is pathognomonic of a specific infection is the intracytoplasmic *Negri body* of rabies (see below).

Necrosis

This may range from selective neuronal necrosis, as in poliomyelitis, to frank infarction of grey and white matter, as in herpes simplex virus encephalitis. Where the necrosis is an integral part of

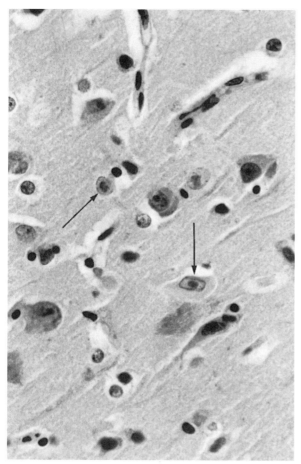

a

b

Fig. 7.5 Virus encephalitis. (a) Intranuclear inclusion bodies (arrows) are present. (b) Intranuclear herpes simplex virus particles in a similar area. ((a) H & E. (b) Bar = 0.1 μm)

the encephalitis, the histological features are those of infarction combined with those of inflammation, as shown by the admixture of lymphocytes, plasma cells and lipid-containing macrophages. This type of necrosis has to be distinguished from terminal changes attributable to hypoxia (see Ch. 3), such as selective neuronal necrosis in susceptible parts of the brain, e.g. the hippocampus or the thalamus, or selective necrosis of Purkinje cells.

INFECTIONS WITH HERPESVIRUSES

Herpesviruses are ubiquitous in both human and animal populations. The human herpesviruses that affect the nervous system are herpes simplex virus (HSV), varicella zoster (VZ), cytomegalovirus (CMV) and Epstein–Barr (EB) virus. B virus of monkeys may also affect the CNS in man. All exhibit the property of remaining latent within the body after primary infection. Latent virus persists for many years – probably throughout life – and in some patients reactivates to cause secondary or recurrent infections.

Herpes simplex virus

There are two types of herpes simplex virus, type 1 (HSV-1) and type 2 (HSV-2). Primary infections are often symptomless but HSV-1 may produce an acute gingivostomatitis. After the primary infection both HSV-1 and HSV-2 become latent in sensory ganglia. When it is reactivated, the virus spreads centrifugally along sensory nerves to the skin and mucous membranes where it is shed and may cause lesions in areas supplied by these nerves, the commonest being the familiar cold sore around the mouth caused by HSV-1. The more important of the viruses with regard to infection of the CNS is HSV-1, but HSV-2 may cause encephalitis in the neonatal period as a result of infection of the fetus during birth, and in immunocompromised individuals.

Infection with HSV-1

This virus affects the CNS in one of three ways, the most important of which is an *acute necrotizing encephalitis* which is the commonest virus encephalitis in western Europe and the commonest non-epidemic viral encephalitis encountered in the USA. Other diseases produced by HSV-1 are an aseptic meningitis, which is a benign and self-limiting infection, and a fulminating disseminated infection that may occur in infants and in immunocompromised individuals.

HSV-1 encephalitis

This is an acute fulminating disease that may occur in any age group, with the exception of infants and young children. In a series of cases encountered in Glasgow, the mortality was 70 per cent, and only some 12 per cent of the patients recovered sufficiently to pursue an independent existence. Fortunately, effective treatment with acyclovir for HSV encephalitis has become available in the last 10 years. Treatment with this agent reduces mortality in the acute stage to about 20 per cent, and serious residual morbidity in the survivors at 1 year to 20 per cent. Considerable controversy exists as to whether the encephalitis is part of a primary infection or is due to reactivation of latent virus because only about a quarter of patients have a history of recurrent cold sores. Another possibility is reactivation of latent virus already in the brain that has gained access via the olfactory tracts or the trigeminal ganglia.

Pathology

This has a highly characteristic pattern, the distinctive feature being widespread and asymmetrical necrosis in the temporal lobes, in the insulae and in the cingulate gyri. In the more severely affected hemisphere there is usually necrosis of all of the temporal gyri, this often being continuous with necrosis in the insula and in the posterior orbital gyri. In the less severely affected hemisphere, necrosis in the temporal lobe tends to be restricted to the parahippocampal and medial temporo-occipital (fusiform) gyri, and there is rarely necrosis in the posterior orbital gyri. The necrosis is not restricted to the cortex, particularly in the more severely affected hemisphere where it spreads to involve the adjacent white matter, the hippocampus, the amygdaloid nucleus and the inferior pole of the putamen (Fig. 7.6).

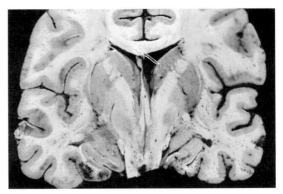

Fig. 7.6 Herpes simplex virus encephalitis. The left temporal lobe is swollen and focally haemorrhagic. Only minor abnormalities are seen in the inferomedial part of the right temporal lobe.

In a patient dying in the acute phase, the more severely affected temporal lobe is soft and swollen, and the swelling is often sufficient to produce a shift of the midline structures and a tentorial hernia. The necrotic tissue may be focally haemorrhagic but, on occasion, it is pale when the necrosis is often not immediately apparent macroscopically, although the affected tissue is softer than normal. If the patient survives the acute stage, the necrotic tissue in the temporal lobes, the insulae and the cingulate gyri characteristically becomes shrunken and cystic (Fig. 7.7).

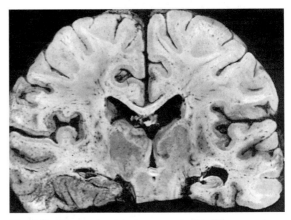

Fig. 7.7 Herpes simplex virus encephalitis. The necrotic tissue in the left temporal lobe and in and adjacent to the left insula is disintegrating. There is only minimal damage in the corresponding parts of the right temporal lobe.

Despite the selective distribution of the necrosis, histological examination of the brain of a patient who has died early in the course of the disease discloses a diffuse meningoencephalitis, as shown by the presence of lymphocytes and plasma cells throughout the subarachnoid space, perivascular cuffing by similar cells in all parts of the CNS, generalized microglial hyperplasia and examples of neuronophagia. In the temporal lobes, in the insulae and in the cingulate gyri there is necrosis in addition to particularly intense inflammatory changes, plasma cells and lymphocytes extending into the brain tissue from the perivascular spaces. Intranuclear inclusion bodies (Fig. 7.5a) may be found within neurons and astrocytes, particularly adjacent to areas of necrosis. In our experience, however, inclusion bodies can only be identified in the minority of cases. Virus particles can usually be identified on electron microscopy, but this is often a time-consuming exercise (Fig. 7.5b). If the patient survives for a week or so, lipid-containing macrophages and reactive astrocytes become numerous in the areas of necrosis.

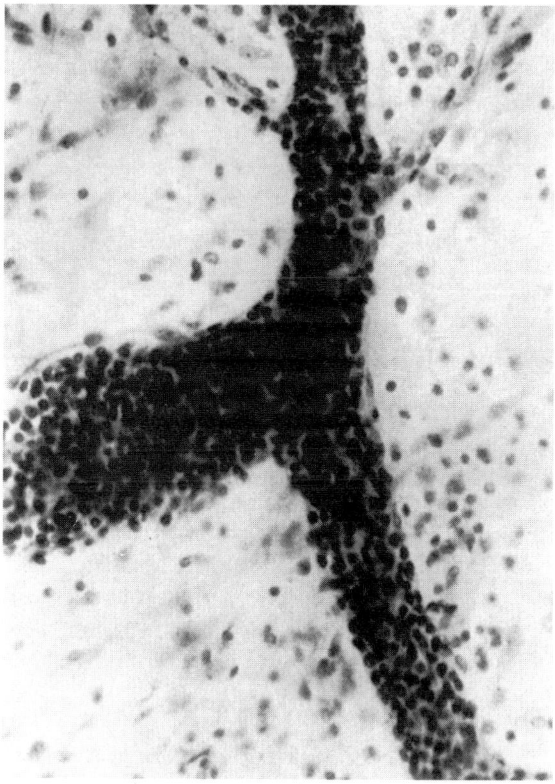

The development of appropriate antiviral agents has made the early diagnosis of HSV-1 encephalitis a matter of some urgency. This can be achieved by a biopsy of the more severely affected temporal lobe: in smears and frozen sections there is perivascular cuffing with lymphocytes and plasma cells, hypertrophied microglia and possibly also the presence of lipid phagocytes (Fig. 7.8), but since very similar appearances may be seen adjacent to a brain abscess, the final diagnosis depends on virological examination. This can be most rapidly established by the immunofluorescent identification of HSV antigen in the tissue. Virus can usually also be isolated from the biopsy, but rarely, if ever, from CSF.

Latency

By immunofluorescence, electron microscopy and autoradiography it has been shown that HSV is latent in the neurons of sensory ganglia. The mechanisms of latency are not fully understood but they involve processes of initiation and maintenance of the latent state, and virus reactivation. Prior viral DNA replication is probably not required for the initiation of latency, and recently a latency-associated HSV RNA transcript (LAT) has been described which may play a role in the control of HSV latency, although such transcripts may have a role in virus reactivation. Immunological mechanisms do play a role in HSV latency, but are much less important than in varicella zoster virus latency.

Varicella zoster (VZ) virus

Primary infection with VZ virus produces varicella (chicken pox). During the period of the cutaneous eruption it is assumed that virus travels centripetally along sensory nerves, where it remains latent in sensory cranial ganglia and posterior root ganglia. When the virus reactivates it produces an acute necrotizing inflammatory response in the affected ganglion and travels down the nerve causing neuritis and, when it reaches

Fig. 7.8 Herpes simplex virus encephalitis. Cuffing of a blood vessel by inflammatory cells in a smear from a brain biopsy. (Toluidine blue.)

the skin, a characteristic vesicular rash. In its commonest form zoster occurs in a dermatome supplied by one posterior root ganglion, most often in the thoracic region. Sometimes more than one dermatome is involved and occasionally involvement may be bilateral. The second commonest nerve involved is the ophthalmic division of the trigeminal nerve, but other branches of the trigeminal nerve may be affected. Cervical and lumbar dermatomes may also be affected. Recurrent zoster is not infrequent, particularly in elderly patients, and post-herpetic neuralgia is a well recognized and distressing sequel. What produces reactivation of the virus is not known, but in a small proportion of cases some precipitating factor, such as physical trauma to the affected region, has been identified. Immunological disturbances may also be involved since zoster is common in patients with malignant lymphoma. In patients undergoing treatment with cytotoxic drugs and corticosteroids, and in immunocompromised individuals, zoster may become disseminated and lead to a generalized varicelliform rash and a fatal multifocal necrotizing encephalomyelitis.

In about 5 per cent of patients with zoster there is also involvement of the corresponding motor nerve. Motor weakness usually develops within 2 weeks of the onset of the rash. Zoster is infectious in that adults with zoster may infect susceptible children, with varicella resulting. Molecular techniques have now confirmed that varicella zoster virus isolates from the same individual with varicella and subsequent herpes zoster are identical.

Pathology

In the acute stage the affected ganglion is swollen and congested, and may be haemorrhagic. On microscopic examination there is intense lymphocytic infiltration, both within and around the ganglion (Fig. 7.9) and in the nerve root. There is usually necrosis of individual neurons and occasionally extensive necrosis throughout the ganglion. The inflammatory process often extends into the posterior nerve root and the ipsilateral dorsal quadrant of the spinal cord, where vessels are cuffed with lymphocytes and plasma cells,

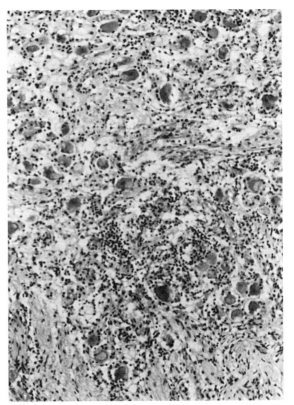

Fig. 7.9 Herpes zoster. There are acute inflammatory changes in this posterior root ganglion. (H & E.)

and there may be a mild lymphoplasmacytic infiltrate in the adjacent subarachnoid space. As the inflammatory reaction diminishes, fibrosis occurs within the ganglion. The death of neurons leads to Wallerian-type degeneration in nerve fibres in the peripheral nerve and in the ascending columns of the spinal cord. In cases of trigeminal zoster infection, the pathological changes in the ganglia are similar to those described in spinal ganglia. The brain stem may also be involved, as may the spinal cord. Arteritis occasionally develops and may lead to infarction. The skin lesions of zoster are identical to those of varicella.

Cytomegalovirus (CMV)

Generalized infection by cytomegalovirus is almost restricted to neonates, the fetus having been infected during a maternal viraemia. In these cases there is hepatosplenomegaly, jaundice, anaemia and thrombocytopenia: death may follow quickly. In 10 per cent of cases there is involvement of the CNS, with mental retardation, deafness and microcephaly. Pathologically there is destruction of the ependyma, focal necrosis of grey and white matter with glial nodule formation and calcification. Cytomegalovirus inclusions measuring up to 15 μm may be seen.

Primary infection with CMV is usually asymptomatic in an otherwise healthy individual, but in adults it may present as a 'glandular fever' type syndrome. In can also be a serious disease in immunocompromised individuals. Infection with CMV is widespread and, where socioeconomic conditions are poor, some 80 per cent of children have antibodies by the age of 4 years. In more affluent societies only 30–40 per cent of preschool children have demonstrable antibodies. Infection of the fetus by CMV secondary to primary infection of the mother, or resulting from reactivation of latent virus, is a significant cause of congenital abnormalities in the CNS (see Ch. 13).

Epstein–Barr (EB) virus

This virus is the major cause of infectious mononucleosis. Neurological complications have an incidence of about 1–5 per cent. Aseptic meningitis has been described and may be due to direct invasion by virus, but the other neurological complications of this infection, such as the Guillain–Barré syndrome, Bell's palsy and transverse myelitis, are delayed immunological responses rather than direct effects of the virus.

Herpesvirus simiae

Often referred to as B virus, this is a natural infection of monkeys and in them behaves in a manner very similar to HSV in man. The virus may be transmitted to man by a monkey bite or by the contamination of a skin wound by saliva or tissues from an infected animal. In man the clinical signs take the form of an encephalitis which is usually rapidly progressive, leading to paralysis of cranial nerves and the respiratory muscles, coma and death within a few days to 3 weeks. The essential pathological feature is a multifocal necrotizing encephalitis affecting grey and white matter, sometimes with a particular predilection for the spinal cord.

INFECTIONS WITH ENTEROVIRUSES

The enteroviruses are a large family of RNA viruses, the most important of which are the polioviruses, the Coxsackie viruses and the Echo viruses. They cause 30–50 per cent of all cases of viral meningitis and most cases of paralytic poliomyelitis. The latter is classically associated with the polioviruses, but is occasionally caused by other enteroviruses. – Coxsackie viruses A4, A7 and B3, Echo viruses 2 and 9, and enterovirus 71.

Enterovirus infections are usually contracted by ingestion of the virus, which then multiplies in the pharynx and in the cells lining the gastrointestinal tract. Within a few days virus is present in adjacent lymphoid tissue and, if the antibody response is inadequate, reaches the CNS via the bloodstream. Faecal excretion of virus continues long after the acute infection.

Acute anterior poliomyelitis

This form of acute encephalomyelitis has a worldwide distribution and, in its classic overt clinical form, is associated with paralysis caused by involvement of the motor neurons in the ventral horns of the spinal cord and in the motor nuclei in the brain stem. There are three types of poliovirus (types 1, 2 and 3); immunity to one type does not protect against the others, but most cases of paralytic poliomyelitis in susceptible populations are caused by type 1 virus. Prior to the introduction of successful immunization programmes, poliomyelitis was probably the commonest acute encephalomyelitis caused by a neurotropic virus; the disease occurred sporadically and also in minor and major epidemics. It also had a seasonal incidence, being particularly common in the late summer months. No intermediate host or significant reservoir has been identified and it is generally accepted that the virus spreads directly or indirectly from individual to individual. The spread of the virus is greatly facilitated by the fact that it may be excreted in the faeces for 2 or 3 months by infected individuals, even if they have not suffered any apparent clinical illness.

Where poliomyelitis was endemic it was a disease that primarily affected young children, hence the term '*infantile paralysis*'. The infectivity rate of poliovirus appeared to be high, but most of those infected developed either no symptoms or only a mild febrile illness, with or without clinical aseptic meningitis. In an infected individual the development of paralysis was influenced by several factors, such as excessive muscular exertion, especially swimming, and by local trauma including tonsillectomy and the intramuscular injection of immunizing agents, especially those containing alum. In countries where higher standards of hygiene had been achieved, primary infection in childhood became less common and individuals tended not to encounter the virus for the first time until they had reached adult life. A particularly unfortunate aspect of this change was that paralytic disease occurs more commonly in adults than in children.

It has been shown experimentally that poliovirus can travel along peripheral nerves, but it is generally accepted that, as in all enterovirus infections, the principal if not the only route by which virus reaches the CNS in natural infections is by the bloodstream. Thus, in chimpanzees fed with virulent poliovirus, the virus multiplies primarily in the mucosa of the throat and ileum and can be isolated from faeces and throat secretions within a few days, i.e. 1–2 weeks before the onset of paralysis. The virus then spreads to regional lymph nodes and, after a further few days, there is a period of viraemia. The virus then multiplies in the CNS, where there is a sharp rise in viral concentration on the day prior to the appearance of paralysis.

Pathology

The virus selectively attacks motor neurons in the ventral horns of the spinal cord, particularly in the lumbar and cervical enlargements, where the medially situated neurons tend to be more severely affected than those in the lateral parts of the ventral horns. The motor nuclei in the brain stem are also often affected – '*bulbar polio*' – when there may be early involvement of the respiratory centre. In a patient dying in the acute stage of the disease, the CNS is often of normal appearance macroscopically. In particularly florid cases, however, there may be foci of haemorrhage in the ventral horns in the spinal cord and in the motor nuclei in the brain stem.

Microscopical examination discloses the typical features of a generalized acute viral encephalitis, with selectively severe involvement of the spinal cord. The most severely involved levels are usually the cervical and lumbar enlargements: the most severe changes are in more medially placed cell groups. Thus there are numerous lymphocytes, plasma cells and macrophages in the subarachnoid space and around small blood vessels within the spinal cord. Neuronophagia (see Fig. 3.14) is conspicuous in the affected nuclei and central chromatolysis is often seen in neurons that have not been destroyed. Elsewhere in the cerebral hemispheres there are varying degrees of perivascular cuffing, and inflammatory changes in the meninges. In some cases central chromatolysis has been observed in the Betz cells of the motor cortex. In cases of bulbar poliomyelitis there are dense cellular infiltrations in relation to motor cranial nerve roots and in the reticular formation. Sensory neurons remain unaffected.

With time, the inflammatory changes subside and at least some of the paralysis may improve. This is not due to regeneration but to recovery of function in neurons that have been only transiently affected by the inflammatory process.

In patients with residual paralysis who die long after the acute stage of the disease, the most striking structural abnormality is atrophy of the ventral horns of the spinal cord. There is loss of neurons in the affected segments (this is often asymmetrical) and there is a fibrillary gliosis. There is also atrophy of the corresponding ventral nerve roots and their motor units, with the result that there are varying degrees of neurogenic atrophy (see Ch. 17) in the affected muscles. If only a few neurons have been destroyed, there will be occasional clearly defined groups of small denervated fibres within the muscle. If there has been severe involvement of the nerve supply to the muscle, it becomes atrophied and fatty. On histological examination there are denervation changes in the great majority of the muscle fibres and a considerable increase in interstitial fat. Muscle spindles, however, are retained.

INFECTIONS WITH ARBOVIRUSES

There is a large number of arboviruses. They are transmitted from host to host by blood-sucking insects (arthropod-borne) and they are all RNA viruses. They give rise to a wide variety of diseases including several named types of encephalitis. An arthropod vector is infected by ingesting blood from a vertebrate reservoir and, after an incubation period, the virus reaches the salivary glands of the arthropod. The virus is then introduced by a bite from the insect into a new host and, after an interval during which viral proliferation occurs, there is a period of viraemia during which a further arthropod may become infected. Arbovirus infections tend to have a seasonal occurrence as climatic factors exert some influence in maintaining the cycle by directly affecting both vectors and hosts. This is probably contributed to by the migration of the natural hosts, usually wild birds. As with other forms of virus encephalitis, only a proportion of individuals infected develop clinical evidence of encephalitis.

Mosquito-borne arbovirus encephalitis

These include St Louis encephalitis, Eastern and Western equine encephalomyelitis and Japanese B encephalitis. The primary reservoir of the arboviruses producing these diseases is probably wild birds. The precise diagnosis can only be made as a result of virological studies.

In the great majority of patients dying in the acute stages, the brain may appear macroscopically normal but there may be some congestion and swelling and, in the Western type of equine encephalomyelitis, there may be frank necrosis, particularly in the white matter and in the basal ganglia. Histological studies show the features of an acute disseminated encephalitis.

Tick-borne arbovirus encephalitis

These viruses are responsible for Russian (Far Eastern) spring–summer encephalitis, Central European encephalitis and louping-ill encephalitis. The natural virus cycle is maintained between ticks and various warm-blooded mammals. The clinical features of the various types of infection range from aseptic meningitis to a frank fulminating encephalitis. Occasionally, some of these diseases may be very similar to poliomyelitis.

The brain often appears normal macroscopically but there may be some congestion and petechial haemorrhages, particularly in the brain stem. Microscopical abnormalities tend to be confined to the precentral cortex, the basal ganglia, the brain stem, the cerebellum and the spinal cord, where there may be neuronal necrosis, neuronophagia, perivascular cuffing with lymphocytes and plasma cells and, occasionally, a necrotizing vasculitis.

RABIES

Rabies, a disease feared in many countries for centuries, is still a major problem in some parts of the world, particularly central and eastern Europe, India and in some parts of North and South America. Its incidence in western Europe is increasing. The great majority of human cases can be traced to the bite of an infected animal, especially the dog. The virus (a rhabdovirus) enters the body via the saliva contaminating the bite and reaches the CNS by travelling along peripheral nerves. The major reservoirs of the virus are the fox, the skunk and the jackal. Vampire bats seem to be important in maintaining the virus in some regions.

The incubation period of the disease varies greatly, its duration being related to the distance of the bite from the CNS. Sometimes it is as short as 2 weeks but, more commonly, it is 1–3 months or even longer. The disease may assume a *restless* type, corresponding to the furious rabies of dogs, or a *paralytic* type. As the old name, hydrophobia, implies, spasm of the muscles of deglutition on attempting to drink water may be the first, or at least a prominent and early, symptom. There may be some paraesthesiae in the neighbourhood of the wound, but once the disease is established there is a most extraordinary sensitivity of the CNS to external stimuli. The lightest touch is painful and any trivial movement may precipitate wide-ranging motor responses which may progress to violent convulsions.

Experimental studies have shown that following intramuscular injection, rabies virus replicates in muscle cells and spreads via neuromuscular and neurotendinal spindles along axons to sensory ganglia and spinal cord. Neurectomy prevents the spread of infection from the periphery to the brain.

Pathology

In a fatal case the brain may appear normal macroscopically, or perhaps slightly congested. Microscopical examination shows the features of a virus encephalitis predominantly affecting grey matter i.e. a polioencephalitis. In addition to perivascular cuffing by lymphocytes, plasma cells and macrophages, there is widespread microglial hyperplasia and neuronophagia. The pathognomonic histological feature of rabies, however, is the *Negri body*. They are seen only after infection by 'street virus' and do not occur after the virus has become 'fixed' by laboratory passage. They are not found in every case but appear as sharply defined, rounded or oval acidophilic intracytoplasmic inclusions varying in size from 1 μm to 7 μm across. They may lie anywhere in the cytoplasm of the cell body or its dendrites, and two or more may be seen in one cell. The largest Negri bodies tend to occur in the pyramidal cells of the hippocampus, in the adjacent temporal cortex and in Purkinje cells. Virus can be identified within the Negri body using immunofluorescent techniques or electron microscopy. However, the virus is not restricted to Negri bodies and occurs widely in various cell types throughout the CNS. Clusters of microglia tend to be particularly conspicuous in rabies, and they have in the past been referred to as Babe's nodules; they are not, however, lesions specific to rabies.

In the rare paralytic form of rabies there is selectively severe involvement of the spinal cord, particularly its lower thoracic and lumbar regions.

ENCEPHALITIS LETHARGICA

This remains one of the fascinating enigmas of the 20th century. The fact that it was the first pandemic encephalitis in modern times, and its sudden appearance, rapid spread and subsequent disappearance, are not the least of its mysterious features, since its cause was never established. It is, however, generally accepted that it was a virus encephalitis, possibly caused by influenza A virus. A small epidemic of encephalitis with a high mortality occurred in Vienna in the winter of 1916–1917. The disease then spread to western Europe and to the UK, and towards the end of 1918 it spread to North America. The epidemic reached its peak in Britain in 1924. Thereafter it became less common and very few cases have been known to occur in Britain since 1926. Most cases occurred during the months of winter and early spring.

The disease was protean in its clinical manifestations but in many cases was characterized by a peculiar somnolent state from which the patient could be wakened easily and completely so as to answer questions rationally, but then would quickly relapse again into sleep.

Pathology

In patients dying in the acute stage, the features were those of an acute virus encephalitis, as shown by perivascular cuffing by lymphocytes and plasma cells. There was also widespread microglial hyperplasia and infiltration of the meninges by lymphocytes and plasma cells. Neuronal necrosis was not a feature of the disease but there was sometimes thrombosis of small blood vessels in the brain.

There was a high incidence of personality disorders and parkinsonism in patients who survived the acute disease. The structural abnormalities had some features in common with those that occur in idiopathic parkinsonism (see Ch. 12).

PERSISTENT VIRUS INFECTIONS

The two infections of the CNS which can most appropriately be classified as persistent infections are subacute sclerosing panencephalitis and progressive multifocal leukoencephalopathy.

Subacute sclerosing panencephalitis

First described as subacute inclusion body encephalitis, and later as subacute sclerosing leuko-encephalitis, subacute sclerosing panencephalitis (SSPE) is a persistent virus infection of the nervous system caused by the measles virus. It is a rare disease, affects young people between the ages of 4 and 20 years of age, and is usually fatal within 6 months of onset. Clinically it is characterized by the insidious onset of behavioural changes, myoclonus, mental deterioration, ataxia and seizures. It occurs some years after an apparently uncomplicated attack of measles, but its pathogenesis is not completely understood. It appears, however, that there is a replication of measles virus which has remained in the brain since the time of the primary infection. There are high levels of both IgM and IgG classes of antibody to measles virus in the blood and CSF. Antibody levels in the CSF are higher than in the serum and on immunoelectrophoresis of the CSF they separate into distinct oligoclonal bands, indicating that there are antibody-producing plasma cells derived from a small number of B lymphocyte clones synthesizing immunoglobulins in the CNS. In a considerable proportion of patients the original measles infection has occurred unusually early in life. This has led to the idea that the existence of some degree of persisting passive immunity inhibits the development of full active immunity. This is apparently sufficient to protect the individual from a second attack of clinical measles but not sufficient to prevent the persistence of measles virus genomic material in certain cells, particularly in the brain.

The first stage of the disease is characterized by personality changes and intellectual deterioration. The second is by periodic involuntary movements that tend to occur at regular intervals, often once every 5–10 seconds. A characteristic EEG occurs in the second stage in a large proportion of cases, there being periodic successions of high-voltage complexes which are usually synchronous with the involuntary movements. Some patients experience repeated grand mal convulsions. The third and final stage is characterized by a progressive profound dementia and decerebration. There is some increase in protein and cells (lymphocytes, plasma cells and monocytes) in the CSF.

There are two main theories of pathogenesis. The first is that particular strains of measles virus cause SSPE, and the second is that there is a defective immune response, in which patients fail to produce antibody to the virus protein M necessary for the release of free virus, most probably because M antigen is not produced.

Pathology

The brain may appear normal externally but it is usually of increased consistency. If the disease has run a protracted course there may be some generalized cerebral atrophy, but in many cases hypoxic brain damage consequent on convulsions is superimposed on the pathology of SSPE, which is basically that of a subacute encephalitis. Thus, inflammatory changes predominate in cases in which the disease has progressed rapidly. The subarachnoid space and perivascular spaces in grey and white matter are infiltrated, often heavily, with lymphocytes and plasma cells. Neuronophagia is common. Type A intranuclear inclusion bodies (Fig. 7.10) are frequently seen in neurons, but they occur also in oligodendroglia. Confirmation of the diagnosis can be achieved by the application of the immunoperoxidase technique using a measles antiserum, or by electron microscopy.

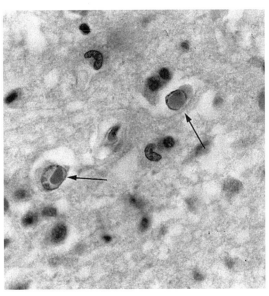

Fig. 7.10 Subacute sclerosing panencephalitis. Large intranuclear inclusion bodies (arrows) are present. (H & E.)

In cases that have pursued a longer course, there is a conspicuous and generalized fibrillary astrocytosis in the white matter, which is the cause of the increased consistency. Even when gliosis is well established in the white matter myelin is usually well preserved, but there may on occasion be some diffuse loss of myelin.

Other types of brain damage reported include loss of neurons from the hippocampus and thalamus, and long-standing hypoxic damage in the cortex, and should be attributed to the convulsions and not to the encephalitis.

Another type of infection caused by measles virus is *measles inclusion body encephalitis* which occurs in immunosuppressed individuals, particularly in children being treated for acute leukaemia. There may be little or no inflammatory response in the brain but eosinophilic intranuclear inclusions are widespread.

Progressive rubella panencephalitis

Usually a late sequel to congenital rubella, this disease is similar to SSPE. It is uncommon and pathologically there is widespread neuronal loss, perivascular infiltration by lymphocytes, vasculitis and focal calcification. Inclusion bodies are not found.

Progressive multifocal leukoencephalopathy (PML)

Since this disease was established as a clearly defined entity in the late 1950s, a great many cases have been reported from all parts of the world. It is a relentlessly, and usually rapidly, progressive disease characterized by multiple foci of demyelination in the brain, associated with which there are several highly characteristic cytological changes.

The disease is caused by a virus belonging to the polyomavirus subgroup of papovaviruses (usually JC virus) and occurs in middle-aged patients with some immunological deficiency. Thus, nearly all of the early cases reported were suffering from some pre-existing malignant lymphoproliferative disease. PML has also been associated with other diseases which involve the lympho-reticular system, such as miliary tuberculosis, widespread sarcoidosis, carcinomatosis, AIDS and leukaemia. It can also occur in patients who are receiving immunosuppressive therapy.

The precise relationship between the papovavirus and PML has not been completely established, but it is possible that the virus frequently produces a latent infection in man and when some other factor is superimposed that causes an immunological deficiency, the virus is activated and attacks the brain. Infection with JC virus is widespread, surveys showing antibodies in about 30 per cent of 10-year-old children rising to 80 per cent later.

Pathology

The most characteristic macroscopic feature is the presence of multiple small grey foci distributed widely but usually asymmetrically through the brain, mainly in white matter but also in the basal ganglia. These foci can coalesce to form large grey areas, which may become frankly cystic (Fig. 7.11).

Histological examination shows multiple foci of demyelination (Fig. 7.12) associated with which there are lipid-containing macrophages, abnormal oligodendrocytes and large bizarre astrocytes (Fig. 7.13). The abnormal oligodendroglia have a particularly characteristic appearance (Fig. 7.14): their nuclei are larger than normal, hyperchromatic and devoid of a normal chromatin pattern; some contain ill-defined intranuclear inclusions of varying density. These oligodendrocytes are particularly numerous at the periphery of the foci of demyelination and in the immediately adjacent brain. Within the smaller foci of

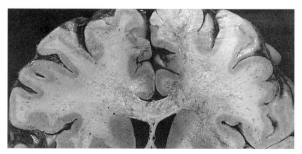

Fig. 7.11 Progressive multifocal leukoencephalopathy. There is multifocal degeneration of deep white matter, including the corpus callosum.

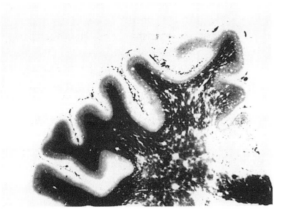

Fig. 7.12 Progressive multifocal leukoencephalopathy. Numerous small foci of demyelination are present in addition to a larger area. (Celloidin section; Heidenhain for myelin.)

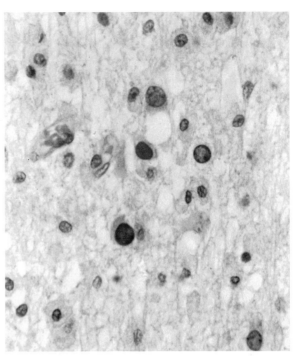

Fig. 7.14 Progressive multifocal leukoencephalopathy. Oligodendroglial nuclei are enlarged and hyperchromatic, and contain ill-defined inclusions. (H & E.)

demyelination there is relative sparing of axons, but in the larger lesions very few axons remain.

On electron microscopy, pseudocrystalline arrays of virions can be regularly found in the abnormal oligodendrocytes (Fig. 7.15). Virus antigen can

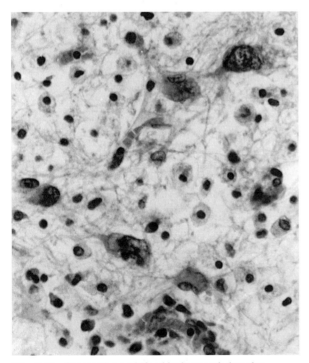

Fig. 7.13 Progressive multifocal leukoencephalopathy. Bizarre astrocytes and lipid-containing macrophages are present in this demyelinated focus. (H & E.)

also be identified with immunofluorescence or immunoperoxidase techniques, or by *in situ* hybridization. Virus has also been cultured.

SLOW VIRUS INFECTIONS (PRION DISEASES)

The association of transmissible agents with progressive non-inflammatory disease of the brain has long been recognized in animals, but in the course of the last 30 years the association has also become recognized in man. The diseases are often referred to as the *spongiform encephalopathies* and include *scrapie, mink encephalopathy* and *bovine spongiform encephalopathy* in animals, and *kuru* and *Creutzfeldt–Jakob* disease in man. Indeed, the discovery and investigation of kuru was one of the most dramatic occurrences in the entire field of diseases of the nervous system.

Unlike the viral encephalitides already described in this chapter, there is no conventional inflammatory response in the CNS.

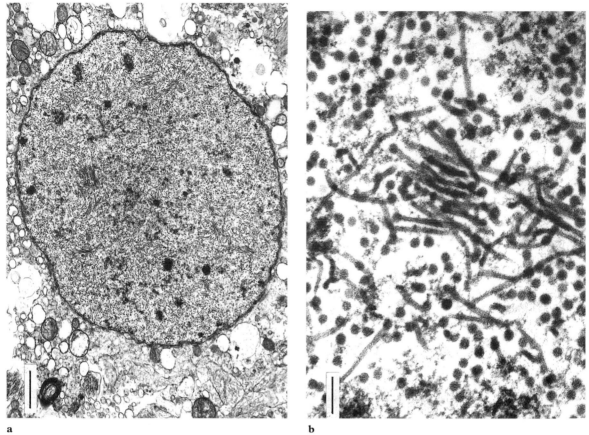

a   b

Fig. 7.15 Progressive multifocal leukoencephalopathy. (a) An oligodendrocyte nucleus showing loss of the normal chromatin pattern. (b) High-power of (a) showing individual polyoma virus particles (40 nm diameter) together with filamentous or rod-shaped structures, probably composed of viral proteins. (Electron micrographs. (a) Bar 10 mm = 1 μm; (b) Bar 10 mm = 0.1 μm.) (a) Reproduced by permission from *Systemic Pathology*, 3rd edn., Vol. 4, *Nervous System, Muscle and Eyes*, edited by R. O. Weller. Edinburgh: Churchill Livingstone, 1990. (b) Courtesy of Professor R. O. Weller, Department of Neuropathology, University of Southampton.)

HUMAN TRANSMISSIBLE SPONGIFORM ENCEPHALOPATHIES

Kuru

This disease has now virtually disappeared, but it occurred in almost epidemic form in the Fore tribe and some of their tribal neighbours in the eastern highlands of New Guinea in the 1950s. It was carefully investigated and reported for the first time in the 1960s. It was a uniformly fatal disease with an average duration of about 1 year, and after a prodromal period characterized by malaise and vague limb pains, affected individuals developed postural instability, ataxia of gait and tremor, i.e. there appeared to be a pro-

gressive subacute cerebellar degeneration. Its pathogenesis remained a mystery until it was suggested that it might be worth seeking some transmissible agent, because kuru had many similarities to naturally occurring and experimental scrapie. Transmission studies were then initiated and the disease was successfully transmitted, first to chimpanzees but now also to several old and new world monkeys and some other smaller mammals. Thus a transmissible agent had been found to be the cause of a naturally occurring progressive, degenerative, non-inflammatory disease of the CNS in man.

It is now generally accepted that the rites of cannibalism were the primary mode of transmission of the agent in kuru, contamination of lesions of the skin with tissue containing the agent being probably more important than ingesting it.

Pathology

The brain may appear macroscopically normal apart from some atrophy of the cerebellum, particularly in the vermis. Histological examination discloses a widespread status spongiosus in grey matter, similar to that seen in Creutzfeldt–Jakob disease (see below), particularly in the limbic system and in the thalamus. Associated with the status spongiosus there is loss of neurons, a great excess of hypertrophied astrocytes and hypertrophied microglial cells, many of which contain lipid. The status spongiosus appears to be due to the enlargement of astrocytic processes. There is often coarse vacuolation of the large neurons in the caudate nucleus and in the putamen. More dramatic histological abnormalities occur in the cerebellum, where there is loss of granule cells and Purkinje cells. Swellings are seen on the axons of many of the surviving Purkinje cells.

A particularly interesting feature is the presence of plaques throughout the brain, mainly in the granule-cell layer of the cerebellum. Each plaque consists of a solid, rather homogeneous core surrounded by a halo of delicate, radially arranged fibrils (see below).

Creutzfeldt–Jakob disease

This is a progressive dementia which runs a subacute or chronic course, most patients dying within 3–12 months of onset. The dementia is frequently accompanied by myoclonus and clinical evidence of cerebellar degeneration. Both sexes are affected equally and the incidence rate is about one per million. About 15 per cent of cases are familial.

Pathology

Because of the rapid progress of the disease, the brain may be of normal appearance macroscopically, but in cases of longer survival there may be evidence of diffuse cerebral atrophy and selectively severe atrophy of the cerebellum. The

classic histological feature is status spongiosus in grey matter, with some predilection for the cingulate gyri, the medial temporal cortex, the thalamus and the molecular layer of the cerebellum. The affected tissue has a spongy appearance brought about by many small, usually rounded or oval, vacuoles in the neuropil (Fig. 7.16). These vacuoles occur in the cell processes of neurons or astrocytes. The smallest vacuoles measure only a few micrometres across but they may coalesce to form larger vacuoles measuring up to 50 μm in diameter. In patients of short survival there may be very little neuronal loss, but it may be conspicuous and widespread in patients of longer survival. Other fairly constant abnormalities are astrocytosis, particularly in the deep grey matter (Fig. 7.17), lipid-containing rod cells in the affected grey matter, axonal swellings on Purkinje cells, large vacuolated neurons in the

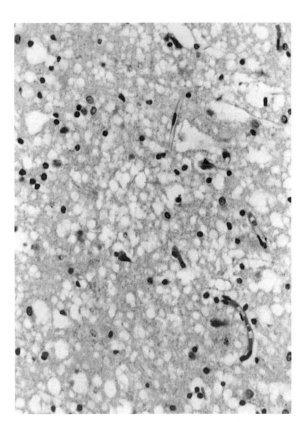

Fig. 7.16 Creutzfeldt–Jakob disease. There are multiple vacuoles within the cerebral cortex: status spongiosus. (H & E.)

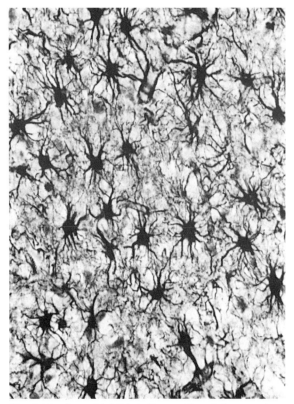

Fig. 7.17 Creutzfeltd–Jakob disease. There is hypertrophy of astrocytes in the putamen. Cajal technique for astrocytes.

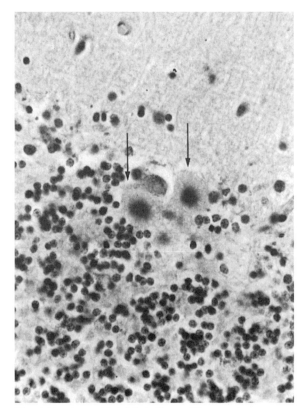

Fig. 7.18 Creutzfeltd–Jakob disease. There are kuru type plaques (arrows) in the cerebellum.

striatum, and a diffuse fibrillary gliosis in white matter. In occasional cases, plaques (Fig. 7.18) identical to those seen in kuru have been described.

Pathogenesis

It has now been clearly established that Creutzfeldt–Jakob disease is caused by an agent similar to that responsible for kuru, that can be transmitted to experimental animals and from man to man. Man to man transmission has occurred as the result of corneal transplants, as a result of electrodes implanted in the brain of a patient with the disease, as a result of the administration of growth hormone extracted from the pituitary gland, and following the use of certain dural grafts. Despite the occurrence of some 'clustering' of cases, it seems unlikely that the disease can be transmitted merely by close contact.

There is no evidence of any increased incidence of the disease in individuals treating, or undertaking post-mortem examinations on, affected patients. If the diagnosis is suspected, however, all involved must be particularly vigilant and take every step to prevent its transmission (see below).

Gerstmann–Sträussler–Scheinker disease

This disease is characterized by cerebellar ataxia, pyramidal signs and dementia. The average age of onset is 40 years and its duration of 5 years is much longer than that of most cases of Creutzfeldt–Jakob disease. The incidence is between 1 and 10 per 100 million. Neuropathologically it is characterized by spongiform change in grey matter and the extensive formation of amyloid plaques, features that are particularly common in the cerebellum. The amyloid does not stain with antibodies against βA4 protein, but does so with antisera raised against prion protein 27–30 (see below). The clinical and pathological features may vary considerably: most cases are familial and appear to be inherited as an autosomal dominant.

Animal-transmissible spongiform encephalopathies

Scrapie

This worldwide disease of sheep affects the CNS of breeding ewes between the ages of 2 and 4 years. Histologically there is vacuolation of neurons in the brain stem, status spongiosus and astrocytosis. There is a complete absence of inflammatory changes. The disease is transmissible, the agent having a number of characteristic features. First, it is transmissible by inoculation, with an incubation period of between 1 and 5 years; secondly, the agent replicates *in vivo*; thirdly, the agent can be recovered in a 410 nm membrane filtrate; and fourthly, the agent is not inactivated by the usual methods of disinfection.

Scrapie can be transmitted (possibly via scrapie-associated fibrils) to both goats and sheep, as well as hamsters. Genetic factors play an important role, the incubation period of experimental scrapie being controlled by a single gene.

Bovine spongiform encephalopathy

The first cases were reported in 1987. In the brains of affected animals there were vacuolation of neuronal processes, principally in the brain stem, astrocytosis and small sparse deposits of amyloid. The disease shows a uniform pattern of CNS involvement, unlike the variability seen with scrapie.

There seems little doubt that cattle in the UK were infected orally by the transmission of the scrapie agent from processed sheep protein. Thus bovine spongiform encephalopathy represents scrapie in cattle. There is no association with breed or sex and it is not a genetic disease. The incubation ranges from 2.5 to 8 years. The onset

of the epidemic in the early 1980s corresponded with substantial changes in the processing of animal foodstuffs.

The disease has been transmitted to mice and the agent appears to cross the species barrier, thereby raising the possibility that it might enter the human food chain.

Other animal-transmissible spongiform encephalopathies

These include *transmissible mink encephalopathy*, an uncommon disease which is thought to be scrapie in mink, and *chronic wasting disease of deer*, which has a scrapie-like pathology in deer and elk.

Prion proteins

The term prion was introduced to describe a proteinacious infectious particle (PrP), first found in scrapie and fundamentally different from conventional viruses. Apparently without nucleic acid, it has been suggested that the protein PrP27–30 alone may cause infection. This protein is found normally on the surface of neurons and is encoded by a single gene localized on the short arm of chromosome 20. PrP27–30 can polymerize into rods which have the electron-microscopical and histochemical features of amyloid: similar rods have now been identified in cases of bovine spongiform encephalopathy and in some human cases of kuru and Creutzfeldt–Jakob disease. A number of isoforms of PrP27–30 have now been isolated and there is increasing evidence that they are responsible for infectivity.

The hypothesis that infection can be propagated by a protein alone is both novel and controversial, although according to the 'nucleoprotein' or 'virion' hypothesis the agent is composed of a small nucleic acid which replicates conventionally, and the PrP coat is then provided by the host cell.

Molecular genetics has revealed a number of mutations associated with inherited human spongiform encephalopathy. For example, mutations include a 144 base-pair insert at PrP codon 53, a substitution of leucine for proline at PrP codon 102, a substitution of valine for alanine at PrP codon 117, and a substitution of lysine for gluta-mate at codon 200.

Safety precautions when dealing with cases of Creutzfeldt–Jakob disease

The nature of the spongiform encephalopathies, their uncertain aetiology and the iatrogenic trans-mission of a few cases has created considerable uncertainty about the safety of carrying out autopsies and handling pathological specimens. However, clear guidelines for *clinical, surgical* and *pathological* practices have now been established.

The brain and other parts of the nervous system are the most infectious, whereas liver, lung and kidneys are less likely to transmit the disease. The causative agent is neither disinfected nor sterilized by heat, formaldehyde, 70 per cent alcohol, UV light or ionizing radiation. Formalin-fixed paraffin-embedded material remains infec-tious: it is now known, however, that treatment with formic acid eliminates the infectious agent completely, while still providing good histological preparation. Autoclaving at 120°C for 60 minutes and the use of 1 per cent hypochlorite containing 10 000 parts per million chlorine are satisfactory for disinfecting instruments and contaminated surfaces. Codes of practice for the handling of this material have been drawn up in departments of neuropathology, and it is strongly recommended that histopathologists who have been requested to undertake autopsies on known or clinically suspected cases of Creutzfeldt–Jakob disease con-tact the nearest such department or, within the UK, the Creutzfeldt–Jakob Disease Surveillance Unit at the Western General Hospital, Edinburgh.

HIV infection of the nervous system and the acquired immunodeficiency syndrome (AIDS)

First recognized in the early 1980s, AIDS has reached epidemic proportions, with major medical, social and economic consequences. Epidemio-logical studies have established that some two-thirds of patients with AIDS are homosexual men, about 20 per cent are intravenous drug abusers, 5 per cent have acquired the infection from a heterosexual activity, a small number have received blood or blood products (after surgery or because of haemophilia), and about 3 per cent are children born to AIDS-infected mothers.

Following a single known exposure, many months may elapse before the subject becomes HIV-positive and an asymptomatic carrier. Many more months or years may elapse before the onset of either the so-called AIDS-related com-plex (ARC) or the lymphadenopathy syndrome (LAS). The clinical features of these syndromes include fatigue, fever, diarrhoea, weight loss, lymphadenopathy, and oral candidiasis. The interval between the appearance of ARC or LAS and full-blown AIDS is again variable, being 3 years in about 11 per cent of cases and 5 years in 30 per cent. The manifestations of disease affecting the nervous system include the development of opportunistic infections, various tumours and the effects of HIV infection upon the CNS itself.

Pathogenesis

The disease is due to a known RNA retrovirus now termed HIV (previously LAV, HTLV-III). The virus produces its main effects on the immune and nervous systems. The effect on the immune system is to induce a progressive and apparently irreversible reduction in the number of CD4 'helper' lymphocytes. These cells possess a membrane receptor to which HIV apparently binds.

Uncertainties about the pathogenesis of HIV *encephalopathy* remain, for example, the mode of entry of the virus into the brain and how it produces its pathogenic effects. Access may be via infected blood monocytes which migrate into the CNS and develop into macrophages and microglia. Apparently, under the influence of HIV gp120 protein multinucleated cells develop which carry the immunohistochemical hallmarks of macrophages. It is not clear how the macrophages and multinucleated cells damage the CNS, but a number of mechanisms have been suggested. For example, there may be a slow release of a low level of infection to other cells, or the induction of various cytokines or the release of neurotransmitter-like substances. Furthermore, the role of other infections on the pathogenesis of AIDS needs to be clarified, particularly Epstein-

Barr virus, hepatitis virus and the herpes viruses, especially as there are aspects of the pathology of AIDS that cannot adequately be explained by the biology of HIV alone.

The diagnosis of HIV infection is made by the identification of specific antibody in serum: there may be a delay of several weeks after exposure before serum conversion develops. Biopsy and autopsy tissues need to be handled with full precautions, as set out in local codes of practice and in recent recommendations.

Pathology of HIV encephalopathy

The brain may appear normal macroscopically, or there may be some atrophy. The most prominent changes histologically are those of diffuse pallor of white matter, focal or diffuse infiltration by macrophages, an astrocytosis, the formation of nodules or clusters of microglia, and vacuolation of white matter. Emphasis has been placed on the presence of relatively small multinucleated giant cells (Fig. 7.19).

Pathology of HIV-associated myelopathy

A small number of patients with AIDS develop a progressive paraparesis, sensory ataxia and incontinence. At autopsy there is a vacuolar myelopathy that affects principally the white matter of the posterior and lateral columns (Fig. 7.20). The appearances are reminiscent of vitamin B_{12} deficiency but serum levels of this vitamin are usually normal. The consensus view is that the pathogenesis of HIV myelopathy is similar to that of HIV encephalopathy.

Other pathologies found in AIDS

Principal among these are the development of opportunistic infections and primary lymphomas. In many patients the infections appear macroscopically as areas of necrosis in different stages of repair. Opportunistic infections by viruses and fungi are common. For example, microscopy may reveal the features of *cytomegalovirus* infection and also *herpes simplex* virus. In some patients the features of *progressive multifocal leukoencephalopathy* may be seen. Infections by mycobacteria

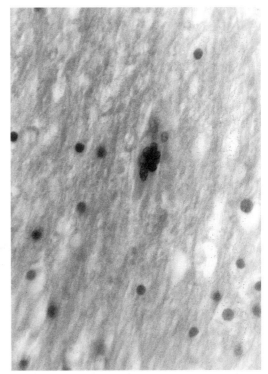

Fig. 7.19 Acquired immunodeficiency syndrome. HIV encephalopathy. There is a multinucleated giant cell in the white matter. (H & E.) (Courtesy of Dr Jeanne Bell, Department of Neuropathology, University of Edinburgh.)

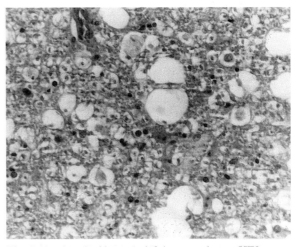

Fig. 7.20 Acquired immunodeficiency syndrome. HIV-associated vacuolar myelopathy. There was spongiform degeneration in both the posterior and lateral columns of the cervical cord. (H & E.) (Courtesy of Dr Jeanne Bell, Department of Neuropathology, University of Edinburgh.)

and toxoplasma are common, and mycotic infections include aspergillus, cryptococcus, nocardia, candida and coccidioides immitis.

There is an increased incidence of malignant tumours in the CNS that include Kaposi's sarcoma and lymphomas. Primary B-cell lymphomas of the CNS are common, and it has been predicted that CNS lymphomas occurring in association with HIV-positive patients will be the most common intracranial tumour by the end of this century.

There is an increased risk of suicide, and both in these cases and in those dying from unrelated disease it may be possible to identify the earliest features of HIV encephalopathy or myelopathy. There is also an increased association with cerebrovascular disease, principal among which are non-bacterial thrombotic endocarditis, thrombocytopenia predisposing to subarachnoid haemorrhage, and intracranial haemorrhage and angiitis.

There is also involvement of the peripheral nervous system (see Ch. 18) and a myopathy (see Ch. 17). Peripheral neuropathy is said to develop in some 90 per cent of cases of AIDS, comprising acute or subacute relapsing demyelinating neuropathy, mononeuritis multiplex, cranial neuropathies and an autonomic neuropathy.

FUNGAL INFECTIONS

Some fungi may produce disease in man in the absence of any obvious predisposing factors but, more often, fungal infections are 'opportunist', occurring in patients where the natural defences of the body are lowered, as in chronic debilitating diseases such as diabetes mellitus or alcoholism, the lymphomas or other disseminated malignant processes, or by the prolonged use of antibiotics, corticosteroids, cytotoxic drugs or immunosuppressive agents. Fungal infections of the CNS are invariably secondary to infection elsewhere in the body, but lesions at the portal of entry may be small and readily overlooked, with the result that the brain may appear to be the only organ involved. It is generally accepted that fungi usually reach the CNS by the bloodstream and that the primary focus is most often in the lung. Faced with what seems an unusual infection of the CNS, material must be taken for culture and sections stained with PAS and methenamine silver.

CRYPTOCOCCUS NEOFORMANS

Cryptococcus neoformans is a pathogenic yeast and infection with it is not restricted to individuals with impaired resistance to infection. It is thought that an important reservoir of the infection is pigeon manure. It gains access to the body through the respiratory tract but pulmonary cryptococcosis is less commonly encountered clinically than infection of the CNS. The commonest clinical presentation in man is as a subacute encephalitis and, unless the diagnosis is made early in the disease, it is usually fatal. Cryptococci may be identified in the CSF but in dried films they may be mistaken for lymphocytes, unless their capsules are sought by the appropriate techniques.

Pathology

There is usually some exudate and sometimes small nodules 2–3 mm in diameter in the subarachnoid space, particularly in the interpeduncular fossa and within sulci. Macroscopically the typical abnormality is the presence of numerous small cysts measuring up to 2–3 mm in diameter in grey matter (Fig. 7.21a). On histological examination encapsulated cryptococci (Fig. 7.21b) are scattered throughout the subarachnoid space, either as isolated units or as small collections. The cysts in the superficial layers of the cortex usually contain masses of cryptococci. Reactive inflammatory changes are often mild, but occasionally there may be a granulomatous reaction similar in many respects to tuberculous meningitis because of the presence of multinucleate giant cells, lymphocytes and plasma cells. Cryptococcosis is the most common type of cerebral mycosis in AIDS, occurring in between 2 and 4 per cent of cases.

COCCIDIOIDOMYCOSIS

This fungus (*coccidioides immitis*) is restricted to regions with a semi-arid climate and occurs particularly in the southwestern USA, Mexico and

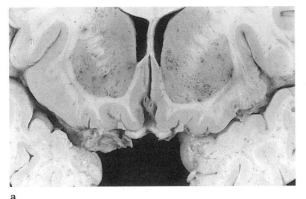

a

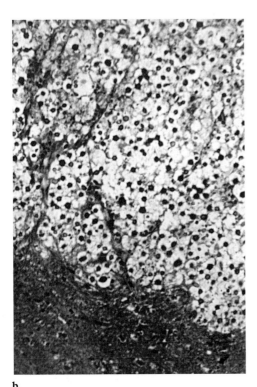

b

Fig. 7.21 Cryptococcosis. (a) There are multiple small cysts in each striatum and in the medial parts of each temporal lobe. (b) There are many encapsulated cryptococci in the subarachnoid space. (Toluidine blue.)

South America. The fungus usually causes only a mild transient febrile illness, but in a small proportion of cases granulomatous lesions appear in the lungs. The fungus may then be carried by the bloodstream to the brain where it produces a granulomatous meningitis. Occasionally granulomas may occur within the brain. Histologically the lesions closely resemble those of tuberculosis, but many of the giant cells contain the fungus, which appears as spherules about 10–60 μm in diameter filled with endospores.

BLASTOMYCOSIS

Blastomyces dermatidis is a fungus that exists as a filamentous growth and as a yeast and is the causal agent of blastomycosis, which occurs particularly in the USA, Canada and Mexico. It may also produce a pulmonary granulomatous process. Spread to the brain results in a granulomatous meningitis in which the yeasts occur free or within macrophages, or as single or multiple abscesses. Involvement of the vertebrae is not uncommon and the resulting extradural spinal granuloma may cause compression of the spinal cord.

HISTOPLASMOSIS

Infections by *Histoplasma capsulatum* are common in the USA, South America and southern Africa. Infection probably usually takes place by the inhalation of spores. Epidemics have occurred as a result of exposure to bird manure. Haematogenous spread to the brain is uncommon: it produces a diffuse granulomatous meningitis characterized by a thick yellow exudate in the subarachnoid space, with occasional discrete greyish-white opacities resembling tubercles adjacent to blood vessels. On histological examination there are macrophages, lymphocytes and plasma cells, and small granulomas. Granulomas may also occur within the brain. The organism appears as a small ovoid and budding body measuring 1–5 μm in diameter. It is PAS-positive.

ACTINOMYCOSIS

In spite of *Actinomyces* now being classified (with *Nocardia*) as bacteria, it remains traditional to continue to consider it as a fungal infection of the CNS.

Actinomycosis normally takes the form of a chronic suppurative disease in the cervical, facial or alimentary regions, and only rarely spreads to the CNS either directly from the former or by the bloodstream. If spread occurs to the brain it usually takes the form of a multilocular abscess within which the delicate branching hyphae can be identified.

OTHER FUNGAL INFECTIONS

These are the classic opportunist infections and they are most commonly caused by *Candida albicans* and *Aspergillus fumigatus*. *Nocardia asteroides*, although no longer classified as a fungus, acts in a similar fashion. All three generally produce abscesses of varying size and often multiple in the brain, and early in the disease process the lesions may resemble haemorrhagic infarcts (Fig. 7.22). With the passage of time they become well-defined abscesses. Histological examination shows varying degrees of infarction, including necrosis of blood vessel walls, and a cellular infiltrate consisting of lymphocytes, plasma cells, neutrophil polymorphs and macrophages. Aspergillus often provokes a granulomatous reaction characterized by the presence of multinucleate

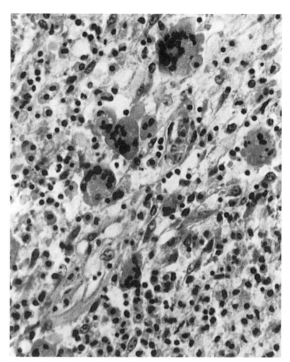

Fig. 7.23 Aspergillosis. There are numerous multinucleate giant cells in the inflammatory reaction. (H & E.)

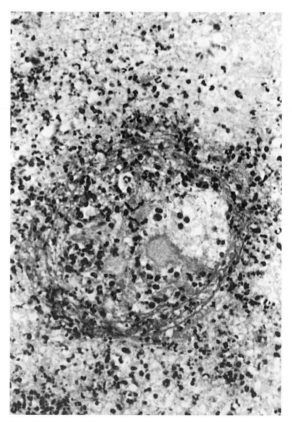

Fig. 7.24 Candidosis. There is necrosis of a blood vessel wall within the fungal abscess.

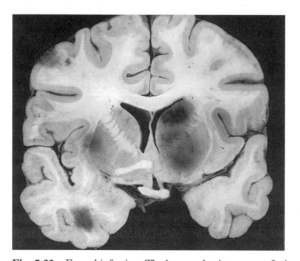

Fig. 7.22 Fungal infection. The haemorrhagic areas are foci of acute inflammation caused by candida.

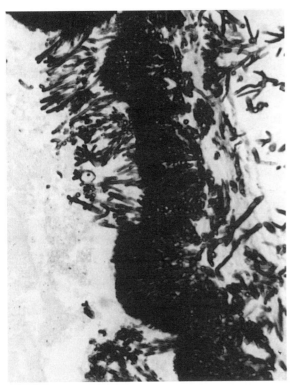

Fig. 7.25 Candidosis. A blood vessel wall is replaced by pseudohyphae and yeasts. (Grocott's methenamine silver.)

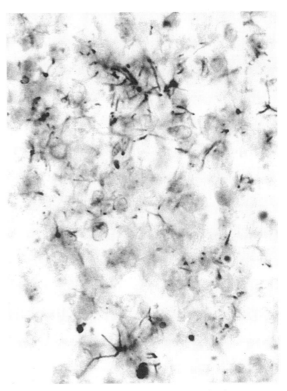

Fig. 7.26 Nocardiosis. Delicate branching hyphae are present. (Grocott's methenamine silver.)

giant cells (Fig. 7.23). Necrosis of blood vessel walls is often a prominent feature with infections with candida (Fig. 7.24). With appropriate stains, candida appears as yeast forms with pseudo-hyphae which may virtually replace necrotic blood vessel walls (Fig. 7.25), aspergillus as branching septate hyphae without yeast forms, and nocardia as rather delicate branching hyphae that readily fragment into coccal and bacillary forms (Fig. 7.26). Precise identification of the fungus cannot be achieved by the histopatho-logist and, as with other infections of the CNS, tissue must be taken for culture.

Another opportunist infection of the nervous system is *mucormycosis*, a clinical term to describe infection with phycomycetes. This fungus has a particular propensity to infect patients with un-controlled diabetes, when the infection tends to start in paranasal air sinuses or in the adjacent skin. It produces a rapidly progressive necrotizing process and spreads through the bone of the base of the skull and the cavernous sinuses to involve the adjacent brain, where it produces an acute necrotizing meningitis and, on occasion, abscess

formation (Fig. 7.27). On microscopical exam-ination there is necrosis of the walls of blood

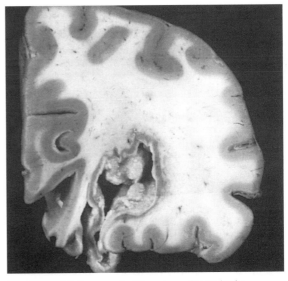

Fig. 7.27 Mucormycosis. There is an abscess in the inferomedial part of the frontal lobe.

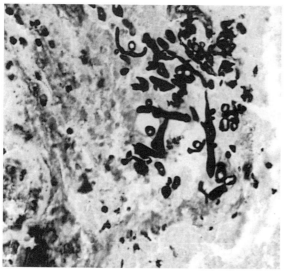

Fig. 7.28 Mucormycosis. There are large branching hyphae in nasopharyngeal tissue.

vessels and tissue, and large branching hyphae (Fig. 7.28).

PROTOZOAL INFECTIONS

TOXOPLASMOSIS

This is probably the commonest protozoal infection of man and is produced by *Toxoplasma gondii*, a coccidian parasite which is a crescentic oval or elongated protozoon consisting of an acidophilic cell body and a polar mass of chromatin. *Toxoplasma gondii* is widespread in nature but its principal life cycle occurs in cats, and infection in man is probably most often acquired by contamination with cat faeces and as a result of consuming infected undercooked meat. Between 30 and 50 per cent of the population have antibodies to *Toxoplasma*, but in the majority of cases the infection is subclinical.

Acquired toxoplasmosis may present as lymphadenopathy alone, lymphadenopathy with involvement of another organ, and generalized toxoplasmosis. Lymph nodes are most often involved, but acute encephalitis has been described in older children infected with the protozoon. Toxoplasmosis, a relatively benign disease in normal adults, is often fatal in patients who are immunosuppressed. With the appearance of AIDS, cerebral toxoplasmosis has become an important cause of an intracerebral mass lesion, toxoplasma abscesses being present in between 10 and 13 per cent of HIV-positive cases.

On CT scan toxoplasmosis appears as multiple bilateral ring-enhancing lesions. Although most of the cases occur in patients 'at risk', this is not always the case and so brain biopsy may be indicated. However, in view of the risks involved and the possibility of false-negative results, biopsy should be limited to patients in whom therapy has failed to produce clinical and radiological improvements after 1–2 weeks.

There may be numerous cysts in the brain (see Fig. 13.26) without there being any associated inflammatory reaction. However, on other occasions in patients with AIDS, toxoplasma may cause an acute multifocal necrotizing encephalitis. Congenital toxoplasmosis is dealt with in Chapter 13.

AMOEBIASIS

This occurs in two principal forms – amoebic meningoencephalitis and amoebic abscess of the brain.

Amoebic meningoencephalitis

This is a relatively recently identified disease caused by free-living amoebae traditionally regarded as being non-pathogenic in man; however, numerous cases have now been described from many parts of the world, including the UK. The amoeba most frequently implicated is *Naegleri fowleri*, and the infection is acquired by swimming in warm lakes or pools contaminated with it. The amoebae spread by the olfactory passages to produce acute meningitis. Recovery is rare because diagnosis early in the course of the disease is not often achieved. Amoebae, however, can be found in the CSF.

Pathology

In fatal cases there is a purulent meningitis and the olfactory bulbs and tracts may be haemorrhagic. On microscopic examination there is a fibrinopurulent exudate in which macrophages are often as numerous as neutrophil polymorphs. The inflammatory cells may extend for a short distance along perivascular spaces into the cerebral cortex, where there may be a necrotizing vasculitis. Amoebae are usually present in large numbers, particularly around the blood vessels.

Amoebic abscess of the brain

This is caused by *Entamoeba histolytica*, a parasite that commonly causes colitis in tropical and subtropical regions. In most cases of amoebic abscess in the brain there is also an abscess in the liver. Cerebral abscess is rare and tends to be a late complication of amoebiasis, and is secondary to haematogenous dissemination of the amoeba.

Pathology

Amoebic abscesses are usually solitary, and the wall of the cavity is poorly defined. On histological examination there is an inner zone of necrotic tissue and a broader outer zone of necrosis and diffuse infiltration by lymphocytes, plasma cells and phagocytic cells. Amoebae can be recognized by their large size and relatively small, usually eccentric, palely stained nucleus. They measure 10–20 μm in diameter. The prognosis is poor.

MALARIA

Cerebral malaria is almost always due to infection with *Plasmodium falciparum*. Unless it is diagnosed early and appropriate treatment instituted, the mortality rate is high, usually some 20–50 per cent of cases. Appropriate early treatment can, however, result in complete recovery. In hyperendemic areas severe infection is limited to children aged 6 months to 5 years, non-immune visiting adults, pregnant women and patients receiving cytotoxic drugs or steroids or on whom splenectomy has been carried out. The mortality is said to be reduced in patients with protein–calorie malnutrition, in subjects with glucose-6-phosphate deficiency and in those who are heterozygous for the sickle-cell gene. Clinically patients may present in coma, with or without focal signs.

Pathology

In fatal cases the most characteristic features are cerebral oedema and the presence of numerous petechial haemorrhages throughout the brain. On histological examination small blood vessels are seen, plugged with red blood cells within which the plasmodia may be identified, and malaria pigment is seen in relation to capillaries. There may also be ball and ring haemorrhages. To what extent the structural abnormalities are related to disseminated intravascular coagulation, to acute haemorrhagic leukoencephalopathy, or to the presence of the parasites, remains unclear.

TRYPANOSOMIASIS

Three trypanosomes may attack the CNS: *T.b. Gambiense*, *T.b. Rhodesiense* and *T.b. Cruzi*. The first two of these occur mainly in Central Africa and produce sleeping sickness, whereas the third is the cause of Chagas' disease in South America. In sleeping sickness the infection results from the bite of a tsetse fly, whereas Chagas' disease is transmitted by house bugs.

Human African trypanosomiasis

Infection with *T.b. Rhodesiense*, a disease of East Africa, usually follows a fairly acute course and a pancarditis is often more conspicuous than an encephalitis. *T.b. Gambiense* is the cause of classic sleeping sickness, a disease found in Central and West Africa, and characterized by subacute encephalitis. Many cases, however, also have a pancarditis. An important cause of morbidity with both forms of trypanosomiasis is an acute reactive arsenical encephalopathy as a result of treatment with trivalent arsenical compounds. This complication of treatment occurs in about 10 per cent of patients, tends to occur around the 10th day after the institution of treatment, and results in a fatal outcome in 2–5 per cent of all patients treated. Many of the patients who develop the encephalopathy experience serial convulsions that may lead to hypoxic brain damage, whereas in others the typical postmortem findings are those of acute haemorrhagic leukoencephalopathy. This disease is endemic in

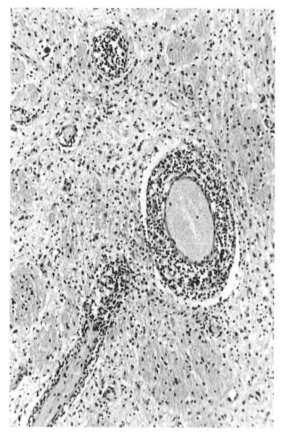

Fig. 7.29 Human African trypanosomiasis. There are numerous cells of inflammatory type within perivascular spaces and in the adjacent brain tissue. (H & E.)

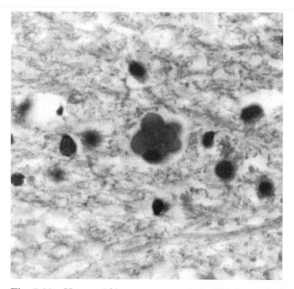

Fig. 7.30 Human African trypanosomiasis. This is a typical morular cell in the white matter. (H & E.)

areas of tropical forest near rivers. The two African species appear in the blood and tissue fluids as flagellate forms measuring 10–30 µm in diameter. Man is the primary reservoir for *T.b. Gambiense* and wild animals for *T.b. Rhodesiense*.

Pathology

In a patient dying as a result of human African trypanosomiasis the brain may be of entirely normal appearance macroscopically. If the disease has pursued a protracted course, however, there may be some generalized cortical atrophy. The histological features are those of a non-specific lymphoplasmacytic meningoencephalitis, the encephalitis being much more severe than the meningitis. The most striking feature is cuffing of blood vessels by lymphocytes and plasma cells and, in the more severe cases, these cells extend into the adjacent parenchyma (Fig. 7.29). The inflammatory reaction is particularly severe in the deep white matter, the basal ganglia, the brain stem and the deep structures in the cerebellum, and tends to be mild in the cerebral and cerebellar cortex. In the more florid cases there are often collections of lymphocytes, plasma cells and microglia in the brain not directly related to blood vessels, and there is usually diffuse microglial hyperplasia in grey matter. So called *morular cells*, plasma cells filled with immunoglobulin, are a common but not diagnostic feature of the disease (Fig. 7.30). In the more chronic cases there are large reactive astrocytes throughout the white matter. Some degree of demyelination has also been reported.

The pancarditis takes the form of diffuse infiltration of the pericardium and endocardium with lymphocytes and plasma cells, and focal collections of such cells within the myocardium.

Trypanosomes are not identifiable. Thus all of the changes are non-specific, with the result that a definitive diagnosis of trypanosomiasis cannot be made on the basis of a post-mortem examination. Confirmation of the diagnosis can only be made by confirming trypanosomal infection during life.

Chagas' disease

This disease is usually acquired in childhood and may be acute in children, or chronic both in

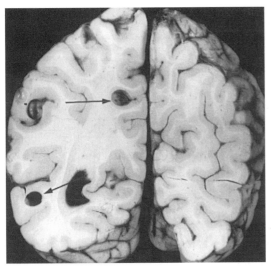

Fig. 7.31 Cysticercosis. Multiple sharply defined cysts (arrows) are present in the left occipital lobe. (Courtesy of Dr Ross Bullock, University of Durban, Republic of South Africa.)

Cysticercosis

This is caused by the pork tapeworm, *Taenia solium*. Man is infected, usually as a result of eating undercooked pork; in the duodenum the shells of the ova are dissolved, the embryos penetrate the wall of the intestine and are then disseminated throughout the body by the bloodstream. Involvement of the brain is common. As the larvae develop, cysts measuring up to about 1 cm in diameter form. They are frequently multiple within the brain (Fig. 7.31). Less frequently, thin-walled racemose cysts develop in the basal cisterns.

children and in adults. The infection may remain dormant for 10–20 years. Encephalitis is more common in acute than in chronic cases, and takes the form of numerous small inflammatory foci consisting of lymphocytes, plasma cells and microglia throughout the brain. They are more commonly seen in white matter than in grey matter. Leishmania-like forms may be seen within glial cells. There is frequently evidence of carditis. About 10 per cent of the acute cases of Chagas' disease evolve into a chronic phase, in which the heart and hollow viscera are principally affected.

OTHER INFECTIONS

Various other infections including *cestodes, trematodes* and *nematodes* may affect the brain, but the reader is referred to appropriate reference books for a detailed account of these rare disorders.

Echinococcosis

Hydatid disease is caused by the larvae of *Echinococcus granulosus*. The adult worm occurs in the dog, and man may be infected by ingesting food contaminated with ova. Hydatid cysts occur most often in the liver, and in many patients with a cerebral hydatid cyst there is also a cyst in the liver. The cerebral cysts are usually single, spherical and unilocular, and can ultimately reach a size of several centimetres in diameter.

Schistosomiasis

The CNS is one of the rarer sites of schistosomal infection. Granulomas are most often found in the brain and are usually caused by *S. japonicum*, but granulomas may also occur in the vertebral canal when they are caused by *S. haematobium* or *S. mansoni*.

Other *parasitic infections* such as toxocariasis and trichinosis rarely affect the CNS, but when they do they produce a non-specific granulomatous reaction.

FURTHER READING

Booss J & Esiri M M (1986) *Viral Encephalitis. Pathology, Diagnosis and Management*. Oxford: Blackwell Scientific Publications.
Brown W J & Voge M (1982) *Neuropathology of Parasitic Infections*. Oxford: Oxford University Press.
Concensus Report. HIV-associated disease of the nervous system: review of nomenclature and proposal for neuropathology-based terminology. *Brain Pathology* 1, 143–213.
Fetter B F, Klintworth G K & Hendry W S (1967) *Mycoses of the Central Nervous System*. Baltimore: Williams and Wilkins.

Johnston R T (1982) *Viral Infections of the Nervous System.* New York: Raven Press.

Kennedy P G E & Johnston R T (eds) (1987) *Infections of the Nervous Ssytem.* London: Butterworths.

Lantos P L (1992) From slow virus to prion: a review of transmissible spongiform encephalopathies. *Histopathology* 20, 1–11.

Sriram S (1991) Neuroimmunology. In: *Neurology in Clinical Practice*, Vol. 1. Edited by W G Bradley, R B Daroff, G M Fenichel & C D Marsden. Oxford: Butterworth-Heinemann.

8. Trauma

In many accidents the most important factor governing the outcome is the damage sustained by the brain or the spinal cord, since such damage is structurally irreversible. In the UK trauma is responsible for more deaths in all age groups under 45 than any other single cause, and head injury is the single most important factor in deaths due to trauma. The precise incidence of head injury is difficult to define but there are some 150 000 admissions to hospital for head injury every year in England and Wales, and in the UK there are some nine deaths from head injury per 100 000 population per year. Spinal injury is a smaller problem, but published reports suggest that in the UK some 1.3–2.7 people per 100 000 population sustain severe paralysis as a result of such an injury. Furthermore, in some 50 per cent of patients hospitalized for paraplegia or quadriplegia, trauma has been the cause. Of these, 45 per cent are a result of a road traffic accident and 30 per cent as a result of a fall, the remainder being due to sporting accidents, missile injuries etc.

Fortunately, the great majority of head-injured patients make an uneventful recovery, but others sustain irreversible brain damage, and a particularly distressing feature is that many people who sustain such damage are adolescent or in early adult life. If thereafter they remain severely or moderately disabled, they are likely to require care in institutions or from their families for many years. Even if the physical disability is not severe, intellectual or psychological problems or changes in personality may impose a great strain on their family. The accumulating population of survivors from head injury has resulted in an estimated prevalence in the UK of 150 per 100 000 population with major persisting handicap. One family in 300 has a member with such a disability.

HEAD INJURY

Head injuries are of two types – *missile* and *non-missile*. The *mechanisms of brain damages* are different in the two types.

In *non-missile head injuries* there is sudden deceleration or acceleration of the head, as a result of which the brain moves within the cranial cavity causing it to come in contact with bony protuberances within the skull, resulting in contusions and lacerations, and engendering various shear strains within the brain. These strains are particularly severe when there is a rotational element in the acceleration/deceleration and lead to subdural haematoma and diffuse axonal injury. It has long been known that a change in velocity of the head is a vital factor in the production of concussion since, when the head is fixed, as in a crush injury, consciousness may be retained even when the skull is fractured. It has also now been established that all of the major types of brain damage seen in man as a result of a non-missile head injury can be reproduced experimentally in the non-human primate by non-impact (inertial) controlled angular acceleration of the head. Thus, nothing needs to strike the head, nor the head to strike anything to produce brain damage in head injury – what matters is the acceleration/deceleration conditions that exist at the moment of injury.

In *missile injuries* brain damage is produced by various types of objects which fall or are propelled through the air. The object often enters the cranial cavity producing focal brain damage, and with slow-velocity missiles the patient may remain conscious. High-velocity missiles, however, impart considerable energy to the skull, and brain damage may be more widespread.

NON-MISSILE HEAD INJURY

This is by far the commoner type of head injury encountered in civilian practice, and much of the account that follows is based on a comprehensive neuropathological assessment of 635 fatal head injuries encountered in the Institute of Neurological Sciences, Glasgow, over the 15-year period 1968–1982 (Table 8.1). The two commonest injuries were road traffic accidents (53 per cent) and falls (35 per cent), and a third of the patients were known to have experienced a

Table 8.1 Data from a consecutive series of 635 fatal non-missile head injuries over a 15-year period (1968–1982) on whom post-mortem examinations were undertaken in the Institute of Neurological Sciences, Glasgow. For definition of types of damage, see text.

Sex 497 males (78%) : 138 females (22%)		
Type of injury	Road traffic accidents	— 335 (53%)
	Falls	— 222 (35%)
	Assaults	— 31 (5%)
	Other	— 47 (7%)
Incidence of		
Fracture of the skull	75%	
Surface contusions[1]	94% (mild in 6%, moderate in 78%, severe in 10%)	
Gliding contusions	31%	
Intracranial haematoma[2]	60%	
Extradural	10%	
Subdural	18%	
Intracerebral	16%	
'Burst lobe'	23%	
Diffuse axonal injury	29%	
Raised intracranial pressure	75%	
Ischaemic brain damage[3]	55%	
Brain swelling	53% (34% unilateral: 17% bilateral)	
Intracranial infection	4%	

[1]Measured quantitatively using the contusion index technique (see Further Reading)
[2]Some patients had more than one haematoma
[3]Cases with damage in *arterial boundary zones*, and of *diffuse type*
Some of the figures are approximate since full histological studies were undertaken in only 434 of the 635 cases.

lucid interval, i.e. they had been able to talk after their injury.

Classification of brain damage

There are two principal approaches to the classification of brain damage in head injury: one is to consider the damage as *focal* or *diffuse*, and the other as *primary* or *secondary*. In hospital departments with a particular interest in head injury, the former classification has much support since, in the current era of CT scanning, the various types of focal brain damage can usually be identified during life: in their absence the clinician can conclude that the patient is suffering from diffuse brain damage, but its precise nature is often obscure. In the account that follows, however, we have adhered to the classification of primary and secondary brain damage with the aim of helping pathologists to reconstruct the sequence of events leading to the fatal outcome. An important factor in reconstructing this sequence is whether or not the patient experienced a lucid interval: if there was a lucid interval – usually defined as the ability to talk soon after the injury – primary brain damage cannot have been severe.

The scalp and the skull may be injured at the moment of injury, but the two principal types of primary brain damage are *cerebral contusions* and diffuse damage to white matter known as *diffuse axonal injury*. The principal types of secondary brain damage are *intracranial haematoma*, brain damage secondary to a *high intracranial pressure, brain swelling, ischaemic brain damage* and *infection*.

PRIMARY DAMAGE

Lesions of the scalp and skull

The scalp may be lacerated or bruised at the time of injury and is the only reliable evidence of the site of impact. Lacerations may bleed profusely and they are a potential route for later infection.

The presence of a fracture of the skull indicates that the impact has had considerable force, but many people with a fracture of the skull do not sustain brain damage. In contrast, only 75 per cent of our series of 635 fatal head injuries had a fracture of the skull (Table 8.1). Most fractures are *fissure* fractures and they often extend into the base of the skull, but impact against a small or irregular object will produce a more localized fracture which is often *depressed*. A depressed fracture is said to be *compound* if there is an associated laceration of the scalp. Fractures of the base of the skull may pass through the middle ear or the anterior cranial fossa, producing a CSF *otorrhoea* or *rhinorrhoea*, and they are potential sources for later infection. Basal fractures are often not identifiable *post mortem* until the dura has been stripped from the skull. The term '*hinge*' fracture is sometimes used for a fracture extending right across the base of the skull, usually in the region of the posterior part of the pituitary fossa: it is indicative of very severe injury. Occasionally, there may be fractures in the roofs of the orbits in association with a fall on the occiput: these are referred to as *contrecoup* fractures. *Growing* fractures occur in infancy, when brain tissue or simply meninges protrude through the fracture, preventing it from healing and indeed even enlarging it.

Patients with a fracture of the skull have a much higher incidence of intracranial haematoma than patients who do not have a fracture.

Cerebral contusions

Although contusions are considered the hallmark of non-missile head injury, a patient may die as a result of the injury without there being any surface contusions, e.g. in association with an acute extradural haematoma, diffuse axonal injury or diffuse hypoxic brain damage. In our series of 635 cases (Table 8.1), surface contusions were absent in 6 per cent. Contusions are a focal type of brain damage that occurs at the moment of injury, and are brought about principally by the surface of the brain coming in contact with bony protuberances in the base of the skull. They therefore have a very characteristic distribution, affecting particularly the frontal poles, the orbital surfaces of the frontal lobes (Fig. 8.1), the cortex above and below the Sylvian fissures (Fig. 8.2), the temporal poles, the undersurface of the temporal lobes and, less

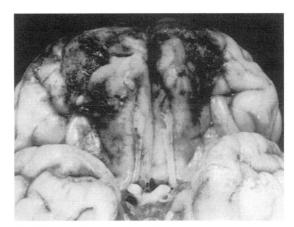

Fig. 8.1 Cerebral contusions. There are acute haemorrhagic contusions on the inferior surfaces of the frontal lobes.

frequently, the inferior surface of the cerebellum. Contusions may also occur in direct relation to a depressed fracture of the vault of the skull. Severe cerebellar contusions occur rarely, unless there is a corresponding fracture in the posterior fossa.

Contusions characteristically occur at the crests of gyri but they often extend into the subcortical white matter. With the passage of time, the contusions come to be represented as brown, shrunken scars which are so characteristic in appearance and distribution that it is possible

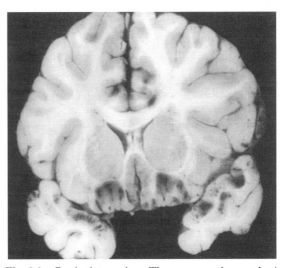

Fig. 8.2 Cerebral contusions. There are acute haemorrhagic contusions above and below the Sylvian fissures.

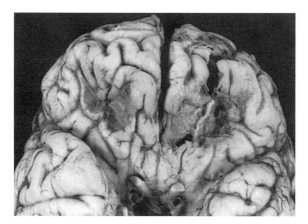

Fig. 8.3 Cerebral contusions. There are old shrunken contusions on the inferior surfaces of the frontal lobes, (cf. Fig. 8.1).

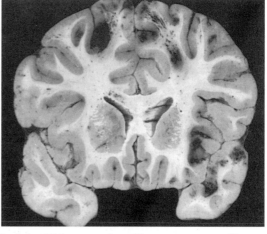

Fig. 8.4 Gliding contusions. These are represented by haemorrhagic foci in the parasagittal regions. Surface contusions are seen affecting the right temporal lobe.

to state with certainty post mortem that a patient has sustained a head injury some time in the past (Fig. 8.3). Since surface contusions are a focal type of brain damage, patients with quite severe contusions may make a remarkably good recovery provided that there has been no diffuse brain damage or complications of the original injury. It is therefore not surprising that healed contusions are a not uncommon incidental finding at autopsy.

Various names have been applied to surface contusions, e.g. *coup* (contusions occurring at the point of impact) and *contrecoup* (contusions occurring diametrically opposite to the site of impact). It has been held in the past that contrecoup contusions are always the more severe and that the distribution of surface contusions can therefore be used to define the site of injury. This is not so: frontal contusions will be severe in association with an occipital impact because of the bony protuberances in the anterior fossa; with a frontal injury, however, there are rarely, if ever, contusions in the occipital region. The term *herniation* contusion is used for foci of haemorrhage in the uncinate processes or in the cerebellar tonsils where they have been injured against the tentorium or foramen magnum respectively at the time of injury.

Gliding contusions are quite different from surface contusions. The term is used to describe haemorrhage into the parasagittal white matter and the adjacent deeper layers of the cortex (Fig. 8.4). They are often bilateral and may enlarge to form a narrow lentiform haematoma. Their pathogenesis appears to be related to the fact that the dorsal angle of each hemisphere is firmly tethered to the dura by arachnoidal granulations, and when the brain moves at the time of injury the subcortical tissue 'glides' more than the cortex.

Contusions of the types described above occur at all ages apart from infancy: non-missile head injury in this age group produces tears at the junction between the cortex and the white matter, particularly in the frontal and the temporal lobes.

Diffuse axonal injury

This in many respects is the most important type of brain damage occurring as a result of a non-missile head injury. Although it occurred in only 29 per cent of our series (Table 8.1), it is a diffuse type of brain damage that occurs at the moment of injury and is the commonest cause of coma in the absence of an intracranial haematoma, and of severe disability after head injury. It also seems likely that milder degrees of this type of brain damage are responsible for concussion and less severe degrees of permanent disability.

In diffuse axonal injury there is widespread disruption of axons attributable to shear and tensile strains affecting axons at the time of an acceleration/deceleration injury, and patients with severe diffuse axonal injury do not experience a lucid interval i.e. they are unable to talk immediately, after their injury. In comparison with patients without this type of brain damage, there is a low incidence of fracture of the skull, intracranial haematoma and raised intracranial pressure, and an increased incidence of gliding contusions and deep intracerebral haematomas. Surface contusions are often minimal. This type of brain damage has become understood relatively recently, and in the past the patients were often said to have sustained *primary brainstem damage*. The structural abnormalities consist of discrete lesions in the dorsolateral quadrant or quadrants of the rostral brain stem and in the corpus callosum, and diffuse damage to axons throughout the brain. The lesions in the corpus callosum and in the brain stem, although often small, can often be seen macroscopically, but the axonal damage can only be recognized microscopically.

When they are apparent macroscopically the lesions in the corpus callosum and in the brain stem are initially haemorrhagic (Fig. 8.5 and

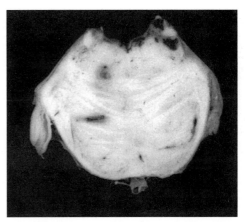

Fig. 8.6 Diffuse axonal injury. There is a haemorrhagic lesion in the dorsolateral quadrant of the pons.

8.6). Although the lesion in the corpus callosum usually lies mainly to one side of the midline in the inferior part of the corpus callosum, it may extend to the midline to involve the interventricular septum and the pillars of the fornix (Fig. 8.5). Rupture of the former may result in intraventricular haemorrhage that is identifiable on CT scanning. Sometimes damage to the corpus callosum is most severe at the level of the splenium (Fig. 8.7). If the patient survives for some weeks, the lesions become soft and rather granular (Fig. 8.8), whereas if survival is for several months, the original lesions come to be represented by shrunken, often cystic, scars

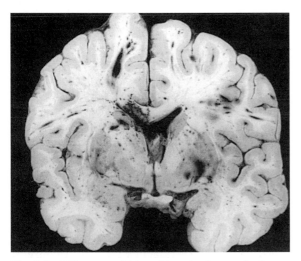

Fig. 8.5 Diffuse axonal injury. There is a haemorrhagic lesion in the corpus callosum to the left of the midline. The interventricular septum has been torn. There are also gliding contusions and a small haematoma in the right basal ganglia.

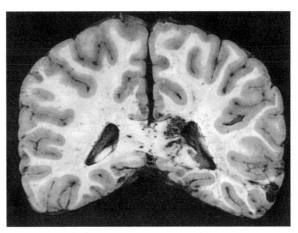

Fig. 8.7 Diffuse axonal injury. There is a haemorrhagic lesion in the splenium of the corpus callosum.

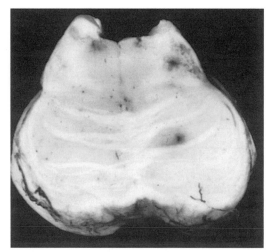

Fig. 8.8 Diffuse axonal injury. There is a slightly discoloured and granular lesion in the dorsolateral quadrant of the pons.

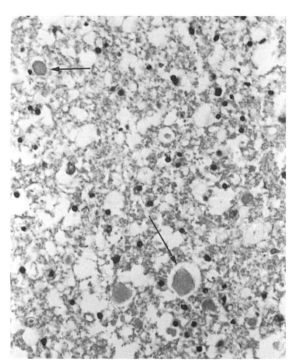

Fig. 8.10 Diffuse axonal injury. In the early stages there are axonal bulbs (arrows) in the white matter. (H & E.)

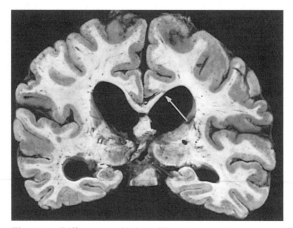

Fig. 8.9 Diffuse axonal injury. There is a small scar (arrow) in the corpus callosum and enlargement of the lateral ventricles.

(Fig. 8.9). By this time, there is moderate ventricular enlargement due to a reduced bulk of the white matter. On histological examination of these focal lesions there is, in the early stages, rarefaction of tissue in addition to haemorrhage. Thereafter, reactive astrocytes, hypertrophied microglia and lipid containing macrophages appear, and in long survivors there is a shrunken, gliosed lesion within which there are usually haemosiderin-containing macrophages.

The diffuse injury to axons can only be identified microscopically. In patients with severe axonal injury who survive for only a short time (days), there are vast numbers of axonal bulbs ('retraction balls') throughout the cerebral hemispheres, brain stem and cerebellum. They can be seen in sections stained by H & E, when they appear as small round eosinophilic masses (Fig. 8.10), but they are more easily seen in sections impregnated with silver (Fig. 8.11). They tend to be particularly numerous in the parasagittal white matter, in the corpus callosum and in certain parts of the brain stem, particularly the superior cerebellar peduncles, the medial lemnisci and the corticospinal fibres. In patients who survive for some weeks after this type of brain damage, the characteristic feature is the presence of many clusters of microglia throughout the white matter (Fig. 8.12). In cases who survive for some months in a vegetative state, there is evidence of degeneration of long tracts in the cerebral hemispheres, the brain stem and the spinal cord. This is most easily seen in Marchi preparations and degeneration tends to be particularly conspicuous in the corticospinal fibres and in the medial lemnisci (Fig. 8.13).

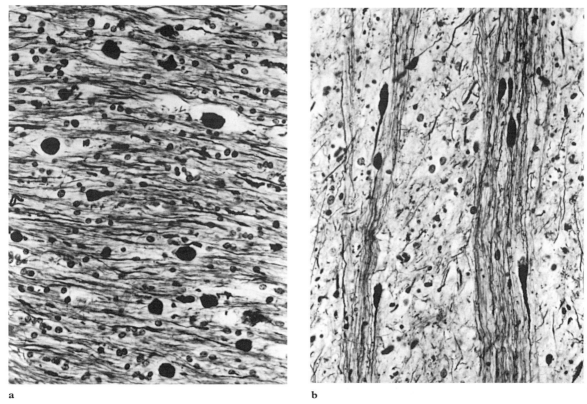

a   b

Fig. 8.11 Diffuse axonal injury. The axonal bulbs are more clearly seen in silver impregnations: (a) in the corpus callosum; (b) in nerve fibres traversing the thalamus. (Palmgren silver technique.)

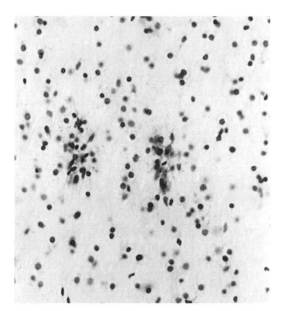

Fig. 8.12 Diffuse axonal injury. There are clusters of microglia in the white matter. (Cresyl violet.)

It is very important for pathologists to have a clear understanding of this type of brain damage. If, at autopsy there is no evidence of intracranial

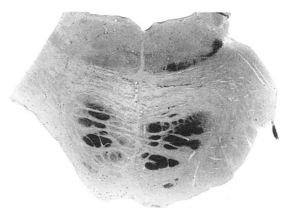

Fig. 8.13 Diffuse axonal injury. There is asymmetrical Wallerian-type degeneration in the corticospinal tracts and in a medial lemniscus. (Marchi preparation.)

haematoma or raised intracranial pressure, and if contusions are absent or minimal, the most likely structural basis of the brain damage is diffuse axonal injury. Furthermore, the lesions in the corpus callosum and in the brain stem may be difficult to identify unless looked for specifically, particularly if the brain is sliced prior to fixation. A further problem is that the axonal injury can only be recognized microscopically, and it has recently become apparent that there are mild degrees of diffuse axonal injury without there being classic focal lesions in the corpus callosum and in the brain stem. Thus, in any head injury where there appears to be a lack of clinico-pathological correlation, it is important to screen the brain for diffuse axonal injury by examining blocks from the corpus callosum, the brain stem and the parasagittal white matter for – depending on the duration of survival – axonal bulbs or clusters of microglia. It has to be emphasized that axonal bulbs are not restricted to head injury, because they occur in any circumstances where axons are disrupted, e.g. at the edge of an infarct.

Three grades of diffuse axonal injury are now recognized: in Grade 1 abnormalities are restricted to scattered axonal bulbs throughout the white matter of the brain; in Grade 2 there is also a focal lesion in the corpus callosum; in Grade 3 there is in addition a lesion in the dorsolateral quadrant(s) of the rostral brain stem. There is a good correlation between these grades and the patient's clinical state, patients with Grade 3 diffuse axonal injury always remaining unconscious or in the vegetative state until death.

Contusions and diffuse axonal injury are common types of primary brain damage in non-missile head injury. They are both brought about by alterations in the velocity of the head and considerable light has been shed on their pathogenesis in experiments on non-human primates. Surface contusions (and intracranial haematoma) are more severe when the acceleration/deceleration period is very short, whereas diffuse axonal injury and gliding contusions are associated with a longer acceleration/deceleration time. This accords well with observations on fatal non-missile head injury in man, where there is an association between the severity of surface contusions and intracranial

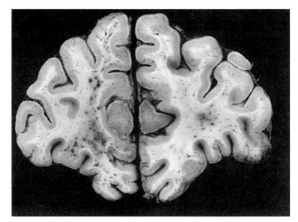

Fig. 8.14 Diffuse vascular injury. There are multiple petechial haemorrhages in the white matter of the frontal lobes.

haematoma with a fall where the period of deceleration is very short, whereas diffuse axonal injury and gliding contusions are commoner in road traffic accidents where the period of acceleration/deceleration is longer. Diffuse axonal injury may occur as a result of a fall from a considerable height, but we have yet to observe it in an individual who has fallen from his own height. This has certain medicolegal implications in that if diffuse axonal injury is identified post mortem, it is unlikely to have resulted from such a simple fall. Diffuse axonal injury may also occur as a result of an assault.

Other types of primary damage

In patients who die within minutes of a head injury, there are often multiple petechial haemorrhages throughout the cerebral hemispheres, particularly in the white matter of the frontal and the temporal lobes, and in the brain stem (Fig. 8.14). This is known as *diffuse vascular injury.* Occasionally there is a *tear in the brain stem* at the pontomedullary junction. Other structures may be torn at the time of injury, such as *cranial nerves,* the cavernous part of the internal carotid artery leading to a *caroticocavernous fistula,* and the *pituitary stalk,* leading to infarction of the anterior lobe of the pituitary gland due to disruption of the long portal hypothalamo-hypophyseal blood vessels. Blows to the upper part of the neck just below the ear may cause rupture of a vertebral artery: this is usually rapidly fatal and the principal finding at autopsy is *massive subarachnoid haemorrhage* within the posterior fossa. Injuries to the neck may also cause dissection of the internal carotid artery, subsequent thrombosis leading to cerebral infarction.

SECONDARY DAMAGE

Intracranial haematoma

This is a frequent complication of a non-missile head injury and is the commonest cause of deterioration and death in patients who have experienced a lucid interval after their injury. A significant haematoma, i.e. one considered large enough to act as an intracranial expanding lesion (> 35 ml), was present in 60 per cent of our series of 635 fatal head injuries (Table 8.1). Many of the haematomas had, however, been evacuated surgically. The incidence of haematoma is much higher in patients with a fracture of the skull than in those who do not have a fracture. It has in the past tended to be assumed that intracranial haematomas developed fairly slowly after head injury, but experimental studies in non-human primates and the increasing use of CT scanning have established that the haematoma may be present very soon after the injury and before it produces clinical deterioration. This is a manifestation of spatial compensation in the presence of an intracranial expanding lesion (see Ch. 4). It would therefore appear that haemorrhage may begin at the time of injury – i.e. it is a *primary* event – but the clinical presentation is usually that of a complication, because of the interval between the onset of haemorrhage and the occurrence of clinical deterioration attributable either to brain swelling adjacent to the haematoma or to a progressive increase in the size of the haematoma. Serial CT scans, however, have established that some haematomas do not develop until 2 or 3 days after the injury: these are referred to as *delayed haematomas* and their pathogenesis remains unknown.

Traumatic intracranial haematomas may be *extradural* or *intradural,* and the latter may be subdivided into *subdural, intracerebral* or a '*burst lobe*' (intracerebral and subdural haematomas in continuity through a surface contusion). Frequently, more than one type of haematoma is present. Subarachnoid haemorrhage almost invariably occurs in a patient who has sustained a severe head injury, but a subarachnoid haematoma sufficiently large to act as a significant intracranial expanding lesion is very rare.

Extradural haematoma

This is basically a complication of a fracture of the skull which disrupts a meningeal artery, but it may occur in young children in the absence of a fracture. The artery most often damaged is the middle meningeal artery as it runs across the squamous part of the temporal bone. The resulting haematoma therefore occurs in the temporoparietal region. Since any meningeal artery can be disrupted by a fracture, extradural haematomas may occur at other sites including the posterior fossa. Occasionally they are bilateral. Extradural haematoma was present in 10 per cent of our series of 635 non-missile head injuries (Table 8.1). The classic clinical history is that of a trivial head injury after which the patient is completely lucid and thereafter deteriorates as the haematoma develops. Extradural haematoma may, however, also develop in patients with more severe damage, and only 50 per cent of the patients in the Glasgow series with an extradural haematoma experienced a lucid interval.

As the haematoma develops it strips the dura from the skull to form a large ovoid circumscribed mass that indents the adjacent brain (Fig. 8.15). If untreated, there is midline shift leading to the formation of internal herniae and compression of the midbrain (see Ch. 4). If the patient has experienced a lucid interval, there may be little or no evidence of other brain damage attributable to the injury.

In fatal cases of burning where the head is charred, blood is sometimes forced into the extradural space. Thus the finding of an extradural haematoma in such a case at autopsy does not necessarily mean that the patient has sustained a head injury prior to the fire.

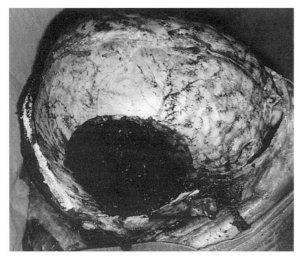

Fig. 8.15 Extradural haematoma. There is a sharply defined haematoma in the extradural space.

Intradural haematoma

Subdural haematoma. Thin smears of blood in the subdural space that are not large enough to act as significant expanding lesions are common in any acute head injury. A subdural haematoma usually arises as the result of rupture of the bridging veins where they run from the dorsal angle of the cerebral hemispheres to the sagittal sinus. The veins rupture because of a sudden change in the velocity of the head, and subdural haematoma is a recognized complication of 'whiplash' injury. In such cases there may be very little other evidence of brain damage attributable to injury, and the patient may have experienced a lucid interval. Subdural haematoma may also be caused by haemorrhage from severe cerebral contusions, and in such cases there is more clinical evidence of primary brain damage.

In contrast to the localized nature of extradural haematoma, haemorrhage into the subdural space spreads diffusely over the affected hemisphere. This, in turn, prevents flattening of the convolutions and narrowing of the sulci. As the haematoma expands, there is progressive shift of the midline structures, internal herniae and compression of the brain stem. Diffuse swelling of the underlying hemisphere is common and, not infrequently, when the haematoma is evacuated, there is little or no reduction in the midline shift (Fig. 8.16). A subdural haematoma was present in 18 per cent in our series of 635 head injuries (Table 8.1).

An *acute* subdural haematoma consists of clotted blood, this state remaining for a few days after the injury. Thereafter there is a mixture of blood clot and fluid blood, when the haematoma is said to be *subacute*. After about 3 weeks the entire haematoma is fluid, this being referred to as a *chronic* subdural haematoma. By this time the haematoma may be encapsulated by a sheet of tissue within which there are fibroblasts, proliferating capillaries and haemosiderin-containing macrophages. This process is so variable, however, that accurate ageing of a subdural haematoma on the basis of the histological findings is not possible.

Chronic subdural haematoma unrelated to an obvious head injury remains a poorly understood problem. The current view is that after a trivial injury, usually in an elderly person, there is haemorrhage into the subdural space and the haematoma progressively increases in size. It also becomes encapsulated in a membrane. Because there is already some pre-existing cerebral atrophy, and because the haematoma enlarges slowly, there may be considerable distortion of the brain before there is any significant increase in intracranial pressure. In untreated cases,

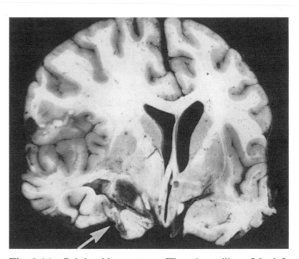

Fig. 8.16 Subdural haematoma. There is swelling of the left cerebral hemisphere deep to an acute subdural haematoma that had been evacuated. There is a broad tentorial hernia (arrow).

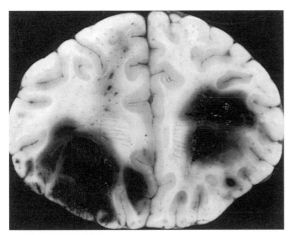

Fig. 8.17 Traumatic intracerebral haematoma. Haematomas are present in both frontal lobes.

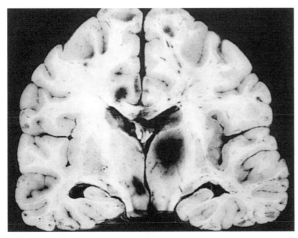

Fig. 8.18 Traumatic intracerebral haematoma. There are bilateral 'basal ganglia' haematomas in the thalami. There are also small gliding contusions and a haemorrhagic lesion in the corpus callosum.

however, death is usually due to brain damage secondary to increased intracranial pressure. Chronic subdural haematoma is not infrequently bilateral. There is an increased incidence of chronic subdural haematoma in patients on anticoagulant therapy.

A *subdural hygroma* is a collection of yellowish-brown fluid in the subdural space and is probably always attributable to a previous head injury and some haemorrhage into the subdural space. It is uncommon in adults but may become large in infants. Such hygromas are frequently found in infants subjected to non-accidental injury ('battered baby' syndrome), when they are often bilateral, and it has been suggested that severe shaking of the infant is a contributory factor.

Intracerebral haematoma. These were present in 16 per cent of our series of 635 head injuries (Table 8.1). They occur in two principal forms. One is a haematoma in a frontal or a temporal lobe in relation to contusions (Fig. 8.17), whereas the other is a deeply seated haematoma not related to contusions (Fig. 8.18): the latter are often referred to as '*basal ganglia haematomas*' and the advent of CT scanning has shown that they are commoner than was previously suspected clinically. They may be multiple and are usually indicative of a severe head injury, since gliding contusions and diffuse axonal injury are often also present. Basal ganglia haematomas were present in 10 per cent of our series of 635 fatal head injuries.

'Burst lobe'. This is the coexistence of subdural haematoma, cerebral contusions and intracerebral haemorrhage, and is usually indicative of severe brain damage. The frontal and temporal lobes are most often affected. A burst lobe was identified in 23 per cent of our series of 635 fatal non-missile head injuries (Table 8.1).

Cerebral oedema and brain swelling

Vasogenic cerebral oedema (see Ch. 4) occurs around contusions and haematomas and may contribute significantly to the effective size of the expanding lesion. Acute congestive brain swelling (see Ch. 4) also occurs in head injury in the form of diffuse swelling in one or both cerebral hemispheres. Its development may be very rapid but occasionally appears to be delayed for 24–48 hours.

Diffuse swelling of an entire cerebral hemisphere occurs in about one-third of patients with an acute traumatic intracranial haematoma, but is particularly common deep to an acute subdural haematoma (see Fig. 8.16). Diffuse swelling of both hemispheres occurs in young children (Fig. 8.19). The original injury may have been apparently trivial or severe. The pathogenesis of either type of brain swelling in head injury is not known, but because of the rapidity with which it

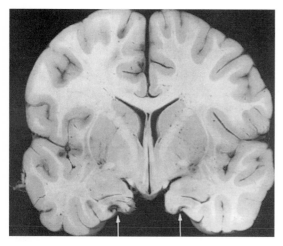

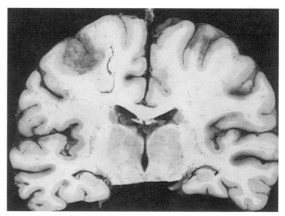

Fig. 8.19 Brain swelling. There is diffuse swelling of both hemispheres. The lateral ventricles are small and there are bilateral tentorial herniae (arrows).

Fig. 8.20 Ischaemic brain damage. Partly haemorrhagic and partly pale infarcts are seen in the boundary zones between the territories supplied by the anterior and middle cerebral arteries.

can appear it seems likely that there must be some vasomotor paralysis and loss of auto-regulation (see Ch. 5).

Brain damage secondary to raised intracranial pressure

This subject has been dealt with in Chapter 4, but it should be clear from the preceding sections that complications of the original head injury often take the form of intracranial expanding lesions. In our series of 635 fatal head injuries there was evidence of raised intracranial pressure in 75 per cent and in 53 per cent there was secondary damage to the brain stem.

Ischaemic brain damage

This is a frequent finding in patients who die as a result of a non-missile head injury. Much of it occurs adjacent to contusions and haematomas, or is clearly secondary to raised intracranial pressure, shift and herniation of the brain, such as infarction in the territories supplied by the posterior cerebral arteries (see Ch. 4). In our series of 635 head injuries, however, there was ischaemic damage in arterial boundary zones (Figs 8.20 and 5.18) in 20 per cent of cases, whereas there was diffuse hypoxic brain damage in 35 per cent. The infarction in arterial boundary zones is sometimes haemorrhagic, when it can be

identified macroscopically. In other cases it can only be demonstrated microscopically, and it has already been emphasized in Chapter 5 that severe diffuse hypoxic damage may defy recognition macroscopically even when it has been present for a few days. With the passage of time, how-ever, reactive changes occur and the affected areas become gliosed and shrunken.

The pathogenesis of ischaemic brain damage resulting from a head injury is not yet established but the available evidence suggests that it occurs soon after injury, and correlations have been established between the presence of hypoxic brain damage and an episode of systemic hypoxia (defined as a systolic blood pressure of <80 mmHg for at least 15 minutes, or a PaO_2 of 50 mmHg or less at some time after the injury) or a high intracranial pressure. The basic cause of ischaemic damage in arterial boundary zones is a transient period of greatly reduced cerebral blood flow, whereas diffuse hypoxic brain damage is frequently brought about by an episode of cardio-respiratory arrest or status epilepticus. These are well known events in a patient with an acute head injury.

It is important that pathologists are aware of the frequent occurrence of ischaemic brain damage in non-missile head injury since, as with diffuse axonal injury, it may only be recognizable histologically.

Infection

Although rare – it occurred in 4 per cent of our series of 635 fatal head injuries (Table 8.1) – *meningitis* is a well recognized complication of a non-missile head injury due to the spread of micro-organisms through an open fracture of the vault of the skull or through a fracture of the base of the skull. If there is only a small defect in the dura of the base of the skull in relation to a fracture, the meningitis may be delayed for some months, and such small traumatic fistulae may be a cause of recurrent episodes of meningitis. Brain *abscess* is more often a complication of a missile head injury (see below).

Fat embolism

Some patients with a head injury have multiple injuries – extracranial fractures were present in 37 per cent of our series of 635 fatal non-missile head injuries. Such patients are at risk of developing systemic fat embolism. The classic feature of cerebral fat embolism is said to be the presence of multiple petechial haemorrhages throughout the brain, particularly in the white matter, but such petechiae are not always present even in patients with fulminating fat embolism, hence the importance of examining frozen sections of the brain, and other organs, for fat embolism in a patient who has died as the result of multiple injuries.

THE AUTOPSY

It should be clear from the foregoing account that there are many subtle types of brain damage in non-missile head injury. Only too often death is certified as being due to a fracture of the skull and cerebral contusions when neither may be the reason for the patient even being in coma. The great majority of patients with a fracture of the skull make an uneventful recovery, and patients with quite severe cerebral contusions may make an excellent recovery if no other type of brain damage is present.

The pathologist must be present when the skull is opened so that it can be clearly established whether an intracranial haematoma is extradural or intradural. The volume of the haematoma should be measured, since haematomas of less than 35 ml are unlikely to have been significant intracranial expanding lesions unless there is also brain swelling. The pathologist should also assess the tightness of the dura, since this is a useful method of determining whether or not intracranial pressure has been high during life. Some comments relating to the autopsy in infants will be found in Chapter 13.

In many severe head injuries the cause of the fatal outcome is immediately apparent, e.g. if there is an intracranial haematoma, evidence of a high intracranial pressure and secondary haemorrhage in the brain stem. But even in these patients there may be other types of brain damage. On the other hand, the pathologist may find a brain of almost entirely normal appearance when the clinical history clearly indicates that the patient has died as a result of a non-missile head injury. The worst thing to do in such circumstances is to slice the unfixed brain, when it may be difficult to identify focal lesions in the corpus callosum or rostral brain stem, or evidence suggestive of hypoxic damage. Furthermore, ventricular size and displacement caused, for example, by swelling, is almost impossible to assess. Even if the brain is sliced unfixed, it must be screened for diffuse axonal injury, ischaemic brain damage and fat embolism. The presence or absence of the last of these can easily be established by taking two or three blocks for frozen section. To establish the presence of diffuse axonal injury or ischaemic brain damage, tissue from the arterial boundary zones, the parasagittal white matter, the corpus callosum, the hippocampi, the cerebellum and several levels of the brain stem must be examined histologically.

If a patient has survived in coma or vegetative for some weeks or months after a head injury, the most likely causes of the brain damage are diffuse axonal injury or ischaemic brain damage, since most patients who sustain secondary damage in the brain stem rarely survive for more than a few weeks. The situation should be clarified by a similar histological survey but, if the patient has survived for more than 2 months after the injury, the importance of looking for long tract degeneration in Marchi preparations has to be emphasized.

Post-traumatic dementia (dementia pugilistica)

There is no convincing evidence that a head injury may cause progressive dementia of the types described in Chapter 14. Individuals subjected to a large number of blows to the head, such as boxers, however, sometimes develop neurological signs and progressive dementia. This condition is often referred to as the *punch-drunk syndrome* and may not develop until years after the last injury. It usually develops in boxers with long careers who have been dazed, if not knocked out, on many occasions. The pathogenesis of the brain damage is not understood, but it is characterized by defects in the interventricular septum, thinning of the corpus callosum, enlargement of the lateral ventricles, degeneration of the substantia nigra and the presence of many neurofibrillary tangles throughout the cerebral cortex and the brain stem. Until recently dementia pugilistica has been regarded as being entirely separate from other common types of dementia because there was no evidence of neuritic plaque formation as demonstrated by silver and Congo red histochemistry (see Chapter 14). It has, however, now been shown that the brains of boxers with dementia pugilistica contain large numbers of diffuse plaques composed of βA4 protein. The presence of these plaques might indicate a long-term consequence of head injury that may predispose to the onset of Alzheimer's disease, mediated through the upregulation of amyloid precursor protein 751/770.

MISSILE HEAD INJURY

This can be defined as depressed, penetrating or perforating. In a *depressed* injury, the missile does not enter the cranial cavity but produces a depressed fracture of the skull. In a *penetrating* injury, the object enters the cranial cavity but does not pass through it. In a *perforating* injury, the object, usually a bullet, traverses the cranial cavity and leaves through an exit wound.

Missile injuries produce focal damage to the brain in the form of lacerations at the site of injury, haemorrhage into the regions of the brain destroyed by the penetration of the object, and varying degrees of oedema around it. Since the damage is focal, there may be no disturbance of consciousness unless some vital structure is damaged by the missile. With a severe missile injury, such as that produced by a bullet, radial displacement forces from the bullet track may cause remote contusions affecting the undersurfaces of the frontal and temporal lobes and the cerebellum. Contrecoup fractures (see p. 135) may also occur in the orbital plates.

With penetrating and perforating injuries there is a high risk of infection, abscess being more common than meningitis (Fig. 8.21), and a higher incidence of post-traumatic epilepsy than

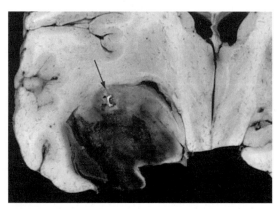

Fig. 8.21 Cerebral abscess. There is an airgun pellet (arrow) in this acute haemorrhagic abscess.

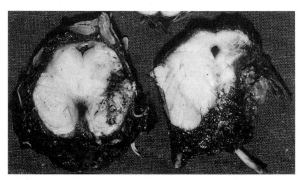

Fig. 8.22 Penetrating head injury. There is direct damage to the upper brain stem as a result of injury by a nail gun.

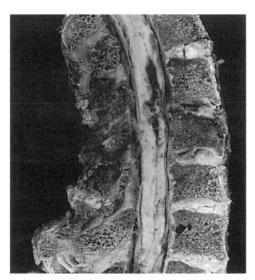

Fig. 8.23 Spinal injury. There is a traumatic haematomyelia in relation to a fracture of the cervical spine.

is brought about by non-missile head injury. Occasionally there may be direct damage to the brain stem in deep penetrating injuries (Fig. 8.22).

SPINAL INJURY

These may also be classified as *non-missile* and *missile* injuries. The former result from sub-luxations and fracture/dislocations of the vertebral column, and are usually brought about by acute flexion or extension injuries. The vertebrae may return to a normal position, when the fracture/dislocation is said to be *stable*. If the damaged vertebrae are still capable of moving, the fracture is *unstable* and thoughtless movement of the injured patient may intensify damage to the spinal cord. Missile injuries are caused by such objects as bullets or missiles, or may be caused by a stab wound.

Evidence of dysfunction of the spinal cord may not be permanent since it may be contributed to shortly after the injury by impaired axonal conduction, oedema or compression by extra-dural or subdural blood. The final outcome therefore depends on the severity of irreversible damage at the level of injury, where there are varying degrees of haemorrhagic necrosis. The affected cord is soft and swollen and there is

often a *traumatic haematomyelia*, which is a collection of blood within the cord. This often extends as a fusiform mass for some distance above and below the level of injury, usually in the posterior columns immediately dorsal to the central canal (Fig. 8.23). Reactive changes in the form of hyperplasia of astrocytes, microglia and blood vessels occur and the dead tissue is ultimately removed. If the spinal cord has been severely damaged it becomes greatly narrowed at the level of injury.

In a patient with traumatic paraplegia there is Wallerian degeneration (see Ch. 3) in ascending tracts above, and in descending tracts below, the level of injury. Immediately above the level of injury there is degeneration of virtually the entire posterior columns and the spinocerebellar tracts. Higher in the cord, however, because of the inflow of sensory fibres from posterior nerve roots above the level of the lesion, normal fibres will be found in the spinocerebellar tracts and in the lateral parts of the posterior columns (the cuneate tracts). The medially situated gracile tracts, however, remain devoid of myelin because there is very little admixture of nerve fibres in the posterior columns (Fig. 8.24). Below the damaged segment of the spinal cord there is descending degeneration in the crossed and uncrossed pyramidal tracts (Fig. 8.25). The latter end in the upper thoracic region but the crossed pyramidal tracts continue down the entire length of the

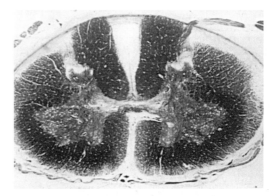

Fig. 8.24 Ascending degeneration in spinal cord. There is loss of myelin in the gracile and spinocerebellar tracts. The cuneate tracts are normal because of the inflow of nerve fibres above the lesion in the lumbar spinal cord. Cf Fig. 3.16b. (Myelin stain.)

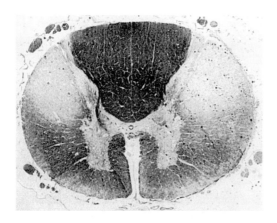

Fig. 8.25 Descending degeneration in spinal cord. There is loss of myelin in the corticospinal tracts below a lesion in the cervical spinal cord. Cf. Fig. 3.16a. (Myelin stain.)

spinal cord. Histological examination of the spinal cord at the level of the injury in long-standing paraplegia often discloses regenerative features in the form of proliferating Schwann cells and axons in the region of the posterior nerve roots.

A delayed – often many years after the accident – result of traumatic paraplegia is the development of *post-traumatic syringomyelia*. This takes the form of a centrally situated cystic cavity which may extend upwards or downwards from the damaged segment. The upward extension produces progressive damage to the cord and increases the patient's neurological disability.

Post-mortem procedures are difficult in this type of case and it is essential to remove a block of the vertebral column extending for at least two or three vertebrae above and below the level of the injury. This block should then be fixed. Thereafter a laminectomy can be done and the spinal cord removed from the vertebral canal, or the specimen can be cut with a band saw in the midline sagittal plane to demonstrate the damaged vertebrae and spinal cord (Fig. 8.23). In long-standing cases of traumatic paraplegia, the damaged segment of the cord may be densely adherent to bone as a result of the formation of scar tissue.

OTHER LESIONS AFFECTING THE SPINAL CORD

This is an appropriate place to summarize such lesions since the majority produce a *transverse lesion* which has many features in common with those produced by trauma, namely varying degrees of paraparesis, ranging from a mild weakness in the legs to paraplegia, and varying degrees of degeneration of long tracts above and below the level of damage to the spinal cord.

COMPRESSION OF THE SPINAL CORD

There are many and varied causes of spinal compression that have essentially similar clinical features affecting to some extent all functions of the spinal cord (motor, sensory and autonomic) below the level of compression, and pain or paraesthesiae and loss of function in the form, for example, of denervation atrophy of muscle at the level of the lesion. The damage to the spinal cord is often partial, leading to the syndrome of hemisection (Brown–Séquard syndrome), namely spastic weakness and loss of vibration and joint position on the same side as the lesion because of involvement of the ipsilateral crossed corticospinal tract and posterior column, whereas involvement of the crossed spinothalamic tract results in disturbances of pain and temperature sense on the opposite side. The clinical effects depend to a considerable extent on the rate of development of the compressive lesion: this may extend over many months, but some of the more rapidly expanding lesions can produce paraplegia within days. If the lesion becomes large enough, it will interfere with the blood supply to the cord at the level of the compression and, if surgery is delayed, there is frequently irreparable structural damage.

Many of the causes of compression of the spinal cord are dealt with in more detail in the appropriate chapters. The lesion may arise in the *vertebral column*, such as a prolapsed intervertebral disc (see below), whereas in patients with a severe kyphoscoliosis, increasing angulation of the vertebral column may interfere with the blood supply to the spinal cord at that level. The majority of lesions causing compression of the spinal cord, however, arise in the *spinal extradural space*, metastatic carcinoma and lymphoma, including myeloma, being the commonest. Other lesions are a subacute pyogenic abscess that is usually caused by staphylococci or coliform bacilli, extension of a tuberculous infection in a vertebral body into the extradural space, vascular malformations and tumours of mesenchymal origin. Spontaneous extradural haemorrhage is a recognized clinical entity but its pathogenesis is not clear. The commonest *intradural extramedullary lesions* are meningioma and schwannoma (Fig. 15.39). *Intramedullary* tumours within the spinal cord may have similar effects.

The structural abnormalities within the spinal cord will depend on the severity of the compression and, as indicated above, may amount to frank infarction. A peculiar histological feature seen in the spinal cord related to less severe compression is coarse vacuolation of white matter, the basic cause of which is not known.

'Transverse myelitis'

This is a clinical rather than a pathological term and is used to describe a transverse lesion in the spinal cord in the absence of a compressive lesion. Causes include infarction, demyelination, caisson disease, infection or haemorrhage (spontaneous haematomyelia).

PROLAPSED INTERVERTEBRAL DISC

This is a common occurrence. The central part of an intervertebral disc consists of soft fibrocartilage (the *nucleus pulposus*), and this is surrounded by a ring of much firmer fibrocartilage (the *annulus fibrosus*). As age advances the nucleus pulposus becomes progressively dehydrated and the annulus wider. The annulus is thicker anteriorly and this presumably accounts for the fact that most disc protrusions occur posteriorly.

A disc may prolapse acutely in an apparently normal spine as a result of sudden physical stress, but more frequently, it occurs secondary to degenerative disease. Most protrusions occur in the lumbar region, the discs most commonly affected being L5/S1 and L4/5. An acute disc prolapse may also occur in the cervical region. Most protrusions are posterolateral (Fig. 8.26a), affecting the related spinal nerve root. The rarer central protrusions are of greater importance

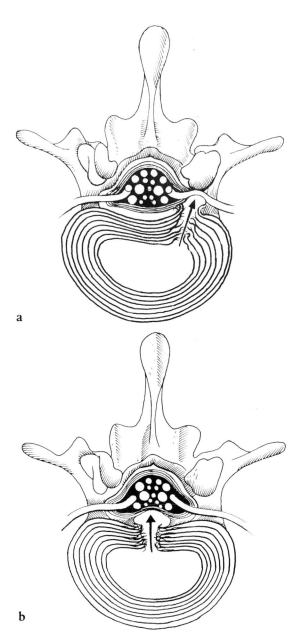

a

b

Fig. 8.26 Prolapsed intervertebral disc. (a) Posteroateral protrusion compressing a nerve. (b) Central protrusion compressing cauda equina.

since they compress the cauda equina (Fig. 8.26b), as a result of which there may be paraparesis and sphincter dysfunction.

Cervical spondylosis

This results from degeneration of intervertebral discs in the cervical region. The disc spaces are narrowed and transverse bars develop in the vertebral canal as a result of posterior protrusion of the annulus. There is also a reactive osteophytosis affecting the neurocentral joints and the intervertebral foramina, and thickening of intervertebral ligaments, leading to compression of nerve roots and fibrosis of the dural root sleeves. As the spondylosis progresses there may, in addition to compression of nerve roots, be interference with the blood supply to the spinal cord, where the vertebral canal is narrowest. There is considerable controversy about the importance of cervical spondylosis, since it can be demonstrated radiologically in some 50 per cent of adults over the age of 50, and in some 75 per cent over 65. It may be, therefore, that secondary ischaemic damage in the spinal cord – *cervical myelopathy* – occurs only in individuals with congenital narrowing of the vertebral canal. The *structural changes* in the spinal cord are a combination of focal infarction and subtotal degeneration of the lateral parts of the posterior columns secondary to damage to axons in the cervical posterior nerve roots. Congenital narrowing of the vertebral canal in the lumbar region – *lumbar stenosis* – may lead to compression of nerves in the cauda equina.

Other bony abnormalities that may affect the spinal cord

Basilar invagination

This is the term applied to abnormal protrusion of the tip of the odontoid process. It may be a developmental malformation but can also occur secondary to osteomalacia or rheumatoid arthritis. As the invagination progresses, the odontoid compresses the upper end of the cervical cord and the lower medulla.

Tuberculosis

Where tuberculosis is common, the vertebral column is not infrequently affected, usually in the midthoracic region. The cord may be com- pressed by granulation tissue within the extra- dural spinal space or as a result of angulation (kyphosis) of the spine.

Paget's disease

When Paget's disease affects the vertebral column there is often some degree of kyphosis, but of greater importance is a general reduction in the size of the vertebral canal leading to compression of the spinal cord.

SELECTIVE LESIONS IN NEUROSURGERY

There are several disease processes where clinical improvement can be achieved by the selective destruction of certain structures within the nervous system. As a result of improved drug treatment, however, these techniques are being used less than they were in the past.

One of the first techniques to be introduced was *prefrontal leucotomy* for patients with severe schizophrenia. The original procedure cut most fibres to and from the frontal poles and caused considerable destruction of brain tissue (Fig. 8.27). More restrictive procedures have now been devised that are directed more selectively at certain fibre tracts. *Thalamotomy* and *pallidotomy* are sometimes undertaken for certain movement disorders, including parkinsonism (Fig. 8.28), while *cordotomy*, which is aimed at destroying the spinothalamic fibres in the spinal cord, is some-

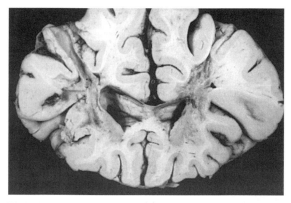

Fig. 8.27   Prefrontal leucotomy. There is considerable long-standing destruction of white matter in the frontal lobes.

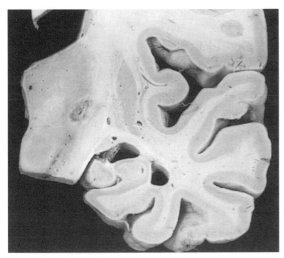

Fig. 8.28 Thalamotomy. There is a sharply defined lesion in the lateral nucleus of the thalamus.

times undertaken in patients with intractable pain. Various techniques are available to produce the brain damage, the commonest being heat or cold. The outcome is a sharply circumscribed focus of tissue destruction. Ultrasound also produces focal brain damage but has been little used in practice.

During the last decade evidence has accumulated that fetal neurons implanted into the brain of adult rats can re-establish damaged connections in the host brain and restore functions lost or damaged as a result of a preceding lesion. The intracerebral grafting of neural tissue has opened up the possibility that at least some types of neurons in the CNS may possibly be replaced by new implanted neuronal tissue. Such grafting techniques have particular relevance in the neurodegenerative disorders of Parkinson's disease and Huntington's disease. Although the possibility that dopaminergic neurons could be grafted to patients with Parkinson's disease has been discussed since the first reports of dopamine neuron grafting in rodents, there still remain many unanswered questions. In an attempt to overcome immunological rejection, and to avoid the ethical implications of using human fetal tissue, alternative sources of catecholamine-containing donor tissue have been sought by genetic engineers. There have already been a number of clinical trials with autografts of adrenal medulla

to the striatum in Parkinson's disease: these studies have shown that the grafting of human dopamine neurons to Parkinson's disease patients is not only feasible but, when used in association with nerve-growth factor, the graft is likely to survive and may result in some functional recovery.

TRAUMA BY NON-MECHANICAL FORCES

Radiotherapy is the mainstay of treatment of malignant brain tumours. The most important complications in the CNS result from the effects of ionizing radiation, and the concept that the human brain is resistant to the effect of therapeutic irradiation is no longer held. The type, frequency and extent of post-radiotherapy complications depend on many factors, which include the total dose of irradiation, the number of fractions, the dose per fraction, the total treatment time, the volume irradiated, the elimination of 'hot spots' by the use of multiple fields and the use of other treatments such as steroids, radiosensitizers or antineoplastic chemotherapy.

The main affect of irradiation on the tumour itself is to produce necrosis. This is particularly true for radiosensitive tumours such as pineal germinoma or lymphoma (see Ch. 15), where large fluid-filled cysts lined with scarred glial tissue can be found following treatment. With less radiosensitive tumours, including gliomas, extensive central necrosis may be produced although peripheral tumour may remain. Tumour irradiation may also lead to a change in tumour cytology. Typically, multinucleated giant cells with irregular hyperchromatic nuclei are found: the number of mitotic figures is reduced. The pathological affects of irradiation on the tumour blood vessels include thickening, hyalinization and occlusion of vessels, with proliferation of collagen in perivascular regions.

Irradiation can cause injury to *scalp and bone*. Although megavoltage irradiation is relatively skin-sparing, the exit dose to the skin must be considered. Skin erythema and hair loss are common. Hair loss may be patchy or extensive and may be permanent. The combination of irradiation with certain chemotherapeutic regimens may exacerbate skin reactions and can increase the risk of permanent hair loss. Necrosis of bone flaps is a potential risk but is not often a clinical problem, but impaired wound healing does occur.

The effects of irradiation upon normal brain

These have been studied according to the time of their manifestations: *acute reactions* occur during the course of irradiation; *early delayed reactions* appear a few weeks to 2–3 months later; and *late delayed reactions* appear from a few months to many years after irradiation. Acute reactions are usually minor with conventional doses and fractionation, particularly when steroids are used. They cause symptoms and signs of raised intracranial pressure. The reaction is dose-related and is probably due to increased oedema, and usually responds to an increase in the dose of steroids. Early delayed reactions are usually transient and disappear without treatment. The clinical features include lethargy, somnolence and an intensification of pre-existing symptoms and signs. Transient somnolence and lethargy has been reported in 80 per cent of children given 25 Gy whole-brain radiotherapy as a prophylactic treatment in acute lymphoblastic leukaemia; it has also been reported in adults given 1.8 Gy daily fractions to a total dose of 60 Gy. Very occasionally early delayed reaction may lead to the patient's death, neuropathological examination then revealing multiple small foci of demyelination with perivascular infiltration by lymphocytes and plasma cells. In some instances there is evidence of damage to blood vessels. The early delayed reaction probably results from injury to oligodendrocytes, the latent interval of clinical recovery being consistent with the time required for myelin replacement.

Late delayed reactions are caused either by diffuse damage to white matter accompanied by ventricular enlargement – a *leukoencephalopathy* – or as a space-occupying gliovascular reaction known as *radionecrosis*. These features tend to occur from about 1 year to many years after treatment, and may be delayed by up to 30 years. There are many reports of radionecrosis after irradiation of intracranial or extracranial tumours,

such as nasopharyngeal carcinoma, parotid carcinoma or basal-cell carcinoma of the scalp. The macroscopic appearances of radionecrosis are similar to those of a malignant glioma. The white matter is expanded and replaced by focally cystic waxy pale yellow tissue in which there may be petechial haemorrhages (Fig. 8.29). In long-standing cases the affected tissue becomes granular and is apt to crumble. Anatomical definition is blurred, but in the main grey matter is spared. Histologically, the process is characterized by appearances that range from coagulative necrosis around which there is no or minimal reactive change, to foci of demyelination, loss of axons and infiltration by lipid-containing macrophages, lymphocytes and plasma cells. The most important change, however, is fibrinoid necrosis and hyalinization of the walls of blood vessels (Fig. 8.30) and proliferation of endothelium, which may be sufficient to cause an obliterative endarteritis and thrombotic occlusion of small vessels. Additional features include the formation of telangiectatic vessels, the proliferation of perivascular fibroblasts, with the formation in some cases of large amounts of relatively acellular collagen, and an associated astrocytosis often with bizarre multinucleated cells. Similar changes may be seen in the spinal cord. Referred to as *radiation myelopathy*, this complication is said to occur in between 1 and 2 per cent of patients who have received irradiation in the corresponding region. Changes in the cerebellum, however, are of a different nature,

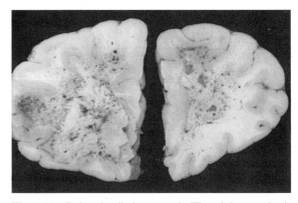

Fig. 8.29 Delayed radiation necrosis. There is haemorrhagic necrosis, mainly in the white matter, in the frontal lobes.

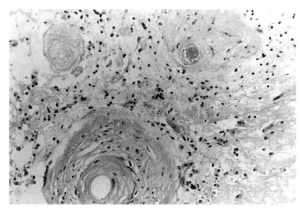

Fig. 8.30 Radionecrosis. There are striking changes in small blood vessels in the form of fibrinoid necrosis and endothelial proliferation. (H & E.)

the only feature consisting of the formation of small cysts in the Purkinje-cell layer of the cortex, with some loss of both Purkinje cells and granule cells with subsequent atrophy of folia, and demyelination and gliosis (Fig. 8.31). Eventually the Purkinje cells are replaced by a series of confluent cystic spaces associated with which there is exudation of fibrin which spreads readily along the molecular layer, hyaline thickening of the walls of blood vessels and focal calcification.

The pathogenesis of radionecrosis remains uncertain: vascular change, a direct effect of

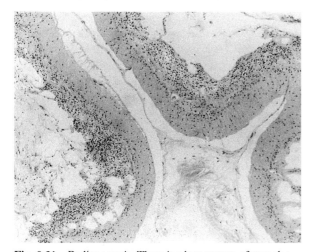

Fig. 8.31 Radionecrosis. There is a lacy pattern of vacuoles between the Purkinje cells and the granular neurons. There is associated atrophy of the folia, demyelination of the white matter and gliosis.

radiation on the glia and immunological mechanisms have all been proposed. The risks of developing radionecrosis are not clearly defined, although there is a general consensus that daily fractions of 1.8 –2 Gy to a total dose of 65–70 Gy would normally be well tolerated, although occasional cases of radiation necrosis will occur. In general the incidence of necrosis is progressively greater with high irradiation doses: below 57 Gy this complication is rarely seen; between 57 and 65 Gy it may develop in up to 3 per cent of patients; and above 65 Gy the incidence may be as high as 18–20 per cent.

A *diffuse leukoencephalopathy*, which may be necrotizing, is also associated with radiotherapy. Most of the reported cases have been treated simultaneously with various chemotherapeutic agents, and it is likely that this disease is primarily a complication of drug treatments. Intellectual deficits may follow irradiation in both children and adults, and various studies in children have suggested that low doses of about 25 Gy produce little or no intellectual disturbance, although mild psychomotor dysfunction and general slowing down may be seen. The complications of radiotherapy are greater in the developing brain, and radiotherapy to the CNS is usually delayed as long as possible in young children. Additional complications include *hypothalamopituitary dysfunction*, especially of growth hormone regulation. Other complications include blindness, which is thought to be secondary to demyelination in the visual pathways, and occasionally radiation-induced damage to both *large extracranial and intracranial arteries* has been described.

An interesting phenomenon is the *induction of brain tumours* as an uncommon complication of cerebral irradiation. The commonest examples are meningeal fibrosarcomas, which have generally been complications of irradiation of pituitary adenomas. Such complications have also been noted following low-dose irradiation for acute lymphocytic leukaemia. Meningiomas can also be induced either by a high dose of radiation for the treatment of intracranial tumours or following low-dose treatment of benign scalp disorders such as ringworm. An increasing number of children are surviving after radiotherapy for intracranial tumours. There have as a result been increasing numbers of reports of further neuroectodermal tumours developing in these children. Doses of radiation have been very wide, ranging from 1.5 to 60 Gy and the latency period has been 5–25 years. Most of these tumours are anaplastic astrocytoma or glioblastoma and have appeared within the first three decades of life.

Chemotherapy

Treatment with antineoplastic agents may be given as a primary treatment or, more commonly, as adjunctive therapy following surgery and/or radiotherapy. Factors that limit the effectiveness of chemotherapy on malignant brain tumours include drug access into the brain by virtue of the blood–brain barrier and low sensitivity to single-agent chemotherapy. However, the sensitivity of normal brain to chemotherapeutic agents is the cause of most complications in the CNS: these include an acute or chronic *encephalopathy* or *myelopathy* and an acute *cerebellar syndrome*. Complications in the CNS are usually due to a direct effect of the drug, although infection in the CNS may occur secondary to the leukopenic effect of treatment. Seizures may complicate treatment with any agent in sufficient dosage, but are most commonly seen with methotrexate, vincristine, nitrosoureas and cisplatin. An acute cerebellar syndrome has been described after treatment with 5-fluorouracil, procarbazine, BCNU and vincristine. The syndrome is reversible on stopping the drug. Pathologically there is loss of neurons in the olivary and dentate nuclei and in the granular layer of the cerebellum.

An *acute encephalopathy* may complicate the intravenous administration of many agents, and has been found in 40 per cent of patients treated with high doses of l-asparginase and 5-fluorouracil. Not uncommonly lethargy, confusion and hallucinations develop, and these are often reversible on stopping treatment, but progressive deterioration to coma and death has been described. A *chronic encephalopathy* has been described following methotrexate administration, and has since been recognized as a *disseminated necrotizing leukoencephalopathy*. The clinical onset is often insidious and may occur months or years after stopping treatment. The characteristic features are confusion, drowsiness, irritability, ataxia, tremor, seizures and dementia. The neuropathological features of this condition are well defined. Macroscopically, abnormalities tend to be limited to white matter, changes varying from grey-pink randomly distributed foci of necrosis to larger areas of creamy-white necrosis in which there may be petechial haemorrhage or cavitation, depending upon the survival time. The histological features are distinctive, comprising foci of disseminated coagulative necrosis that appear to be unrelated to blood vessels. There is loss of myelin, extensive damage to axons with bulb formation and astrocytosis, but all in the apparent absence of either an inflammatory cell or macrophage response. These changes may occur in the absence of any vascular damage: on the other hand, the features of irradiation with fibrinoid necrosis may be seen in the blood vessels in the larger lesions. In some instances the lesions may become chronic, when they are characterized by periventricular cavitation in the white matter, calcification in the centrum semi-ovale and compensatory enlargement of the ventricles. Is is now clear that this condition can be brought about by other treatment regimens. These include intra-arterial and intraventricular chemotherapy and chemotherapy plus opening of the blood–brain barrier.

Intrathecal or intraventricular methotrexate can cause a severe leukoencephalopathy characterized by demyelination and necrotizing lesions in the periventricular white matter bilaterally. Encephalopathies have also been described after intracarotid perfusion of other agents, such as BCNU. Other complications of antineoplastic agents include gliosis in white matter, diffuse cortical atrophy, sclerosis of the cerebellum, neuroaxonal dystrophy, peripheral neuropathy and spinal myelopathy.

FURTHER READING

Adams J H, Doyle D, Graham D I *et al.* (1985) The contusion index: a reappraisal in human and experimental non-missile head injury. *Neuropathology and Applied Neurobiology* **11**, 299–308.

Adams J H, Doyle D, Ford I *et al.* (1989) Diffuse axonal injury: definition, diagnosis and grading. *Histopathology* **15**, 49–59.

Adams J H & Graham D I (1984) Diffuse brain damage in non-missile head injury. In: *Recent advances in Histopathology*, 12. Edited by P P Anthony & R N M MacSween. Edinburgh: Churchill Livingstone, pp. 241–257.

Adams J H, Graham D I, Murray L S et al (1982) Diffuse axonal injury due to non-missile head injury in humans: an analysis of 45 cases. *Annals of Neurology* **12**, 557–563.

Becker D P & Povlishock J T (eds) (1985) *Central Nervous System Trauma Status Report 1985*. Washington, USA: NINCDS.

Cooper P R (ed) (1992) *Head Injury*, 3rd edn. Baltimore: Williams & Wilkins.

Gennarelli T A, Thibault L E, Adams J H *et al.* (1982) Diffuse axonal injury and traumatic coma in the primate. *Annals of Neurology* **12**, 564–574.

Jane J A, Anderson D K, Torner J C & Young W (eds) (1991) *Central Nervous System Trauma Status Report 1991*. Washington, USA: NINCDS.

Jennett B & Teasdale G (1981) *Management of Head Injuries*. Philadelphia: F A Davis.

9. Demyelinating diseases

These disorders of the CNS are characterized by the destruction of myelin with the relative preservation of axons, a process referred to as *periaxial demyelination*. They therefore differ from genetic disorders of myelin formation – *leukodystrophy (dysmyelination)* (see Ch. 10) – and from diseases causing breakdown of myelin due to destruction of neurons or their axons – *Wallerian degeneration* (see Ch. 3). The group of periaxial demyelinating diseases is further subdivided into *primary demyelination*, in which the demyelination is the only pathological process, and *secondary demyelination*, in which the demyelination is associated with another disease process. The former group is by far the more important and includes a spectrum that ranges from acute conditions – *acute disseminated (perivenous) encephalomyelitis* and *acute haemorrhagic leukoencephalitis* – to chronic disorders, the most important of which is *multiple (disseminated) sclerosis*. Demyelination in peripheral nerves is dealt with in Chapter 18.

Myelin in the CNS is formed by the modification and compaction of the cell membranes of interfascicular oligodendrocytes (see Ch. 3). Each oligodendrocyte gives rise to a number of processes, which form a segment of the myelin sheath of several axons. Primary demyelination may therefore be due to damage to the parent oligodendrocyte and its processes, damage to the myelin sheath *per se* or damage to both the oligodendrocyte and the myelin sheath. Minimal damage is therefore represented by periaxial demyelination limited to a single internode, in contrast to a lesion which involves many oligodendrocytes, when the result will be an area in which there is complete demyelination.

PRIMARY DEMYELINATION

Acute disseminated encephalomyelitis

This monophasic and generally self-limiting disease occurs mainly in older children and young adults after measles, mumps, chicken pox or rubella (postinfectious encephalitis). It is often of rapid onset, and develops about 4–14 days after the clinical onset of the initial infection. Recovery is generally good, but the condition is associated with a 10–20 per cent mortality following measles or rubella. There is also an association with upper respiratory tract infections, presumed to be viral in nature, and with primary vaccination against smallpox (post-vaccinial encephalitis) and antirabies inoculation. An association with pertussis vaccine remains controversial. The incidence of acute disseminated encephalomyelitis has been markedly reduced by changes in immunization programmes – the discontinuation of vaccination against smallpox and the institution of immunization against measles virus before the age of 2 years. Indeed, the condition is now most frequently seen after non-specific upper respiratory tract infections.

Pathology

The brain and spinal cord may look normal, or there may be some congestion and oedema. This contrasts with widespread histological changes in the white matter of the centrum semi-ovale, but also in the ventral half of the pons, in the deep layers of the cerebral cortex and in the thalami. In these areas there is cuffing of small blood vessels (probably venules) by inflammatory cells

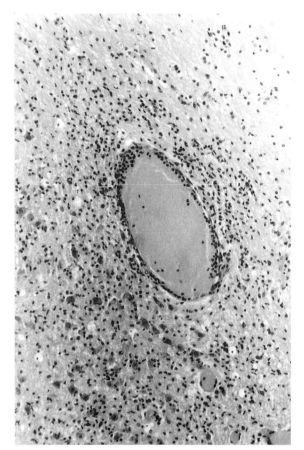

Fig. 9.1 Acute disseminated encephalomyelitis. There is a diffuse inflammatory process in which lymphocytes and some monocytes are seen around a small vessel (probably a venule) and white matter. (H & E.)

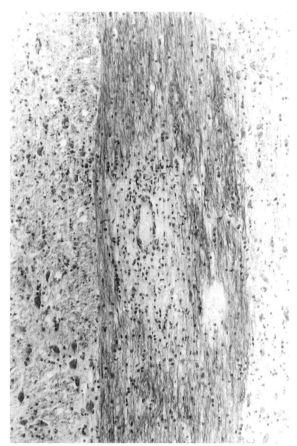

Fig. 9.2 Acute disseminated encephalomyelitis in the pons. There is perivascular demyelination. LFB/CV.

(Fig. 9.1) and perivenular demyelination (Fig. 9.2). Early in the disease neutrophil polymorphs are seen around small blood vessels, but these are soon replaced by lymphocytes and lipid-containing macrophages. With recovery, gliosis develops in the demyelinated areas and in all stages of the disease there is preservation of axons. Occasionally the demyelinating lesions become confluent, particularly in the spinal cord.

Aetiology

Because of the clinical similarities between acute disseminated perivenous encephalomyelitis and acute viral encephalitis, it was initially thought that both were due to the presence of virus in the CNS. However, the clinical course of the disease, the inability to isolate any virus consistently from the brain, and the appreciation that both the character and distribution of structural abnormalities are quite different in the two conditions, soon led to the conclusion that acute disseminated encephalomyelitis is not infectious in nature but represents a delayed hypersensitivity reaction. The possibility of an immune reaction against virus or virus-infected cells, however, cannot be ruled out completely. Either mechanism could produce damage by an associated immune response. Available evidence suggests that, as the condition complicates certain acute infections of childhood, vaccination and immunization procedures, and can be transferred to healthy animals by the injection of sensitized lymphocytes from an affected animal, the disease is due to autoallergy in which a host-mediated response is directed against antigen in the CNS.

Acute haemorrhagic leukoencephalitis

This disease is a distinct clinical and pathological entity characterized by a rapid and dramatic onset, a short clinical course and, usually, a fatal outcome. Most cases arise as a sequel to any one of several possible viral infections, and some have been described in association with diseases presumed to be autoallergic, e.g. thrombotic thrombocytopenic purpura, acute glomerulonephritis and asthma. It may also occur after sensitization to drugs, e.g. sulphonamides and oxyphenarsine, and has also occurred after pertussis immunization and the administration of antitetanus serum. More recently, it has been shown to complicate septic shock.

Pathology

The brain is swollen and there are multiple petechial haemorrhages, particularly in the white matter (Fig. 9.3a). The petechiae may become confluent to produce extensive and sometimes quite sharply defined haemorrhagic areas (Fig. 9.3b), and they may also occur to a lesser extent in the cerebral cortex, the basal ganglia, the brain stem and the cerebellum. Histologically, the condition is characterized by necrosis of blood vessel walls and exudation of fibrin into and through the vessel walls into their perivascular spaces (most of these blood vessels appear to be venules); perivascular 'oedema' which tends to become confluent and to affect fairly large areas of the white matter; infiltration of the abnormal areas by neutrophil polymorphs in the early stages, and later by monocytes and lymphocytes, zones of perivascular demyelination which, in cases of short survival, are associated with enlarged microglial cells and in the later stages with lipid-containing macrophages; and ball and ring haemorrhages, some of which are related to necrotic blood vessels (Figs 9.4a and b). Because of the severity of the vascular lesions, microinfarction is a common sequel.

Aetiology

Although the aetiology is unknown, the condition is thought to be a hyperacute variant of acute disseminated encephalomyelitis and to be caused by the deposition of immune complexes and the activation of complement. It seems likely that both conditions have an allergic basis and form part of a pathological continuum. Corroborative evidence for this is obtained from the animal model of experimental allergic encephalomyelitis (see below) and in the kidneys of patients dying from acute haemorrhagic leukoencephalitis complicating Gram-negative septicaemia in the form of

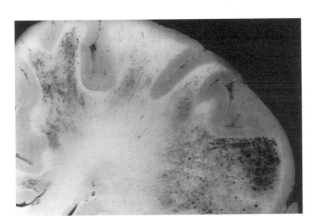

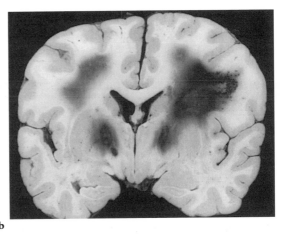

a   b

Fig. 9.3 Acute haemorrhagic leukoencephalitis. (a) There are numerous petechial haemorrhages, mainly in white matter. (b) There are confluent petechial haemorrhages in the deep white matter including the internal capsules, and in the lentiform nuclei.

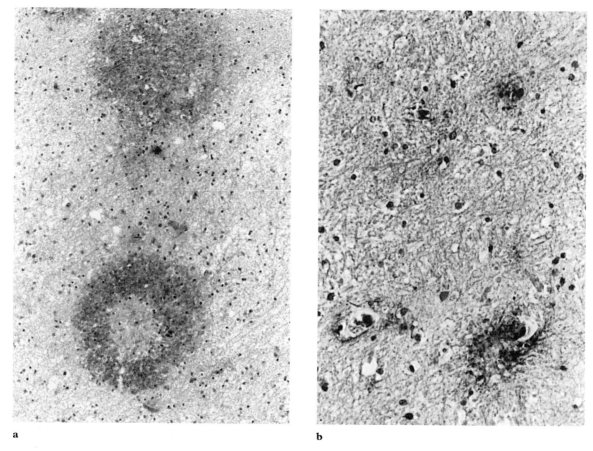

a   b

Fig. 9.4 Acute haemorrhagic leukoencephalitis. (a) Ring and ball haemorrhages. (b) Small blood vessels in which there is fibrinoid necrosis. ((a) H & E; (b) Martius scarlet blue.)

disseminated intravascular coagulation with tubular necrosis and, in some, appearances indistinguishable from membranoproliferative glomerulonephritis.

Multiple (disseminated) sclerosis

This is the most common of the primary demyelinating diseases. Its incidence varies with latitude, ranging from 30 per 100 000 in a band of high frequency that girdles the earth between the 40th and 60th parallels, to less than 10 per 100 000 in lower latitudes. The disease virtually disappears at the equator. These gradients occur both north and south of the equator. Very high prevalence rates have been found in the Orkney and Shetland Islands (about 300 and 180 per 100 000 respectively). It is more common in

women than men, and its incidence increases from early adolescence, with a peak in the third and fourth decades. Few cases occur after the age of 60. It is a chronic disease, and in its classic form is characterized by relapses and remissions, and about two-thirds of patients ultimately show continuous deterioration. The early symptoms are usually those of focal lesions in the CNS or in the optic nerves (optic neuritis), whereas the later clinical picture is often one of progressive neurological deterioration, often with ataxic paraplegia. Cognitive function may be impaired in the late stages of the disease. With improved nursing care and antibiotics many patients have a full lifespan, despite severe disability.

The exact basis of the clinical symptomatology is not fully understood. Many can be explained in anatomical terms but the cause of the remitting/ relapsing nature of the disease and the fluctuations of symptoms and signs is obscure. Experimental and clinical work using conduction studies and MRI confirms the importance of demyelination as a cause of the symptoms. It is, however, difficult to explain why a plaque in the region of the entry of the sensory root of the Vth cranial nerve should cause pain, in contrast to the apparent lack of symptoms and signs as a result of the many lesions that are often found around the ventricles. There is no doubt that reversible neurological deficits may be caused by secondary phenomena such as breakdown of the blood-brain barrier, oedema, perivascular inflammation and astrocytosis.

Pathology

The principal feature is that of foci of demyelination (*plaques*) irregularly distributed throughout the brain and spinal cord. In patients who die after a short clinical history or in relapse, *acute* plaques appear as well defined yellowish-white soft lesions (Fig. 9.5) in which there is histological evidence of periaxial demyelination, as shown by destruction of myelin, the presence of lipid-containing macrophages and the preservation of axons. Oligodendrocytes are greatly reduced in number, and there is often cuffing of blood vessels within the plaque by lymphocytes, plasma cells and macro-

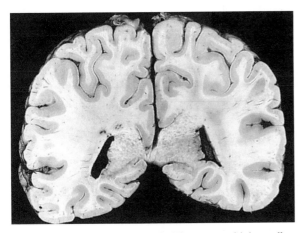

Fig. 9.5 Acute multiple sclerosis. There are multiple small areas of grey discoloration in the splenium of the corpus callosum.

phages (Fig. 9.6a & b). Immunohistochemical techniques have shown that the majority of the lymphocytes are T cells and that the plasma cells contain immunoglobulin. The macrophages play an active role in both the stripping of myelin from the intact axons and the phagocytosis of the myelin debris.

In *chronic* multiple sclerosis, which is the common type encountered in clinical practice, there are firm grey and slightly translucent lesions ranging from 2 to 10 mm in diameter throughout the CNS. Large subpial plaques in the brain stem – particularly the pons – and in the spinal cord may produce a grey translucent indrawing of the overlying pia-arachnoid, such that it is sometimes possible to make the diagnosis before dissection of the brain (Fig. 9.7). On the other hand, quite large plaques within the brain stem and the spinal cord may only be identifiable histologically. Some 75 per cent of the plaques occur in the deep white matter, some 5 per cent in the cortical mantle, and the remainder at either the junction between cortex and white matter or in the deep grey matter. Within the cerebral hemispheres a characteristic situation is adjacent to the ventricles, either at the dorsal angles of the bodies of the lateral ventricles (Fig. 9.8) or in relation to the frontal, temporal or occipital horns. Plaques also occur in the optic nerves (Fig. 9.9a), in the brain stem (Fig. 9.9b), particularly in relation to the aqueduct, and in the cervical portion of the spinal cord (Fig. 9.9c). In some patients these sites are selectively affected, there being none or only a few plaques within the cerebral hemispheres. Plaques are irregularly distributed and are not limited to particular fibre tracts or vascular territories.

On histological examination, *chronic* plaques appear as sharply defined areas of demyelination. The plaque may be centred on a small blood vessel (usually a venule). If it involves grey matter, neurons within the demyelinated area are preserved. This contrasts with an infarct, where there is loss of neurons and myelin. Oligodendroglia are reduced in number. In relatively recent plaques there are many large fibrillary astrocytes, but in old plaques there is simply a dense network of astrocytic fibres. The edges of the plaque are usually well demarcated because of the complete demyelination. There may, however, be a transition between complete loss of

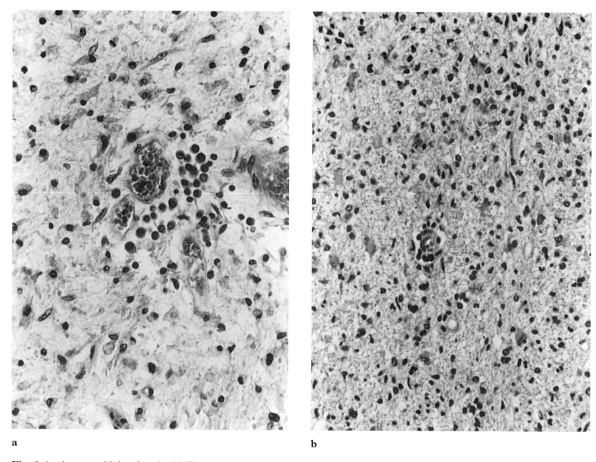

a   b

Fig. 9.6   Acute multiple sclerosis. (a) There is perivascular cuffing by lymphocytes and plasma cells. (b) In the foci of demyelination there are lipid-containing macrophages and reactive astrocytes. (H & E.)

myelin and normal myelination (shadow plaque), an appearance that has been attributed to a mixture of normally myelinated, demyelinated and remyelinated fibres. Apart from occasional perivascular lymphocytes, inflammatory cells are absent. Occasionally, there is histological evidence of both active and inactive demyelination *post mortem*, so that a whole spectrum of change may be seen that ranges from the inflammatory infiltration of the active phase, through subacute (where there is evidence of demyelination and residual mild inflammatory cell infiltration) to chronic plaques. Although axons are normally preserved within plaques, they may ultimately be destroyed if they are affected at several levels, particularly in the spinal cord. Commonly, therefore, in long-standing cases, there is ultimately Wallerian

degeneration in ascending and descending tracts within the spinal cord.

Electron microscopy has confirmed the importance of macrophages in the uptake and degradation of myelin, but has not resolved what constitutes the initial process involved in the breakdown of myelin.

Diagnosis

This can only be confirmed beyond doubt at autopsy, as there is no single laboratory test on which a definitive diagnosis can be established. However, by combining the clinical features, various electrophysiological studies and examination of the CSF, the diagnosis of multiple sclerosis can be achieved with varying degrees of certainty

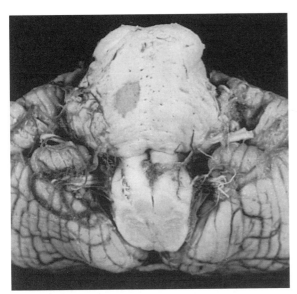

Fig. 9.7 Chronic multiple sclerosis. The leptomeninges have been removed to reveal a well-defined grey plaque in the pons.

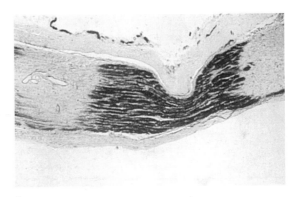

a

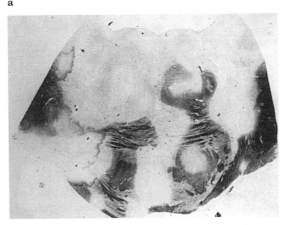

b

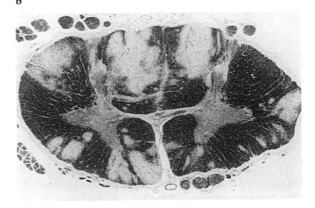

c

Fig. 9.9 Chronic multiple sclerosis. (a) Two plaques are seen in the optic nerve. (b) There are large and small plaques in the pons. (c) There are multiple plaques in the spinal cord. ((a), (b) and (c) Luxol fast blue/cresyl violet.)

that range from possible or probable to definite. Thus, the presence of clinically silent lesions may be suggested if conduction times with evoked responses are increased: high-resolution CT and MRI scanning of the brain and spinal cord may help in the identification of plaques, and in the majority of patients with multiple sclerosis there is an increase in the γ-globulin/albumin ratio and

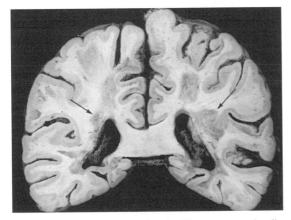

Fig. 9.8 Chronic multiple sclerosis. There are several well-defined grey plaques of demyelination (arrows) adjacent to the ventricles. Smaller areas of demyelination are present in the digitate white matter and at the corticomedullary junction.

oligoclonal bands of γ-globulin when CSF is examined by electrophoresis on agarose or polyacrylamide. Although oligoclonal bands are not specific to multiple sclerosis (they are present in other diseases such as subacute sclerosing panencephalitis and neurosyphilis) they are present in 85–95 per cent of patients with definite multiple sclerosis. With rare exceptions these immunoglobulin bands are IgG. Destruction of white matter releases myelin basic protein into the CSF of patients with multiple sclerosis, but this is also seen in patients with other disorders, such as 'stroke' and following trauma.

Aetiology

Many events may immediately precede the onset of the disease and have been considered as precipitating factors, although their mode of action is not known. These include viral infections, surgical operations and the extraction of teeth. Both genetic and environmental factors appear to be of importance. Thus, genetic factors may provide an explanation as to why multiple sclerosis is common in the temperate latitudes of northern Europe but is uncommon in Japan. Furthermore, Caucasian patients with multiple sclerosis have a higher proportion of histocompatibility types HLA–A3, B7, DW2, DR2 than the normal population, and these types tend to be more common within the ethnic groups living at higher latitudes. However, the HLA associations are different in patients with multiple sclerosis from other parts of the world. Twin studies have shown that the risk of developing multiple sclerosis for a patient's monozygotic twin is 533 times that of the normal population, and for a dizygotic twin 259 times. These findings are again suggestive of a genetic background, but one that is not sufficient to produce the disease.

Epidemiological studies on individuals migrating from areas of high incidence to areas of low incidence suggest that an environmental factor interacting with genetic factors may be important. Thus, people born in low latitudes appear to carry their lower attack rate with them if they move to higher latitudes after the age of 15. Conversely, people migrating after the age of 15 from northern Europe to, for example, South Africa and Israel, retain the high risk of their country of origin, whereas those leaving at a younger age seem to be relatively protected. There is also a 15–20 times increased incidence of multiple sclerosis in the families of patients with the disease, but it is not known whether this is attributable to genetic or

environmental factors, or to a combination of both. Another epidemiological observation suggests that an environmental agent is involved in the pathogenesis of multiple sclerosis. Before the Second World War, multiple sclerosis was virtually unknown in the sparsely populated and largely isolated Faroe Islands. After the war, multiple sclerosis is alleged to have become quite common on the islands, this outbreak being attributed to the occupation by British troops or to the introduction of dogs on to the islands.

Although these studies might suggest an infective aetiology, there is no convincing evidence yet for this theory. Multiple sclerosis has not been transferred to experimental animals by inoculation of serum, CSF or brain tissue, and no viral agent has been consistently isolated from the brain tissue of patients with multiple sclerosis, although virus-like particles have been identified by electron microscopy in such tissue. It is possible that with DNA viral probes a virus may yet be identified, particularly as many studies have demonstrated an increased titre of antibodies (particularly to measles, and less consistently to vaccinia, rubella and herpes simplex) in the sera of patients with multiple sclerosis. The recent demonstration of antibodies to the retrovirus HTLV–1 in patients with tropical spastic paraparesis has raised the possibility that a retrovirus might be implicated in multiple sclerosis. However, there is no evidence of a common aetiology. The meaning of these increased titres is not clear, but it may well be that a non-specific, increased B-cell response explains the antibody titres, although the possibility of continual stimulation due to viral persistence cannot be excluded as it has not been possible to relate the specific antibodies to the oligoclonal bands of immunoglobulin in the CSF. It is also pertinent to note that the disease does not resemble any known persistent or slow virus infection of the CNS in man or animals (see Ch. 7). The concepts of viral persistence, latency and reactivation are of possible significance and could explain the viral antibody response and the relapsing/remitting nature of the disease. With the advent of viral molecular techniques in future studies, it should be possible to determine whether or not viral genomic sequences are present.

Interactions between viruses and the immune

system are complex, and genetically determined host factors and the viral genome are of importance. Genetic background and immune function must therefore be taken into account.

There is considerable evidence now for an immune reaction in the pathology of multiple sclerosis. Certainly the presence of lymphocytes and plasma cells in acute plaques is in keeping with such a theory, and recent work has shown that in patients with acute attacks of multiple sclerosis there is a marked decline in the activity of suppressor T cells in the peripheral blood, the activity rising again after an attack. Multiple sclerosis may therefore be a disorder of immune regulation, the loss of suppressor cells permitting autoimmune reactions that would ordinarily be suppressed. In support of an autoimmune aetiology, antibodies, which together with complement cause demyelination of cultures of neural tissue, have been detected in the serum of patients with multiple sclerosis, but such antibodies have also been found in various non-demyelinating diseases. In spite of considerable effort, the antigen(s) under immune attack is not yet known. One suggestion is that some patients with multiple sclerosis have an increased cell-mediated immunity against myelin basic protein. This might perhaps have been anticipated, as it is still not known whether the target containing the antigen is the oligodendrocyte or the myelin sheath, or a combination.

Experimental autoallergic encephalomyelitis (EAE)

This is a condition that has been extensively studied as a potential model for multiple sclerosis. It can be produced in various species of animal by the injection of brain extract or myelin basic protein of the same or a different species, emulsified in Freund's adjuvant. The disease develops some 8–10 days later and is thought to be due to the development of an immune response to antigens from the CNS in the inoculum and a subsequent immunological reaction with the animal's own CNS. Although the role of antibody is unclear, there is good evidence that the lesions result from a delayed autohypersensitivity reaction in which sensitized lymphocytes and possibly macrophages act directly with the antigenic component of myelin.

Within species, different strains of animal show a marked variation in susceptibility to EAE. For example, strain 13 guinea pigs are highly susceptible to EAE, whereas strain 2 are comparatively resistant. Similarly, Lewis rats are highly susceptible whereas Brown Norwegian rats are resistant.

In some species the pathological changes are similar to those of acute disseminated encephalomyelitis in man (see p. 157) and may be caused by a similar immunological reaction. Acute perivenous encephalomyelitis and EAE are, however, monophasic illnesses, whereas multiple sclerosis is essentially a chronic relapsing condition. Nevertheless, the analogy between EAE and multiple sclerosis has become greater with the development of chronic models of EAE. Recently a relapsing and remitting form of EAE has been produced in strain 13 guinea pigs and SJL mice by the inoculation of autologous spinal cord homogenized in complete Freund's adjuvant. This disease shares many histological and clinical features with multiple sclerosis and, in the future, should prove very useful in the better understanding of immune-mediated demyelination.

Variants of multiple sclerosis

These include *sudanophilic diffuse sclerosis, neuromyelitis optica (Devic's disease)* and *Balo's disease (concentric sclerosis)*.

Sudanophilic diffuse sclerosis

This uncommon condition is not to be confused with a *leukodystrophy* (see Ch. 10), as the disorder is not one of abnormal formation of myelin but one in which extensive demyelination occurs in apparently normally formed myelin. The brain may be somewhat atrophic, and there is widespread symmetrical loss of myelin in the central portions of each cerebral hemisphere, particularly in the occipital lobes (hence the common occurrence of early visual impairment), but any part of the cerebral hemispheres, the cerebellum or brain stem may be affected (Fig. 9.10). Characteristically, however, there is preservation of the subcortical U-fibres, which stand out as a conspicuous white band in the affected areas. In addition to the diffuse demyelination, there are usually also well-defined

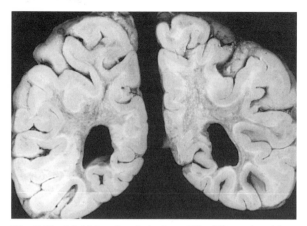

Fig. 9.10   Multiple sclerosis (sudanophilic diffuse sclerosis). There is extensive demyelination in the deep white matter of the occipital lobes, with characteristic preservation of subcortical 'U' fibres.

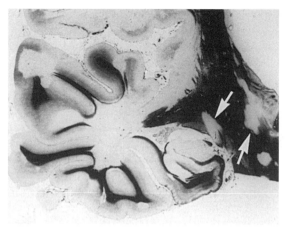

Fig. 9.11   Multiple sclerosis (sudanophilic diffuse sclerosis). In addition to the diffuse demyelination there are several well defined plaques typical of chronic multiple sclerosis (arrows). Celloidin, Heidenhain for myelin.

plaques typical of multiple sclerosis, i.e. cases are encountered that appear to be transitional between classic multiple sclerosis and this condition (Fig. 9.11). Within the affected areas there are many sudanophilic lipid-containing macrophages, some loss of axons and a reactive astrocytosis. Inflammation is not a feature.

Neuromyelitis optica (Devic's disease)

This is an acute illness of adults, presenting with blindness and paraplegia due to demyelination of the optic nerves and the spinal cord: death occurs in 50 per cent of patients within months, whereas in the remainder there may be complete or partial recovery. This condition is relatively rare in northern Europe and North America, being more common in the Far East. Although the constellation of signs and symptoms may be due to a variety of disease processes, such as syphilis or systemic lupus erythematosus, the term neuromyelitis optica is restricted to cases due to rapid demyelination, often combined with acute disseminated encephalo-myelitis or multiple sclerosis.

At autopsy there is partial or complete demyelination of the optic nerves and spinal cord. With survival the cord – most often the upper dorsal segments – is thinned and there is marked gliosis and thickening of the meninges. Demyelination by Schwann cells is often seen in the posterior root entry zone.

Concentric sclerosis (Balo's disease)

This rare form of multiple sclerosis is characterized by plaques in the white matter formed by alternating concentric rings of myelinated and demyelinated tissue. Of variable size, the lesions may be found in the deep white matter of the cerebral hemispheres, but also in the brain stem. The significance of this pattern of demyelination is not known. In some cases, concentric sclerosis is found in association with neuromyelitis optica.

SECONDARY DEMYELINATION

There are a number of systemic conditions and intoxications that produce demyelination with relative preservation of axons and neurons.

Central pontine myelinolysis

This condition usually occurs in middle-aged patients who are alcoholic, chronically debilitated or malnourished. It has also been described in association with cirrhosis of the liver, uraemia, leukaemia and chronic lung disease. It is characterized by symmetrical demyelination in the central portion of the pons, impinging on the tegmentum but not reaching the pial or ventricular surfaces (Fig. 9.12). Histologically there is a sharply defined

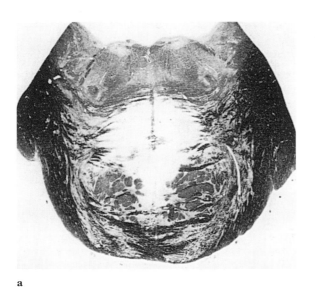
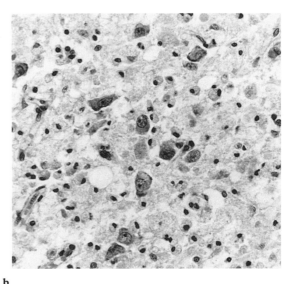

a   b

Fig. 9.12   Central pontine myelinolysis. (a) There is a centrally placed symmetrical area of demyelination in the pons. (b) Same case to show sparing of neurons in the demyelinated region. ((a) Luxol fast blue/cresyl violet; (b) H & E.)

area of loss of myelin, in which there is preservation of neurons and axons, thus distinguishing the condition from an infarct in the pons. Its aetiology is not known, but is thought to be related to a metabolic disturbance involving a fluid – electrolyte imbalance. In particular there appears to be a strong association with hyponatraemia, and it has been suggested that demyelination is caused by the too-rapid therapeutic correction of the plasma sodium to normal levels. This view is supported by experimental evidence in which demyelination has been induced in laboratory animals following rapid correction of hyponatraemia.

Marchiafava-Bignami disease

This is condition in which there is demyelination of the central portions of the corpus callosum and often of the anterior and hippocampal commissures. It was first described in chronically alcoholic Italian men who drank crude red wine. Cases have now been described, however, in non-Italians, females and in alcoholics with a preference for other than red wine. The features of Wernicke's encephalopathy (see p. 191) and pellagra may be present. Histologically, the appearances range from periaxial demyelination to cavitating lesions

in which there is loss of myelin, oligodendrocytes and axons. The aetiology is not known, but the condition is usually associated with alcoholism and malnutrition. Not all cases, however, have a history of alcohol abuse. Similar lesions can be produced by chronic cyanide and chronic methyl alcohol intoxication.

Toxic demyelination

Demyelination with relative preservation of axons may be produced by various agents, such as *hexachlorophane, tin* and *cuprizone*.

Carbon monoxide myelinopathy

The clinical signs and symptoms of carbon monoxide poisoning are most commonly due to hypoxic damage to grey matter (see Ch. 5). In some patients, however, who often appear to have recovered from the acute episode, there is progressive clinical deterioration some days to a week or so later. In these cases the most conspicuous feature is demyelination, which may be either focal and perivascular, or more generalized with a butterfly-like distribution across the corpus callosum. The pathogenesis of the demyelination is not known, but many studies have stressed the importance of systemic circulatory factors and have attributed the demyelination to a combination of the cytotoxic effect of carbon monoxide and a moderate reduction in cerebral blood flow.

Virus diseases

Demyelination is a feature of certain viral diseases such as *progressive multifocal leukoencephalopathy* (see p. 116) and *subacute sclerosing panencephalitis* (see p. 114).

FURTHER READING

Adams C W M (1989) *A Colour Atlas of Multiple Sclerosis and other Myelin Disorders*. London: Wolfe Medical.
Blakemore W F (1982) Myelination, demyelination and remyelination in the CNS. In: *Recent Advances in Neuropathology*, Vol 2. Edited by W T Smith & J B Cavanagh. London: Churchill Livingstone, pp. 53–81.
Hallpike J F (1990) Animal models of demyelination. *Current Opinion in Neurology and Neurosurgery* 3, 218–222.
Kermode A G, Thompson A J, Tofts P *et al.* (1990)

Breakdown of the blood–brain barrier precedes symptoms and other MRI signs of new lesions in multiple sclerosis. *Brain* **113**, 1477–1489.
Mathews W B (ed) (1991) *McAlpine's Multiple Sclerosis*. Edinburgh: Churchill Livingstone.
Raine C S (1990) Demyelinating diseases. In: *Textbook of Neuropathology*, 2nd edn. Edited by R L Davis & D M Robertson. Baltimore: Williams and Wilkins, pp. 535–620.

10. Metabolic disorders

Although uncommon, *primary (inherited) metabolic diseases* make a considerable contribution to morbidity and mortality in children. Many are inherited as autosomal recessive diseases, although in a few there is X-linked recessive inheritance. Inherited metabolic defects involve many substances, e.g. lipids, carbohydrates, mucopolysaccharides, amino acids and trace metals. Depending on the particular disease, structural changes may or may not be present in the CNS and, although the onset of clinical symptoms may not become apparent until adult life, the majority appear during childhood and frequently in the first few days of life.

The metabolic complexity of the CNS makes it dependent upon the functional integrity of other systems in the body for the adequate provision of essential nutrients and hormones, the maintenance of proper electrolyte and pH status and the elimination of potential toxins. It is therefore not surprising that various *metabolic* effects on the nervous system are *secondary* to systemic disease. In many instances the clinical features are reversible and there are minimal morphological changes, both occurrences supporting the belief that many of the disorders are attributable to biochemical derangement rather than a structural abnormality. It is only when the metabolic disorder has been profound and prolonged that structural changes occur, thus accounting for the permanent clinical neurological deficits that some of these patients manifest. Such secondary (acquired) CNS manifestations of systemic disease occur at all ages.

INHERITED METABOLIC DISEASE

Many of these disorders are due to deficiencies of particular *lysosomal enzymes*, which play an essential role in the degradation of various normal metabolites or the breakdown products of cells. As a result the undegraded material accumulates in, and causes enlargement of, the lysosomes of certain cells. The distribution of structural abnormalities depends on the particular enzyme deficiency, some of the disorders affecting the CNS, others the peripheral nervous system or muscle and others both the nervous system and visceral organs such as liver, spleen and lymph nodes. The affected cells become enlarged and have a ballooned appearance (Fig. 10.1) – hence the previous term of neuronal storage disorders. The stored material can be detected histochemically: frozen sections are essential because lipids dissolve in alcohols and mucopolysaccharides in water. The stains required include Oil red O and Sudan black B for lipids; Luxol fast blue, which is traditionally regarded as a stain for complex lipids; PAS with and without diastase for glycogen and other carbohydrate-containing constituents; toluidine blue or acidified cresyl violet for metachromatic leukodystrophy; and toluidine blue for mucopolysaccharides. A range of histochemical techniques, both non-specific and highly specific, is now available for the identification of the stored materials. It is, however, often necessary to correlate the histochemical findings with the clinical and morphological features in order to identify a clinicopathological pattern of a particular disease. In many instances, the precise diagnosis can be made on a block of unfixed tissue frozen for biochemical analysis, including thin-layer and gas-liquid chromatography, and enzyme assays. Electron microscopy is also essential since this will demonstrate grossly enlarged lysosomes

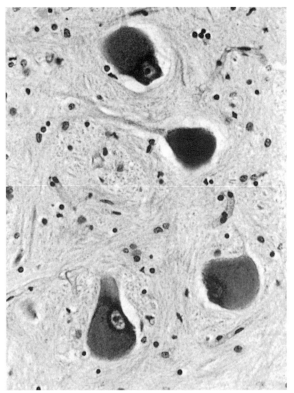

Fig. 10.1 Mucopolysaccharidosis. The neurons are greatly distended by stored material. (PAS.)

containing non-metabolizable residue. At one stage it was considered that the distinctive ultra-structural features of some disorders were such that morphology could be used to diagnose a specific disorder: this is now known not to be so.

It is generally agreed that there are racial differences in the incidence of certain forms of mental retardation and, in particular, that Tay–Sachs' and Niemann–Pick disease and the adult form of Gaucher's disease are more common in Jews than in non-Jews. Although reservations have been expressed about the validity of this in view of the genetic heterogeneity of 'Jews' and the probability that the incidence of these disorders has been underestimated in Gentiles, there is now considerable evidence that these disorders are more common among patients with Ashkenazi Jewish ancestry. For example, as determined by enzyme assay, the carrier rate of Tay–Sachs' disease is about 1 in 30 in Ashkenazi Jews, compared with a frequency of about 1 in 300 in other races.

The metabolic disease leads first to dysfunction but the affected cells often ultimately die, and in many of the conditions that affect the CNS there is atrophy of the brain, with gliosis in grey and white matter; on the other hand, there may be megalencephaly, as in the early stages of Tay–Sachs' disease. In Tay–Sachs' and Niemann–Pick disease the immediate postnatal course is often normal, but in the first 12 months the infant fails to thrive, there is retardation or progressive deterioration of mental and motor functions, spastic or flaccid paralysis, epilepsy and ultimately coma and death. The affected children often develop a cherry-red spot in the retina because the photo-receptors (cone cells) of the macula die, leaving a defect in the retina through which the choroid is visible.

Many of the diseases can be diagnosed by assay of lysosomal enzymes in blood, urine, leuco-cytes, amniotic fluid and cultured skin fibroblasts. Histological examination of bone marrow, liver, rectum, muscle, peripheral nerve or brain may, however, be required to establish the diagnosis.

With the appreciation that enzymes are not usually specific for a single substance, the lyso-somal theory of storage disorders has been modified. It is now recognized that the concept of a single enzyme defect requires to be modified, in that defective enzyme activity may result from a variety of causes, each having its own individual genetic control.

LYSOSOMAL DISORDERS

DISORDERS OF LIPID METABOLISM

Principal among these are the *sphingolipidoses* (with abnormalities of ganglioside, cerebroside, sulphatide, sphingomyelin and ceramide metabolism) and *Batten's disease* (neuronal ceroid-lipofuscinoses – Table 10.1).

The sphingolipidoses

This is probably the most important group of metabolic disorders that affects the nervous system. The sphingolipids include gangliosides, cerebrosides, sulphatides and sphingomyelins, all of which are important constituents of the normal cell. The interrelationship between lipid com-

Table 10.1 Principal lysosomal disorders

Disorder	Enzyme defect	Disorders of lipid metabolism	
		Substances stored	Staining methods and other tests
Sphingolipidoses			
GM1-gangliosidosis (two types)	β-galactosidase	GM1-ganglioside oligosaccharides ceramide tetrahexoside	PAS; β-galactosidase; LFB; TLC; EM
GM2-gangliosidosis (several types including Tay–Sachs' and Sandhoff)	hexosaminidases	GM2-ganglioside ceramide trihexoside	PAS; LFB; TLC; EM
Cerebrosidosis (Gaucher's disease (3 types))	β-glucocerebrosidase	glucocerebroside	PAS; TLC; EM
Sphingomyelinosis (Neimann–Pick) groups 1 and 2	sphingomyelinase (in group 1 only)	sphingomyelin, cholesterol	PAS; Sudan black B; acid haematein; TLC; EM
Batten's disease (neuronal ceroid lipofuscinosis)	not known	lipofuscin-like substances	PAS; Sudan black B; autofluorescence; EM
		Disorders of glycosaminoglycan metabolism	
Mucopolysaccharidoses			
Hurler (MPSI-IH)	α-L-iduronidase	acid mucopolysaccharides (heparan sulphate, chondroitin sulphate, keratan sulphate and several gangliosides)	Toluidine blue; PAS; LFB; Sudan black B; EM
Hunter (MPS II)	sulphoiduronate sulphatase		
Sanfilippo (MPS III) (4 types)	various		
Morquio (MPS IV) (2 types)	various		

PAS = Periodic acid–Schiff; LFB = Luxol fast blue; EM = electron microscopy; TLC = Thin-layer chromatography
(Reproduced in modified form with permission of author and publisher from Lake, B. D., Metabolic disorders of the central and peripheral nervous system. In: *Histochemistry in Pathology*. Eds. M. I. Filipe & B. D. Lake. Edinburgh: Churchill Livingstone, 1983, pp. 53–69.)

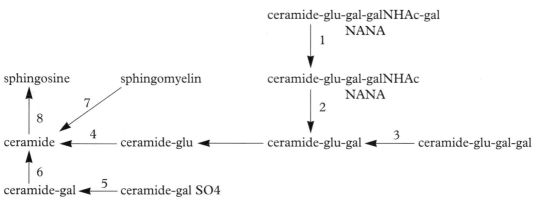

Fig. 10.2 Interrelations between lipid components and enzyme deficiencies in the lipid storage diseases.
1. β-galactosidase; G_M-gangliosidosis. 2. β-hexosaminidase A; G_{M2} gangliosidosis (Tay–Sachs'); 3. α-galactosidase; Fabry; 4. β-glucocerebrosidase; Gaucher; 5. arylsulphatase A; metachromatic leukodystrophy; 6. galactocerebrosidase; Krabbe leukodystrophy; 7. spingomyelinase; Niemann–Pick; 8. ceramidase; Farber.
gal = galactose; glu = glucose; galNHAc = N-acetylgalactosamine; NANA= *N*-acetylneuraminic acid (sialic acid).
(Reproduced with permission of author and publisher from Lake, B.D. Metabolic disorders of the central and peripheral nervous system. In: *Histochemistry in Pathology*. Eds. M. I. Fulipe & B. D. Lake. Edinburgh: Churchill Livingstone, 1983, pp. 53–69).

ponents and enzyme deficiencies in the lipid storage diseases is shown in Fig. 10.2.

Gangliosidosis

Gangliosides are composed of ceramide, hexose molecules, sialic acid and hexosamine. There are two main types – GM1 and GM2 – both of which contain one sialic acid residue per molecule.

GM1-gangliosidosis may present in infants (type 1), in children (type 2) and, rarely, in adults. GM1 accumulates in the brain and viscera because of a deficiency of β-galactosidase. In type 1 the clinical course is rapid, with failure to thrive, hepatosplenomegaly and psychomotor retardation at or soon after birth. Characteristically, these patients show many of the clinical and radiological features of mucopolysaccharidosis (see p. 174), with coarse facial features, abnormally thick and misshapen bones and hepatosplenomegaly. The type 2 form of the disease has a slower clinical course and usually does not become manifest until the end of the first year of life, progressing thereafter to spastic quadriplegia and dementia by about 10 years. The diagnosis can be achieved by staining for β-galactosidase.

There are several types of *GM2-gangliosidosis* resulting from deficiencies of the isoenzymes hexosaminidase A and B. The most common type is *Tay–Sachs' disease* (type B) in which hexosaminidase A is deficient. Hexosaminidase has now been shown to be made up of α and β subunits and that hexosaminidase B has only β subunits. In type B Tay–Sachs' disease there is no synthesis of the α subunit, resulting in deficient hexosaminidase A activity. The β subunit is not present in type O (Sandhoff disease), in which neither hexosaminidase A nor B activity is present. The diagnosis may be established prenatally by amniocentesis and carriers may be detected by examining leucocytes.

Pathology. At autopsy, depending on the duration of survival, the brain may be enlarged or normal (short survival), or small and firm with atrophic gyri (long survival). The white matter may appear swollen or have a greyish discoloration as a result of loss of myelin (Fig. 10.3). The cerebellum and optic nerves are often atrophic. The brain stem and spinal cord are usually

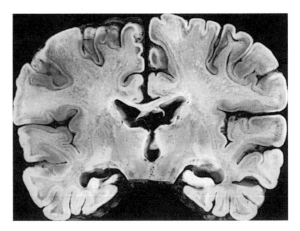

Fig. 10.3 GM2-gangliosidosis. (Tay–Sachs' disease). There is greyish discoloration of the white matter due to loss of myelin.

normal. Evidence of neuronal storage is seen throughout the central and peripheral nervous systems. The stored neuronal material in frozen sections stains positively with PAS and Luxol fast blue, but poorly with the Sudan dyes. Similar

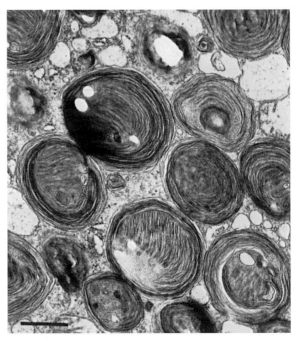

Fig. 10.4 GM2-gangliosidosis. (Tay–Sachs' disease) Membranous cytoplasmic bodies in a neuron. (*Courtesy of Dr I. More, Department of Pathology, University of Glasgow.*)

material is also seen in astrocytes and macrophages. Electron microscopy shows membranous cytoplasmic bodies (Fig. 10.4) which, although identical ultrastructurally in the GM1 and GM2-gangliosidoses, are biochemically distinct. In longer surviving cases there is loss of neurons, an astrocytosis and a progressive loss of myelin.

Cerebrosidosis

The two main disorders of cerebroside metabolism are Gaucher's disease and Krabbe's disease (see p. 177).

Gaucher's disease, a systemic lipidosis, may present in adults (type 1), infants (type 2) or juveniles (type 3). The most common is the adult (type 1) form of the disease, the patients presenting with hepatosplenomegaly, bone pain and hypersplenism: there is no neurological involvement. Hepatosplenomegaly with hypersplenism and neurological symptoms predominates in the infantile and juvenile forms of the disease. The basic defect is a deficiency of β-glucocerebrosidase (one of the β-glucosidases). An association between Gaucher's disease and leukaemia, lymphoma and gliomas has been reported.

Pathology. The brain in the adult form of the disease is usually normal, both macroscopically and microscopically. In contrast, the brain in the infantile and childhood forms is often smaller than normal. There is atrophy of the cortex and basal ganglia and an unusually sharp demarcation between grey and white matter. Neuronal storage is particularly evident in the deep grey matter, the cerebellum and the brain stem: affected neurons are moderately distended with PAS-positive material. Perivascular PAS-positive cells are also seen throughout the neuraxis. There may be typical Gaucher cells (20–100 µm in diameter, with a small nucleus and cytoplasm with the appearance of crinkled tissue paper), non-specific lipid-laden cells or multinucleated macrophages (the latter cells resemble those seen in Krabbe's disease). There is neuronal loss and an astrocytosis affecting both the cortical mantle and the subcortical grey matter, especially the dentate nucleus and the tegmentum of the brain stem. Myelin is preserved.

Sphingomyelinosis

Principal among the disorders of sphingomyelin metabolism is *Niemann–Pick disease* in which there is storage of large amounts of sphingomyelin, a normal component of myelin, and of cell membranes. Two main types are recognized: Group I in which there is sphingomyelinase deficiency, and Group II in which sphingomyelinase activity is essentially normal. Both groups are further subdivided into neurovisceral and visceral forms. In Group I, the neurovisceral form, which at least in its early stages is very similar to Gaucher's disease, presents early with hepatosplenomegaly, failure to thrive and mental retardation, whereas the visceral form is characterized by hepatosplenomegaly and haematological problems in the absence of neurological involvement. Group II cases present with various symptoms and signs which tend to be similar in any one family: these include failure to thrive, hepatosplenomegaly and severe prolonged neonatal obstructive jaundice.

Pathology. The most striking abnormality in Group I post mortem is gross hepatosplenomegaly. There may be some atrophy of the brain. The histological features are very similar to those of a gangliosidosis, the stored material in neurons staining positively with PAS, Oil red O, Sudan black B, Luxol fast blue, acid haematein and by the ferric-haematoxylin method. Foamy cells are seen in the meninges, the choroid plexus, around blood vessels and in their endothelium, sites which help to distinguish this condition from the gangliosidoses. With time, there is neuronal loss, an astrocytosis and pallor of myelin staining. Systemically, the characteristic feature is the foam cell, or Niemann–Pick cell, which measures between 20 and 90 µm in diameter and may be uni- or multinucleated; it is present in most tissues of the body and has a 'mulberry-like' appearance due to multiple small cytoplasmic vacuoles.

In cases with Group II disease there is often some degree of cerebral atrophy: myelin is preserved, although there is an astrocytosis. Ballooning of neurons is seen in all regions and is accompanied by axonal swellings. On electron microscopy there are membrane-bound cytoplasmic bodies that measure 3 µm across and contain loosely, packed lamellae.

Other types of sphingolipidoses

These include *Farber's lipogranulomatosis*, in which there is an accumulation of ceramide in both the central and peripheral nervous systems due to a deficiency of the enzyme acid ceramidase, and *Fabry's disease* (angiokeratoma corporus diffusum), which is a rare X-linked inherited disorder due to a deficiency of α-galactosidase A.

Batten's disease

This group of disorders, formerly designated as types of *amaurotic familial idiocy*, is characterized by progressive hereditary neurological illnesses associated with blindness (amaurosis). They are divided by clinicopathological criteria into five main categories: infantile (Hagberg–Santavuori), late-infantile (Bielschowsky–Jansky), early-juvenile (Lake–Cavanagh), juvenile (Spielmeyer–Vogt; Batten–Mayou), and adult (Kufs).

In all forms of Batten's disease the brain is atrophic, there being thinning of the cerebral cortex and loss of myelin. In contrast with the gangliosidoses, neurons are not ballooned, although their cytoplasm is filled with a mixture of lipofuscin and ceroid-like material, both of which are polymers of lipids. Lipofuscin is the pigment that accumulates with increasing age as an indigestible end-product of lysosomal activity. Different parts of the brain normally contain variable amounts of this pigment. The term ceroid was used initially to describe a pigment in cirrhotic rat livers, and has also been used in reference to the material that accumulates in several neuronal storage diseases. In Batten's disease the lipopigment is found within lysosomal-like bodies in neurons and in the retina, as well as in many extraneural tissues. The stored material stains positively with PAS, and Sudan black B and shows strong autofluorescence. Ultrastructurally, the lipopigment granules are pleomorphic, electron-dense, membrane-bound and acid phosphatase-positive. They often have a characteristic appearance, such as curvilinear or fingerprint bodies, but a considerable degree of overlap exists, especially in the brain.

DISORDERS OF GLYCOSAMINOGLYCAN METABOLISM (MUCOPOLYSACCHARIDOSES)

This group of disorders is due to genetic deficiencies of enzymes involved in the catabolism of mucopolysaccharides which share in common the accumulation of glycosaminoglycans in tissues and their excessive excretion in urine. The glycosaminoglycans are large polysaccharide molecules that are found predominantly in skin, cartilage, bone, blood vessels, heart valves and tendons. They are made up of repeating disaccharide units, either glucosamine or galactosamine, usually linked to a hexuronic acid. Classification is based on specific enzyme defects and analysis of urinary glycosaminoglycans. Clinically, these diseases of children are characterized by coarse facial features (*gargoylism*), multiple organ involvement and multiple skeletal abnormalities. Death from respiratory tract infections or heart disease within the first decade of life is usual (Table 10.1).

Hurler's disease is an autosomal recessive disorder due to a deficiency of α-L-iduronidase, which is required for the degradation of both heparan sulphate and dermatan sulphate. The same deficiency is found in the Scheie and Hurler/Scheie subtypes of mucopolysaccharidosis.

Pathology. At autopsy the brain tends to be rather small due to loss of both grey and white matter. The ventricular system is enlarged and there are often prominent perivascular spaces in the white matter (Fig. 10.5). Neuronal storage of gangliosides is seen to a variable extent in all areas, the material staining with PAS, the Sudan dyes, and Luxol fast blue. Associated features include loss of neurons, an astrocytosis and partial loss of myelin. A well recognized but non-specific feature in neurons on electron microscopy is an inclusion called the zebra body, which consists of irregular arrays of transverse lamellae of alternating dense and clear lines, with a periodicity of 5–7 nm, enclosed by a single membrane (Fig. 10.6). Hepatocytes and Kupffer cells store variable amounts of acid mucopolysaccharide in all forms of mucopolysaccharidosis.

Hunter's disease resembles Hurler's disease but is generally less severe. It is the only known

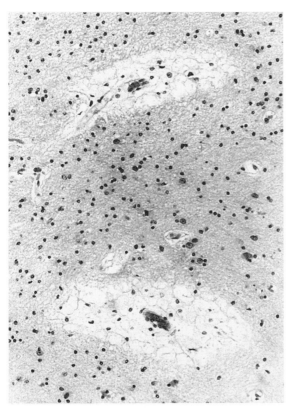

Fig. 10.5 Mucopolysaccharidosis. (Hurler's disease). Perivascular spaces are distended with cells containing water-soluble mucopolysaccharides. (H & E.)

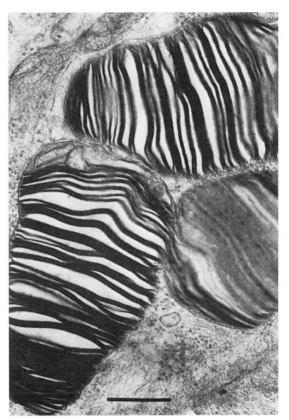

Fig. 10.6 Mucopolysaccharidosis. Membrane-bound collections of lipid lamellae (zebra bodies) are present in the cytoplasm of an astrocyte. (*Courtesy of Dr I. More, Department of Pathology, University of Glasgow*). (Bar = 0.5 μm)

X-linked recessive mucopolysaccharidosis. Both dermatan sulphate and heparan sulphate are excreted in large amounts and the deficient enzyme is sulpho-iduronate sulphatase.

Other types of mucopolysaccharidosis include the *Sanfilippo* and *Morquio syndromes*.

THE LEUKODYSTROPHIES

These are a complex group of uncommon disorders which have in common *diffuse symmetrical loss of myelin and gliosis* of the white matter of the cerebral hemispheres (*diffuse cerebral sclerosis*), and sometimes also of the cerebellum, the brain stem and the spinal cord. There are several different types of leukodystrophy (Table 10.2), most of which are genetically determined and occur in childhood. They are therefore regarded as *dysmyelinating diseases*, in the belief that the myelin is biochemically abnormal before it

degenerates, in contrast to the primary demyelinating disorders (see Ch. 9) in which myelination is thought to be normal prior to the onset of demyelination. Whereas *metachromatic leukodystrophy* and *Krabbe's disease* are primary leukodystrophies due to identified disorders of lipid metabolism, the enzyme defects in the other (idiopathic) types of leukodystrophy are not known.

Metachromatic leukodystrophy

This, the most common of the leukodystrophies, can be divided by age of onset and clinical presentation into three main types, late infantile (onset before 2 years), intermediate (onset 4–6 years) and, juvenile (onset 6–10 years): adult cases also occur. In general, however, the disease pursues a relentless clinical course over a period of 1–2

Table 10.2 Principal types of leukodystrophy

Disorder	Enzyme defect	Substances stored	Staining methods and other tests
Metachromatic	Arylsulphatase A	Sulphatides	Acidified cresyl violet; TLC
Krabbe's	Galactocerebroside β-galactosidase	Galactocerebroside	PAS; TLC; EM
Adrenoleukodystrophy	Not known	Very long-chain fatty acid esters	ORO; EM; GLC
Alexander's	Not known	Fibrillary material in astrocytes (Rosenthal fibres)	Immunohistochemistry for glial fibrillary acidic protein; LFB; EM
Spongiform	? ATPase	? oedematous fluid	—
Pelizaeus–Merzbacher	Not known	Not known	—
Cockayne's	Not known	Not known	—

TLC = thin-layer chromatography; EM = electron microscopy; GLC = gas-liquid chromatography; PAS = Periodic acid–Schiff; ORO = Oil red O; LFB = Luxol fast blue
(Reproduced in modified form with permission of author and publisher from Lake, B. D. Metabolic disorders of the central and peripheral nervous system. In: *Histochemistry in Pathology*. Eds. M. I. Filipe and B. D. Lake. Edinburgh: Churchill Livingstone, 1983, pp. 53–69.)

years. There is an accumulation of metachromatic material within both the central and peripheral nervous systems. This autosomal recessive disease is a systemic lipidosis due to a deficiency of arylsulphatase A, an enzyme that is responsible for cleaving the sulphate radicle from sulphatide. Myelin in this condition is not broken downinto neutral fat or cholesterol esters but into metachromatic material containing sulphatides.

Pathology

At autopsy the brain may appear normal externally; on section it is firm and the white matter may be somewhat greyer and more translucent than normal (Fig. 10.7). Histologically there is widespread loss of myelin in the white matter, including the subcortical arcuate fibres, and the fibre tracts which mature last are the most severely affected. Within the demyelinated areas there are large amounts of both intracellular (prominent in oligodendrocytes and astrocytes) and extracellular metachromatic granules that measure 15–20 μm in diameter (Fig. 10.8); smaller amounts are seen within neurons and in perivascular macrophages. The macrophages contain cerebroside sulphate (sulphatide), which is responsible for the metachromasia in frozen and cryostat sections when stained with acidified cresyl violet. The metachromatic lipid is also seen in peripheral nerves and other tissues, such as the liver, pancreas and kidney. Electron microscopically, some of the cytoplasmic inclusions have a characteristic pattern – a herringbone appearance in longitudinal section and a honeycomb structure in cross-section.

Initial screening can be easily done by the examination of urinary sediment for metachromatic deposits. Confirmation can be achieved by enzyme assay in white blood cells, cultured fibroblasts or urine, or by sural nerve biopsy.

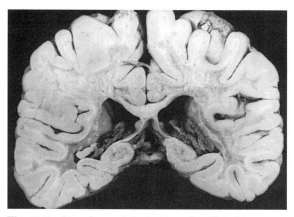

Fig. 10.7 Metachromatic leukodystrophy. The white matter is grey due to demyelination.

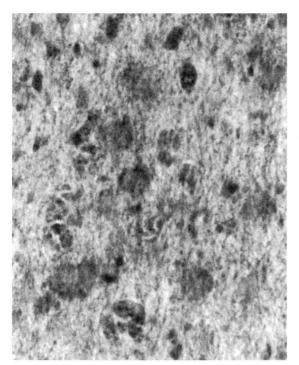

Fig. 10.8   Metachromatic leukodystrophy. Cryostat section showing metachromatic macrophages in the white matter. (Acidified cresyl violet.)

Bone marrow transplantation has been carried out to retard the onset of neurological deterioration.

Krabbe's disease

This autosomal recessive disease occurs mainly in infants, and is due to a deficiency of galactocerebroside-β-galactosidase.

Pathology

The brain is generally small and has a normal external appearance. On section the white matter, with the exception of the subcortical arcuate fibres, is greyish in colour and firm. Histologically, the cortex is normal but there is widespread loss of myelin, with more or less preservation of axons and an astrocytosis. The characteristic feature is perivascular clusters of multinucleated globoid cells within the areas of loss of myelin. The globoid cells measure some 20–50 μm in diameter and are thought to develop from smaller

mononuclear (epithelioid) macrophages that become filled with galactocerebroside (Fig. 10.9). The cytoplasm is moderately positive with PAS but stains only weakly with Oil red O and Sudan black B. As the loss of myelin becomes more severe, a point is reached where there is marked loss of axons, an intense astrocytosis and only a few scattered clusters of globoid cells. The diagnosis can be established by enzyme assay of leucocytes or cultured fibroblasts.

A disorder very similar to human Krabbe's disease occurs in dogs, and experimental work has shown that globoid cells may be produced by injecting cerebrosides into the cerebral white matter or spleen of rats.

Adrenoleukodystrophy

This is an X-linked recessive disorder that occurs most commonly in children, occasionally in adult life, and is characterized by a variable increase in pigmentation of the skin, atrophy of the adrenal glands and progressive cerebral sclerosis.

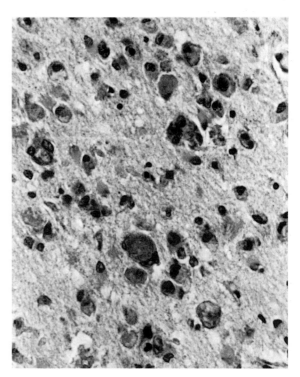

Fig. 10.9   Krabbe's leukodystrophy. There are globoid cells in the white matter. (H & E.)

Pathology

There is extensive loss of myelin, particularly in the posterior portions of the hemispheres, the abnormal tissue having a grey, rather translucent, appearance. Histologically the cortex is normal apart from mild gliosis. In the most affected areas of white matter there is almost complete demyelination, loss of axons and oligodendrocytes, and a dense astrocytosis. Occasional PAS, Oil red O and Sudan black B positive macrophages occur in perivascular spaces. At the margins of the most severely affected areas there is a zone of partial loss of myelin, numerous lipid-laden macrophages and a prominent infiltrate of lymphocytes and plasma cells. By light microscopy the macrophages often have a striated appearance, the typical ultrastructural feature of which is the presence of abundant cytoplasmic membrane-bound inclusions consisting of distinctive curvilinear membranous profiles with two 2.5 nm wide electron-dense lines separated by a clear space. Similar inclusions occur in Schwann cells, in ballooned vacuolated cells of the zona fasiculata and zona reticularis of the atrophic adrenal gland, and in presumptive Leydig cells of the testes. A possible pathogenic factor is cellular toxicity due to saturated fatty acids, very long-chain fatty acids (VLCFA), abnormal cholesterol esters or gangliosides. Consequently, these substances accumulate (VLCFA in oligodendrocytes and Schwann cells, and cholesterol esters in adrenal and Leydig cells) and become toxic. Loss of myelin results and the liberation of immunogenic lipids excites a delayed hypersensitivity reaction.

It is now considered that the overwhelming majority of males thought to have sudanophilic leukodystrophy (see Ch. 9) are in fact examples of adrenoleukodystrophy, and that patients with this type of dysmyelination in whom the adrenal glands are normal are suffering from a variant of multiple sclerosis. The term *Schilder's disease* has been used in the past for leukodystrophy of sudanophilic type. If the term has to be retained, it should be restricted to cases of adrenoleukodystrophy.

Adrenomyeloneuropathy

This condition, characterized by a slowly progressive spastic paraparesis, a distal symmetrical polyneuropathy, Addison's disease and hypogonadism, is now considered to be linked to adrenoleukodystrophy and to be caused by the same mutant gene. Morphological studies have demonstrated cytoplasmic inclusions in the nervous system, adrenal glands and interstitial cells of the testes, similar to those described in adrenoleukodystrophy. Similar biochemical abnormalities have also been described, and some clinical benefit has been derived by the dietary restriction of very long-chain fatty acids.

A family in which adrenoleukodystrophy and adrenomyeloneuropathy coexisted has been reported. There was again some clinical improvement with dietary restriction of very long-chain fatty acids.

Alexander's disease

This is a rare disorder of infancy characterized clinically by mental retardation with progressive megalencephaly.

Pathology

At autopsy the brain is heavy and appears enlarged; on section there may be hydrocephalus, the cortex is ill-defined and the white matter is soft and grey. Histologically, the most striking feature is the presence of large numbers of homogenous elongated hyaline bodies measuring up to 200 μm long (Rosenthal fibres) arranged radially around blood vessels and at right-angles to both the surface of the brain beneath the pia and the ependyma. The Rosenthal fibres stain red with H & E, dark purple with PTAH and blue with Luxol fast blue; immunohistochemistry has shown that their peripheral portions are made up of glial fibrillary acidic protein. Their central portions do not stain and, on electron microscopy, consist of non-fibrillary and densely osmiophilic masses without limiting membranes. There is continuity of the filaments with the granular masses. The relationship between Rosenthal fibres and glial fibres is therefore uncertain. In general the number of Rosenthal fibres correlates with the severity of myelin loss, but the cause of the demyelination in a disease process that principally affects astrocytes is not known.

Spongiform leukodystrophy (Canavan's disease: Canavan–Van Bogaert–Bertrand spongy degeneration)

In some children spongiform degeneration of the white matter is the only abnormality: such cases, if familial, are termed spongiform leukodystrophy. Congenital, infantile and juvenile types have been described and are characterized clinically by mental deterioration and megalencephaly.

Pathology

At autopsy, the white matter is soft and 'oedematous'. Histologically, the most striking feature is spongy change in white matter, loss of myelin, relative preservation of axons and a reactive astrocytosis. Sudanophilic macrophages are seen and there are many Alzheimer type 2 astrocytes in the cerebral cortex and subcortical grey matter. Neurons are normal in the early stages of the disease. Ultrastructural studies have shown that the spongy change is due to vacuolation of myelin sheaths and swelling of astrocytic cytoplasm, the latter frequently containing greatly enlarged mitochondria with a peculiarly arranged matrix and cristae. This suggests that the disease may be a metabolic disturbance of the mitochondria of astrocytes, although the basic biochemical defect remains unknown. In some cases the diagnosis can be established by finding abnormal mitochondria in a muscle biopsy.

A defect in ATPase has, however, been suggested, especially as ouabain, a powerful inhibitor of sodium potassium-activated ATPase, produces vacuolation of white matter similar to that seen in this disease in experimental preparations. Status spongiosis of the nervous system can also be induced experimentally by a number of other agents, namely isonicotinic acid hydrazide, triethyltin poisoning and cuprizone. Similar spongy degeneration of white matter is also a feature of phenylketonuria and certain aminoacidopathies.

Other types of leukodystrophy

Sudanophilic (orthochromatic) leukodystrophies are a heterogeneous group of disorders which share in common the sudanophilic nature of the lipid material found in white matter. The term is therefore applied to leukodystrophies that cannot be classified as inflammatory demyelinating disease, those without metachromatic substances and those without other distinguishing features. Examples include X-linked *Pelizaeus–Merzbacher disease*, which is characterized by progressive loss of myelin with intact residual myelin islets (tigroid demyelination), and *Cockayne's syndrome*.

OTHER LYSOSOMAL DISORDERS AFFECTING THE NERVOUS SYSTEM

These include *mannosidosis* due to a deficiency of α-mannosidase, *fucosidosis* due to a deficiency of α-fucosidase and *aspartyl-glycosaminuria* due to a deficiency of aspartyl glycosylamine amidohydrolase.

OTHER INBORN ERRORS OF METABOLISM

Although not common, these conditions are important because some can be detected by screening tests in infants, and brain damage can be prevented or reduced either by replacement therapy or by excluding precursor substances from the diet.

DISORDERS OF AMINO-ACID METABOLISM

There are many different types of disorder due to specific enzyme deficiencies which result in an increase in the amount of specific amino acid. This may be accompanied by systemic acidosis, hypoglycaemia and hyperammonaemia. Although some are potentially treatable, many are associated with mental retardation. In general, they are characterized by status spongiosus of white matter, partial loss of myelin and an astrocytosis. The peripheral nervous system is generally spared.

Phenylketonuria

This is the most common type of amino-aciduria (1 in 12 500 live births) and is characterized genetically by autosomal recessive inheritance, clinically by mental retardation, seizures and decreased hair pigmentation, and biochemically by the excretion of large amounts of phenyl-pyruvic acid. It is not a single disease entity and encompasses nine subtypes, the most common of which is impaired hydroxylation of phenylalanine to tyrosine due to defects in the activity of phenylalanine hydroxylase and, in some rare cases, a deficiency of the cofactor, tetrahydro-biopterin. The relationship between mental retardation and the biochemical findings, and the occasional occurrence of spongiform change in white matter is not clear, but there is general agreement that increased amounts of phenyl-alanine retard the development of the nervous system. Once maturation of the CNS is complete, elevated levels of phenylalanine do not affect intellectual capacity. Screening programmes for the detection of phenylketonuria depend on the recognition of a raised concentration of phenyl-alanine in the blood in the first few days of life. The aim of treatment is to lower the circulating level of phenylalanine to a level just slightly higher than that found in normal individuals by dietary restriction of protein and by using synthetic substitutes.

Other types of amino-aciduria

These include *maple syrup urine disease* in which abnormalities of leucine, isoleucine and valine metabolism occur, *homocystinuria* in which there is a deficiency of cystathionine β-synthase and *Hartnup* disease, which is due to defective renal transport of monoaminomonocarboxylic acids.

DISORDERS OF CARBOHYDRATE METABOLISM

Principal among these are *galactosaemia*, the *glycogen storage diseases* and *disorders of fructose metabolism*. Some cause hypoglycaemia and severe metabolic acidosis, both of which may lead to brain damage.

Galactosaemia

This is a treatable cause of mental retardation and is due to deficient activity of galactose-1-phosphate uridyltransferase. Affected infants are normal at birth but fail to thrive, develop vomiting, become jaundiced and are found to have hepatosplenomegaly and cataracts. If not recognized and treated, affected individuals are likely to be mentally subnormal and develop cirrhosis of the liver. The only effective treatment is exclusion of galactose (and therefore lactose and milk) from the diet; otherwise galactose, galactose-1-phosphate and galactitol accumulate in neural tissue.

Glycogen storage disorders

Deficiency of enzymes involved in the synthesis and degradation of glycogen can present in many ways, namely, brain damage or as disorders primarily of the liver, heart or musculoskeletal systems. All are rare and mostly of autosomal recessive inheritance. There are eight major types (Table 10.3) of which types II and rarely IV primarily affect the brain, and types II, IV, V and VII affect muscle (see Ch. 17). Brain damage is most likely caused by the severe recurrent bouts of lactacidosis and hypoglycaemia. New feeding

Table 10.3   Glycogen storage disorders

Type	Enzyme defect	Major organs involved
I (Von Gierke's)	Glucose-6-phosphatase	Liver, kidney
II (Pompe's)	Acid-1:4-glucosidase	Liver, muscle, CNS
III (Forbes')	Amylo-1:6 glucosidase (debranching enzyme)	Liver
IV (Andersen's)	Amylo-1, 4 1,6 transglucosylas (branching enzyme)	Liver, muscle; rarely CNS
V (McArdle's)	Myophosphorylase	Muscle
VI	Liver phosphorylase kinase	Liver
VII (Tarui's)	Phosphofructokinase	Muscle
VIII	Hepatic phosphorylase kinase	Liver

regimens have resulted in considerable improvement in the clinical state and outcome. Inheritance is autosomal recessive except for type VIII which is X-linked.

Type II (Pompe's disease) is due to a deficiency of α-1,4-glucosidase (acid maltase). The infantile form is rapidly progressive and fatal, death usually occurring by the age of 2 years. It is a generalized condition and there is profound hypotonia, cardiomegaly and sometimes hepatomegaly. Juveniles present with the symptoms and signs of muscular dystrophy, and adults with weakness of respiratory and other skeletal muscles. Excessive amounts of glycogen can be demonstrated in dorsal root ganglia, in neurons in the ventral horns of the spinal cord and in motor nuclei in the brain stem. There may be limited involvement of other nuclei in the brain stem. This stains positively with PAS and methenamine silver, and is sensitive to salivary amylase. Skeletal muscle is affected in all forms of the disease (see Ch. 17). In the infantile form the heart is enlarged, and all fibres are vacuolated and contain excess glycogen. Similar changes are seen in hepatocytes and in Kupffer cells, and in cells of the lympho-reticular system. Ultrastructurally, glycogen accumulates in greatly distended lysosomes.

Disorders of fructose metabolism

Hereditary fructose intolerance arises from a deficiency of fructose-1-phosphate aldolase activity. The symptoms do not become manifest until sucrose is introduced into the diet. The onset of symptoms and signs is therefore delayed by breast feeding.

DISORDERS OF TRACE METAL METABOLISM

Principal among this group of disorders are *Wilson's disease (hepatolenticular degeneration)* and *kinky hair (Menkes') disease*.

Wilson's disease

This is a genetically determined disorder (autosomal recessive) that usually presents in young adults as an extrapyramidal syndrome or hepatic insufficiency. Copper is deposited in the liver (cirrhosis), in the cornea (Kayser–Fleischer rings), in the kidneys (impaired tubular absorption and transport), and in the CNS. The enzymatic deficiency is not known but the copper-binding protein ceruloplasmin is low and increased amounts of copper are excreted in the urine.

Pathology

In rapidly progressive fatal cases there is cavitation in the lenticular nuclei. In the commoner chronic form there is atrophy and often light-brown discoloration of these nuclei. Histologically there is neuronal loss, an astrocytosis and haemosiderin – containing macrophages in the basal ganglia and distinctive changes in the protoplasmic astrocytes. These changes also occur in the cerebral cortex and dentate nucleus and take two forms, namely Alzheimer type 1 and type 2 astrocytes. Alzheimer type 1 cells, which are much less frequent than type 2, consist of hyperchromatic irregular nuclei often having a rim of

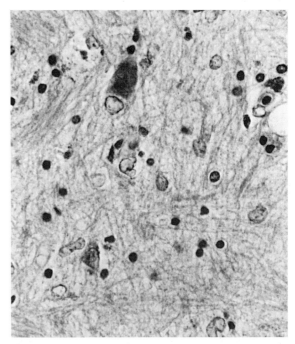

Fig. 10.10 Alzheimer type 2 astrocytes. The nuclei are swollen and vesicular, and usually contain prominent nucleoli. (H & E.)

pink cytoplasm studded with small yellow-brown (with H & E stains) or green (with Nissl) granules. Alzheimer type 2 astrocytes have enlarged vesicular nuclei due to the accumulation of glycogen; prominent nucleoli are often seen and cytoplasm is conspicuously absent (Fig. 10.10). Another feature of Wilson's disease is the presence of Opalski cells in the same locations as Alzheimer type 2 cells, but particularly in the globus pallidus. The cells are globoid, measure up to 35 μm in diameter and have a slightly foamy cytoplasm and an eccentric nucleus. An origin from degenerating neurons and macrophages has been suggested, but recent evidence suggests that they are derived from Alzheimer type 2 astrocytes. The latter are not unique to Wilson's disease since they occur in non-Wilsonian hepatic encephalopathy.

Liver damage is a presenting, and often fatal, feature in many cases, patients dying before any neurological changes are seen. Chelation of copper produces marked clinical improvement, particularly in the early stages of the disease.

Kinky hair (Menkes' disease)

This very rare disease of male infants is an X-linked recessive disorder characterized by severe systemic neurological abnormalities associated with erect undulating and fragile colourless hair. The disorder is secondary to impaired absorption of copper in the gastrointestinal tract and there is decreased activity of copper-dependent enzymes, including cytochrome oxidase. In some cases there is atrophy and cystic degeneration of the brain, particularly in the cerebellum. Abnormalities are also seen in the elastica of blood vessels, possibly due to dysfunction of the copper-dependent lysyl oxidase.

DISORDERS OF PURINE AND PYRIMIDINE METABOLISM

The Lesch–Nyhan syndrome, an X-linked recessive disorder of male infants, is characterized clinically by mental retardation, spasticity, movement disorders and compulsive self-mutilation. The deficient enzyme is hypoxanthine guanine phosphoribosyl transferase which results in the systemic accumulation of uric acid and the development of the clinical features of gout. There are no specific abnormalities in the brain, suggesting that the disorder is due to changes in functional balance between GABA, dopamine and acetylcholine neurons.

DISORDERS OF PIGMENT METABOLISM

Porphyria is a group of uncommon inborn or acquired metabolic disorders of porphyrin metabolism. Porphyrins are pigments normally present in haemoglobin, myoglobin and cytochromes. Classification is based on clinical and biochemical features. The most common is the acquired type (precipitated by drugs or intoxicants) in which there is moderate cutaneous photosensitivity and increased uroporphyrin and coproporphyrin in the faeces at all times. On the other hand, patients with acute intermittent porphyria which has a dominant mode of inheritance present with episodic attacks (often following the use of barbiturates or sulphonamides) of emotional instability, sleepiness, severe abdominal pain and vomiting, but no cutaneous photosensitivity. The metabolic abnormality is due to a breakdown in the mechanism (aminolaevulinic acid synthetase) controlling the rate of haem synthesis in the liver, which results in the accumulation of porphobilinogen and aminolaevulinic acid. Similar neurological manifestations occur in the main forms of porphyria. The most constant finding is that of chromatolysis of neurons in the anterior horns of the spinal cord, in motor nuclei and in dorsal root ganglia secondary to a peripheral neuropathy.

DISORDERS OF ENDOCRINE METABOLISM

Addison's disease

Patients with Addison's disease may present with clinical signs and symptoms of raised intracranial pressure due to diffuse swelling of the brain. As in cases of adrenoleukodystrophy there is a variable increase in skin pigmentation and atrophy of the adrenal glands (see p. 177).

Hypothyroidism

Congenital hypothyroidism can be detected from

a single heel stab between 6 and 14 days of life. If untreated, the infant fails to develop normally (possibly due to faulty dendritogenesis) and becomes cretinous. Features of hypothyroidism in adults include peripheral mononeuropathy due to entrapment of nerves, psychotic signs and symptoms (myxoedematous madness), impairment of higher neurological functions (myxoedematous dementia), and cerebellar ataxia.

Calcium metabolism

Perivascular mineralization (primarily calcium, phosphorus and iron) is commonly seen histologically in the basal ganglia, hippocampus and dentate nucleus in normal subjects over the age of 40. Larger amounts of calcification, again in the basal ganglia of asymptomatic subjects, may be seen by CT scanning. Occasionally, the amount is so great that it may be seen on plain X-rays of the skull, and in over 50 per cent of these cases there is an associated deficiency of parathyroid hormone. On slicing the brain, small amounts of calcification impart a gritty resistance to the knife, whereas larger concretions ('brain stones') are dislodged and appear as solid lumps with an irregular rough surface. Calcification is seen to be more widely distributed histologically than the macroscopic appearances would suggest: it consists of rows of small calcospherites lying along the walls of capillaries and as tubular deposits in the medial coats of medium-sized arteries and veins. Brain stones appear to develop by coalescence of these pericapillary deposits.

MISCELLANEOUS METABOLIC DISORDERS

Subacute necrotizing encephalomyelopathy of Leigh

This disease was originally thought to be inherited as a mendelian recessive, occurring more commonly in infant males than females. It is now realized that sporadic cases occur and that the condition may present in adolescence and adulthood. Clinically, there is often psychomotor retardation, difficulties in swallowing, weakness, ataxia and visual disturbances. There appear to

be a number of different metabolic defects that can produce this disease: inhibition of thiamine pyrophosphate–ATP phosphoryltransferase, defective activation of pyruvate decarboxylase or dehydrogenase, and deficiency of liver pyruvate carboxylase, or cytochrome C oxidase in muscle. Most of these relate to mitochondrial dysfunction but none is sufficiently specific to provide a biochemical basis for the disorder.

Pathology

The neuropathological findings are very similar in nature to Wernicke's disease (thiamine deficiency). Typically there are bilateral symmetrical lesions, predominantly in the grey matter of the diencephalon (especially putamen and thalamus), and in the tegmentum of the brain stem (especially the periaqueductal grey matter (Fig. 10.11) and substantia nigra) but sparing the mamillary bodies. The earliest change histologically is vacuolation of the neuropil (Fig. 10.12), which may proceed to microcystic degeneration (status spongiosus). This is associated with loss of myelin, prominent proliferation of capillaries and astrocytes, and relative sparing of neurons and their axons.

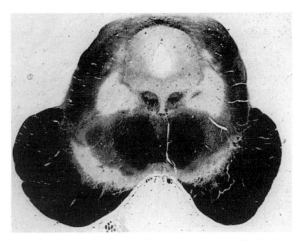

Fig. 10.11 Leigh's disease. There are symmetrical lesions in the tegmentum of the midbrain, with loss of myelin. (Celloidin; Heidenhain for myelin.)

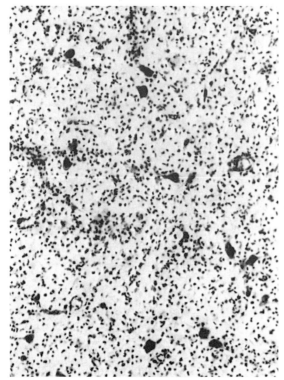

Fig. 10.12 Leigh's disease. There is endothelial proliferation, macrophage formation with loosening of the neuropil, and a reactive astrocytosis with relative preservation of neurons. (Celloidin; cresyl violet.)

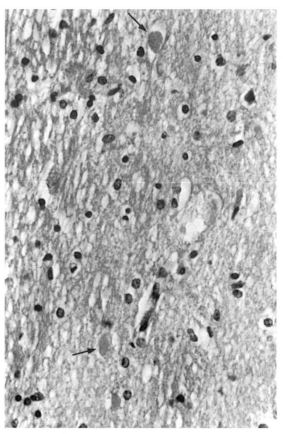

Fig. 10.13 Neuroaxonal dystrophy. There are several large oval or round bodies (spheroids—arrows) and a reactive astrocytosis. (H & E.)

Neuroaxonal dystrophies

There are a number of neurological diseases in which focal swellings (*spheroids*) develop on dystrophic axons throughout the nervous system (Fig. 10.13). Their pathogenesis is unknown, but it is thought that they are due to several different mechanisms which cause dysfunction of axoplasmic transport. One suggested mechanism is vitamin E deficiency due to malabsorption. They are usually classified according to age of onset, the topographical distribution of the spheroids and the presence or absence of pigmentation in the lentiform nucleus and the substantia nigra. The pigment is strongly PAS-positive and stains with Perl's reaction. The two most common are *infantile neuroaxonal dystrophy* and *Hallervorden–Spatz disease* (see Ch. 12).

MANIFESTATIONS OF SYSTEMIC DISEASE IN THE NERVOUS SYSTEM

METABOLIC ENCEPHALOPATHIES

Hypoxic encephalopathy, including brain damage due to carbon monoxide poisoning and hypoglycaemia, has already been discussed (see Ch. 5), as has the role of altered serum sodium in the genesis of central pontine myelinolysis (see Ch. 9). In this section the encephalopathies associated with hepatic and renal disease and with diabetes mellitus will be described in greater detail. Kernicterus is considered in Chapter 13.

Hepatic encephalopathies

A metabolic encephalopathy invariably accompanies severe liver failure. Cases of massive hepatic necrosis, whether viral or drug-induced, are accompanied by an *acute hepatic encephalopathy* characterized by rapidly developing coma. On the other hand, in cases of liver disease with cirrhosis, particularly when there is portal-systemic shunting of blood, *chronic hepatic encephalopathy* develops. Both types are potentially reversible so the patients often present an episodic and relapsing course; they may, however, become chronic and progressive.

There may be no histological abnormalities in the CNS in cases with acute fulminant hepatic encephalopathy. In some, however, Alzheimer type 2 astrocytes (see Fig. 10.10) may be present, and a not uncommon finding is diffuse cerebral oedema, which may be sufficient to cause tentorial or tonsillar herniation. The cause of the cerebral oedema is unclear but it has been shown experimentally that there may be alterations in the blood–brain barrier in acute hepatic encephalopathy. Alternatively, the cerebral oedema may be secondary to complications of the acute liver failure, such as hypoglycaemia and hypotension.

Pathology

The principal histological finding in *chronic hepatic encephalopathy* is the presence of Alzheimer type 2 astrocytes (see p. 181) in the deeper layers of the cerebral cortex and in the basal ganglia. In cases of portal-systemic shunting or portocaval anastomosis, the nuclei of the Alzheimer astrocytes become lobulated, particularly in the globus pallidus, substantia nigra and dentate nucleus. In general, glial fibrils cannot be demonstrated in their cytoplasm. Although a prominent feature, morphometric studies have failed to reveal any increase in the total number of glial nuclei in hepatic encephalopathy. Alzheimer type 2 cell change is not pathognomonic of hepatic encephalopathy, similar cells being found in patients dying as a result of hypoxaemia and uraemia. They are also seen in the brains of children with hyperammonaemic syndromes due to genetically determined enzyme defects in the urea cycle.

Acquired (non-Wilsonian) hepatocerebral degeneration sometimes occurs as a result of repeated bouts of hepatic encephalopathy, when rather softened grey/tan areas of discoloration may be

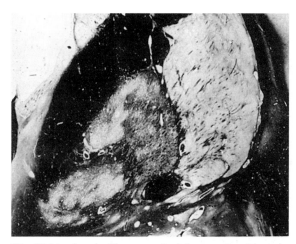

Fig. 10.14 Acquired hepatocerebral degeneration. There are rarefied areas in the globus pallidus. (Celloidin; Heidenhain for myelin.)

seen in the deeper layers of the cortex and in the lentiform nucleus (Fig. 10.14). On histological examination there is spongy degeneration (Fig. 10.15) and many Alzheimer type 2 astrocytes, loss of neurons and degeneration of myelin and axons. Reactive changes are minimal. The struc-

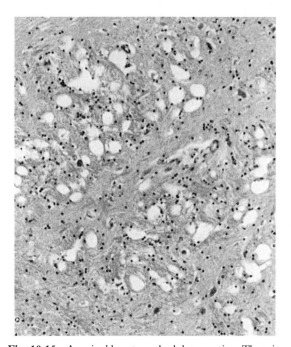

Fig. 10.15 Acquired hepatocerebral degeneration. There is spongy degeneration in the globus pallidus. (H & E.)

tural abnormalities are very similar to those seen in Wilson's disease (see p. 181). For example, Alzheimer type 1 astrocytes and Opalski cells, which were traditionally regarded as specific features of Wilson's disease, are also found in acquired hepatocerebral degeneration.

Patients with a portal-systemic shunt of blood may occasionally develop *hepatic myelopathy*, in which there is symmetrical demyelination of the lateral corticospinal tracts.

It is generally thought that hepatic encephalopathy is due to an accumulation of neurotoxic substances in the blood which have an origin in the gastrointestinal tract. Normally, these substances are metabolized by the liver, but in cases of hepatic necrosis or of portal-systemic shunting of blood, they are not detoxified. In general, there is a correlation between the clinical symptoms and the level of blood ammonia, but other substances such as amino acids, biogenic amines (false neurotransmitters) and free fatty acids have also been incriminated in the pathogenesis of the encephalopathy.

Reye's syndrome

This is an acute non-inflammatory encephalopathy of children characterized by diffuse cerebral oedema and very severe microvesicular fatty change in the liver. Hyperammonaemia is the rule and hypoglycaemia may also be present. The mortality rate is about 20 per cent, and many survivors are disabled with mental impairment, epilepsy and neurological deficit. The pathogenesis is not known, but it is thought that it might be due to injury to mitochondria, resulting in deficiencies of carbamylphosphate synthetase and ornithine transcarbamylase, leading to impaired liver synthesis of urea. There appears to be an association between various viral illnesses such as varicella and influenza, the ingestion of salicylates and contamination of food by aflatoxin, a metabolic product of *Aspergillus flavus*. It is likely that there is a spectrum of heritable defects in the conversion of ammonia to urea which becomes manifest following exposure to various agents, including viruses, drugs and toxins.

Pathology. The brain is swollen and there may be evidence of herniation and secondary damage

to the brain stem. Histologically, depending on the degree and duration of the hepatic failure, there are variable numbers of Alzheimer type 2 astrocytes. In many cases there is histological evidence of widespread ischaemic brain damage.

Uraemic encephalopathy

This is a well recognized complication of renal failure. The symptoms, however, correlate poorly with any single laboratory test, although the level of the blood urea nitrogen is often a useful index of its severity. The condition is reversed by dialysis, suggesting that it is due to low molecular weight compounds. Recent evidence suggests that a parathyroid-like hormone may play a role. Because patients with renal failure frequently have coexisting diseases such as hypertension, diabetes mellitus, collagen diseases etc., and are subject to intercurrent conditions, it is not surprising that most of the neuropathological findings are thought to be non-specific and not to be the cause of the encephalopathy *per se*.

Complications associated with dialysis and renal transplantation

Disequilibrium syndrome

This normally self-limiting condition occurs typically at the end of dialysis. It is more common in children than in adults and is thought to be due to osmotic gradients between brain and blood that result in cerebral oedema and an elevation in the intracranial pressure.

Dialysis encephalopathy (dialysis dementia)

Certain patients with renal failure who have been dialysed for at least 10 years develop a distinct syndrome characterized by dysarthria, dyspraxia of speech, myoclonus and dementia. At first the condition is reversible but later it becomes progressive, although it may be reversed by renal transplantation. Death usually occurs within 18 months. There is an association between this condition and the accumulation of aluminium in blood and brain. The aluminium is derived from the frequent use of phosphate-binding aluminium gels and from the water used in the dialysis bath. The pathogenic role of the aluminium, however, has not been universally accepted.

Dialysis may also be complicated by subdural haematoma, which is presumably due to anti-coagulation and clotting abnormalities associated with renal failure rather than to the haemodialysis *per se*.

Renal transplantation

As a result of immunosuppressive treatment, transplant patients are susceptible to a variety of opportunist infections of viral (cytomegalovirus or herpes simplex), bacterial, fungal (Candida and Aspergillus) and protozoal origins. Microglial nodules (see Ch. 7) are the most common microscopic abnormality in the brain, and they have been ascribed to infection by either cyto-megalovirus or herpes simplex virus. Some 70–90 per cent of transplant patients surviving more than 2 months show virological and immu-nological evidence of infection by cytomegalo-virus, and this presumably accounts for the occurrence of inclusion bodies in the brain. The lack of a florid inflammatory cell response is attributed to an impaired immune response.

Neoplasia is another important complication of transplantation, the risk of developing a *de novo* tumour being approximately 100 times greater than in equivalent age- and sex-matched con-trols. Malignant lymphoid tumours are particu-larly prone to develop, and have a propensity for the CNS. There is also an association with car-cinoma of the skin, lips and cervix. The interval between transplantation and the development of tumour varies between 5 and 46 months. Poss-ible mechanisms for this increased incidence are impairment of the immunological surveillance system, the effects of repeated antigenic stimu-lation from the transplanted kidneys and acti-vation of an oncogenic virus. In some patients the possibility that the tumour was present at the time of transplantation cannot be completely ruled out.

A further complication of renal transplantation is the development of central pontine mye-linolysis (see Ch. 9).

Encephalopathy of diabetes mellitus

Complications of diabetes mellitus in the CNS are usually attributable to *cerebrovascular disease* (see Ch. 5). Clinical and epidemiological studies have shown that hypertension and atheroma occur at an earlier age and with greater severity in diabetic than in non-diabetic patients. It is also thought that the poorer outcome in diabetics with cerebral infarction is due to the high glucose levels and the associated increase in lactate production.

Diabetic ketoacidotic coma

Although this may be due to β-hydroxybutyric acid and acetoacetate, it is more likely due to the severity and duration of osmotic dysequilibrium between blood and brain, with a contribution from the vascular changes of the disseminated intravascular coagulation syndrome, rather than to the degree of ketoacidosis. The initial favour-able response to treatment of diabetic ketoacid-osis in young patients is occasionally followed by sudden deterioration and evidence of raised intracranial pressure. A sudden drop in glucose following insulin therapy is believed to be the cause of *cerebral oedema*. Whether or not cerebral oedema complicates the treatment of non-ketotic hyperosmolar diabetic coma is controversial.

Demyelination

A common histological finding is demyelination of the posterior columns of the spinal cord. The changes can be so marked that the cord acquires a distinctive shape, referred to as *'pseudotabes'* (see Ch. 6). Demyelination of the lateral columns has been reported as diabetic *amyotrophic lateral sclerosis*. The pathogenesis of the demyelination is not known; possibilities include primary de-myelination, a toxic metabolic factor or a micro-angiopathy due to thickening of the basement membrane and changes in the blood–brain barrier.

Neuropathy of peripheral, autonomic and cranial nerves is also common in patients with diabetes mellitus (see Ch. 18).

Infection

About 80 per cent of cases of mucor (rhizopus) infections of the nose, orbits and the base of the brain occur in diabetics (see Ch. 7).

Pancreatic encephalopathy

Patients with acute pancreatitis may develop neurological dysfunction as a result of various complications that include electrolyte imbalance, hypocalcaemia, liver disease, hypotension, hypoglycaemia and haemorrhagic shock. However, a syndrome apparently independent of these metabolic changes has been described, characterized by acute delirium, seizures and multiple focal neurological signs occurring between the second and fifth day after the onset of acute pancreatitis.

Neuropathological findings include petechial haemorrhages, perivascular oedema and astrocytosis, particularly in the basal ganglia and periventricular structures. These findings have been attributed to toxic vasoactive peptides, hormones and enzymes produced during the acute pancreatitis. A similar mechanism may cause CNS complications of the pancreatitis caused by mumps.

NON-METASTATIC (REMOTE) EFFECTS OF CARCINOMA

The nervous system is frequently involved by malignant tumours arising elsewhere in the body. Metastases may occur in the brain, the spinal cord and peripheral nerves, or the cord may be compressed by extradural deposits of tumour. Many tumours, however, particularly carcinoma of the bronchus and lymphoma may have indirect (remote) effects upon neurons, myelin, the myoneural junction and muscle. The central or peripheral nervous systems may be affected at various levels, singly or in combination. The various neurological syndromes are not rare and an incidence of 6 per cent has been estimated in all patients with carcinoma. There is no constant relationship between the course of the neurological disorder and that of the carcinoma. They may develop concurrently, but the neurological disorder may antedate objective evidence of

tumour. Furthermore, the severity of the neurological disease is not related to the size of the tumour.

There are five main categories of disorder:

1. *Metabolic syndromes.* In some cases these are due to disease of the liver – *acquired hepatocerebral degeneration*, or the kidneys – *uraemic encephalopathy*. Others are of a hormonal nature and include the ectopic ACTH syndrome (*Cushing's syndrome*), release of a parathyroid hormone-like substance (*hypercalcaemia*), release of an antidiuretic hormone-like substance (*water intoxication and hyponatraemia*), release of thyroid-stimulating hormone-like substance (*thyrotoxocosis*) and release by the tumour of 5-hydroxytryptamine serotonin, (*carcinoid syndrome*). *Hypoglycaemia* has also been described in association with malignant tumours, usually large fibrosarcomas, but occasionally in patients with bronchial carcinoma. The likely cause of the hypoglycaemia is either the production by the tumour of a substance with an insulin-like action or increased glucose uptake by the tumour. Other endocrinopathies undoubtedly await discovery.

2. *The neuromuscular syndromes.* The most common is a *peripheral neuropathy*, which may be predominantly motor or sensory or of mixed type. The most conspicuous histological abnormalities in the cases with sensory symptoms are loss of neurons in the dorsal root ganglia and degeneration of the dorsal nerve roots, the posterior columns of the spinal cord and peripheral nerves. In predominantly motor neuropathies, histological changes are usually slight, although there may be various degrees of neurogenic atrophy of muscle and central chromatolysis in neurons in the ventral horns of the spinal cord. Other conditions in this group are *motor neuron disease*, an *amyotrophic lateral sclerosis-like syndrome*, a *myasthenic syndrome* (Eaton–Lambert syndrome), a *myopathic syndrome* and *dermatomyositis/ polymyositis*, fuller details of which are given in Chapter 17.

3. *Encephalomyelitic syndromes.* In this group of disorders the principal features are the presence of lymphocytes and some plasma cells around small blood vessels within the CNS, and small aggregates of microglia (Fig. 10.16). Grey matter

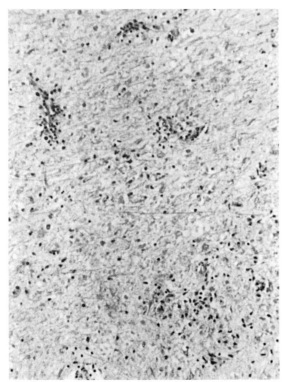

Fig. 10.16 Non-metastatic effects of carcinoma: cerebellum. There is light perivascular cuffing by lymphocytes, clusters of microglia and a reactive astrocytosis. (H & E.)

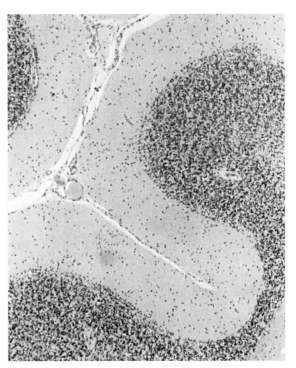

Fig. 10.18 Subacute cerebellar degeneration. There is loss of Purkinje cells. (H & E.)

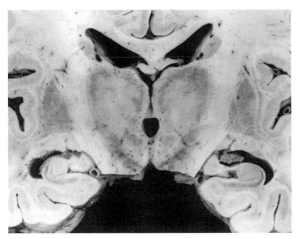

Fig. 10.17 Limbic encephalitis. There is discoloration of the Ammon's horns.

is affected more than white matter and the inflammatory changes are associated with loss of neurons and Wallerian degeneration. Various subdivisions exist based on the clinical features and the distribution of the lesions. For example, in *limbic encephalitis* involvement of the medial parts of the temporal lobes, including the hippocampi (Fig. 10.17) and amygdaloid complex, results in selective impairment of recent memory. In other cases the *encephalomyelitis* is localized principally to the brain stem, the cerebellum and the spinal cord. Other forms include *subacute cerebellar degeneration* in which there is extensive degeneration and loss of Purkinje cells (Fig. 10.18) and, to a lesser extent, of the granule cells, and a *subacute necrotizing myelopathy*. A combination of the various subdivisions is often found.

Many suggestions have been put forward about the pathogenesis of these neurological syndromes. They include toxins, infection, autoimmune processes, and metabolic and endocrine disorders. The presence of inflammatory lesions in the nervous system similar to those seen in virus infections certainly suggests the possibility that a neurotropic virus is the cause of the encephalomyelitides. An alternative explanation is that of an antigen–antibody reaction following the discovery of specific circulating antibodies against neural tissue.

Posterior root ganglia may be selectively affected, when there is loss of ganglion cells and proliferation of satellite cells leading to the formation of residual nodules of Nageotte. Secondary Wallerian degeneration results in loss of myelinated nerve fibres in the sensory nerve roots, the posterior columns of the spinal cord and peripheral nerves.

4. *Vascular syndromes.* Patients with thrombocytopenia, particularly if due to leukaemia, may present with intracranial haemorrhage. There is also an association between cerebral infarction and various carcinomas, mediated either through the disseminated intravascular coagulation syndrome or as a result of embolism from cardiac vegetations.

5. *Syndromes secondary to therapy.* These include *steroid psychosis, radiation necrosis of the brain* and *encephalopathies due to chemotherapy* (see Ch. 8).

Infections

These occur most commonly in patients with lymphoma, and include infections due to bacteria (meningitis due to *Listeria monocytogenes*), viruses (herpes simplex encephalitis and progressive multifocal leukoencephalopathy), fungi (cryptococcal meningitis, aspergillosis, and mucormycosis encephalitis) and parasites (toxoplasmosis).

FURTHER READING

Glew R H, Basu A, Prence E M et al (1985) Lysosomal storage disorders. *Laboratory Investigation* 53, 250–269.
Henson R A & Urich H (1982) *Cancer and the Nervous System.* New York: McGraw-Hill.
Lake B D (1989) Metabolic disorders – general considerations. In: *Pediatric Pathology*, 2nd edn. Edited by C L Berry. Berlin: Springer Verlag.
Lake B D (1990) Metabolic disorders of the central and peripheral nervous system. In: *Histochemistry in Pathology*.

Edited by M I Filipe & B D Lake. Edinburgh: Churchill Livingstone, pp. 109–128.
Scriver C R, Beaudet, A L, Sly W S, & Valle, D (eds) (1989) *The Metabolic Basis of Inherited Disease*, 6th edn. New York: McGraw-Hill.
Stanbury J B, Wyngaarden J B, Fredrickson D S, Goldstein J L & Brown M S (eds) (1983) *The Metabolic Basis of Inherited Disease*, 5th edn. New York: McGraw-Hill.

11. Deficiency disorders and intoxications

Deficiencies of vitamins and protein-calories are responsible for various neurological disorders. In the developed countries of Europe and North America many cases of vitamin deficiency are due to alcoholism, less commonly to malabsorption from gastrointestinal tract disease and, rarely, to food faddism. In contrast, the deficiency syndromes that are common in certain underdeveloped countries are usually due to an inadequate food supply. Malnutrition may cause irreparable brain damage at certain critical periods of both prenatal and postnatal development. There is considerable evidence now that children with low birth weights, including infants of malnourished mothers and children who survive protein–calorie deficiency (kwashiorkor), remain disadvantaged for life.

Interest in the effect of toxins on the nervous system has been growing rapidly, not only because of increased public concern about the effects of chemicals and toxins on health, but also because the nervous system is particularly vulnerable to chemical insult. Toxic disorders of the nervous system may occur as a result of exposure (deliberate or unintentional) to a host of substances that include therapeutic drugs, pest-control products, industrial chemicals, chemical warfare agents, food additives, heavy metals, the products or components of living organisms and other substances that include, for example, ethanol, inhalants or narcotics.

DEFICIENCY DISORDERS

VITAMIN A

A carotene, this substance is the precursor of the light-sensitive pigment rhodopsin which is present in the rods of the retina. Vitamin A is also necessary in the synthesis of active sulphate and the formation of myelin. Experimental deficiency in laboratory animals has caused raised intracranial pressure.

VITAMIN B$_1$ (THIAMINE)

This water-soluble vitamin plays an important part in the metabolism of carbohydrates, thiamine being a coenzyme in the glycolytic pathway and the citric acid cycle. Deficiency of thiamine impairs the oxidation of pyruvic acid, thereby raising pyruvate and lactate levels and reducing the amount of transketolase in red blood cells. The vitamin, which is not synthesized in the liver and is only stored in small quantities in the body, is found in many foods and is absorbed through the small intestine. Thiamine deficiency in the western hemisphere is usually due to chronic alcoholism and is responsible for *Wernicke's disease* and *beriberi*. Deficiency of thiamine may also be a contributory factor in *nutritional amblyopia*.

Wernicke's encephalopathy

Although found most commonly in malnourished chronic alcoholics, this condition also occurs as a result of excessive vomiting and malabsorption due to gastrointestinal tract disease, and in association with certain tumours such as leukaemia and lymphoma. It is characterized clinically in the acute stage by disturbances of consciousness, extraocular muscle palsies and nystagmus. The incidence of Wernicke's encephalopathy found post mortem in Perth, Western Australia, between 1973 and 1976 was 1.7 per cent; in Cleveland, Ohio, USA, the incidence post mortem between 1968 and 1973 was 2.7 per cent. In a more recent prospective study in Sydney, Australia, there was an incidence of 2.1 per cent in patients over the age of 15 years.

The disease may be acute, subacute or chronic, and the principal structures affected are the mamillary bodies, the walls of the third ventricle, the anterior nucleus of the thalamus, the peri-aqueductal tissues in the midbrain and the floor of the fourth ventricle. In less fulminant cases, abnormalities are restricted to the mamillary bodies.

Pathology

In acute or subacute Wernicke's encephalopathy, the brain is usually of normal appearance externally. On section there is vascular engorgement and petechial haemorrhage in the affected areas (Fig. 11.1). On the other hand, in patients who have survived an acute episode, the mamillary bodies are characteristically small and on section are often tan/grey in colour and granular in appearance (Fig. 11.2).

The histological changes depend on the duration and severity of the condition and are similar in all of the regions affected. In acute cases there is rarefaction of the neuropil and haemorrhage, but with preservation of neurons and axons (Fig. 11.3). Within a short time the changes become subacute,

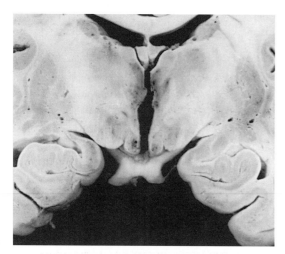

a

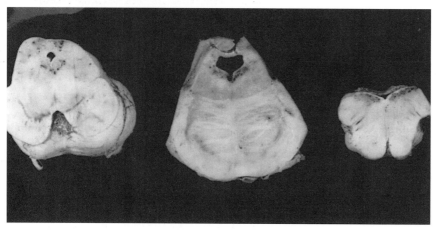

b

Fig. 11.1 Wernicke's encephalopathy. There are multiple petechial haemorrhages (a) in the mamillary bodies and in the walls of the third ventricle, and (b) around the aqueduct and in the floor of the fourth ventricle.

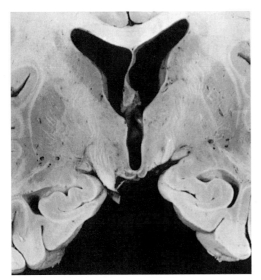

Fig. 11.2 Chronic Wernicke's encephalopathy. The mamillary bodies are small.

as shown by hyperplasia of capillary endothelial cells. In chronic cases there is loss of myelin in the central portions of the mamillary bodies,

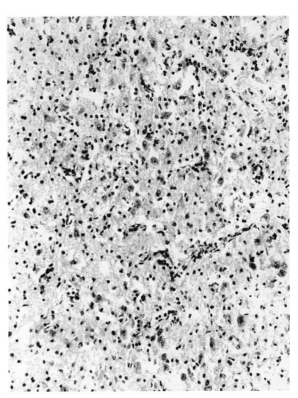

Fig. 11.4 Chronic Wernicke's encephalopathy. There is loss of myelinated fibres and prominence of capillaries in the central part of a mamillary body. There are also lipid-laden macrophages, some of which contain haemosiderin, and a prominent reactive astrocytosis. (H & E.)

gliosis and more normal-looking blood vessels (Fig. 11.4). Evidence of previous haemorrhage is frequently seen in the form of haemosiderin pigment in macrophages. In some 25 per cent of cases structural abnormalities can only be seen histologically. If the Wernicke's encephalopathy is due to chronic alcoholism, there is commonly atrophy of the superior vermis of the cerebellum (Fig. 11.5) and peripheral neuropathy. Coexisting disease of the liver may give rise to the histological features of hepatic encephalopathy (see Ch. 10).

The acute lesions of Wernicke's encephalopathy is due to thiamin deficiency. In alcoholics there may be decreased intake, reduced absorption, malutilization or increased excretion. The lesions of Wernicke's encephalopathy may develop only after prolonged alcohol abuse, but not all alcoholics are necessarily equally at risk.

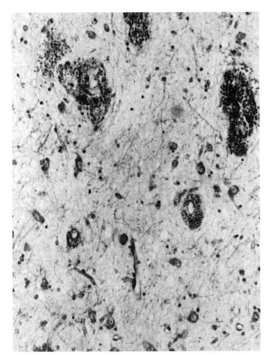

Fig. 11.3 Wernicke's encephalopathy. There are petechial haemorrhages in a mamillary body. Neurons are preserved. (H & E.)

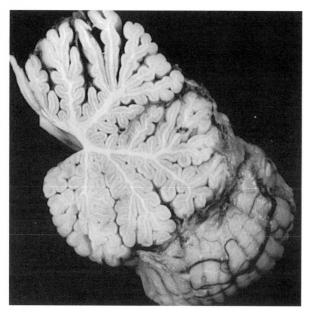

Fig. 11.5 Chronic alcoholism. There is atrophy of the superior vermis of the cerebellum.

The term *Korsakoff's psychosis* refers to an amnestic syndrome and is usually secondary to Wernicke's encephalopathy, when it is referred to as the Wernicke–Korsakoff syndrome. The condition can occur with other disease processes that involve the diencephalon or the medial structures of the temporal lobe. The cause of Korsakoff's psychosis is uncertain, although there appears to be a correlation with structural abnormalities in the dorsomedial nucleus of the thalamus. It is perhaps not surprising, therefore, that the prognosis of Korsakoff's psychosis is unpredictable. For example, even when appropriate treatment has been given to cases of alcoholic origin, only 25 per cent make a complete recovery and 50 per cent a partial recovery. The remainder make no improvement at all. In the past it was thought that lesions in the mamillary bodies were responsible for the amnesia, but this appears not to be the case.

Beriberi

This is endemic among rice-eating people. The form known as wet beriberi is characterized by heart failure and oedema that result from changes in the heart that are specifically due to lack of thiamine. Dry beriberi is characterized by a peripheral and central neuropathy (see Ch. 18). A disorder similar to dry beriberi can be produced in pigeons by feeding them polished rice; the affected birds recover rapidly when given thiamine. The disease in horses known as the 'staggers' is due to thiamine deficiency caused by the animals eating fodder contaminated with bracken; it too is quickly cured by treatment with thiamine.

VITAMINS OF THE B$_2$ GROUP

The association of *pellagra* (dermatitis, diarrhoea, dementia) in various parts of the world with poverty and subsistence on a diet predominantly of maize has been known for many years. It is caused by a dietary deficiency of nicotinic acid (niacin) itself, or of tryptophan, the amino acid precursor of nicotinic acid. Although nicotinic acid itself is important in the diet, it may also be biosynthesized in the intestines. People whose diet was based almost wholly on maize were therefore liable to suffer from nicotinic acid deficiency, but this has now become rare, largely as a result of enriching common foods. Circumstances under which the condition is now found include the modification of the normal bacterial flora of the intestines by certain antibiotics or other drugs, in chronic diarrhoea and in alcoholism.

The principal histological abnormality in the CNS is the occurrence of central chromatolysis (see Fig. 3.15) in Betz cells, in various nuclei in the brain stem, in the anterior horn cells of the spinal cord, in Purkinje cells and in the pyramidal cells of the hippocampus. In some cases there is degeneration of the gracile, the spinocerebellar, and the crossed and uncrossed corticospinal tracts of the spinal cord. There may also be a peripheral neuropathy. As many pellagrins also have other nutritional deficiencies, it is possible that at least some of the features of pellagra are due to deficiencies other than tryptophan-nicotinic acid, e.g. pyridoxine.

VITAMIN B$_6$

Deficiency of vitamin B$_6$ (pyridoxine, pyridoxal

and pyridoxamine) may be the cause of the peripheral neuropathy that sometimes occurs in patients taking drugs that interfere with the normal metabolism and utilization of vitamin B_6. These drugs include isoniazide, hydralazine and penicillamine.

There are many pyridoxine phosphate-dependent enzyme reactions in the nervous system, of particular importance being their role in the decarboxylation of amino acids and also the formation of amines such as adrenaline, noradrenaline, dopamine and serotonin. It has been suggested that the neuropathy associated with acute intermittent porphyria may be due to deficiency of pyridoxal phosphate as a result of its overuse by D-aminolaevulinic acid. In under-developed countries where there is widespread malnutrition, convulsions in children have been attributed to vitamin B_6 deficiency.

VITAMIN B_{12}

Man cannot synthesize this essential vitamin, which must be obtained from dietary sources, principally meats and dairy products. Vitamin B_{12} (cyanocobalamin) is absorbed in the distal ileum after combining with intrinsic factor which is secreted by the parietal cells of the gastric mucosa. Deficiency is almost always due to inadequate absorption, which most often results from inadequate production of intrinsic factor in patients with pernicious anaemia. Other, rarer, causes include impaired absorption from the small bowel as a result of various malabsorption syndromes, or competitive uptake of the vitamin due to fish tapeworm infestations or bacterial overgrowth in blind loops and diverticulae of the small bowel. In vegans, deficiency may be due to dietary insufficiency.

Deficiency of vitamin B_{12} affects particularly the haemopoietic tissue, epithelial surfaces and the nervous system. The vitamin is known to be involved in the conversion of L-methylmalonyl-CoA to succinyl-CoA mutase and methylation of homocysteine to methionine by methionine synthetase, but the biochemical basis for the various deleterious effects of this particular deficiency upon the nervous system is not known. Lesions in the spinal cord similar to those found in human B_{12} deficiency have been produced in monkeys exposed to nitrous oxide, which is thought to inactivate one of the vitamin B_{12}-dependent enzymes, thereby causing a depletion of methionine and a deficiency of the methyl group. There may also be a link between vitamin B_{12} deficiency and cyanide poisoning, since treatment with this vitamin leads to an improvement in tobacco amblyopia. Recently a number of cases have been reported in which the basis of the clinical signs and symptoms has been a hereditary disorder of cobalamin metabolism.

The principal structural abnormalities in vitamin B_{12} deficiency are found in the spinal cord, the optic nerves and the peripheral nerves. The best known is *subacute combined degeneration* of the spinal cord, when there are degenerative changes in the lateral and posterior columns, particularly in the mid-thoracic region. In the cervical region there is more severe involvement of the posterior columns, whereas the lateral columns are more affected in the lumbar region. In early cases there is focal swelling and ballooning of myelin sheaths; these lesions progressively enlarge, thereby imparting a characteristic spongy appearance to the affected white matter (Fig. 11.6). Eventually there is some loss of myelin, degeneration of axons and phagocytosis of the debris by macrophages. Wallerian degeneration ensues and there is an astrocytosis, the degree of which is said to correlate with the duration of the disease. In long-standing severe cases there may be atrophy and discoloration of the posterior and lateral columns.

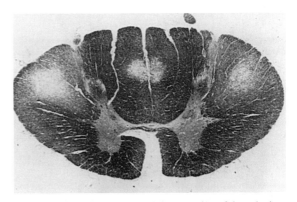

Fig. 11.6 Subacute combined degeneration of the spinal cord. There is focal pallor of myelin staining in the posterior and lateral columns. Luxol fast blue/cresyl violet.

Similar histological appearances are occasionally seen in the deep white matter of the cerebral hemispheres and, more rarely, in the optic nerves. There is also often an associated peripheral neuropathy.

Folic acid and vitamin B_{12} are commonly discussed together as both are related to DNA metabolism. Deficiency can result from an inadequate diet, from the ingestion of certain anticonvulsant drugs such as phenytoin, or from treatment with anti-folate drugs such as methotrexate.

VITAMIN E

This vitamin has an important role in the maintenance and function of the nervous system, and its role as an antioxidant preventing the peroxidation of phospholipids has been suggested.

Conditions causing chronic malabsorption or reduced concentration of bile salts in the small intestine may lead to vitamin E deficiency. An inborn error of vitamin E metabolism has also been described, associated with which is a degenerative neurological disorder. Vitamin E deficiency occurs in abetalipoproteinaemia, in which there is a failure of synthesis of apoprotein B, an essential component of chylomicrons. The electrophysiological appearance and neuropathology are those of a distal axonopathy affecting both central and peripheral axons of sensory ganglion cells. Experimental studies in rats and monkeys confirm that vitamin E deficiency produces a 'dying back' neuropathy in both central and peripheral sensory neurons.

PROTEIN–CALORIE DEFICIENCY

The effects of serious malnutrition have been described in young children in many of the underdeveloped countries. They are thought to be more profound and lasting on the developing CNS than in the mature adult CNS. Most of the changes are thought to be secondary to vitamin deficiencies, but the developing CNS is also vulnerable to a deficiency of protein-calories, since post-mortem studies on malnourished children have shown a reduction in the weight of the brain, in the number of neurons and in the amount of myelin in the CNS. Long-term consequences are a product of disturbed neuronal maturation, myelin formation and synaptogenesis.

Tobacco amblyopia

The cause of this condition remains unknown but it is possibly due to more than one nutritional deficiency, or a combination of nutritional deficiencies. Neither alcohol nor tobacco is primarily responsible for the condition, since well documented cases of this type of amblyopia have occurred in patients who neither smoked tobacco nor drank alcohol. The disorder is probably the result of a deficiency of several vitamins.

Neurological complications of steatorrhoea and related gastrointestinal disorders

The neuropathological findings in *coeliac disease* (gluten-induced enteropathy) are different from those associated with Wernicke's encephalopathy, subacute combined degeneration, Vitamin E deficiency or pellagra. About 10 per cent of patients with coeliac disease develop neurological complications attributed to focal neuronal loss and associated reactive changes in the cerebellum, the basal ganglia, the nuclei of the brain stem and the spinal cord. A peripheral neuropathy is not uncommon. The aetiology of the neurological involvement in this disease is not known, but nutritional, toxic, infective, autoimmune and genetic factors have been implicated. Peripheral neuropathy may also be a feature of *post-gastrectomy states* after surgery for peptic ulcer.

Neurological complications also occur in *Whipple's disease*, a disorder in which PAS-staining granular material is present in macrophages in the wall of the small bowel; focal collections of similar cells are also found in the brain. The PAS-positive material has been shown by ultrastructural studies to be bacterial in nature, but there is no agreement as to its precise type.

INTOXICATIONS

TOXIC GASES

Carbon monoxide

The clinical features of acute carbon monoxide

intoxication can be correlated with the concentration of carboxyhaemoglobin in the blood, which in turn is a product of the duration of exposure to and the concentration of carbon monoxide in the environment. A previously healthy individual will experience severe headache and dizziness with 20–30 per cent saturation; impaired vision, hearing and mental function at 40–50 per cent saturation; coma and convulsions at 50–60 per cent saturation; and cardiorespiratory failure and death at over 70 per cent saturation. The outcome is often influenced by pre-existing cardiovascular disease, many of the acute deaths resulting from myocardial dysfunction.

Pathology

When death occurs within a few hours, the blood, brain, muscles, skin and viscera have the pink/red colour characteristic of carboxy-haemoglobin. The brain and leptomeninges are usually congested and petechial haemorrhages are frequently seen in white matter, particularly in the corpus callosum. If the patient survives in coma for a few days, macroscopic evidence of necrosis may be seen in the cerebral cortex, the hippocampi and in the basal ganglia, particularly in the globus pallidus (Fig. 11.7). The pattern of damage is very similar to that seen in other types of ischaemic brain damage (see Ch. 5). In contrast, alterations in the white matter may result from carbon monoxide intoxication, and

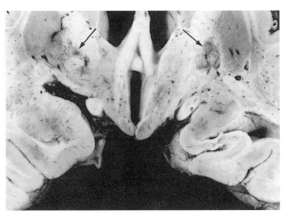

Fig. 11.7 Carbon monoxide poisoning. There are foci of necrosis in each globus pallidus (arrows).

their extent is not necessarily proportional to the damage in grey matter, so the latter may appear normal even when there is extensive myelin breakdown. White matter damage takes the form of *periaxial demyelination* (see Ch. 9) and is a well recognized feature of the brains of patients presenting with delayed onset neurological symptoms following an acute episode of intoxication. The pathogenesis of carbon monoxide encephalopathy is multifactorial, and includes the high affinity of carbon monoxide for the ferrous haem of haemoglobin and its binding to brain cytochromes, and various vascular mechanisms due to systemic circulatory factors. The concentration of damage in white matter is thought to be due to a local cytotoxic effect of carbon monoxide, with an additional reduction in blood flow.

Nitrous oxide

Nitrous oxide, as with other inhalation anaesthetics, may occasionally lead to accidents during which the patient becomes hypoxic. If resuscitation is successful, then the patient may manifest various degrees of disability as a result of ischaemic brain damage (see Ch. 5).

Prolonged exposure to nitrous oxide, particularly in dental personnel, occasionally causes *myeloneuropathy*, the clinical features of which are similar to subacute combined degeneration of the spinal cord. It has been suggested that nitrous oxide produces the myeloneuropathy by inactivating methionine synthetase, a vitamin B_{12} dependent enzyme. Confirmation of the similarity between chronic exposure to nitrous oxide and subacute combined degeneration of the cord has been obtained in monkey models.

Malignant hyperthermia (or hyperpyrexia) is an uncommon but often fatal complication of general anaesthesia and, in over three-quarters of reported cases, is characterized by a dramatic rise in core temperature and generalized muscle rigidity (see Ch. 17). It has been associated with exposure to a variety of anaesthetic agents, including nitrous oxide, and is more common when succinylcholine is used as premedication. A positive family history is present in about 30 per cent of patients. Malignant hyperthermia, however, has also been reported in certain muscle diseases, such as

Duchenne muscular dystrophy, myotonia congenita and central core disease.

Cyanides

The effects of the cyanide ion are due to the inhibition of cytochrome oxidase, the terminal enzyme in the respiratory electron transport chain which utilizes the oxygen derived from dissociation of oxyhaemoglobin. There is no essential difference between the neuropathological effects of sodium and potassium cyanide, hydrocyanic acid and cyanogen chloride. In acute intoxication, death from respiratory failure ensues rapidly and is often preceded by convulsions. The brain may be congested and occasional petechial haemorrhages are seen, but there are no significant microscopic changes. If death is delayed, there may be pathological evidence of alterations in both grey and white matter. Experimental studies have shown that cyanide can damage myelin sheaths after administration by any route. Grey matter may also be damaged, but only after cardiorespiratory complications, including epilepsy, have occurred.

ALCOHOL

Ethanol

After absorption by the small intestine into the blood, ethyl alcohol is rapidly distributed to all parts of the body and equilibrates with body water compartments. Eventually, most of the alcohol is oxidized in the liver through acetaldehyde to acetic acid; a small proportion – less than 10 per cent – is excreted unchanged from the lungs, kidneys and skin. An average adult can metabolize about 10 ml of pure ethyl alcohol hourly. Blood alcohol levels above 100 mg per 100 ml are usually associated with signs of intoxication in a non-habituated person: levels above 400 mg per 100 ml are associated with stupor or coma, regardless of the degree of tolerance, and levels above 500 mg per 100 ml are often fatal.

The pathological effects of chronic alcohol abuse on the liver are well established, yet in many instances abnormalities in the nervous system are not due to a direct toxic effect of alcohol but rather to an associated nutritional deficiency. A wide range of histological changes have been attributed to alcoholism, but most are now regarded as non-specific. There are, however, a number of conditions that fall within the domain of the neuropathologist.

Acute alcohol intoxication and the withdrawal syndrome

There are no specific neuropathological features, but head injury and subarachnoid haemorrhage due to rupture of a saccular aneurysm are more common in intoxicated than sober individuals, and there is an increased risk of cerebral infarction after an alcoholic 'binge'. There are no characteristic features in fatal cases of *delirium tremens* or *withdrawal seizures* other than those associated with terminal hypoxia and electrolyte imbalance.

Nutritional diseases of the nervous system associated with alcoholism

Principal among these are the *Wernicke– Korsakoff syndrome*, *optic neuropathy*, *pellagra* and *peripheral neuropathy*.

Other lesions found in association with alcoholism

Cerebral atrophy may occur in patients with chronic alcoholism and there may be a global deterioration in intellect known as *alcoholic dementia*. The frequency, severity and relation of the atrophy to the alcoholism is controversial, but there is increasing evidence from CT scans and autopsy studies that both cerebral atrophy and ventricular enlargement are common in alcoholic patients, even in the absence of significant hepatic disease. Post-mortem studies have suggested that the cerebral atrophy is not due to loss of grey matter but rather to a reduction in the volume of the deep white matter. The abnormalities may be reversed by abstinence from alcohol. Perhaps an appropriate term for the reversible abnormalities would be 'thiamine dementia'.

There is often selective atrophy of the anterior

portion of the superior vermis of the cerebellum in chronic alcoholics. This atrophy may be an isolated finding or may be associated with other alcohol-related diseases, such as Wernicke's encephalopathy and cerebral atrophy. Microscopically, within the atrophic cerebellar cortex there is loss of Purkinje cells, a variable loss of granule cells, and associated reactive proliferation of Bergmann astrocytes and an isomorphic fibrillary gliosis in the molecular layer. Clinicopathological studies have shown that these changes correlate with the truncal instability, leg ataxia and widebased stance and gait that are often seen in chronic alcoholics. The cerebellar degeneration has been attributed to the direct toxic effects of alcohol, but a more likely explanation is that it is secondary to nutritional deficiency, particularly as similar atrophy is seen in malnourished patients in whom there is no history of alcohol abuse.

There is an association between chronic alcoholism and *central pontine myelinolysis*, *Marchiafava-Bignami disease, peripheral neuropathy* and *myopathy*.

Fetal alcohol syndrome

The incidence of this is reported as 1 in 600 births in France, the USA and Sweden, and the syndrome is now regarded as one of the leading causes of birth defects associated with mental retardation. The degree of maternal alcoholism, and the critical stage in gestation for the development of this disorder, are not known, and it is still unclear whether it is the alcohol *per se*, one of its metabolites or an associated nutritional deficiency that is the actual cause of the teratogenic effects. The most common abnormality is microcephaly. Hydrocephalus, agenesis of the corpus callosum, generalized disorganization of neuronal migration, hypoplasia of the midface and limb malformations have also been reported. In several animal experimental studies there has been impaired maturation of cortical neurons and a decreased number of dendrites in the progeny of mothers given ethyl alcohol throughout pregnancy.

Neurological disorders secondary to alcohol-induced cirrhosis of the liver portal-systemic shunt

These include *hepatic encephalopathy* and *chronic hepatocerebral degeneration* (see Ch. 10).

METHANOL

There is considerable variation in individual susceptibility to ingested methanol, either in the form of cheap intoxicants or products such as solvents. The more serious sequelae, however, are produced by its catabolites, formaldehyde and formic acid. Blindness occurs frequently in methanol intoxication and has been attributed either to degeneration of the retinal ganglion cells and photoreceptors, or to swelling of the optic disc, thought to be due to swelling of axons in which there is stasis of axoplasmic flow, possibly related to the diffusion of formic acid from choroidal vessels. The neuropathological features in acute deaths are nonspecific, but in patients who survive, necrosis of the basal ganglia and of the deep white matter of the cerebral and cerebellar hemispheres has been described. It has been suggested that the changes in the white matter and in the optic nerves represent a toxic form of loss of myelin caused by formates.

Ethylene glycol

This dihydroxyalcohol is widely used as a solvent and as a component of certain antifreezes and coolants. Intoxication is encountered most often when it is consumed as an ill-advised substitute for ethanol, or is used as a means of suicide. The minimum lethal dose is thought to be in excess of 100 ml. Ethylene glycol is progressively oxidized into a series of toxic compounds, including glycoaldehyde, glycolic acid and glyoxylic acid; a small proportion is oxidized eventually to oxalic acid. In fatal cases there is swelling, congestion and occasional petechial haemorrhages in the brain. Histologically, there is an infiltration by neutrophil polymorphs in the meninges and in relation to the parenchymatous blood vessels. Deposits of crystalline calcium oxalate may be seen in and around the blood vessels of the meninges, the brain and choroid plexus: they are best seen with polarized light.

DRUGS AND DIAGNOSTIC AGENTS

PHENYTOIN (DIPHENYLHYDANTOIN)

Manifestations of toxicity include drowsiness, nystagmus, cerebellar ataxia, encephalopathy and peripheral neuropathy. Some appear in relation to high serum drug levels and resolve when the levels are decreased. Occasionally, however, the symptoms and signs do not resolve even after withdrawal of the drug, and this has led to the long-standing controversy about the pathogenesis of the *cerebellar syndromes* attributed to atrophy of the cerebellum brought about by diffuse loss of Purkinje cells (Fig. 11.8). Opinions differ about the role of phenytoin in their pathogenesis because the cerebellum is particularly sensitive to hypoxia, and epilepsy alone may be a cause of loss of Purkinje cells. Even experimental studies of phenytoin neurotoxicity have yielded conflicting results, and although there is considerable evidence to suggest that phenytoin *per se* can cause cerebellar degeneration, no definite conclusion can be reached.

The administration of anticonvulsants, including phenytoin, to pregnant women has been implicated in the production of various congenital anomalies, namely the so-called *fetal hydantoin syndrome*. The spectrum of malformations of the CNS includes hydrocephalus, microcephaly and defects of the neural tube. It is necessary, however, to consider a whole variety of possibilities, such as the effects of maternal infections and possible prenatal exposure to other teratogens before directly attributing any fetal abnormalities to anticonvulsants.

AMPHETAMINE-RELATED COMPOUNDS

Stimulant drugs of abuse include amphetamine derivatives and cocaine. These agents cause hypertension, hyperthermia with convulsions, cardiac fibrillation and eventual circulatory collapse. Intracranial haemorrhage is a common finding post mortem, and has been attributed to pharmacologically induced hypertension, as many of these cases occur in young adults in whom there is no evidence of cerebrovascular disease. The distribution of the intracranial haemorrhage is typical of that of primary intracerebral haemorrhage, i.e. in the thalamus and basal ganglia. Sometimes, however, bleeding occurs into the subarachnoid and subdural spaces.

The chronic abuse of amphetamine analogues may be complicated by a necrotizing angiitis, the histological features of which are indistinguishable from polyarteritis nodosa.

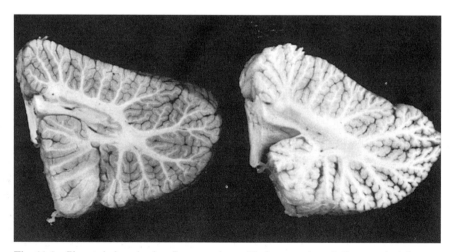

Fig. 11.8 Phenytoin intoxication. In comparison with the normal cerebellum on the left, there is atrophy of folia in the cerebellum on the right.

OPIATES

Important drugs associated with opiate addiction include morphine, heroin and the synthetic alkaloid methadone. Neuropathological studies on fatal cases of opiate abuse indicate that there is a fairly consistent pattern of ischaemic damage in the globus pallidus, the cerebral cortex, the hippocampus, the deep white matter of the cerebral hemispheres and, occasionally, the thoracic part of the spinal cord. These changes have been attributed to one or more bouts of perfusion failure, and might be due to respiratory depression caused by opiates. Other findings include the effects of trauma and infections, such as bacterial endocarditis, meningitis, viral hepatitis with encephalopathy, malaria and tetanus. A vasculitis has been observed in some opiate abusers but the current evidence suggests that it is probably due to concurrent amphetamine abuse.

NEUROLEPTICS

Drugs such as the phenothiazines and butyro-pherones are important in the long-term treatment of psychosis. An untoward complication is that of *tardive dyskinesia*: this is more common in females and increases with age, the duration of treatment and with the total dose of the agent given. Neuropathological studies in these patients have shown that there is an increase in the amount of neuronal loss, satellitosis and increased neuronal lipofuscin in the basal ganglia, substantia nigra and midbrain compared with age-matched controls.

BARBITURATES

In spite of the obvious pharmacological effects produced by the barbiturates on the CNS, there are no descernible structural abnormalities in the brain that can be attributed to this class of drug *per se*. The pattern of damage, however, that can be identified in patients who survive an acute overdose but are left with residual neurological deficits is that of hypoxic brain damage due to the known depressive effects of barbiturates on the respiratory and cardiovascular systems.

CLIOQUINOL

This drug has been used for many years in the treatment for intestinal amoebiasis. It has also been used less discriminately for a variety of chronic non-specific diarrhoeas and 'travellers diarrhoea'. There is considerable circumstantial evidence that it may cause *toxic encephalopathy, isolated optic atrophy* and *subacute myelo-optic neuropathy (SMON syndrome)*. The toxic syndrome has, for reasons unknown, been restricted almost exclusively to the Japanese. Post-mortem studies in human cases of the SMON syndrome have revealed lesions in the spinal cord, spinal nerve roots, dorsal root and autonomic ganglia, optic and – less severely – peripheral nerves. There is axonal degeneration in the gracile tracts and, to a lesser extent, in the spinocerebellar and the distal parts of the corticospinal tracts of the spinal cord. Neuronal loss and proliferation of satellite cells in the dorsal root ganglia, with evidence of both axonal degeneration and demyelination in the posterior spinal roots and in peripheral nerves, are also seen. Similar changes are seen in the optic nerves. Experimental studies have produced similar changes in the CNS and in the optic nerves. There is distal degeneration of centrally directed fibres of dorsal root ganglia cells, with sparing of peripheral fibres.

ANTIBIOTICS, ANTIVIRAL AND ANTIFUNGAL AGENTS

The antibacterial agents *dapsone, nitrofurantoin* and *chloramphenicol* are recognized but rare causes of peripheral neuropathy in man. On the other hand, *isoniazid* may cause peripheral neuropathy in some 30–40 per cent of cases, depending on dose and genetic factors: it causes a disturbance of vitamin B_6 metabolism, which can produce distal axonal degeneration. Pyridoxine supplementation reduces the incidence of the neuropathy. Neurotoxicity, manifested by ototoxicity, encephalopathy and psychosis, has also been associated with the use of *gentamicin*.

Neuropathological studies have demonstrated widespread central chromatolysis and necrosis of neurons in the brain stem of patients treated with *adenine arabinoside*, following treatment of herpes simplex encephalitis and disseminated varicella zoster infections.

Dementia and akinetic mutism have followed the intravenous use of amphotericin B for the treatment of fungal infections. The principal findings are those of a diffuse cerebral leukoencephalopathy with relative preservation of axons. Experimental studies have confirmed that the methyl ester of the drug is particularly neurotoxic.

ANTINEOPLASTIC AGENTS

Various neurological complications may occur as a result of systemic or intrathecal chemotherapy with various antineoplastic agents. Of particular interest have been those associated with *methotrexate*, a widely used folic acid antagonist. Methotrexate neurotoxicity may take several forms, principal among which are a *chemical arachnoiditis* and a *disseminated necrotizing leukoencephalopathy* (see Ch. 8). Occasionally the intracarotid infusion of a high dose of methotrexate has been associated with multiple haemorrhagic infarcts in the brain. Of particular concern has been the delayed encephalopathies which most often follow a combination of high-dose long-term systemic and/or intrathecal methotrexate therapy and cranial irradiation in children with leukaemia. Several patterns of damage have been identified. The best-known is a disseminated necrotizing leukoencephalopathy which consists of multiple well-circumscribed yellowish-grey granular lesions in the white matter of the cerebral hemispheres, the brain stem and the spinal cord. Histologically, the lesions consist of focal areas of coagulative necrosis with loss of myelin, axons and oligodendrocytes. There is no inflammatory cell infiltrate and lipid-containing macrophages are sparse. Axonal swellings, some of which may be mineralized, are frequently seen at the periphery of the lesions in association with vacuolation of the white matter and a reactive astrocytosis (Fig. 11.9). In many cases there are no vascular changes but in some there is fibrinoid necrosis of small blood vessels (Fig. 11.10). The aetiology of this condition is unknown, as most patients with necrotizing leukoencephalopathy have received both methotrexate and irradiation to the CNS. The neuropathological features, however, are not those typically associated with radiation necrosis, and it may be that the radiation, by damaging the blood–brain barrier, permits methotrexate to diffuse into the brain to produce damage to white matter. Milder cases of encephalopathy have also been described in which there is CT scan evidence of cerebral atrophy, with ventricular dilatation and intracerebral calcification.

Acute encephalopathies, degeneration of the cerebellum and necrotizing encephalomyelopathy have all been described after treatment with various antineoplastic agents that include *cytosine arabinoside, 5-fluorouracil, nitrogen mustard, cyclophosphamide* and various nitrosourea compounds. On the other hand, the *vinca alkaloids* vincristine and vinblastine, which are mitotic spindle inhibitors, are particularly associated with peripheral neuropathy. A rare complication of vincristine neurotoxicity is myeloencephalopathy, when it has accidentally been administered intrathecally. Histologically, there are marked changes in the neurons of the brain stem and spinal cord, consisting of large amounts of interwoven neurofilaments with loss of microtubules and the formation of crystalline masses. The changes have been attributed to the action of the alkaloids on microtubule protein (tubulin) and consequent changes in axoplasmic transport mechanisms.

AGENTS USED IN DIAGNOSTIC NEURORADIOLOGY AND IN NEURORADIOTHERAPY

Non-ionic contrast media are extensively used for diagnostic neurological studies. Complications include seizures and encephalopathy, thought to result from the inhibition of hexokinase. Histological abnormalities consist of an inflammatory cell infiltrate in the meninges or the ventricles.

Complications of the *nitroimidazoles* and *metronidazole*, which are used as potentiating agents in radiotherapy, include encephalopathy and seizures, but in particular a peripheral neuropathy. Both the structural abnormalities and their topography resemble those found in thiamine-deficient rats although the effects of the intoxications in man are not prevented by the administration of thiamine.

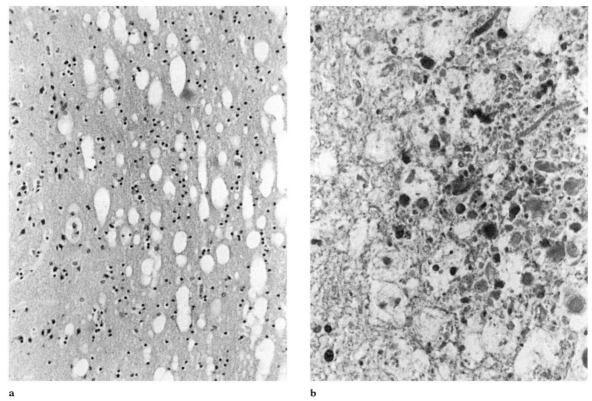

a   b

Fig. 11.9   Disseminated necrotizing leukoencephalopathy. (a) Vacuolation of the white matter and an astrocytosis. (b) Multiple axonal swellings, focal calcification and vacuolation of white matter. (H & E.)

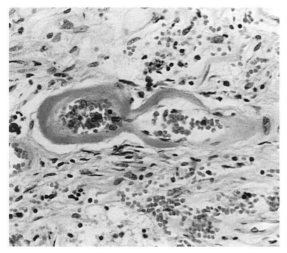

Fig. 11.10   Disseminated necrotizing leukoencephalopathy. Fibrinoid necrosis of a small blood vessel. (H & E.)

INDUSTRIAL TOXINS

CARBON DISULPHIDE

Exposure is an occupational hazard in the production of viscose rayon and film. Fortunately, acute toxicity no longer occurs, and attention is now directed to complications of long-term exposure to low concentrations of carbon disulphide – it is, for example, a consituent in fumigants used for treating grain – which include peripheral neuropathy and an increase in cardio-vascular disease. Pathologically the changes are consistent with a central–peripheral distal axonopathy which closely resembles the hexacarbon neuropathies. It has been suggested that carbon disulphide acts by binding with neurofilament protein, thereby affecting axoplasmic transport.

Carbon disulphide is a metabolite of disulfiram, a drug used in the treatment of chronic alcoholism and occasionally associated with a toxic neuropathy. The neurotoxicity of disulfiram is probably due to its conversion in the body to carbon disulphide.

SOLVENTS

Toluene is both an important solvent in many different industries and an important base compound in the synthesis of other substances. It is a prominent substance in solvent abuse. It is readily absorbed from the lungs, and rapidly distributed through, and metabolized in, the body. Acute toxicity depends upon the concentration and duration of exposure. Chronic exposure produces cerebellar ataxia and a peripheral neuropathy.

Carbon tetrachloride, a common solvent, has been used in certain types of fire extinguishers. Acute intoxication results in damage to the CNS, liver and kidneys. In cases where there is hepatic or renal failure, the neural dysfunction may be secondary to a metabolic encephalopathy. In addition, there are changes in the white matter referred to as carbon tetrachloride-induced vasculopathy.

Another important solvent is *trichloroethylene* used in dry-cleaning procedures. Acute intoxication produces multiple cranial nerve palsies, particularly of the Vth and VIIth nerves.

The hexacarbon compounds *n-hexane* and *methyl n-butyl ketone*, have been employed extensively as organic solvents in the production of adhesives and cement. These two substances and their common metabolite 2,5-hexanedione, produce a distinctive form of peripheral neuropathy which may occur in 'glue-sniffers' as well as a result of industrial exposure. Histologically, the hexacarbon neuropathies are characterized by the formation of focal swellings on axons prior to degeneration of the more distal regions of the affected nerves. These swellings tend to develop proximal to nodes of Ranvier, and are filled with masses of neurofilaments. Their formation may be related to impairment of axoplasmic transport due to inhibition of a glycolytic enzyme or, alternatively, through a reaction of hexacarbons with amino groups of neurofilaments, causing them to form aggregations. Similar axonal enlargements have been seen in other forms of intoxication, namely *acrylamide* and *carbon disulphide*. In hexacarbon neuropathy there is distal axonal degeneration in both the central and peripheral nervous systems, and changes are therefore found in the gracile, corticospinal and spinocerebellar tracts.

TOXIC OIL SYNDROME

Following the ingestion of contaminated rapeseed oil in 1981 there was an outbreak of a new toxic syndrome in Spain that affected 25 000 people. Clinically there was a multisystem illness that included respiratory symptoms and involved the skin and muscles. Nerve and muscle biopsy revealed an inflammatory vasculitis and at autopsy there was chromatolysis of anterior horn cells in the spinal cord and of brain-stem nuclei. The cause is not known.

ORGANOPHOSPHORUS COMPOUNDS

Exposure to organophosphates occurs in the manufacture and formulation of the compounds, and in large-scale spraying operations with insecticides. Acute poisoning results in the accumulation of endogenous acetylcholine in neural tissue and effector organs because of the inhibition of cholinesterase, with subsequent signs and symptoms that mimic the muscarinic, nicotinic and CNS actions of acetylcholine. These can usually be controlled and there are no long-term effects. Some organophosphates, however, cause a delayed peripheral neuropathy which develops between 1 and 3 weeks after a single dose. One such agent, triorthocresyl phosphate (TOCP), is used as a plasticizer and lubricant and has been responsible for accidental neurotoxicity, well documented cases occurring in 'ginger jake paralysis' which followed the consumption of alcoholic extracts of ginger contaminated with TOCP during prohibition in the USA, and after contamination in Morocco of cooking oil by aircraft lubricating oil. TOCP causes distal degeneration of peripheral nerves, particularly affecting the longest and largest fibres; long fibre tracts in the cord are also involved. Degeneration gradually progresses towards the parent cell body. It was originally suggested that this 'dying back' type of neuropathy was caused by some impairment of perikaryal metabolism, whose effects would be most marked upon the largest and longest fibres. Experimental studies with another organophosphorus compound, di-isopropylfluorophosphonate (DFP), however, have shown focal and non-terminal fibre changes, which suggest a direct effect upon the axon rather than on the perikaryon.

MISCELLANEOUS NEUROTOXINS

Botulism is caused by intoxication with the protein neurotoxin produced by the organism *Clostridium botulinum*. Foodborne botulism is caused by ingestion of the neurotoxin preformed in foods contaminated with the organism. The illness is now relatively rare in most developed countries, although outbreaks continue to be reported, largely caused by home-processed foods or improperly cooked or uncooked marine meats. Botulinum toxins block transmission at cholinergic synapses by preventing the release of acetylcholine. There is no effect on the conduction of impulses along the axon into the presynaptic nerve terminal and no effect on the excitability of muscle fibres themselves. Morphological studies demonstrate binding of labelled toxin to the presynaptic membrane. Wound botulism is now very rare and occurs when wounds become contaminated by the microorganism.

In spite of widespread immunization programmes, *tetanus* continues to occur and has a high mortality. The toxin is a protein produced by *Clostridium tetani*, the primary clinical manifestations of which are caused by a blockade of inhibitory input to spinal motor neurons. The toxin probably gains access via retrograde axonal transport along nerve fibres, and perhaps along the endoneurium as well, originating at the portal of entry. The effects of the toxin may remain localized to the motor neuron pool supplying the affected muscles (local tetanus), e.g. 'lockjaw' or 'risus sardonicus'; however, the effect becomes generalized if enough toxin is present to enter the bloodstream and affect the nervous system diffusely, resulting in generalized muscle spasms.

Diphtheria is now an uncommon illness in most parts of the world as a result of widespread active immunization. It is due to a protein neurotoxin released by *Corynebacterium diphtheriae*, which is believed to act by preventing the elongation of polypeptide chains. The condition may be life-threatening because of either the local pharyngeal infection or from systemic intoxication, which primarily affects the heart and nervous system. The predilection of diphtheria toxin for the peripheral nervous system is unexplained, but it has been shown to inhibit synthesis of myelin proteolipids and basic proteins, causing a segmental demyelinating neuropathy.

Lathyrism occurs when large amounts of the seeds of *lathyrus* are eaten, usually at times of drought and famine. The characteristic clinical feature is spastic paraplegia, which neuropathologically is due to symmetrical degeneration of the corticospinal tracts. The substance at present considered most likely to be responsible is B-N-oxalylamino-L-alanine (BOAA), the neurotoxicity of which is similar to another plant-derived amino-acid, L-B-methylaminoalanine (BMAA).

NEUROTOXIC METALS

More than 25 metals can be detected in human tissues, but of these only 13 are considered to be 'essential'. Deficiency of certain of the essential elements may lead to neurological dysfunction, the basis of which is often the absence of the metal in critical metalloenzymes, loss of stabilization of membranes or impaired release of neurotransmitters. On the other hand, certain of the essential and non-essential metals, if given in sufficient concentration and appropriate form, are known to be toxic, affecting multiple systems in the body including the nervous system.

ALUMINIUM

Aluminium was for a long time considered to be a non-absorbable, non-toxic element the health hazard of which was restricted to the occupational inhalation of aluminium-contaminated dust. In recent years, however, it has been implicated as an aetiological factor in *dialysis encephalopathy* (see Ch. 10). The source of the increased levels of aluminium in the brains of these patients was originally identified as the aluminium-containing phosphate binders, but later studies have suggested that there is a relationship between the encephalopathy and the aluminium content in the water used to prepare the dialysis fluid.

Aluminium has also been implicated as a factor in the pathogenesis of dementia of Alzheimer type (see Ch. 14). The neurofibrillary tangles that can be produced in experimental animals by aluminium, however, are quite different electron-microscopically from the paired helical filaments seen in the naturally occurring Alzheimer's neurofibrillary tangles in man; furthermore, senile plaques, granulovacuolar degeneration and amyloid angiopathy are not seen. The significance of the increased amounts of aluminium in the brain is also uncertain, as accumulation of this element takes place with increasing age. The deposits are in the form of aluminium silicate in neurons within which there are neurofibrillary tangles. Opinions differ as to whether or not the deposition of aluminium is a secondary event and therefore unimportant, or whether it plays a role in the pathogenesis of the disease.

ARSENIC

Toxicity can be caused by exposure to a variety of arsenic-based compounds used as pesticides, mordants, paints, wood preservatives and medical agents. Both inorganic and organic arsenical compounds may be toxic.

Acute inorganic arsenic poisoning manifests first as a gastrointestinal disturbance, and thereafter by circulatory collapse and hepatic and renal failure. There may then be a transient encephalopathy. Peripheral neuropathy is a well known and often disabling sequel of both acute and chronic arsenical intoxication. Occupational exposure to inorganic arsenic occurs mainly in the smelting industry and in the manufacture and application of arsenic-based pesticides. Patients with mild sensory–motor disturbances recover completely and quickly, but recovery from an acute attack or after cessation of exposure during chronic poisoning may take as long as 3 years, and residual disability is to be expected in those severely affected initially.

Organoarsenic toxicity in the form of an *acute haemorrhagic encephalopathy* was a serious complication of the treatment of syphilis with organic arsenicals (arsenobenzene derivatives). The problem was recognized soon after the introduction of arsphenamine and its wide use in the 1930s and 1940s, about 10 per cent of patients developing an acute neurological illness. It is also currently a major problem in the treatment of human African trypanosomiasis ('sleeping sickness'). The clinical onset of organoarsenic encephalopathy is rapid, and the mortality rate is over 50 per cent. Post mortem there are multiple haemorrhages of varying size, particularly in the white matter of the brain. Microscopy shows varying degrees of endothelial damage and occasional thrombi in venules and capillaries: perivascular infiltrates are rare. There may be focal demyelination. The pathogenesis of this condition is unclear, although a direct toxic effect of arsphenamines on the endothelial cells is possible. There are, however, similarities between arsphenamine encephalopathy and acute haemorrhagic leukoencephalitis (see Ch. 9). There is, however, no evidence that organoarsenic encephalopathy is an immune response, and it seems more likely that, particularly with trivalent forms of arsenic, the encephalopathy is related to the binding of arsenic to thiol groups.

GOLD

Medicinal gold salts have been used in the treatment of rheumatoid arthritis and psoriatic arthritis. Toxicity affects multiple systems, including both the central and peripheral nervous systems. Gold-induced peripheral neuropathy is well recognized. The pathological basis of gold encephalopathy has not been clearly defined, and ranges from psychosis or encephalopathy to loss of myelin with necrosis of white matter.

LEAD

There is no known biological requirement for lead and it must therefore be viewed purely as a toxicant. Lead poisoning has afflicted man since antiquity, and although many of the occupational and domestic environmental sources have been eliminated or reduced, raised blood levels still occur in large numbers of children, especially among lower socioeconomic groups. Lead can enter the body through the gastrointestinal and respiratory tracts and occasionally through the skin: many systems of the body are affected adversely by an excessive amount of lead. Most modern-day exposure is from industrial sources in the manufacture of organo-leads, such as fuel additives, or the manufacture of lead-based pigments, solder or batteries. There is also a potential source from deteriorating housing with lead furnishings and lead-based paint. It is also a consequence of the consumption of lead-contaminated alcohol.

Inorganic lead poisoning

The systemic pathological features of *plumbism* include basophil stippling of red cells, lead lines in the metaphases of long bones in children and lead-containing intranuclear inclusion bodies in the proximal tubules of the kidney. By contrast, the changes in the CNS in acute lead encephalopathy are less specific. There may be generalized swelling of the brain, diffuse vascular congestion and petechial haemorrhages in both grey and white matter. Histologically, capillaries may be dilated, necrotic or occluded by thrombus, and around many there is a protein-rich exudate which stains positively with PAS and often appears as discrete perivascular PAS-positive droplets, which appear to be within astrocytic processes. A similar proteinaceous exudate may also be seen in the meninges. Endothelial proliferation and/or enlargement also occurs, and within the affected areas there are enlarged astrocytes, changes in neurons that are difficult to distinguish from hypoxia, and macrophages. These changes are particularly marked in the cerebellum: they are more frequently seen and severe in children than in adults. Experimental studies suggest that lead causes selective damage to capillary endothelial cells. Developing blood vessels appear to be particularly susceptible. Recent evidence suggests that there is an association between chronic lead poisoning and mineralization of the dentate nuclei of the cerebellum (see Ch. 10).

Of contemporary concern is the possibility of subclinical neurological manifestations of lead toxicity and, in particular, the potential consequences of low-level lead exposure on the mental development of infants and children. Certainly, there are clinical studies that suggest a correlation between undue lead burdens during the postnatal period, and learning and behaviour disorders. The potential for low levels of lead to cause latent brain dysfunction or minimal brain damage is a contentious issue, possible sources of the lead being the breathing of vehicular exhaust fumes and ingestion of domestic water conveyed in lead pipes. The biochemical basis for lead toxicity and neurotoxicity is not known, although there is some evidence that lead affects enzymes involved in oxidative phosphorylation and in haem formation, and for lead possibly replacing such biologically important divalent cations as calcium. It is also known that lead, by its inhibition of aminolaevulinic acid dehydrogenase, creates a pool of δ-*aminolaevulinic acid* which, because of its structural similarity to γ-*aminobutyric acid*, may act as a putatative neurotransmitter. Other proposed mechanisms of lead encephalopathy are related to the effects of the vasculopathy.

Peripheral neuropathy is now an uncommon manifestation of lead neurotoxicity in the adult. Before improvements in industrial conditions, however, lead caused a remarkably pure motor neuropathy, often selectively severe in the radial nerve. Experimental studies show species variation in the type of neuropathy: guinea pigs and rats generally develop demyelination, whereas in rabbits an axonal type of neuropathy occurs. In man the neuropathy appears to be of a demyelinating type. Endoneurial oedema is a conspicuous feature of lead neuropathy.

Organic lead

Organolead poisoning is usually due to either tetraethyl or tetramethyl lead compounds, which are either inhaled or absorbed through the skin. Most cases of organolead toxicity are industrial, exposure occurring in workers wearing inadequate protective clothing when cleaning out petrol storage tanks when tetraethyl lead has been added to the petrol as an anti-knock agent.

Acute toxicity is characterized by brain swelling, congestion and petechial haemorrhages. Repeated episodes of acute organolead toxicity are the basis of chronic petrol-sniffing encephalopathy, in which the neuropathological findings are similar to those seen in acute encephalopathy with the additional feature of atrophy of the cerebellar folia. In experimental studies, neuronal loss has been identified in neurons of the limbic system. Unlike inorganic lead, organic lead does not damage capillaries or myelin.

MANGANESE

This is an occupational hazard of mining and processing manganese-containing ores. Manganese is absorbed through the lungs and may induce psychiatric disturbances ('*manganese madness*') and parkinsonian-like extrapyramidal dysfunction. Once the chronic stage develops, the neurological dysfunction is irreversible, but cessation of exposure at this stage does stop the progression of the disease. In patients with an extrapyramidal syndrome, there is neuronal loss in the lentiform and subthalamic nuclei and, to a lesser extent, in the substantia nigra. Both the clinical and pathological features identified in man can be reproduced in experimental animals. Biochemical studies suggest that, at high concentrations, manganese ions act as powerful synaptic transmission inhibitors producing release of norepinephrine from synaptic nerve endings and the release of acetylcholine at the neuromuscular junction.

MERCURY

Together with lead and cadmium, mercury is among the most toxic of the heavy metals. It is used in a large number of industrial processes and, depending upon its form, has many commercial uses. The organic compounds, such as methyl mercury and ethyl mercury, have biocidal properties, methyl mercury being a cheap and effective fungicide. Inorganic mercury is a waste product of some industrial processes, most notably in the manufacture of paper and in the chloralkaline industry. Factory effluent is sometimes discharged into nearby rivers or into the sea. Some micro-organisms in the water have the capacity to convert inorganic mercury salts into methyl mercury. This compound then enters the food chain and accumulates in fish to an extent that, if eaten, they become toxic to man or animals.

Inorganic mercury poisoning

Acute mercury poisoning is characterized clinically by gastrointestinal disturbances and acute renal failure. On the other hand, neurotoxicity is a prominent manifestation of chronic inorganic mercury poisoning, the initial symptoms often consisting of bizarre behavioural changes called 'erethism'. Occasionally, patients develop a peripheral neuropathy, which is also one of the major manifestations of 'pink disease', a disorder that is thought to result from chronic mercury poisoning from teething powders and antihelminthic agents. There is also now thought to be a potential danger to dentists preparing amalgam for filling teeth. There is atrophy of the cerebellum, with loss of granule cells and some Purkinje cells.

Organomercury poisoning

Cases are generally due to methyl mercury or ethyl mercury intoxication. Methyl mercury is a fungicide and is particularly useful in treating wheat seed to produce a healthy crop. The first recognized outbreak of disease due to methyl mercury resulted from industrial effluent and occurred in Minamata in Japan in the early 1950s, when 56 people were affected, of whom a third died. There was also an episode of poisoning in Iraq in 1971, where over 6000 people were affected and at least 500 died when treated wheat seed was mistakenly eaten. There is a triad of clinical signs which is unique to adults with methyl mercury poisoning, namely, paraesthesiae around the mouth and in the extremities, ataxia and concentric constriction of the visual fields. Congenital methyl mercury neurotoxicity may occur from exposure *in utero*, affected children then presenting with psychomotor retardation. Whatever the route of administration, the neuropathological changes are consistent, comprising severe focal atrophy in the calcarine and precentral cortex, and less severe atrophy in the postcentral and temporal cortex. In these areas there is neuronal loss, especially from the outer cortical layers, and an astrocytosis. The cerebellar cortex is always affected, there being selective loss of granule cells, particularly in the depths of sulci. Purkinje cells are usually spared but axonal swellings (torpedoes) may develop. There is an astrocytosis.

In experimental studies on organic and inorganic mercury neurotoxicity, similar ultrastructural changes affecting ribosomes are found, suggesting a common mechanism of toxic action affecting protein synthesis. One possible mechanism is impaired phosphorylation of uridine, leading to inhibition of RNA synthesis.

PHOSPHORUS

White or yellow phosphorus is used as a rodenticide, as a component of phosphorescent paints and as the flammable component in match heads. The systemic pathology of phosphorus poisoning includes degeneration of multiple organs, particularly the liver, kidney and heart, and is characterized histologically by fatty change that may progress to frank cell necrosis. In acute cases the brain is often swollen, and on section there are petechial haemorrhages and multiple small foci of necrosis. Histologically there is loss of neurons and a severe 'fatty change' in others, which is thought to represent an accentuated accumulation of lipofuscin pigment. The foci of necrosis are thought to be vascular in nature.

THALLIUM

The use of thallium sulphate as a rodenticide and antkiller presents a most serious hazard for accidental, suicidal and homicidal poisonings. The clinical effects are dose-dependent. A single large dose in rodents may cause death due to gastroenteritis, shock and dehydration; smaller doses result in a peripheral neuropathy associated with severe pain and extreme restlessness. An early and characteristic sign is dark pigmentation of hair roots, followed some weeks later by alopecia. The mode of action of thallium is uncertain but, like other metals, may combine with sulphydryl compounds. Neuropathologically, in acute cases there is cerebral oedema and, with survival, there is a peripheral neuropathy and chromatolysis of motor neurons.

TIN

Inorganic tin is not known to be neurotoxic. Of the many *organotin* compounds known, only two have neurotoxic properties. The neurotoxicity of triethyltin became only too evident in the early 1950s as a result of an outbreak of medical intoxication in France. A total of 290 people were poisoned and 110 died after using an oral preparation containing diethyltindiodide and *triethyltin*. At autopsy there was diffuse swelling of the white matter of the cerebral hemispheres. Histologically there is a characteristic form of intramyelinic oedema due to separation of the myelin lamellae at the intraperiod line. With long-term exposure, demyelination may occur in association with a reactive astrocytosis. Experimental studies have established that peripheral nerve myelin is less susceptible to vacuolation than is central myelin.

Intoxication with *trimethyltin* produces an entirely different type of brain damage. Unlike triethyltin, trimethyltin is not myelinotoxic, but mainly causes neuronal loss in the pyriform cortex, specific regions of the hippocampal formation and the amygdaloid nuclei.

FURTHER READING

Blum K & Manzo L (eds) (1985) *Neurotoxicology*. New York: Dekker.

Cavanagh J B (1979) Metallic toxicity and the nervous system. In: *Recent Advances in Neuropathology*, Vol. 1. Edited by W T Smith & J B Cavanagh. Edinburgh: Churchill Livingstone, pp. 247–275.

Dobbing J (ed) (1987) *Early Nutrition and Later Achievement*. London: Academic Press.

Galli C L, Manzo L & Spencer P S (eds) (1988) *Recent Advances in Nervous System Toxicology*. New York: Plenum Press.

Lapresle J & Fardeau M (1967) The central nervous system and carbon monoxide poisoning. II. Anatomical study of brain lesions following intoxication with carbon monoxide (22 cases). In: *Progress in Brain Research*, Vol 24. Edited by H Bour & I McA. Ledingham. Amsterdam: Elsevier, pp. 31–74.

Pallis C A & Lewis P D (1974) *The Neurology of Gastrointestinal Disease*. London: W B Saunders.

Scriver C F, Beaudet A L, Sly W S & Valle D (eds) (1989) *The Metabolic Basis of Inherited Disease*, 6th edn. New York: McGraw-Hill.

Spencer P S & Schaumburg H H (eds) (1980) *Experimental and Clinical Neurotoxicology*. Baltimore: Williams and Wilkins.

Victor M, Adams R D & Collins G H (1989) *The Wernicke–Korsakoff Syndrome and Related Neurological Disorders Due to Alcoholism and Malnutrition*, 2nd edn. Philadelphia: Davis.

12. System disorders

With increasing knowledge about the aetiology of specific diseases, such as metabolic defects and enzyme deficiencies, and diseases caused by viruses and other transmissible agents, so the number of conditions for which there is no known aetiology becomes smaller. The remainder, commonly referred to as 'system disorders' are a diverse group of disorders; many are familial, have a hereditary basis, and are characterized by a progressive degeneration of neurons and their processes (*abiotrophy*) within anatomically and functionally defined regions or systems, but usually sparing the cerebral cortex. Patients may therefore present with the clinical features of disease of the sensory or motor systems, or with cerebellar ataxia, alone or in combination with other neurological dysfunction. In most there are features of involvement of more than one system, the so-called *multiple system atrophies*, whereas a disease normally affecting very few systems presents a fairly uniform clinical picture. The current classification of these conditions is therefore somewhat confusing and is often based on the clinical features, which vary both within and between affected families and are due to differences in the distribution and extent of the lesions.

These disorders are characterized histologically by neuronal loss and gliosis, and in some there are cytoplasmic inclusions, namely, Lewy bodies in Parkinsons's disease and neurofibrillary tangles in supranuclear palsy.

DISEASES OF THE BASAL GANGLIA

Huntington's disease

This is a progressive hereditary form of chorea associated with mental deterioration, starting in middle life (see Ch. 14). Biochemical studies of tissues have consistently shown decreased amounts of γ-amino butyric acid, glutamic acid decarboxylase, choline acetyltransferase and substance P in the basal ganglia, but it is not clear whether these abnormalities are the result or the cause of the structural changes within the basal ganglia. An important recent observation has been the demonstration of a restriction enzyme marker which indicates that a Huntington's disease gene is located on chromosome 4.

Hallervorden–Spatz disease

This rare genetic disorder is characterized clinically by progressive rigidity, abnormal movements, dysarthria and mental deterioration. Three types: late infantile (3 months to 6 years), classic (7–15 years) and adult or late, have been recognized.

The brain may appear normal externally but on section there is shrinkage and a characteristic rust-brown discoloration of the globus pallidus and the pars reticularis of the substantia nigra. Histologically there is yellowish-brown pigment in these structures which stains positively for iron (Fig. 12.1). Other features are axonal spheroids, loss of neurons and gliosis. The nature of the spheroids remained uncertain until electron microscopy established that they are swollen axons and are widely distributed throughout the CNS.

The disease is now classified among the neuroaxonal dystrophies. Their pathogenesis is not known, particularly as similar spheroids occur in normal ageing human and animal brains, and in a variety of pathological and experimental conditions, when they are thought to represent a

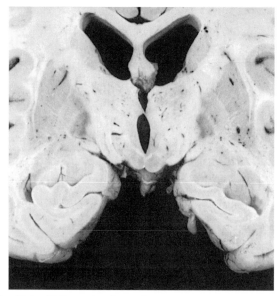

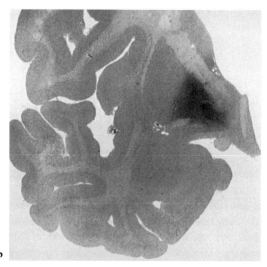

a   b

Fig. 12.1   Hallervorden–Spatz disease. (a) There is discoloration of the medial segments of globus pallidus. (b) The abnormal tissue stains heavily for iron. (Perls' stain.)

non-specific reaction to injury. The diagnosis of neuroaxonal dystrophy can be made by ultrastructural examination of biopsies taken from sensory or autonomic peripheral nerve, skin, conjunctiva or rectal mucosa.

DISEASES OF THE SUBSTANTIA NIGRA AND RELATED SYSTEMS OF NEURONS

Parkinson's syndrome (parkinsonism)

Parkinson's syndrome is a disturbance of motor function characterized by slowing of emotional and voluntary movement, akinesia, muscular rigidity, and tremor. The syndrome is brought about by damage to, or malfunction of, the nigral system. The majority of cases are idiopathic (Parkinson's disease, paralysis agitants or idiopathic parkinsonism), but types of parkinsonism with known aetiologies include the postencephalitic and drug-induced types, and intoxication or poisoning. Closely related disorders are the parkinsonism–dementia complex of Guam, striatonigral degeneration and progressive supranuclear palsy.

Parkinson's disease

This world-wide, slowly progressive disorder affects both sexes and usually commences in the sixth decade with a peak in the seventh.

Pathology. The brain may appear normal externally unless there are coincident senile changes. The striking feature is depigmentation of the zona compacta of the substantia nigra (Fig. 12.2). There is loss of neurons and an astrocytosis in the substantia nigra and in the locus ceruleus. Neuromelanin is seen in macrophages and free in the neuropil. Surviving neurons often contain Lewy bodies – intracytoplasmic eosinophilic bodies with a halo (see Fig. 3.22). Electron microscopy has established that the core of the Lewy body is composed of filaments and granular material that are positive for neurofilaments and ubiquitin by immunocytochemical techniques.

It is generally agreed that Lewy bodies are to be found in nearly all cases of Parkinson's disease; exceptions include cases of postencephalitic parkinsonism and occasionally 'control' material. They may be found not only in the pigmented cells of the substantia nigra, locus ceruleus and dorsal vagal nucleus, but also in the substantia innominata (basal nucleus of Meynert), various nuclei in the brain stem, the neocortex and the grey matter of the spinal cord. Neuronal loss is an associated feature in all of these areas.

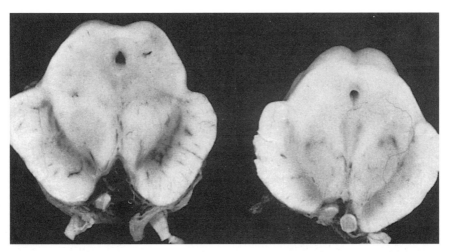

Fig. 12.2 Parkinson's disease. In comparison with the normally pigmented substantia nigra on the left, there is depigmentation of the substantia nigra on the right in a case of Parkinson's disease.

A recently described disorder is that of diffuse Lewy body disease in elderly patients who present initially with dementia and later develop parkinsonism with severe rigidity. The Lewy bodies are distributed widely. The relationship between the two disorders is not clear: they may represent two distinct disorders or parts of a continuum.

It is generally accepted that parkinsonism is due to depletion of the dopamine-synthesizing neurons of the substantia nigra that project to the striatum. Immunohistochemical studies have shown a 75 per cent loss of pigmented tyrosine hydroxylase-containing neurons from the substantia nigra. There is also variable neuronal loss in other catecholamine-containing neurons in the brain stem. Dopamine is an inhibitory neurotransmitter in the striatum, where it acts on cholinergic neurons. Normally there is a balance between the inhibitory nigrostriatal dopaminergic pathway and the striatal cholinergic neurons. Relative deficiency in the dopaminergic system results in parkinsonism.

Idiopathic Parkinson's disease associated with dementia

Mild dementia is common in patients with idiopathic Parkinson's disease, and it cannot be explained by the changes associated normally with Alzheimer's disease because the cortex in patients with Parkinson's disease is usually normal. The explanation for this type of *subcortical dementia* may therefore be degenerative changes in the substantia nigra and corpus striatum, features that are commonly present in other types of multiple system atrophy. On the other hand, the severe dementia that may occur in patients with Parkinson's disease is probably due to Alzheimer's disease. The association of idiopathic Parkinson's disease and severe dementia certainly appears to be more common than in age-matched controls. At present it is not clear whether this represents a combination of two separate, but not uncommon, diseases, or some unknown common interlinking aetiological factor which can produce these abnormalities in the same patient.

Postencephalitic parkinsonism

Many survivors of the pandemic of encephalitis lethargica between 1919 and 1924 developed parkinsonism (see Ch. 7).

Pathology. Pathological studies on patients who died of the acute illness in the 1920s showed the histological features of a viral encephalitis. In patients who recovered from the encephalitis there is, as with idiopathic parkinsonism, depigmentation of the substantia nigra, loss of pigmented neurons and gliosis. Lewy bodies, however, are not seen. Instead, many of the surviving neurons contain neurofibrillary tangles similar to those seen in Alzheimer's disease and composed principally of paired helical filaments.

Parkinsonism–dementia complex of Guam

Among the indigenous Chamorro population of Guam there is a high incidence of parkinsonism, often accompanied by progressive dementia. The disease accounts for some 5–10 per cent of adult deaths. There is a higher incidence among males and many of the patients present features of both the parkinsonism–dementia complex and a Guamanian variant of amyotrophic lateral sclerosis (ALS).

Pathology. There is a variable degree of cerebral atrophy, especially of the frontal and temporal lobes, and of the globus pallidus and the thalamus. There is depigmentation of the substantia nigra, and widespread neuronal loss and an associated astrocytosis. The pathology in the ALS variant is that of loss of motor neurons in the cervical and lumbar enlargements of the spinal cord and the hypoglossal nuclei, degeneration of the corticospinal tracts and widely distributed neurofibrillary tangles in the brain. Neurofibrillary tangles are found throughout the brain but there are no senile plaques or Lewy bodies. The aetiology of the parkinsonism–dementia (ALS) complex of Guam is unknown but intoxication, especially by the cycad seed or by heavy metals, may be implicated. There is also a high incidence of the Guam type of motor neuron disease in other areas of the Western Pacific.

Other causes of parkinsonism

These include *arteriosclerosis, trauma*, various toxins and poisons such as *manganese, carbon monoxide, carbon disulphide* and *mercury*, and drugs, such as *reserpine, phenothiazines* and *butyrophenones*.

The recent demonstration that *N*-methyl-4-phenyl-1, 2, 3, 6-tetrahydropyridine (MPTP) induces the clinical and pathological features of Parkinson's disease has raised the possibility that environmental factors may play a role in the aetiology of idiopathic parkinsonism. MPTP is a byproduct in the synthesis of meperidine-related opiate marketed illegally as synthetic heroin. Numerous cases of severe parkinsonism have been reported among individuals who have injected themselves with this drug, and animal experiments have confirmed that MPTP produces selective destruction of the nigrostriatal dopamine pathway. If industrial pollutants are responsible, then there are a number of pyridines similar in general structure to MPTP that exist in the environment. For example, 4-phenylpyridine has been commercially marketed as a herbicide and the well known weed killer paraquat structurally resembles MPTP. It is possible that in the general population clinical features only develop as a consequence of long-term exposure to small amounts of certain neurotoxins that accelerate the normal age-related changes that take place in the nigrostriatal system.

MPTP acts as a substrate for monoamine oxidase B, resulting in the formation of 1-methyl-4-phenylpyridinium (MPP+), which has been shown to be more neurotoxic than MPTP. MPP+ is thought to act by interfering with mitochondrial energy metabolism or by the generation of superoxide radicals.

Striatonigral degeneration

This uncommon condition is virtually indistinguishable clinically from idiopathic parkinsonism. It differs pathologically, however, in that there is neuronal loss and gliosis in the striatum, particularly in the putamen, as well as in the substantia nigra and locus ceruleus. Neither Lewy bodies nor neurofibrillary tangles are seen. Although the condition has been regarded as a distinct entity by some, it may be related to other system degenerations since many patients with pontocerebellar atrophy also show the features of clinical parkinsonism.

Progressive supranuclear palsy

This condition, of gradual onset between the fifth and seventh decades, affects men more commonly than women, and is characterized clinically by the features of parkinsonism together with a supra-nuclear ophthalmoplegia and, frequently, dementia. There is widespread symmetrical neuronal loss, with gliosis, involving the globus pallidus, the subthalamic nucleus, the red nucleus, the substantia nigra, the periaqueductal grey matter and the dentate nucleus. A characteristic feature is the presence of neurofibrillary tangles without associated neuritic plaques in the same regions and in the nuclei of the brain stem. Electron-microscopical studies have shown that the neurofibrillary tangles are composed of bundles of straight filaments approximately 15 nm in diameter. The aetiology of this condition is not known.

CALCIFICATION OF THE BASAL GANGLIA

This is a common feature without associated symptoms in the brains of elderly subjects. Occasionally calcification is more extensive and in many of these cases there is thought to be a deficiency of parathyroid hormone. Small concretions are present at the junction of cortex and white matter at the depths of sulci and in the cerebellum. In more severe cases calcification occurs in the basal ganglia and may amount to 'brain stones'. Histologically small calcospherites lie along capillaries or as tubular deposits in the media of small to medium-sized arteries. As the lesions coalesce neuronal tissue is destroyed, but in the absence of gliosis or inflammation. The nature of the biochemical disturbances responsible for the calcification is not known.

DISEASES OF THE CEREBELLUM, BRAIN STEM AND SPINAL CORD

The spinocerebellar degenerations are a group of rare inherited disorders in which there is a loss of groups or systems of neurons in the brain stem, the cerebellum and the spinal cord. The principal signs and symptoms depend on the specific structures affected, although there are marked variations in the clinical and pathological findings due to the variable expressions of these disorders. Their aetiology remains unknown.

Friedreich's ataxia

Although the most common of the hereditary ataxias, this is an uncommon progressive degenerative disease occurring in some 2 per 100 000 of the population, usually with an autosomal recessive mode of inheritance: the abnormal gene has been localized to chromosome 9. It presents before the age of 25 years and is characterized clinically by slowly progressive ataxia, loss of deep sensation, dysarthria, skeletal deformities and cardiac abnormalities.

Pathology

There is combined degeneration of the posterior columns in the spinal cord, and the corticospinal and spinocerebellar tracts. Structural abnormalities, however, are not constant, variations occurring within and between families so that the pattern of spinal involvement may be associated with conditions in which there is degeneration of the cerebellum, the brain stem or peripheral nerves. In typical cases the spinal cord is small and there is partial atrophy of the posterior nerve roots and ganglia. Degenerative change in the posterior columns (particularly the gracile tracts) and in the spinocerebellar tracts is particularly marked in the upper dorsal and cervical regions, whereas the changes in the corticospinal tracts are more marked in the lower spinal cord (Fig. 12.3). There is variable loss of neurons in the dorsal root ganglia, in Clarke's column of the spinal cord, in the motor cortex and in the dentate nucleus of the cerebellum. Occasionally there is degeneration of the retina, the optic nerves and tracts, and the lateral geniculate bodies.

There are similarities between Friedreich's ataxia and Marie's hereditary cerebellar ataxia. The two conditions sometimes overlap and there are intermediate forms. Friedreich's ataxia is frequently associated with a chronic progressive myocarditis in which focal coagulative necrosis of the muscle fibres is followed by replacement fibrosis.

Cerebello-olivary degeneration of Holmes

This is a rare autosomally inherited progressive degeneration of the cerebellar cortex associated

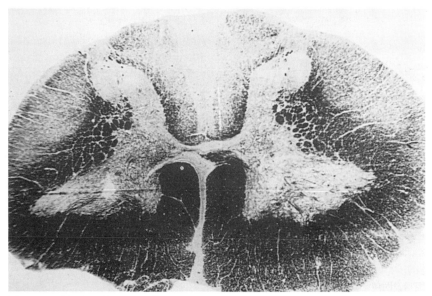

Fig. 12.3 Friedreich's ataxia. There is degeneration in posterior and lateral columns. (Weigert–Pal for myelin.)

with retrograde degeneration in the inferior olives. The clinical features are an ataxic gait, dysarthria and tremor of the limbs. The onset is usually in the fourth decade.

Pathology

There is pronounced atrophy of the cerebellum and less pronounced atrophy of the olives. There is almost complete loss of Purkinje cells and an associated astrocytosis. There is considerable loss of granule cells, and the loss of myelinated fibres is commensurate with the degree of atrophy. Any remaining Purkinje cells are shrunken or swollen and sometimes contain vacuoles: there may be fusiform dilatations (torpedoes) on surviving axons in the granule cell layer (Fig. 12.4). There is atrophy of the inferior and accessory olives associated with the loss of olivocerebellar fibres. The condition is thought to be due to a primary degeneration of the cerebellar cortex with retrograde trans-synaptic degeneration in the neurons of the olives. There is some similarity between this condition and the cerebellar degeneration seen in chronic alcoholics.

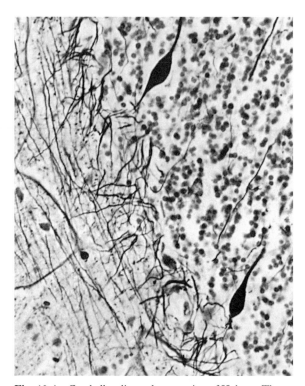

Fig. 12.4 Cerebello-olivary degeneration of Holmes. There are torpedo-like swellings on the axons of degenerating Purkinje cells. (Palmgren technique for axons.)

Olivopontocerebellar degeneration

This dominantly inherited disorder is sometimes referred to as the Menzel, or Déjérine–Thomas type of cerebellar atrophy. It presents in late middle age and is characterized by slowly progressive limb ataxia, dysarthria and, occasionally, dementia and postural hypotension.

Pathology

The ventral part of the pons is atrophic and there is atrophy of the cerebellar cortex, the middle cerebellar peduncles and the olives. The spinal cord and nerve roots are usually normal. There is loss of neurons in the nuclei pontis and loss of the transverse pontine fibres (Fig. 12.5). In the cerebellum there is moderate atrophy of the lateral portions of the hemispheres, with relative sparing of the vermis. Within the affected areas there is loss of Purkinje cells with lesser involvement of the granule cells: loss of cerebellar white matter is commensurate with the reduction in the number of Purkinje cells. The dentate nuclei and the superior cerebellar peduncles are well preserved but there is atrophy due to loss of neurons and an astrocytosis in the inferior olives. Microscopic changes are frequently seen in the long tracts of the spinal cord especially in the posterior columns and spinocerebellar tracts. Involvement of the

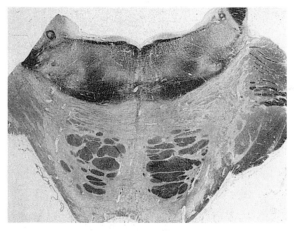

Fig. 12.5 Olivopontocerebellar degeneration. There is loss of myelin in the transverse fibres of the pons and in the middle cerebellar peduncles, and preservation of the tegmentum and pyramidal tracts. (Luxol fast blue/cresyl violet.)

corticospinal tracts and neuronal loss in Clarke's column and in the anterior horns have also been reported. In some cases there is variable neuronal loss in the substantia nigra, the red nucleus, the thalamus and the basal ganglia. The distribution and severity of the changes in this condition, even within a single family, vary considerably.

Ataxia–telangiectasia (Louis–Bar syndrome)

This familial disease of children is characterized by a progressive cerebellar ataxia, with symmetrical telangiectases of the skin and conjunctiva. It is of autosomal recessive inheritance, an affected child appearing normal at birth only for progressive ataxia to appear in infancy; by the second decade the patient is chairbound and grossly dysarthric. Telangiectases develop several years after the onset of ataxia. There is a strong tendency to develop a malignant lymphoma. Recurring chest infections are common and immunological studies have shown a deficiency of IgA, a defect of delayed hypersensitivity, aplasia or hypoplasia of the thymus and a decreased response by lymphocytes to mitogens. Pathologically the thymus is absent or rudimentary and lymphoid tissue is reduced. In the CNS the constant feature is atrophy of the cerebellar cortex, with extensive loss of Purkinje and granule cells. In many cases there is also degeneration of the posterior columns of the spinal cord and atrophy of the posterior root ganglia. This condition is sometimes classified as a phakomatosis (see Ch. 13).

Hereditary spastic paraplegia (Strumpell)

This slowly progressive disorder of adolescence or adulthood is more common in males than in females, and is characterized by weakness of the legs that progresses to a spastic paraplegia.

Pathology

There are no macroscopic abnormalities. There is, however, degeneration of the lateral corticospinal tracts, particularly in the lower part of the spinal cord. There is also degeneration of the posterior columns, particularly of the gracile tracts in the cervical region; the spinocerebellar tracts may also be affected. In some cases there is also a distal form of neurogenic muscular atrophy. The pathogenesis is unknown, although the basic morphological features are those of a distal axonopathy affecting central pathways.

Hereditary posterior column ataxia (Biemond)

This very rare condition appears to be inherited as an autosomal dominant. It is characterized clinically by numbness of the hands and feet that later progresses to total absence of posterior column sensation. The spinal cord is atrophic due to degeneration of the posterior columns and partial degeneration of the posterior nerve roots.

Motor neuron disease

This is a progressive, occasionally familial, degenerative disorder of motor neurons that presents clinically with wasting, weakness and eventually paralysis of muscles. The external ocular muscles are not affected and sensation is preserved. It tends to occur in middle and late adult life, and is more common in males than in females. The disease is usually fatal in 2–3 years, but occasionally patients die in less than a year, whereas others may survive for 10 years or more. Death is usually due to respiratory failure.

Motor neuron disease occurs worldwide and has an incidence of approximately 1 per 1000 deaths. There is a particularly high incidence among the native Chamorro population of Guam. The aetiology is unknown, although suspected causes include genetic disorders, viral infection possibly related to poliomyelitis, and intoxication with heavy metals.

Three variants are recognized depending on the distribution of the disease process. The commonest is *progressive muscular atrophy*, when there is selectively severe involvement of the cervical region of the spinal cord as a result of which there is fibrillation and then atrophy of the small muscles of the hand, which soon assumes a characteristic claw-like form. Involvement then spreads to the muscles of the arm and shoulder girdle. The term *amyotrophic lateral sclerosis* is used when upper motor neurons are also affected,

leading to degeneration of the corticospinal tracts and spastic paraparesis. Occasionally there is selectively severe damage to the motor nuclei in the lower brain stem, the process then being referred to as *progressive bulbar palsy*, resulting in progressive wasting and paralysis of the muscles of the tongue, lips, jaw, larynx and pharynx.

Pathology

There is severe neurogenic atrophy of the affected muscles which are pale and shrunken (see Ch. 17). The most conspicuous macroscopic abnormality in the CNS is atrophy of ventral spinal nerve roots, which become grey and of reduced size: this is most obvious in the cervical region and in the cauda equina (Fig. 12.6). The ventral horns of the spinal cord appear smaller than normal and, in the great majority of cases, the lateral and ventral columns of the spinal cord are rather grey in colour, in contrast to the striking preservation of the white colour of the posterior columns. The most important microscopic change is a loss of motor neurons. This is most easily seen in the ventral horns of the cervical and lumbar segments

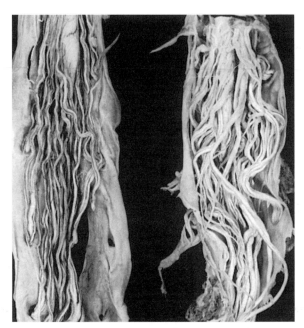

Fig. 12.6 Motor neuron disease. Compared with the normal cauda equina on the right, there is atrophy of ventral nerve roots on the left in a patient with motor neuron disease.

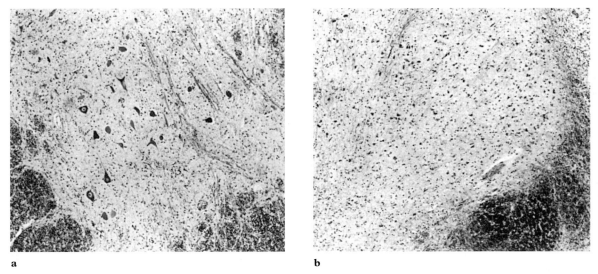

Fig. 12.7   Motor neuron disease. (a) Normal ventral horn. (b) Loss of ventral horn neurons in a case of motor neuron disease. (Luxol fast blue/cresyl violet.)

of the spinal cord (Fig. 12.7) and in the hypoglossal nuclei of the lower brain stem (Fig. 12.8). In contrast, the nuclei of the oculomotor,

trochlear and abducent nerves are rarely affected. In general, it is the large motor neurons that are affected, the smaller and intermediate-size cells

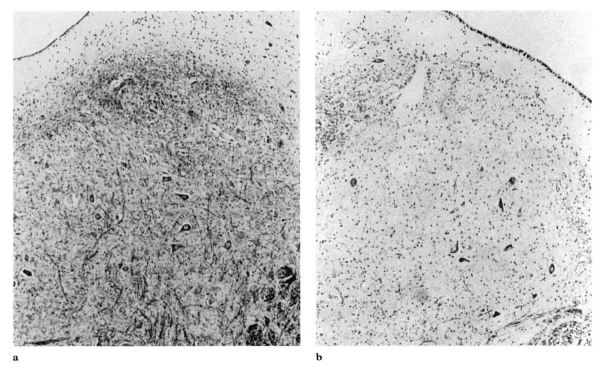

Fig. 12.8   Motor neuron disease. (a) Normal hypoglossal nucleus. (b) Loss of motor neurons in hypoglossal nucleus in a case of motor neuron disease. (LFB/CV.)

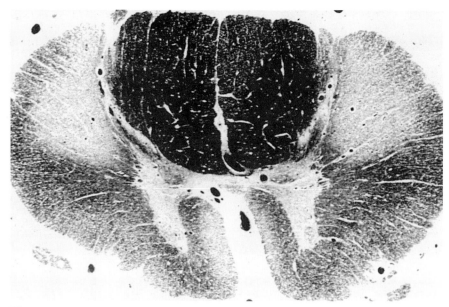

Fig. 12.9   Motor neuron disease. There is degeneration in the lateral, and to a lesser extent in the anterior columns, and preservation of the posterior columns. (Heidenhain for myelin.)

tending to be preserved. Various changes are seen in surviving neurons, ranging from simple atrophy to the less common findings of ghost-cell formation, chromatolysis, the appearance of occasional small eosinophilic inclusions (Bunina bodies), spheroid formation and neuronophagia. Changes in the white matter of the spinal cord are variable. The most common is degeneration of the pyramidal tracts (Fig. 12.9) which, when severe, may be traced upwards into the white matter of the cerebral hemispheres. In other cases it may be undetectable above the medulla.

The changes in the pyramidal fibres usually start first and are most marked at their lower extremities, the process then extending upwards. Detailed analysis of the motor cortex is difficult, but in severe cases there is some loss of Betz cells. Although the corticospinal tracts are the principal tracts affected, there is often a diffuse loss of stainable myelin in the anterior and lateral columns. Sensory changes are rare in motor neuron disease and routine microscopy does not reveal obvious changes in sensory ganglia, sensory nerves or the posterior columns. The cause of motor neuron disease remains unknown, the identification of genetic, metabolic, infectious or environmental causes being unsuccessful. There is no convincing evidence of risk factors

associated with poliomyelitis, heavy metal intoxication or trauma.

Reference has been made earlier in this chapter to the parkinsonism–dementia complex which occurs in Guam and which is characterized by diffuse neuronal loss and neurofibrillary tangles in the cerebral cortex, the deep grey structures, the substantia nigra and the brain stem. The Guamanian Parkinson's dementia complex associated with Guamanian motor neuron disease appears to be quite different from both idiopathic parkinsonism associated with dementia and with sporadic motor neuron disease. The principal feature is that, in addition to the changes of either idiopathic parkinsonism associated with dementia or sporadic motor neuron disease, there is widespread neuronal loss and the formation of neurofibrillary tangles in the brain, brain stem and spinal cord.

Familial forms of motor neuron disease

In 10–15 per cent of cases there is an apparently autosomal dominant mode of inheritance. In many such cases the features are indistinguishable from the usual sporadic examples although in some there is pathological evidence of involvement of the posterior columns and the spinocerebellar tracts.

Familial spinal muscular atrophy

This condition, caused by degeneration of the lower motor neuron due to autosomal recessive inheritance, is characterized by delayed motor development, weakness and hypotonia that begins at or shortly after birth. The most severe form is spinal muscular atrophy type 1 (SMA 1, infantile spinal muscular atrophy or Werdnig–Hoffmann disease). At the other end of the clinical spectrum are those cases of spinal muscular atrophy type 3 (SMA 3, Wohlfart–Kugelberg–Welander disease) which have a benign chronic clinical course (see Ch. 17).

It has been suggested that *arthrogryposis multiplex congenita*, a condition characterized by deformed and rigid joints associated with muscle wasting, is due to paralysis of or interference with muscular activity in the fetus. The causes are various but include spina bifida (see Ch. 13) and Werdnig–Hoffmann disease.

DISEASES OF THE AUTONOMIC NERVOUS SYSTEM

There is a distinctive type of orthostatic hypotension that results from an idiopathic degeneration of neurons in many parts of the nervous system, especially those in the intermediolateral cell columns of the spinal cord. It is known as the *Shy–Drager syndrome* and appears to be more common in males than in females and has an average age of onset in the sixth decade. There is postural hypotension, an atonic bladder, loss of sphincter tone and loss of sweating, in addition to abnormalities suggestive of a widespread multisystem disorder. Pathologically the changes are somewhat variable, but consist principally of neuronal loss from the intermediolateral columns of the spinal cord in association with either Lewy bodies, as for example in Parkinson's disease, or multiple system atrophy, particularly of the striatonigral variety.

FURTHER READING

Martin J E, Swash M & Schwartz M S (1990) New insights in motor neuron disease. *Neuropathology and Applied Neurobiology* **16**, 97–110.

Oppenheimer D R (1983) Neuropathology of progressive autonomic failure. In: *Autonomic Failure: a Textbook of Clinical Disorders of the Autonomic Nervous System.* Edited by R Bannister. Oxford: Oxford University Press, pp. 266–283.

Oppenheimer D R & Esiri M M (1992) Diseases of the basal ganglia, cerebellum and motor neurons. In: *Greenfield's*

Neuropathology, 5th edn. Edited by J H Adams & L W Duchem. London: Edward Arnold, pp. 266–283.

Rowland L P (ed) (1991) *Amyotrophic Lateral Sclerosis and other Motor Neuron Diseases. Advances in Neurology*, Vol 56. New York: Raven Press.

Streifler M B, Melamed E, Korezyn A D & Youdin M B H (eds) (1990) *Parkinson's Disease: Anatomy, Pathology, and Therapy. Advances in Neurology*, Vol 53. New York: Raven Press.

13. Developmental and perinatal disorders

DEVELOPMENTAL ABNORMALITIES

DEVELOPMENT OF THE CENTRAL NERVOUS SYSTEM

The section on Development (pp. 223–226) was written by Dr M.T. Isaac, holder of a MRC Special Training Fellowship in Neuropathology in the Department of Neuropathology, University of Glasgow.

Developmental neurobiology has burgeoned over the past 10–15 years, and many would regard it as a separate division of the neurosciences. Current trends include the application of the latest techniques in molecular biology, the exploitation of new animal models of development and a resurgence of classic methods of manipulative embryology. The fundamental problems may be stated in a variety of ways, but in terms of embryological mechanisms, the question remains 'why do cells move when they move, go where they go, and stop where they stop'? It has to be stressed that the hardest experimental evidence has been derived from animal studies, and that direct evidence from human material has of necessity been limited to observation, epidemiology and the consideration of naturally occurring malformations.

The central nervous system (CNS) is derived from embryonic *ectoderm*. The process by which the primitive two-dimensional *neural plate* forms the axial neural tube is known as *neurulation*, and has been particularly well worked out in amphibia. The original axial neural plate forms cranially from Hensen's node on the dorsal surface of the embryo. The lateral edges of the plate develop *folds*, which increase in size and thickness, bend towards the midline and fuse in a rostrocaudal direction. Meanwhile, the mesodermal *notochord* develops ventral to the neural ectoderm, and the mesodermal *somites* develop laterally and segmentally. The notochord and somites form, *inter alia*, the vertebral column later on. The *neural crest* develops dorsolaterally to the neural tube and migrates widely to participate in the formation of elements of the peripheral nervous system, skull and meninges. The picture is completed by localized rostral thickenings which form ectodermal *placodes*, which participate in the formation of the eyes and ears.

Neural tube defects result not simply from failure of the neurulation process. Their pathogenesis is altogether more complex, and a somewhat stylized section of the embryonic spinal cord at this stage is shown in Fig. 13.1. Although this section is a useful prototype of CNS morphogenesis, differentiation is regionally heterogeneous from the beginning, due primarily to differences in cell proliferation which also occurs in a ventral-to-dorsal gradient. Within the

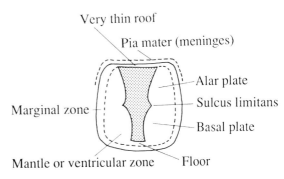

Fig. 13.1 Embryonic spinal cord. Cross-section of 'typical' segment. Note the thin roof of the central canal.

developing cord, *neurogenesis*, neuronal *migration* and subsequent *differentiation* occur sequentially. The neural epithelium is pseudostratified at this stage and cell division occurs in the inner regions of the *mantle* zone. Glial development occurs synchronously and, in particular, radial arrays of glia may provide 'guidewires' for migrating primitive neurons. Cell division usually ends for most prospective neurons at this time, but secondary germinal centres occur in the more rostral parts of the developing CNS. Failure of appropriate migration is the cause of *heterotopia*, but this of course begs the question 'why does migration fail?'

Extensive unequal rostrocaudal growth in the developing CNS, together with hydrostatic effects, results in the appearance of *flexures*. Ventral flexion occurs (Fig. 13.2) at the *spinomedullary* and *mesencephalic* flexures, whereas lateral dorsal flexion occurs at the level of the developing pons. The CNS is thus divided longitudinally into several regions (Fig. 13.3): the *spinal cord*, the *rhombencephalon* (so called because of the diamond-shaped deformation of the thin roof of the neural tube when flexed dorsally), the

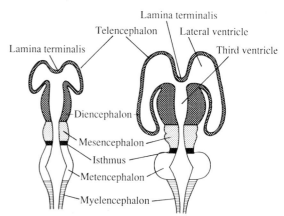

Fig. 13.3 Regional development of the brain. Sketches of two stages (longitudinal section).

metencephalon and the *prosencephalon*, itself divided into the rostral *telencephalon*, which gives rise to the cerebral hemispheres, and the *diencephalon* from which the thalamus, hypothalamus, epithalamus and optic nerves ultimately form.

The horizontal axis of the *lamina terminalis* (Fig. 13.3) forms the centre of the spiral described by the growing cerebral hemispheres as they reach their final positions. As the hemispheres expand, they become connected across the midline by *commissural tracts* of nerve fibres, and already there is some regional variation of the cerebral cortex in respect of the varying complexity of *cortical lamination* (Fig. 13.4). The development of cortical folds – *foliation* – from

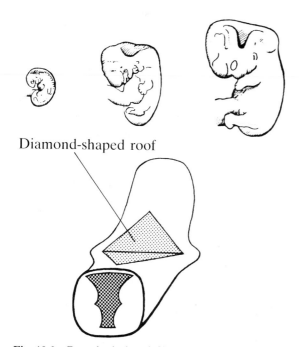

Fig. 13.2 Rostral spinal cord. Sketch of the dorsal aspect following dorsal flexion of the neural tube.

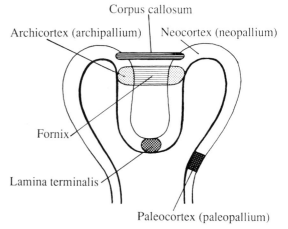

Fig. 13.4 Telencephalon. View showing the development of the commissures (cf. Fig. 13.3).

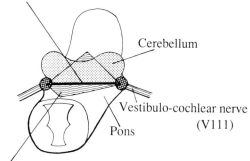

Thickened flocculo - nodular lobe of cerebellum

Cerebellum

Vestibulo-cochlear nerve
(VIII)

Pons

Thin ruffled roof of what is now the fourth ventricle

forming the tela choroidea of the choroid plexus

Fig. 13.5 Spinal cord. Sketch of the dorsal aspect to show further development of the rhombencephalon (cf. Fig. 13.2).

the original smooth, *lissencephalic* surface takes place gradually. The main lobes (frontal, parietal, temporal and occipital) are seen by 3.5 months *in utero*, the lateral (Sylvian) fissures by about 5 months, and the central sulci by 7 months. Most convolutions are complete by birth, although the deep insular cortex remains exposed.

The cerebellum develops in the rostral half of the roof of the rhombencephalon in close contact with the vestibular nuclei and vestibulocochlear nerve (Fig. 13.5). Foliation occupies the period between just under 3 months *in utero* to just over 7 months, and shows the adult pattern at 2 months *post partum*.

The sequence in which myelin is laid down in the main tracts is shown in Table 13.1. Particular note should be taken of those tracts, generally

Table 13.1 Sequences of myelination from the 20th gestational week

Structure	Myelination	
	Begins	Ends
Motor roots	20 i.u.	1 p.p.
Sensory roots	24 i.u.	14 p.p.
Vestibulocochlear nerve	24 i.u.	32 i.u.
Striatum	3 p.p.	24–36 + p.p.
Medial lemniscus	26 i.u.	14 p.p.
Pyramidal tracts	36 i.u.	26 p.p.
Corpus callosum	3–4 p.p.	10 years p.p.
Corticocortical association fibres, neuropil etc.	3–4 p.p.	Middle age, perhaps older

i.u. = *in utero* (weeks); p.p. = *post partum* (months)

held to be phylogenetically the most recent, which are myelinated after birth.

To summarize, the development of the normal brain can be subdivided into phases. Following closure of the neural tube, a glial framework is laid down which acts as a guide for migrating neuroblasts. The first half of pregnancy is termed the phase of *neuronal proliferation*, in which large numbers of neuroblasts are formed in the subependymal germinal matrix plate. In the second half of pregnancy (from about 20 weeks' gestation), proliferation of neuroblasts ceases although *migration* continues throughout the remainder of pregnancy. It is in the second half of gestation that astrocytes and oligodendrocytes are formed. There is very little myelination in the cerebral hemispheres at birth, although some myelin is present in the spinal cord from about 16 weeks.

Developmental abnormalities of the brain are among the most common of all malformations, and a knowledge of them has assumed increasing importance because of better diagnostic procedures and counselling. Whereas severe defects frequently result in spontaneous abortion, stillbirth or obvious malformations at birth, other defects may not become clinically manifest until late infancy, childhood or even adulthood.

It has been estimated that in the UK malformations of the CNS are present in 3–4 per cent of early spontaneous abortions and in approximately 0.6 per cent of births.

In over 50 per cent of cases the aetiology of congenital malformations remains undetermined. Important factors, however, include, either singly or in combination, *genetic factors* (e.g. micrencephaly), *chromosomal abnormalities* such as trisomy 21, the incidence of which is linked to advanced maternal age, and various *environmental factors* including maternal infections such as rubella and cytomegalovirus, irradiation to the pelvis during the first 4 months of pregnancy, the fetal alcohol syndrome (see Ch. 11), pharmaceutical drugs, tobacco smoking and, possibly, vitamin deficiencies.

The nature of a malformation in the brain is largely determined by the stage of development at which either a genetic defect prevents normal expression, or a teratogen operates. The CNS is susceptible throughout its various phases of development but the exact target of the teratogen varies with the time of gestation. Thus, the same teratogenic environmental insult acting at different times in gestation will produce different malformations. In general, a teratogenic agent acting early in development produces more damage than the same insult later in development, because an organ is more sensitive to damage while it is being formed and least sensitive when mature. The teratogenic effects of an agent depend on its nature, the gestational stage at which it acts and the genetic background of the individual. An appreciation of the embryology and postnatal growth of the brain is therefore essential for understanding the basis of these abnormalities. Once the basic structure of the CNS has been established, there are stages of cell *proliferation, migration* and *differentiation*, and teratogens may disrupt any of these depending on whether they act *in utero* or after birth.

Aborted fetuses, stillbirths and children dying in infancy should be examined systematically with accurate and full notes and photography. Karyotyping should be carried out: some 50 per cent of spontaneous abortuses in the first and second trimesters have chromosomal abnormalities.

NEONATAL AUTOPSY

Because of the nature of the disease process presenting in the neonatal period, as well as the physical characteristics of the brain and skull at this time, the procedure for removal and handling of the brain requires a separate comment. Basically, the aim is to allow *in situ* inspection of the brain, dura and great vessels, to establish the sites of traumatic tearing or haemorrhage, and to allow assessment of any developmental abnormalities in the relationship of brain, skull and meninges.

The calvaria is opened with scissors along the sutures. The sagittal suture is opened on each side of the midline and the cuts are extended laterally into the lambdoid and coronal sutures. Towards the base of the skull these cuts are then curved towards each other so that the flaps of skull and dura can be sprung out, petal-like. Gentle manipulation of the head and brain can then disclose the great vessels and the dura and its reflections. The frontal bones can be sprung out by scissor cuts made in the midline and base, and greater exposure obtained. The brain is then removed in the sequence described for the adult after dividing and freeing the falx. In suspected abnormalities of the posterior fossa, the foramen magnum and the cervical spine, and in hydrocephalus, the posterior fossa and cervical spine require to be opened first.

As the neonatal brain is so soft, great care is required in its handling and removal. This can be accomplished by an assistant positioning the head upright during removal, care being taken to support the brain at all times. Removal of the brain under water has some supporters. After removal, handling should be kept to a minimum, and the brain should be weighed after immersion in a previously weighed container of fixative. As suspension by the basilar artery is inappropriate for neonatal brains, several flotation methods have been devised to overcome distortion. These include fixation in 10 per cent formalin using a mattress of cotton wool, flotation in 20 per cent formalin, and fixation in 10 per cent formalin to which glacial acetic acid has been added until the brain begins to float. The last method has the advantage of providing a firmer brain for ultimate dissection and does not jeopardize routine staining procedures.

AETIOLOGY OF HUMAN MALFORMATIONS

Genetic factors

These may contribute to about 30 per cent of all malformations, although there are only a few caused by simple mendelian inheritance. Examples include some forms of micrencephaly, holoprosencephaly and tuberous sclerosis. The exact role of genetic factors in anencephaly, spina bifida and hydrocephalic malformations which sometimes run in families is not clear, but suggests an interplay between genetic and environmental factors.

Chromosomal abnormalities

Chromosomes may be lost or gained during

meiosis: loss is the more serious, leading in almost all cases to fetal death *in utero*. The clinically important disorders in which there is extrachromosomal material and which are characterized by mental retardation include trisomies 21, 18 and 13. The severity of the phenotypic abnormality is related to the size of the extra chromosome, being least in trisomy 21 and greatest in trisomy 13. Although non-specific phenotypic features, such as low-set or misshapen ears and hyper- or hypotelorism, may be present in these trisomies, the same features when associated with anomalies of digits and of skin creasing, and of major developmental malformations of the heart and viscera, may form a constellation of abnormalities that comprise a specific condition. Deletions in which there is loss of part of one chromosome may be seen in conditions such as the '*Cri du Chat*' syndrome. Mosaicism may also be found in patients with mental retardation.

Abnormalities of sex chromosomes include Klinefelter's syndrome (XXY) and Turner's syndrome (XO), and many are associated with mental retardation. Most cases of Turner's syndrome who survive to adult life show no cerebral abnormalities; by contrast, most XO fetuses undergo spontaneous abortion and these often show gross malformation.

Antenatal detection of chromosomal abnormalities is possible, and is based on culture of fetal cells obtained by chorionic villus sampling or by amniocentesis. Since women over the age of 40 years are at considerably greater risk than younger women, they should be advised to have amniocentesis. However, the impact of antenatal diagnosis in the prevention of chromosomal abnormalities at birth in the community has been small because of the small contribution by this age group to the total number of babies born (reduction of about 10 per cent). The association of fetal trisomy with lower than normal levels of maternal serum α-fetoprotein (c.f. neural tube defects, p. 228) has been recognized recently, and this may prove a useful additional screen.

The risk of recurrence of any trisomy is about 1 per cent. Another inherited form of mental retardation, which is the focus of much current research, is that found in association with the so-called 'fragile-X' syndrome. The CNS pathology has not been exhaustively studied as yet.

It is important that the paediatric pathologist and the neuropathologist are aware of the possibility of chromosomal disorders so that the finding post mortem of multiple abnormalities, microencephaly and heterotopias of the cerebellum, singly or in combination, should alert the pathologist to the need for cytogenetic studies.

Down's syndrome – trisomy 21

The incidence of Down's syndrome is 1.4 per 1000 live births and accounts for 30 per cent of all cases of developmental malformations due to chromosomal abnormalities. The extra chromosomal material may be gained in three ways: 95 per cent are due to straightforward trisomy of chromosome 21 as a result of non-disjunction at meiosis; 4 per cent to translocation between chromosome 21 and one of the D or G chromosomes; and 1 per cent are mosaics in which the affected individual has a mixed population of normal and trisomic cells.

The incidence of Down's syndrome in babies born to women over the age of 40 is about 1 per cent, and increases with age. In these cases, the trisomy is usually due to non-disjunction of chromosome 21. Down's syndrome in the children of mothers younger than 25 years, however, is usually due to translocation of part of chromosome 21; this is a familial disorder and some subsequent children will have the syndrome. There is an increased risk of autoimmune disease, diabetes mellitus, thyroiditis and malignant disease.

Pathology

The brain is usually small, often weighing about 1000 g, and its shape is abnormally foreshortened with small frontal lobes and flattened occipital lobes. The cerebellum and brain stem are disproportionately small compared with the cerebral hemispheres. The gyral pattern is often simplified, and in about half of the cases the superior temporal gyri are small. On histological examination there are no specific abnormalities, although neuronal loss in layer III of the cortex has been reported, as has a reduction in the complexity of the dendritic spines demonstrated by Golgi stains.

A characteristic feature in cases with Down's syndrome aged more than 40 years is the presence of large numbers of Alzheimer neurofibrillary tangles and plaques. Quantitative comparison of the tangles and plaques in the hippocampi of patients with Down's syndrome, normal ageing and Alzheimer's disease have revealed marked similarity in their regional topography. Ultrastructurally the neurofibrillary tangles are identical with those seen in typical cases of Alzheimer's disease. Recent studies have shown that the gene encoding for the β-amyloid peptide in neuritic plaques in both Alzheimer's disease and Down's syndrome has been localized to the proximal portion of the q-arm of chromosome 21.

Other trisomies

The rare *Edward's syndrome* (trisomy 17–18) occurs in 1 in 6500 live births and is associated with a shorter life expectancy than Down's syndrome because of associated defects.

Patau's syndrome (trisomy 13–15) is also rare and is associated with severe abnormalities of the CNS incompatible with life, particularly with cyclopia and holoprosencephaly (see p. 231).

Fragile X syndrome

This is the second most frequent chromosomal disorder associated with developmental disability, with an incidence of 1 per 1000 liveborn males. It is, therefore, the most common familial form of mental retardation.

DEFECTS IN THE NEURAL TUBE

The term 'neural tube defect' is applied to a group of disorders in which some part of the neural tube or its coverings has either failed to close or has opened after closing. They are often referred to as *dysraphic malformations*. If the abnormality is limited to defective fusion of the posterior vertebral arches, there may be no abnormality of the overlying skin or meninges (*spina bifida occulta*), whereas if the lesion is more extensive, more of its coverings may be defective (*spina bifida cystica* – meningocele or myelomeningocele). The range of neural tube defects includes *anencephaly*, in which the vault of the skull is absent, and anencephaly with complete spina bifida (*craniorrhachischisis*). Rarer forms include *encephalocele*, which may or may not be part of an inherited condition (*Meckel–Gruber syndrome*) and *iniencephaly*.

The incidence of neural tube defects in the UK varies from 0.1 to 1.0 per cent of live births. There is a familial tendency and the risk of recurrence after one affected child is about 5 per cent, and after two affected children is about 13 per cent. In situations where the fetus is 'at risk' by virtue of a family history, defects of the neural tube may be diagnosed prenatally by the presence of raised α-fetoprotein levels in blood and amniotic fluid, and by ultrasonography. By these means a very effective screening programme has been established.

Defects of the neural tube are induced by damage occurring during the fourth week of fetal development and are thought to result from a combination of genetic and environmental factors. The genetic component is suggested by the higher risk in first-degree relatives. There are, however, marked variations in prevalence rates in different ethnic groups (between black and white Americans), and geographically (Belfast has an approximately threefold greater incidence than London). Many agents have been proposed as potential teratogens, including nitrates and nitrites and blighted potatoes. Nutritional deficiencies, particularly of vitamins, have also been incriminated and an increased prevalence in the low socioeconomic groups has been noted. No one single causative factor, however, has been identified. Nevertheless, the prevalence of neural tube defects appears to be declining.

Anencephaly

The incidence varies between 1 and 6 per 1000 live births: affected infants rarely survive more than a few hours. Three-quarters of anencephalic infants are female and the appearance is striking. The head is retroflexed and appears to sit on the shoulders. The cranial vault is missing and the base of the skull is flattened and small, due to a decrease in size of the anterior and middle cranial fossae. The face is usually formed but, because the orbits are shallow, the eyes tend to protrude. The cervical spine is usually abnormal and there is often an associated spinal defect that ranges from limited to complete rachischisis.

Pathology

The brain is represented by a small disc-shaped disorganized mass of glia, malformed brain and choroid plexus, the *area cerebrovasculosa*, which sits on the base of the skull and is usually covered by a thin smooth membrane (Fig. 13.6). The hypothalamus is abnormal and the posterior pituitary is absent: the anterior lobe of the pituitary, however, is usually present. The lower cranial nerves are sometimes recognizable and the spinal cord is usually slender. The spinal nerves, dorsal root ganglia and peripheral muscles are usually normal.

In many cases of anencephaly the adrenal glands are small, and there may be defects in other organs.

Defects of the spinal neural tube

Defects limited to the spine with failure of fusion of the neural arches are called *spina bifida*. The majority occur in the lumbosacral region, their severity depending upon the relative involvement of ectoderm, mesoderm and neural structures.

Spina bifida cystica

There are two main severe forms of spina bifida, termed *spina bifida cystica*. In some 80–90 per cent of these the lesion is a *myelomeningocele* (Fig. 13.7), in which both the meninges and spinal cord herniate through a large defect in the vertebrae. The fluctuant mass consists of a meningeal sac which is filled with CSF and covered by a thin membrane or by skin. The spinal cord may be closed, or floating on the posterior surface of the sac. In other cases, known as *myelocele*, the malformation appears as

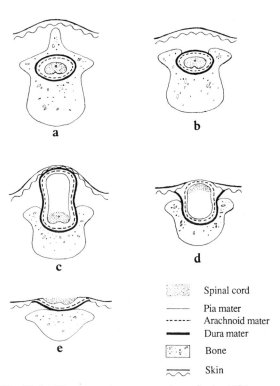

Spinal cord
Pia mater
Arachnoid mater
Dura mater
Bone
Skin

Fig. 13.7 Diagrammatic representations of spina bifida. a = normal; b = spina bifida occulta; c = meningocele; d = myelomeningocele; e = myelocele.

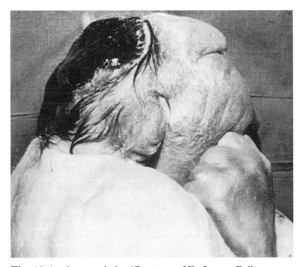

Fig. 13.6 Anencephaly. (Courtesy of Dr Jeanne Bell, Department of Neuropathology, University of Edinburgh.)

a flat open lesion, with CSF leaking on to the exposed area. The abnormal cord is exposed (*area medullovasculosa*) by a defect in skin, vertebral arches and meninges. Examination of the spinal cord both in and around the cystic lesion discloses various abnormalities that include dilatation of the central canal (*hydromyelia*), *syringomyelia* (see p. 236), *diastematomyelia* (see p. 237) or *duplication* of the cord. Most individuals with a myelomeningocele also have the Arnold–Chiari malformation (see p. 233). In the remaining 10–20 per cent of cases the lesion is a *meningocele*, which involves only meninges, vertebral arches and skin, when the cord is virtually normal.

The quality of life in most of those who survive with myelomeningocele is generally poor. The sequelae include incontinence of urine and faeces, flaccid areflexic weakness of the legs with sensory loss, and lumbar kyphosis. Many suffer from moderate or severe mental retardation. Even when early surgical closure of the defect is attempted, most of the patients die of infection in the first few weeks of life.

Spina bifida occulta

The least severe and probably the most common form of spina bifida is *spina bifida occulta* (Fig. 13.7), said to occur on average in 17 per cent of normal adults as determined by the absence of one or more spinous processes radiologically. Limited to the lumbosacral region, the dysraphic abnormality is covered by skin which may show abnormal pigmentation, a hairy patch or dermal sinus; there may be an associated intraspinal lipoma. There is also an association between spina bifida occulta and diastematomyelia (see p. 237).

Spina bifida occulta is in many cases asymptomatic. Neurological disturbances may, however, develop in adult life in the form of incontinence or retention of urine, and slowly progressive weakness and sensory disturbances in the lower limbs. The abnormality can be seen radiologically. A family history of spina bifida occulta increases the risk of spina bifida cystica.

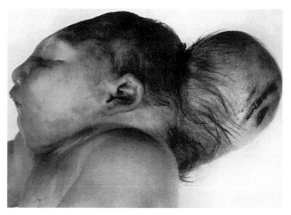

Fig. 13.8   Occipital encephalocele. (Courtesy of Dr A.A.M. Gibson, Department of Pathology, Royal Hospital for Sick Children, Glasgow.)

Encephalocele

This condition is a hernia of brain tissue and meninges through a midline defect in the cranial cavity; it is therefore analogous to spina bifida. Females are more commonly affected than males and in western Europe some 80 per cent occur in the occipital region, where the encephalocele protrudes through either the foramen magnum or the squamous occipital bone (Fig. 13.8). In contrast, frontal encephaloceles, which are relatively common in southeast Asia, present through a defect of the nasion or forehead and usually include olfactory tissue and a portion of frontal lobe. There are often associated facial deformities, with broadening of the face and hypertelorism. Large encephaloceles are usually incompatible with life and have only an incomplete covering of skin, whereas small encephaloceles are usually completely covered by skin.

Pathology

Varying amounts of brain tissue are found in encephaloceles, and large occipital encephaloceles may contain portions of the cerebellum, the brain stem and the cerebral hemispheres. As the herniated brain tissue enters the encephalocele through an opening narrower than the diameter of the encephalocele, varying degrees of haemorrhage, infarction and scar tissue develop. There may be associated abnormalities of the cerebral

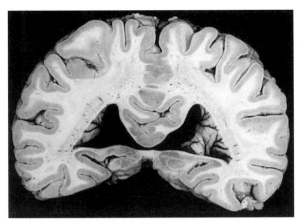

Fig. 13.9 Holoprosencephaly. The telencephalon has not separated into hemispheres or recognizable lobes and there is a single large ventricle and no corpus callosum.

hemispheres within the cranial cavity which include hydrocephalus, distortion of the brain stem and cerebellum and defective development of the corpus callosum.

In the Meckel–Gruber syndrome, an inherited autosomal recessive disorder, polydactyly and renal cystic dysplasia are associated with an encephalocele.

Holoprosencephaly

This complex malformation includes a large spectrum of anomalies ranging from cyclopia to agenesis of one olfactory bulb. In severe forms the base of the skull is usually short and narrow, the crista galli and lamina cribrosa are absent, the sella turcica is absent or shallow and there are varying degrees of hypoplasia of the nasal bones: the falx and sagittal sinus are usually missing. The brain is small, and the forebrain is represented by a single vesicle which has not separated into hemispheres or recognizable lobes. A single cerebral ventricle is present, and this may balloon dorsally in the form of a cyst (Fig. 13.9). There are coexistent facial abnormalities, which vary from hypotelorism with cleft lip to cyclopia, in which the orbits are fused, and the eyes are either set very close together or are completely fused. Holoprosencephaly is often, but not invariably, associated with trisomy 13.

Both recessive and dominant pedigrees have been described. Associations with maternal diabetes, toxoplasmosis and rubella, and the fetal alcohol syndrome have been suggested. It results in severe mental retardation and a reduced lifespan.

Arhinencephaly is a related abnormality which varies in severity from mere absence of the olfactory bulbs and tracts to gross disturbance of the limbic system. Like holoprosencephaly, arhinencephaly may be associated with chromosomal abnormalities.

Arachnoid cysts

These are developmental abnormalities due to the splitting of the arachnoid membrane. They occur most commonly in the Sylvian fissure, in the cerebellopontine angle, over the lateral convexity and at the base of the brain.

ANOMALIES IN THE FORMATION OF CONVOLUTIONS

Malformations of the gyri and sulci in the cerebral hemispheres result from a combination of either failure of adequate cell proliferation in, or failure of cell migration from, the subependymal plate to the cortex, failure of maturation once they have reached the surface of the hemispheres or, in some instances, of increased cell death. However, the aetiology, of these disorders is unclear, for although they may be 'developmental' certain features suggest that they may be caused by hypoxia or viral infections.

Agyria (Lissencephaly)

This malformation is uncommon. It may be sporadic or familial: in 50 per cent of cases chromosome analysis has demonstrated deficiency of band 17p13. The brain is small and has a smooth agyric cortex and a short oblique Sylvian fissure with an exposed insula. The condition therefore resembles that of the immature fetus. Lesser degrees of the condition are referred to as *pachygyria* in which there are reduced numbers of broadened gyri and shallow gyri.

Pathology

On section the cerebral cortex is abnormally thick and may extend almost to the ventricular wall. There is a corresponding reduction in the amount of white matter. The lateral ventricles are enlarged, often with nodules of heterotopic grey matter in the ventricular wall. Histologically, the cortex may appear simply as a rather thick homogeneous layer of neurons in which it is difficult to identify laminae or, less commonly, the affected cortex may be seen to be formed of only four layers. The heterotopic neurons do not elaborate extensive dendritic trees and do not develop normal intraneuronal connections. Severe mental retardation results.

In the *cerebello-ocular dysplastic* syndrome, which is a variant of agyria, there is a combination of complex cerebral and ocular malformations and muscular dystrophy.

Polymicrogyria

More common than pachygyria, polymicrogyria may also be focal or diffuse. It consists of large numbers of small closely packed gyri, the surface appearance of which has been likened to 'cobblestones' or 'Moroccan leather' (Fig. 13.10). The condition is commonly associated with other malformations. The histological appearances are variable, ranging in some areas from a two- to a four-layered cortex. The lamination in these areas, however, is disordered and many of the neurons themselves appear dysplastic or immature. The extent of the lesion varies greatly: it may be bilateral and symmetrical and may correspond to a particular arterial territory. The pathogenesis remains uncertain. Recent theories include either interference with migration or postmigrational necrosis. However, polymicrogyria has been associated with intrauterine infection and certain metabolic and peroxisomal disorders.

Heterotopias

These consist of masses of neurons in the white matter, apparently arrested in their path from the germinal matrix to their final destination in the cortex. They occur most commonly close to the walls of the lateral ventricles (Fig. 13.11), although they may also be seen in both deep and digitate white matter. They may also be seen in the white matter of the cerebellum and in

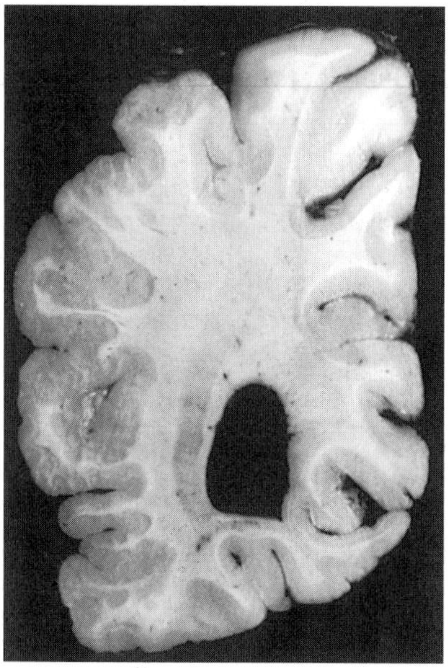

Fig. 13.10 Polymicrogyria. The gyri on the lateral surface of the occipital lobe are broadened and wrinkled due to the presence of large numbers of miniature convolutions.

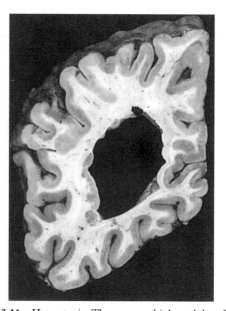

Fig. 13.11 Heterotopia. There are multiple nodules of subependymal ectopic grey matter.

conjunction with other malformations such as polymicrogyria and pachygyria, and in association with trisomy D and E.

Cortical dysplasias and all forms of migration defects have been described in the *cerebrohepatorenal syndrome of Zellweger*.

MALFORMATIONS OF THE CEREBELLUM

There are a number of malformations of the cerebellum that include the *Chiari malformations*, the *Dandy–Walker syndrome* and migration disorders similar to those described above.

Chiari malformations

Chiari originally described three types of malformation affecting the cerebellum, the brain stem and the base of the skull. There is some evidence that not all these malformations are of 'developmental' origin and that arachnoiditis in the posterior fossa may contribute in some cases. The *type 2* lesion is also known as the *Arnold–Chiari* malformation.

Pathology

In the type 2 malformation there is an abnormality of the hindbrain and cerebellum associated with a lumbar myelomeningocele and with hydrocephalus. There are two major components of the hindbrain abnormality. First, there is displacement of the inferomedial part of the cerebellum through the foramen magnum into the upper portion of the spinal canal, and secondly there is caudal displacement of the medulla, which appears narrow, S-shaped and elongated, much of it lying below the level of the foramen magnum (Fig. 13.12). The herniated cerebellar tissue lies on the dorsal surface of the lower medulla and upper segments of the cervical cord, firmly bound to them by fibrous adhesions and including choroid plexus. As a result of the downward displacement of the brain stem into the cervical canal, the lower cranial nerves and cervical nerve roots run a cephalad course from their point of origin. These features are particularly evident if the malformation is exposed at

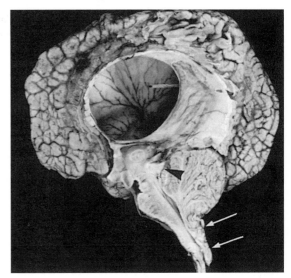

Fig. 13.12 Arnold–Chiari malformation (Chiari type 2). There is protrusion of the inferior part of the cerebellum (arrows) through the foramen magnum, elongation of the medulla, and a beaklike deformity of the quadrigeminal plate (arrowhead). Hydrocephalus is severe. There was also a myelomeningocele.

autopsy by posterior laminectomy and suboccipital craniotomy (see Fig. 1.6). Such an approach will display the additional features of a shallow malformed posterior fossa, low insertion of the tentorium and thickened fibrotic meninges in relation to both the herniated tissue and the exit foramina of the fourth ventricle. Hydrocephalus is almost invariably present, since the exit foramina of the fourth ventricle lie within the spinal canal; as a result of this the foramen magnum is obstructed by the displaced cerebellar vermis and CSF cannot re-enter the cranial cavity where it is normally absorbed. Ascending spinal meningitis may thus produce a pyocephalus, whereas the cerebral subarachnoid space is spared. Other causes of hydrocephalus include obstruction of the aqueduct. Other developmental anomalies include beaking of the tectum (Fig. 13.12), cerebral heterotopias and, frequently, focal polymicrogyria.

Because of the complexity and associated defects of the Chiari type 2 malformation, its pathogenesis remains uncertain. None of the existing theories is satisfactory but they include (i) a disturbance in the normal growth of the contents of the posterior fossa relative to the development of the fossa itself; (ii) a postulated tethering of the lower spinal cord by the myelomeningocele that produces traction on the hindbrain and displaces it caudally; and (iii) the presence of fetal hydrocephalus, which increases hydrostatic pressure in the ventricles.

In the *type 1* malformation there is herniation of the cerebellar tonsils through the foramen magnum and there is minimal displacement of the brain stem. This type of malformation is not usually identified until adult life, when the patient presents with cerebellar ataxia or signs of high cervical compression. It has, however, also been noted in connection with sudden unexpected death in infancy and sleep apnoea. Spina bifida is not usually present but there may be an associated hydrocephalus or syringomyelia. These associations suggest an important if not a primary role for occipital dysplasia in the pathogenesis of the Chiari type 1 malformation.

In the *type 3* malformation there is spina bifida in the cervical region and herniation of the cerebellum through the bony defect forming an encephalocele. It is very rare and is best considered as a form of rostral neural tube defect.

Dandy–Walker malformation

This uncommon malformation develops at or before the end of the first trimester. Its aetiology is uncertain, but it may be due to failure of the foramen of Magendie to perforate, leading to enlargement of the fourth ventricle, which subsequently becomes a large cyst in the posterior fossa and often of the lateral ventricles. However, the finding that the foramina are patent in most cases suggests that a more likely cause involves a disturbance in the development of the rhombic lips and the roof of the fourth ventricle.

Pathology

The disorder is associated with malformation of the cerebellar vermis (Fig. 13.13); there may also be hypoplasia of the cerebellar hemispheres. Histologically the wall of the cyst comprises an outer layer of thickened meninges and an inner layer of glia, occasionally including cerebral

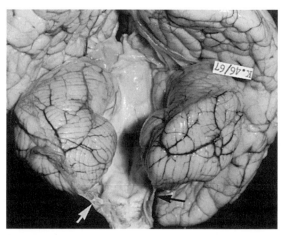

Fig. 13.13   Dandy–Walker malformation. There is absence of the cerebellar vermis, and a large cavity in continuity with the fourth ventricle. The cyst wall (arrows) is in continuity with the cerebellar hemispheres.

vascular remnants. The inner layer is made up of attenuated ependyma covering the deep white matter of the cerebellar hemispheres laterally and whose floor is the dorsum of the brain stem. The posterior fossa is enlarged, with elevation of the torcula, the tentorium and the lateral and straight sinuses. In some two-thirds of cases there are associated anomalies in the cerebral hemispheres, particularly agenesis of the corpus callosum, occipital encephalocele and midline hamartomas. The pathogenesis is uncertain, but an acceptable explanation is a developmental arrest of the hindbrain, which would help explain the associated atretic foramina and brain-stem abnormalities and the occasional involvement of the cerebellar hemispheres.

Other malformations of the cerebellum

These include a variety of conditions in which there is *agenesis of the vermis, hypoplasia of the cerebellar hemispheres* in association with a *small pons* or degeneration of *anterior horn cells, aplasia of the granule-cell layer* and various *heterotopias*.

An uncommon condition is that of *Lhermitte–Duclos disease*, a sporadic disorder that presents in the second or third decade with the features of raised intracranial pressure. It is characterized pathologically by broadening of folia enveloping a central cavity; histologically there is a thick outer layer containing myelinated axons but no Purkinje dendrites. The inner layer adjoining the cavity consists of large neurons with rounded nuclei and peripheral Nissl bodies. Following surgical resection the prognosis is good, suggesting that it is a compact hamartoma rather than a simple hypertrophy.

DISORDERS OF THE CEREBRAL AQUEDUCT

There is considerable variation in the anatomy of the aqueduct but, because of its short length and narrow calibre, it is a frequent site of obstruction to the circulation of the CSF, leading to hydrocephalus. There are four main intrinsic disorders that produce obstruction of the aqueduct, namely stenosis, forking or atresia, membrane formation and gliosis.

Stenosis – one form of which is inherited as a sex-linked recessive disorder – appears to be due simply to a decrease in the diameter of the aqueduct. Indeed, the aqueduct may appear to be absent macroscopically, but microscopically clusters of ependymal cells may be seen forming short channels around the stenosed and narrowed aqueduct. There is no associated gliosis. Obstruction due to forking of the aqueduct is a condition in which there is more than one channel. The ventral channel is usually a slit, whereas the dorsal canal is forked: the channels may communicate with each other or may enter the fourth ventricle separately. Obstruction may also be due to septum formation at the caudal end of the aqueduct: some of the septi have been associated with infections. Reduction of the lumen of the aqueduct associated with gliosis is thought to be due to infection.

MICROCEPHALY AND MEGALENCEPHALY

These conditions are commonly the end result of many disease processes related to genetic, chromosomal and environmental factors.

Microcephaly

Microcephaly, which is a reduction in the size of the head, should strictly speaking be differentiated from microencephaly, which denotes a brain that weighs less than 1000 g in adults and less than two standard deviations below the mean normal weight for the age and sex of the patient. As the small size of the head is usually secondary to an abnormality of the brain, the terms tend to be used synonymously. Although true microcephaly may be seen in apparently normal individuals, most are mentally retarded.

Microcephaly may result from diverse disorders that include degenerative, destructive or congenital conditions. For example, it may follow congenital infections such as rubella, toxoplasmosis, and cytomegalic inclusion body disease, toxins, irradiation, phenylketonuria or Tay–Sachs' disease. It is also common in chromosomal abnormalities and there may often be an association with *intrauterine growth retardation* due to malformations and infections, multiple pregnancy and placental insufficiency with maternal toxaemia or renal diseases. Other associations include *phenylketonuria* and *the fetal alcohol syndrome.*

In contrast to these secondary forms of microcephaly, there is a form of primary malformative microcephaly in which the frontal and temporal lobes are particularly small and the gyral pattern may be either simplified or more complex than usual. The white matter of the cerebral hemispheres is reduced in amount but the basal ganglia are generally unaffected, thereby appearing disproportionately large. In some cases of familial microcephaly the adult brain may weigh less than 600 g and there is extensive calcification in the basal ganglia.

Megalencephaly

This term generally refers to a brain that in the adult weighs more than 1700 g, and more than 2.5 standard deviations from the mean normal for the age and sex of the patient, and individuals so affected are usually mentally retarded. Primary megalencephaly may be an isolated finding or associated with achondroplasia and endocrine disorders, or it may be familial. Secondary megalencephaly may be due to metabolic disorders (see Ch. 10), such as Tay–Sachs' disease in its early stages, the Hunter–Hurler type of muco-polysaccharidosis, Alexander's disease and Canavan's disease. There is also an association with tuberous sclerosis (see p. 239). Other examples appear to be due to malformative conditions that include disorders of migration, such as polymicrogyria and heterotopias.

MALFORMATIONS OF THE SPINAL CORD

Spina bifida has already been discussed under neural tube defects (see p. 228). To be considered here are *syringomyelia* and *diastematomyelia*.

Syringomyelia

This is a cyst-like space (syrinx) or spaces that develop within the cervical cord (syringomyelia) or lower brain stem (syringobulbia). Not infrequently there is an associated Chiari type 1 malformation (see p. 234).

Pathology

The cavity contains clear CSF-like fluid and extends over a distance of several centimetres: it usually lies immediately dorsal to the central canal but may extend eccentrically into one or both dorsal horns of the grey matter (Fig. 13.14). Occasionally it communicates with either the fourth ventricle or the central canal. As the syrinx enlarges, the cord becomes swollen. Occasionally, syringomyelia occurs in association with intradural spinal tumours and vascular malformations, and after spinal injuries.

Histologically, the wall of the cavity consists of enlarged astrocytes and coarse glial fibrils, and there are sometimes nests or rosettes of ependymal cells, which is further evidence of communication between the cavity and the central canal of the cord. Part of the wall may be lined by a thin layer of collagen.

The effects are due principally to destruction of the cord by the enlarging cavity. This usually begins during the second or third decade and the first fibres to be affected are the decussating sensory fibres conveying the sensations of heat and pain. This results in *dissociated anaesthesia*, which is a selective insensibility to heat and pain in the region corresponding to the involved segments of the spinal cord. A neuropathic arthritis similar to that seen in tabes is common,

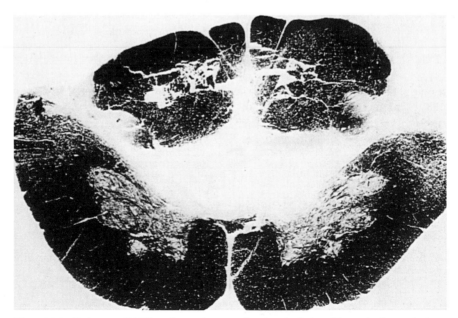

Fig. 13.14   Syringomyelia. There is a cavity extending into both dorsal horns in the cervical cord. (Weigert–Pal for myelin.)

but as syringomyelia usually occurs in the cervical region, the joints of the upper limbs are chiefly involved. Trophic lesions also occur in the skin. As the cavity enlarges, it ultimately affects the lateral white columns leading to spastic paraparesis, the ventral grey horns leading to neurogenic atrophy of muscles, and the posterior white columns leading to even greater disturbances of sensation.

There is considerable controversy about the nature of syringomyelia and its pathogenesis. Traditionally, it has been distinguished from hydromyelia – dilatation of the central canal of the spinal cord – on the basis that syringomyelic cavities first appear dorsal to the central canal. There is, however, evidence that in at least some cases syringomyelia is caused by CSF being propelled through a valve-like opening between the caudal extremity of the fourth ventricle and the central canal. An alternative hypothesis is that syringomyelia is a form of dysraphism in which there has been instability in the lines of junction of the alar and basal laminae with each other. In other words, the cavity is a greatly distended central canal. In syringobulbia the cavities extend cephalad into the medulla, passing ventrolaterally from the floor of the fourth ventricle or along the median raphe between the pyramid and the inferior olive.

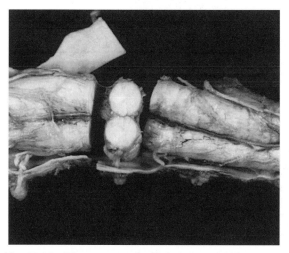

Fig. 13.15 Diastematomyelia. There are two hemicords within a single dural sac, separated by a fibrovascular septum.

Diastematomyelia

This is the term applied when the cord is split by either a bony or fibrous septum projecting into the vertebral canal. There is a variable degree of separation which, in turn, determines whether each half of the cord has its own pial and dural sheath or whether these investments are shared (Fig. 13.15).

This form of spinal cord dysraphism occurs predominantly in the thoracolumbar spine and is often associated with other anomalies, such as spina bifida occulta and the Arnold–Chiari malformation. There is usually a localized kyphoscoliosis at the site of the lesion.

DESTRUCTIVE LESIONS OFTEN RESEMBLING PRIMARY MALFORMATIONS

This group of disorders is due to the destructive action of agents that act on the brain after its initial period of organogenesis. They therefore resemble 'developmental' abnormalities but are in fact acquired *in utero*. Causative agents include drugs or their metabolites, ionizing radiation, and infections such as cytomegalovirus, toxoplasmosis and rubella. Some of the lesions appear to be due to failure of cerebral perfusion, either from disease of the placenta or hypotension in the mother.

Porencephaly

This term was originally used to describe a malformation in which a cyst lined by ependyma extended from the surface of the brain to the ventricle of one or both cerebral hemispheres (Fig. 13.16), but it is now generally used for similar cysts not lined by ependyma. Many appear to be ischaemic in origin, i.e. old infarcts, as the cyst is usually within the territory supplied by a middle cerebral artery.

The convolutional pattern around the edge of a porus is often abnormal: microscopically there may be either irregular islands of grey matter or polymicrogyria. A variety of malformations may be seen elsewhere in the brain. When bilateral porencephalic defects are very extensive, only a

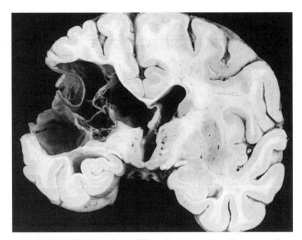

Fig. 13.16 Porencephaly. There is a large cyst that extends from the surface of the left cerebral hemisphere to the ventricle.

thin central area of tissue may connect the occipital and frontal parts of the brain, giving the appearance of a basket with a high handle (the so-called 'basket brain').

Hydranencephaly

This is a more severe form of porencephaly in which there is virtual absence of the cerebral hemispheres except for the basal ganglia and thalami, and the temporal and occipital lobes. There is a large fluid-containing membranous cavity which may or may not communicate with the ventricles. The wall of the membrane consists of pia-arachnoid and a thin layer of cortex in which there is an astrocytosis. Aetiological factors include fetal hypoxia and a history of maternal intoxication or attempts at suicide with domestic gas or butane. There is a strong association with twinning – particularly monozygotic twins – and various intrauterine viral infections have been implicated.

HYDROCEPHALUS

Although this topic has already been covered (see Ch. 4), the causes of hydrocephalus in neonates and infants will be summarized here.

Obstructive hydrocephalus is often due to abnormalities in the posterior fossa, and is commonly present in association with the Arnold–Chiari malformation and spina bifida cystica. Further causes include aqueduct stenosis and tumours. Obstruction may also occur as a result of incomplete development of the exit foramina of the fourth ventricle, as seen for example in the Dandy–Walker syndrome. Whereas the latter is associated with enlargement of the posterior fossa, there are conditions in which ventricular enlargement is associated with either a flattened posterior fossa (platybasia) or a malformed basiocciput, as for example in the Arnold–Chiari malformation and myelomeningocele.

Developmental hydrocephalus occurs typically in *holoprosencephaly*, in which the cerebral vesicles fail to develop laterally from the prosencephalon.

Communicating hydrocephalus is due to failure of proper reabsorption of CSF over the convexity of the brain and along the nerve roots. It may occur as a result of subarachnoid haemorrhage due to birth trauma that results in haemosiderosis and fibrosis of the meninges. A similar effect may be found after meningitis.

Hypersecretory hydrocephalus may be caused by papillomas of the choroid plexus (see Ch. 15).

PHAKOMATOSES

This group of mainly familial disorders is characterized by malformations of the neuraxis together with multiple small tumours which involve neuroectodermal structures. The skin, the eyes and some internal organs, such as the kidneys, are also commonly involved. There are six main types of phakomatoses, of which von Recklinghausen's neurofibromatosis is the commonest.

Neurofibromatosis

There are two separate disorders. The commoner is von Recklinghausen's neurofibromatosis (peripheral neurofibromatosis) when patients may present with mental retardation, epilepsy or spinal root compression. The other is central neurofibromatosis when bilateral acoustic neurofibromas are common.

Neurofibromatosis is a relatively common disease (1 in 3000) which is inherited as an autosomal dominant with a high degree of penetrance but variable expression. The mutation rate is high, accounting for new cases. The responsible gene has been located on the long arm of chromosome 17, linked to the locus encoding for nerve-growth factor.

In its mildest form expression of the condition is limited to cutaneous café-au-lait pigmentation and cutaneous neurofibromas. Visceral lesions and elephantiasis may be present. Between 10 and 30 per cent of plexiform neurofibromas (see Ch. 15) may undergo sarcomatous change.

Central neurofibromatosis

This disease has a prevalence of 0.1 per 100 000. There is a gene deletion on chromosome 22 associated with which there is a deficiency of glial growth factor activity. Patients present with multiple intracranial and intraspinal tumours which are mainly schwannomas and meningiomas. Bilateral acoustic schwannomas are common: in such cases skin lesions are uncommon.

Pathology

In the central form of the disease abnormalities such as megalencephaly, pachygyria, polymicrogyria, heterotopias, syringomyelia and hydrocephalus due to stenosis of the aqueduct may occur. Tumours are common, and include multiple meningiomas, gliomas of the optic nerve, pilocytic astrocytomas of the third ventricle and gliomatosis cerebri (see Ch. 15). Bilateral acoustic schwannomas are common (Fig. 13.17) and the prognosis is better when they are the only manifestation of the disease.

Hamartomatous changes are also a feature and include schwannosis in the form of invasion of the dorsal root entry zones of the spinal cord by Schwann cells, meningiomatosis, angiomatosis, and glial nodules in the cortex and white matter. There is also an association with tumours of the kidney, pancreas and adrenals. Phaeochromocytoma may also occur.

The underlying cause of neurofibromatosis is not known, although there is clearly generalized involvement of derivatives of the neural crest. It has recently been suggested that the abnormality may be due to increased amounts of nerve-growth factor.

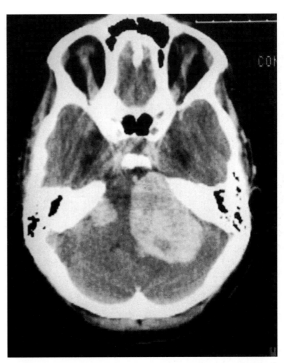

Fig. 13.17 Neurofibromatosis. CT scan showing bilateral acoustic schwannomas. (Courtesy of Dr Peter Macpherson, Department of Neuroradiology, Institute of Neurological Sciences, Glasgow.)

In contrast to the peripheral form of neurofibromatosis, the cutaneous abnormalities in patients with the central form of the disease are often slight. This inverse relationship, however, is not invariable.

Tuberous sclerosis (Bournville's disease)

This familial disease, transmitted as a mendelian dominant, occurs in 1 per 10 000 subjects. About 80 per cent are mutations of the gene which is linked to an oncogene on the long arm of chromosome 9. Seizures are common, and skin manifestations consisting of facial adenoma sebaceum (angiofibromas), shagreen patches, fibromas and café-au-lait spots occur in over 90 per cent of cases. A characteristic lesion is the retinal hamartoma (phakoma). Rhabdomyomas of the heart (Fig. 13.18) occur in one-third of cases and other manifestations include angiomyolipomas of the kidney, pulmonary lymphangiomyomatosis, haemangiomas of the spleen and liver, and fibrous dysplasia in bone.

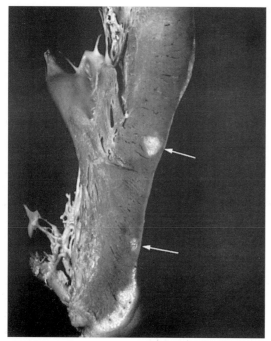

Fig. 13.18 Tuberous sclerosis. There are multiple pale and somewhat translucent rhabdomyomas (arrows) in the myocardium.

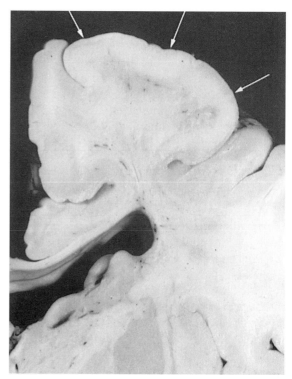

Fig. 13.19 Tuberous sclerosis. A tuber (arrows) has expanded a gyrus and obscured the junction between grey and white matter. There are also several subependymal nodules (candle guttering) bulging into the ventricle.

Pathology

The brain may be small, normal or of increased size. The most characteristic feature is the presence of pale firm tubers in the cerebral cortex (Fig. 13.19). They may be single or multiple and involve one or more gyri, their size varying from 2 to 30 mm in diameter. Nodular protuberances are present in the walls of the lateral ventricles, giving rise to the characteristic 'candle-guttering' appearance (Fig. 13.19). They may become calcified and, although slowly growing, may obstruct the foramen of Monro and cause hydrocephalus.

Histologically, the tubers consist of disordered cortex in which there are glial fibres, bizarre multinucleated hypertrophied astrocytes and groups of large plump cells with numerous short processes which contain vimentin but not usually GFAP. These cells are thought to be immature astrocytes. However, ultrastructural studies have suggested neuronal features indicating that they may be pluripotent. Similar microscopical appearances are seen in the ventricular nodules, changes that are very similar to the phakoma of the retina. The nodules are usually benign, but occasionally astrocytomas may supervene in the deep central portions of the brain.

As in the other phakomatoses, various malformations may be present in the CNS, such as heterotopias and polymicrogyria.

Encephalofacial angiomatosis (Sturge–Weber syndrome)

In this uncommon non-familial disease there are facial and intracranial haemangiomas. The facial lesion consists of an extensive, usually unilateral, facial cutaneous angioma (port wine stain). There is also extensive ipsilateral leptomeningeal angiomatosis. There is often atrophy and calcification in the cortex related to the angiomatosis.

Von Hippel–Lindau disease

In this condition haemangioblastomas (see Ch. 15)

develop in the retina and in the cerebellar hemispheres, but occasionally also around the brain stem and spinal cord. Cysts may occur in the pancreas, kidneys and lungs. Sometimes the tumours, which are usually benign, secrete an erythropoietic substance that causes a raised haematocrit and increased red-cell mass. The disease is dominantly inherited.

Neurocutaneous melanosis

Melanin-containing cells derived from the neural crest are normally present in the meninges on the ventral surface of the brain stem. Rarely, the melanin-containing cells of the meninges and skin may both proliferate. In the Touraine syndrome, inherited as a mendelian dominant, patches of pigmentation are visible macroscopically in both the pia mater and in cutaneous pigmented naevi. Occasionally the meningeal component may become a melanoma.

PERINATAL NEUROPATHOLOGY

In addition to the primary malformative lesions of the brain there are various disorders (traumatic, haemorrhagic, ischaemic, metabolic and inflammatory) that contribute to the overall problem of brain damage in the neonatal period. For the recognition of these disorders the neuropathologist requires a working knowledge of the normal growth and development of the brain and, particularly, of the changes that take place between the 24th week of gestation and the first 28 days of life.

MECHANICAL BIRTH INJURY

Some of the lesions are unique to the perinatal period, almost never occurring beyond this time, e.g. matrix zone haemorrhages, subpial haemorrhages, ischaemic necrosis of the brain stem and thalamus, gliosis of white matter and kernicterus.

Bleeding into the deeper layers of the scalp is common and is almost invariable following the use of a vacuum extractor or forceps. It is generally resorbed.

In some 2.5 per cent of all births there is a *cephalohaematoma*, i.e. a collection of blood between the surface of a calvarial bone and its pericranial membrane. It is usually parietal in location and in a very small percentage of cases is associated with a fracture of the skull. *Fractures of the skull* are usually found only in association with prolonged labour, abnormal presentations and forceps deliveries. Intracranial *extradural haematoma* is uncommon in the neonatal period, largely because the dura mater is firmly adherent to the inner surface of the skull. *Subdural haematoma*, however, may occur in the absence of a fracture when, at full term, it is usually due to either a tear in the falx cerebri or in the tentorium cerebelli, or rupture of the superficial veins of the cerebral convexity during a difficult or breech delivery. Careful autopsy technique is required to identify tears which may extend into the dural sinuses and the great vein of Galen. Subdural haemorrhage may also occur in premature infants. This is most likely to occur during breech presentation, a high forceps delivery or excessive distortion and overlapping of the parietal and occipital bones during passage of the fetal head through the birth canal.

The incidence of subdural haemorrhage has fallen considerably in the last decade or so to less than 2 per cent of live births. The amount of blood varies from a few millilitres to 1.0 cm or more in thickness; it may be unilateral or bilateral and occurs most commonly over the posterior two-thirds of the cerebral hemispheres. Associated lesions may include haemorrhage at other sites or hypoxic/ischaemic damage.

Variable amounts of focal or diffuse *subarachnoid haemorrhage* are common in both premature and full-term infants. It may be due to rupture of blood vessels within the subarachnoid space, in the cerebral hemispheres, to direct extension from the fourth ventricle after intraventricular haemorrhage, or to a tear of the falx or the tentorium. The blood may be particularly conspicuous in the wide Sylvian fissures or in the basal cisterns. Occasionally there is a localized subarachnoid haematoma that may measure up to 10 mm in depth. Subarachnoid haemorrhage may be of traumatic origin in cases of forceps or vacuum extraction, or may result from asphyxia.

Other causes include venous occlusion, rupture

of vascular malformations, sepsis, trauma and coagulopathy.

Injury to the spinal cord during forcible breech extraction or mid and high forceps extraction with cephalic delivery may result in damage to the cervical segments of the cord and the spinal nerve roots.

CEREBRAL HAEMORRHAGE

Babies of low birth weight (less than 2500 g body weight) are prone to intracranial haemorrhage, and those of very low birth weight (below 1000 g) are particularly at risk. This may be localized to the subarachnoid and/or subpial spaces, but of greater importance is bleeding into the *germinal matrix* or *subependymal plate* (Fig. 13.20). This is a normal structure found in the upper pole of the caudate nucleus of the developing brain: it has largely disappeared by the 32nd–33rd week of gestation. It is the source of primitive cells that differentiate into either neurons or glia. It is a soft grey structure that lacks a supporting stroma, a factor that is thought to account for the high incidence of subependymal haemorrhage in the brains of premature infants between the 24th and 26th weeks of gestation. The blood vessels of the subependymal plate also undergo changes between 13 and 35 weeks that may well contribute

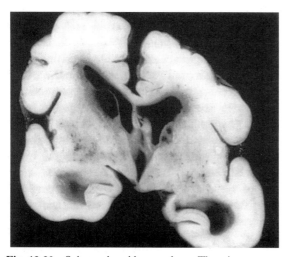

Fig. 13.20   Subependymal haemorrhage. There is asymmetrical haemorrhage into the subependymal matrix layer of each cerebral hemisphere.

to their fragility. Such haemorrhage may be unilateral or bilateral and of variable size, although when large it commonly ruptures through the overlying ependyma into the lateral ventricles to cause *intraventricular haemorrhage* (IVH). Haemorrhage into the germinal matrix plate is found commonly in autopsies on low birth-weight infants, and its true incidence in those who survive is now being determined by ultrasound and CT scanning. The incidence of subependymal haemorrhage in nursery infants weighing 1500 g or less, or of 34 weeks' gestational age or less as determined by CT or ultrasonography, can be as high as 80 per cent: the incidence drops to between 1 and 3 per cent at the gestational age of 37 weeks or more, and there is evidence to suggest that the overall incidence of subependymal haemorrhage is declining. A grading system for subependymal haemorrhage and IVH has been proposed: I. haemorrhage in the matrix; II. IVH without dilatation; III. IVH plus dilatation; IV. IVH plus intraparenchymal haemorrhage. This classification is useful, although it refers only to the extent of the bleeding. In general, however, grades I and II have a better prognosis than grades III and IV. The prognosis following intraventricular haemorrhage is worse than for subependymal haemorrhage.

Infants with subependymal haemorrhage often have the respiratory distress syndrome and disturbances of cardiorespiratory function. It is now accepted that impairment of autoregulation of cerebral blood flow plays a role in the pathogenesis of these haemorrhages: once bleeding has started, it is suggested that high fibrinolytic activity in the matrix zone may contribute to its spread.

In patients dying within a few days of bleeding it is easy to identify the haemorrhage by microscopy: macrophages appear within a few days and siderophages are a striking feature by 2–3 weeks. Cavities may be present by 2–6 months.

Posthaemorrhagic hydrocephalus is the most commonly recognized complication. However, the hydrocephalus either arrests or regresses spontaneously and so any associated mental handicap is likely to be due to additional lesions. The degree of ventricular enlargement varies, the ependymal surfaces may be rust-brown in colour and there may be residual intraventricular clot.

The incidence of matrix zone and intraventricular haemorrhage in the full-term neonate is much less and is of more diverse origin, including rupture of blood vessels in the choroid plexus, trauma, rupture of vascular malformations and venous thrombosis.

Intraventricular haemorrhage in the absence of haemorrhage into the germinal matrix may originate from the choroid plexus.

Compared with other types of intracranial haemorrhage, *intracerebral* and *intracerebellar haematomas* are far less common. They may be small or large, single or multiple, and may or may not be associated with the other types of haemorrhage. Their aetiology is unclear, but in the neonate thrombocytopenia, haemolytic disease, haemophilia and vitamin K deficiency may be responsible for the bleeding. Other risk factors include cardiac malformations and sepsis.

HYPOXIC–ISCHAEMIC AND VASCULAR LESIONS

Hypoxic–ischaemic brain damage in the fetus and newborn infant accounts for a high proportion of children with cerebral palsy, mental retardation and epilepsy. The lesions, which may affect grey and white matter, may be focal or diffuse and occur singly or in combination. They are usually due to hypoxia, the pattern of damage being influenced in part by the maturity of the brain. Indeed several patterns of brain damage seen in neonates are similar to those that can be produced in fetal monkeys, these experiments serving to emphasize that there are many factors, such as changes in cerebral blood flow, blood levels of glucose, the degree of lactacidosis and hypoxaemia, that determine the range and severity of brain lesions in the brains of preterm and term babies. A variety of maternal and placental abnormalities may initiate damage to the fetal brain at any stage of gestation. Those occurring during the first trimester are usually fatal, whereas hypoxic insults at a later stage tend to damage selective areas of the brain. It is now appreciated that a range of lesions may be induced, including combinations of what have been thought to be both of a destructive and malformative nature.

There is now clear evidence that the pathophysiology and the pattern of selective vulnerability of the immature brain to hypoxia are different from those of the mature brain (see Ch. 4). In general there is sparing of the immature necortex; there are many instances when the cortical ribbon is normal, lesions being restricted to thalamus and the white matter. There may also be abnormalities in the brain stem. Nevertheless, it is still customary to describe the hypoxic–ischaemic encephalopathies in terms of involvement of either grey or white matter. The identification of hypoxic neuronal damage in the immature brain is difficult, and the more immature the infant the greater the difficulty. In many instances it is not possible to identify the classic features of the ischaemic cell process (see Ch. 3), neuronal damage being recognizable simply by virtue of nuclear karyorrhexis. Neuronal damage is followed by a macrophage response and, later, by an astrocytosis.

Lesions in grey matter

Cortical lesions may be focal or diffuse, and are usually accentuated in layers III and V in the depths of sulci. Necrosis of the hippocampus is common and there is variable damage in the basal ganglia and thalami. In the brain stem, the inferior colliculi, the nuclei of the cranial nerves and the neurons of the reticular formation and pontine nuclei are often affected. Necrosis of Purkinje cells and of the dentate nuclei is often seen in the cerebellum and there may be lesions in the spinal cord. Four different patterns of hypoxic brain damage are recognized: (i) brain-stem–thalamus; (ii) basal ganglia; (iii) cortex; and (iv) pontohippocampal. They may be unilateral or bilateral and may occur in any combination in any one brain. Whereas in short survivors there may be no macroscopic abnormalities, in long-term survivors the affected gyri are small, white and firm and there is loss of definition between cortex and white matter. Histologically, the architecture of the cortex is abnormal, with residual clumps of surviving neurons separated by abnormal bundles of myelinated axons and glial fibres which radiate through the cortex more or less perpendicular to the surface.

The pathogenesis of these lesions is probably similar in both premature and full-term infants, being a consequence of some hypoxic episode. Such hypoxia may result from maternal factors, e.g. hypotension, abnormalities of the placenta – praevia or abruptio; fetal factors, e.g. prolapse of the umbilical cord; difficult and prolonged delivery; abnormalities of growth *in utero*, and postnatal factors such as apnoea, respiratory distress syndrome and convulsions.

These various patterns of damage have been reproduced in fetal non-human primates by total or partial asphyxia, compression of the umbilical cord and carbon monoxide poisoning.

Lesions in white matter

A common abnormality is *periventricular leukomalacia*. The incidence varies according to the population under study and may occur in up to 35 per cent of low birth-weight high-risk cases. It may be solitary or multiple, unilateral or bilateral, and consists of rather ill-defined white spots in the pale, soft unmyelinated periventricular white matter. Although often small, these may extend to the cortex: with survival, the lesions become outlined by a chalky-white ring and eventually undergo cavitation (Fig. 13.21). Histologically, the initial changes are those of coagulative necrosis and their boundaries are easily seen as positively staining coronas in PAS-stained sections: polymorphonuclear leukocytes and lymphocytes are not seen. Axonal bulbs appear after 24–36 hours and by 14 days macrophages, reactive astrocytes and new blood vessels are present. Later on, microscopy shows debris encrusted with calcium and iron salts. In some cases necrotic lesions are also found in the related ependyma and in grey matter.

Periventricular leukomalacia is a common autopsy finding (up to 20 per cent) in the brains of preterm infants. It is widely accepted as infarction of white matter due to failure of

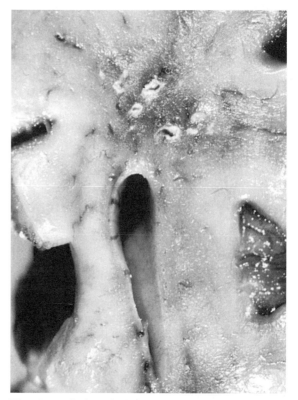

Fig. 13.21   Periventricular leukomalacia. There are white foci in the periventricular region. (Courtesy of Dr. Eleanor Allibone, Department of Pathology, St James's University Hospital, Leeds.)

perfusion along the boundary zones between the centripetal and centrifugal arteries within the brain. Prolonged apnoea or peripheral circulatory failure in the preterm infant probably leads to severe hypotension: autoregulation of cerebral blood flow is deranged and cerebral hypoxia ensues. Additional features include a change from aerobic to anaerobic metabolism, followed by lactoacidosis. With improved neonatal care, the mortality and morbidity and especially the neurological disabilities of low birth-weight infants have decreased significantly.

Hypoxic–ischaemic encephalopathies also occur in full-term neonates, particularly if labour has been difficult or if there have been antecedent obstetric problems. The risk of serious hypoxia has been greatly reduced by better antenatal care and the general use of fetal heart rate monitoring. However, examples, of severe

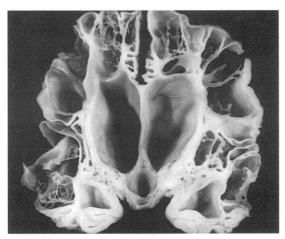

Fig. 13.22 Hypoxic–ischaemic encephalopathy. There is thinning of the cortex and cavitation of white matter.

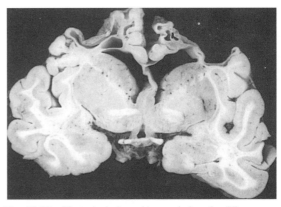

Fig. 13.23 Hypoxic–ischaemic encephalopathy. The ischaemic damage is maximal in the superomedial parts of each cerebral hemisphere, i.e. in the boundary zones between the territories supplied by the anterior and middle cerebral arteries.

hypoxic–ischaemic encephalopathy still occur. The neonate under these circumstances tends to be hypotonic at birth, has an Apgar score of less than 3, and requires both resuscitation and mechanical ventilation. Seizures are common. Fortunately, severe neurological deficit due to such brain damage is now uncommon. However, in those who survive, and die, subsequently the structural changes are variable, ranging from extensive disintegration and liquefaction to a multicystic honeycomb appearance of the white matter and, to a lesser extent, of the cortical mantle (Fig. 13.22). In some cases neuronal loss and poor myelination in the gyri result in *ulegyria*, when the convolutions become thinned and the sulci widened. Ischaemic damage (*granular atrophy*) may be limited to the cortex along the arterial boundary zones between the distribution of the anterior and middle cerebral arteries (Fig. 13.23). The basal ganglia may have a characteristic abnormal appearance – *état marbré* or *status marmoratus* but, more commonly, there is cavitation and gliosis. Status marmoratus consists of whitish spots or streaks resembling the pattern of marble in the lateral portion of the corpus striatum and, to a lesser extent, in the thalamus. Histologically, the appearances are due to an abnormal distribution of myelinated fibres rather than to derangement of myelination.

A second entity is *white matter gliosis*, which may be found in both preterm and term infants. Hypoxia–ischaemia probably plays a role in its pathogenesis, since it is associated with conditions such as the respiratory distress syndrome, congenital heart disease and perinatal asphyxia. The condition needs to be separated from white matter gliosis and delayed myelination that occur in association with nutritional deficiency and congenital rubella. A third category of white matter damage in the immature brain is *subcortical leukomalacia*, in which the lesions lie predominantly in relation to the depths of sulci.

Cerebrovascular disease of the types seen in the adult are uncommon in the neonatal period but thromboembolic phenomena may occur in association with congenital heart disease or nonbacterial endocarditis. Severe dehydration and nutritional disorders may result in cerebral phlebothrombosis and, occasionally, occlusion of one of the major venous sinuses. Although defects in the arteries are common at birth, saccular aneurysms are rare. Arteriovenous malformations are also uncommon, although when present they may cause sufficient shunting of blood through the malformation for the infant to develop congestive heart failure. Aneurysmal malformation of the vein of Galen is the most frequent form seen in the neonate. Lesions due to ischaemia may result in porencephaly or hydranencephaly (see p. 237).

METABOLIC DISORDERS

The principal metabolic disorders in this age group are bilirubin encephalopathy (kernicterus) and hypoglycaemia. Others are considered in Chapter 10.

Bilirubin encephalopathy (kernicterus)

Kernicterus is the name given to selective yellow staining of certain parts of the brain in jaundiced babies when the plasma level of unconjugated bilirubin exceeds 250 µmol/l. The most common cause has been rhesus incompatibility, but hyperbilirubinaemia is also found in other haemolytic conditions such as ABO incompatibility and incapacity of the liver to conjugate an overload of bilirubin, as may occur in septicaemia and as a result of absorption of large haematomas, the administration of certain drugs or a deficiency of glucose 6-phosphate dehydrogenase. Exceptionally there may be a primary hepatic enzyme insufficiency, such as in Crigler–Najjar disease, an autosomal recessive defect. Yellow staining of the brain has also been described in premature asphyxiated neonates with low levels of serum bilirubin (170–205 µmol/l).

Pathology

After fixation the yellow discoloration may be difficult to see, but is most evident in the pallidum, the subthalamic nuclei, the hippocampi, the dentate nuclei and the inferior olivary nuclei. Some cranial nerve nuclei may also be involved. It is therefore the phylogenetically older parts of the brain that are principally affected, although rarely there may be microscopic pigmentation in the newer parts of the brain. On microscopical examination, the neuropil in the affected areas is vacuolated and spongy, and there is cytoplasmic microvacuolation of neurons, loss of Nissl substance and changes in the cytoplasmic and nuclear membranes. The yellow pigment within the neuronal cytoplasmic vacuoles can always be seen in unstained and stained frozen sections, and in many cases is seen in paraffin-embedded material stained with H&E.

Granular mineralization of the neuronal cytoplasmic membrane has also been described and serves as a useful histological marker in infants who survive weeks or months after kernicterus.

The mechanism by which bilirubin enters the brain and damages certain groups of neurons is not fully understood. Recent studies, however, have suggested that asphyxia might injure endothelium and alter the blood–brain barrier, thus allowing bilirubin access to neurons. Indeed, in newborn non-human primates the infusion of unconjugated bilirubin produces kernicterus only when the animals are first made hypoxic. On the other hand, kernicterus in infants with septicaemia may be due not only to damage to the blood–brain barrier, but also to increased haemolysis. In children who survive for some time the discoloration disappears, although the neuronal changes, loss of myelin and gliosis can be readily identified.

Bilirubin encephalopathy due to severe haemolytic disease of the newborn has virtually disappeared since the introduction of anti-D prophylactic measures and the widespread use of exchange transfusion. There remains, however, the problem of kernicterus in low birth-weight infants in whom prevention, diagnosis and treatment remain unsatisfactory.

In contrast to perinatal tissue, the blood–brain barrier in the adult brain does not allow the passage of bilirubin and, with the exception of the choroid plexus, the pineal gland and the area postrema in the fourth ventricle, is not stained, although the patient may be deeply jaundiced. However, in cases where the blood–brain barrier is deficient due to infarction, tumour or abscess, bilirubin becomes extravasated and stains the tissue.

Hypoglycaemia

If the level of blood sugar falls below about 20 mg/dl, structural damage in the brain similar to that seen in hypoxia may ensue. Within the perinatal period this is most likely to occur when there is a delay in initial feeding in 'small for dates' infants, in infants of diabetic mothers and in infants with haemolytic disease of the newborn, hypothermia and inborn errors of carbohydrate metabolism.

Alpers' disease (progressive cerebral poliodystrophy)

Although traditionally considered with the various types of hypoxic–ischaemic brain damage of the fetus and newborn, this condition is probably of heterogeneous origin, ranging from a mitochondrial encephalopathy to the possibility of an infantile form of Creutzfeldt–Jakob disease.

HEXACHLOROPHANE

This chlorinated biphenol is incorporated as an antimicrobial agent in soaps, liquid detergents and cosmetics. It is effective against Gram-positive cocci and has been widely used in neonatal units to prevent staphylococcal skin infections. It is absorbed through normal skin but especially through damaged skin (burns etc.), mucous membranes and the skin of premature infants. It is metabolized in the liver by conjugation with glucuronide. Occasionally, sufficient hexachlorophane is absorbed to cause an *acute encephalopathy* characterized by marked swelling of the brain, the spinal cord and the optic nerves; occasionally the changes are limited to the brain stem or optic nerves. Microscopically there is status spongiosus of the white matter which, as established by electron microscopy, is due to widespread intramyelinic oedema. Neither neurons nor their axons are affected; there is, however, periaxial demyelination (see Ch. 9). Peripheral nerves are also affected.

INFLAMMATORY DISORDERS

Within the perinatal period infections by *T. pallidum, Toxoplasma gondii, cytomegalovirus* and *rubella* are particularly important. Infection of the mother is a prerequisite for fetal infection and usually results from infections of the blood of sufficient magnitude and duration to allow passage across the placenta. Differences in the structure of the placenta at various stages of gestation are also important determinants of fetal infection.

Most pregnancies are accompanied by non-specific 'viral-like' illnesses which do not have an obvious effect on fetal development. Sero-conversion of the mother is not therefore necessarily associated with damage to the fetus. However, if an infection does cross the placenta, then its effects will depend on the developmental stage of the fetus. For example, if the fetus becomes infected early in pregnancy, then a generalized destructive process often leads to fetal death or severe retardation and microcephaly. In contrast, infection acquired at a later stage may result in an apparently normal neonate, only for the congenital nature of the disease to become manifest in childhood or adolescence. Knowledge of the natural history of the infection in mother and fetus thus allows decisions about termination of the pregnancy and the establishment of programmes of prevention.

Congenital syphilis

In the primary and secondary stages in the mother, the fetus becomes heavily infected and usually dies *in utero*. If pregnancy occurs following the secondary stage, the baby may be born alive with lesions of congenital syphilis, namely a generalized petechial rash, hepatosplenomegaly, thrombocytopenia and jaundice. Disease of the nasal bones and mucosa leads to the 'snuffles' and later on a characteristic deformity appears in the incisor teeth (Hutchinson's teeth). Still later, neurosyphilis, corneal opacity and blindness may develop. The longer the interval between secondary syphilis and pregnancy, the more likely the child is to appear healthy at birth and to develop syphilitic lesions later during childhood or adolescence.

Pathology

Infection in early pregnancy may result in malformations, in meningovascular syphilis in early postnatal life, in juvenile congenital general paralysis of the insane, or, less commonly, in juvenile congenital tabes dorsalis between the ages of 6 and 21 years.

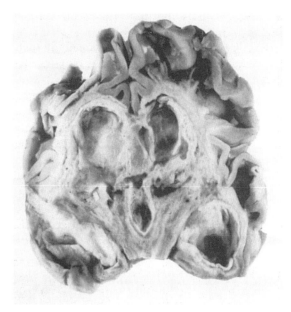

Fig. 13.24   Congenital toxoplasmosis. There is extensive cystic gelatinous degeneration of the cerebral hemispheres, and hydrocephalus.

Congenital toxoplasmosis

Prospective studies of mothers known to have acquired *toxoplasma* infection during pregnancy have shown that in some 30 per cent of cases infection is transmitted to the fetus. The incidence of congenital *toxoplasma* infection is about 1–2 per 1000 live births, and it does not occur in women who already have antibodies to the infection. Depending upon the time of the infection and its severity, there are two main forms of congenital toxoplasmosis. One form is characterized by jaundice, hepatosplenomegaly, a cutaneous rash, myocarditis and pneumonia. Death often occurs within days or weeks. In the other there is a subacute/chronic meningoencephalitis, which is the basis of the classic tetrad of congenital toxoplasmosis, namely hydrocephalus, megalencephaly, chorioretinitis and cerebral calcification.

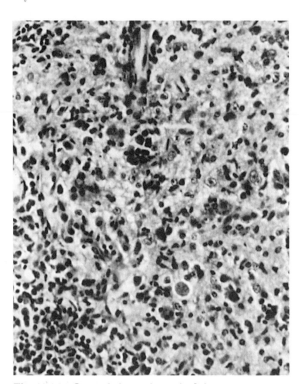

Fig. 13.25   Congenital toxoplasmosis. Subacute meningoencephalitis.

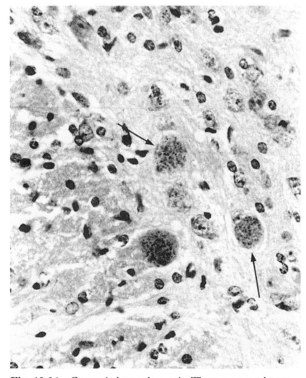

Fig. 13.26   Congenital toxoplasmosis. There are toxoplasma cysts (arrows) in the brain.

Pathology

In severe cases there may be extensive destruction of tissue with cavitation (Fig. 13.24). Histologically, there is a meningoencephalitis characterized by monocytes, lymphocytes and plasma cells in the subarachnoid space and around small blood vessels within the brain (Fig. 13.25). There are also inflammatory focal lesions of varying size within the brain. The smallest foci consist of collections of microglia, whereas the larger lesions may appear as granulomas or areas of necrosis with cyst formation. Necrosis appears to be due to vascular changes, and in some areas there is fibrinoid necrosis of blood vessels. Depending upon the severity of the reaction and the duration of the infection, there is variable calcification in the affected areas and attempts at repair with gliosis. The inflammatory process is particularly severe around the aqueduct of Sylvius, which may be partially or completely occluded, thereby resulting in hydrocephalus. Inflammatory lesions also occur in the eye. Whether in biopsy or autopsy material, the diagnosis of toxoplasmosis is easily made if the specimen contains a *toxoplasma* tissue cyst (Fig. 13.26). The cysts are easily stained with PAS and, interestingly, they are not usually associated with an inflammatory cell infiltrate. In the absence of a cyst, it is difficult to find organisms when they are lying free in brain tissue or in macrophages, although identification using immunohistochemistry has greatly aided the search.

It is now apparent from prospective studies that, although children born to mothers who have seroconverted during pregnancy may appear normal clinically, many will subsequently develop neurological sequelae or chorioretinitis. The incidence of congenital *toxoplasma* infection is lower than that of congenital infection with cytomegalovirus, and is equal to, or greater than, that of congenital rubella infection (see below). Congenital toxoplasmosis therefore appears to be a significant contributor to mental subnormality.

Cytomegalovirus

Cytomegalovirus has been claimed to be the commonest cause of fetal infection. One per cent of all newborns have serological and virological evidence of fetal infection, but only 1–5 per cent of these have cytomegalic inclusion body disease. Over 95 per cent of neonates with congenital cytomegalovirus infection appear normal at birth. However, up to 20 per cent of the clinically silent infections lead to hearing loss or mental retardation, which makes cytomegalovirus the commonest known infective cause of mental retardation.

Pathology

Florid cytomegalic inclusion body disease of the newborn presents with hepatosplenomegaly, jaundice, petechiae and disease of the brain and eyes. Involvement of the brain commonly results in microcephaly, cyst formation and intracerebral calcification. In surviving children, the hepatic and haematological features of the disease usually resolve, the illness then being manifest by epileptic seizures and mental retardation. Deafness is common and chorioretinitis may result in blindness. Only some 15 per cent of survivors of cytomegalic inclusion body disease are normal later in childhood.

There may be microcephaly, microgyria, cerebellar polymicrogyria and, less frequently, hydrocephalus. There is widespread inflammation, particularly in the periventricular white matter; clusters of microglia and granulomas are also seen. Foci of necrosis that result in cyst formation and calcification are common. The key histological feature of cytomegalovirus infection is the presence of inclusions: they are generally round or oval, acidophilic intranuclear bodies measuring up to 15 μm in diameter and are separated from the nuclear membrane by an unstained clear halo. Inclusion bodies may be seen in ependymal cells, neurons and glia.

Rubella syndrome

The association between maternal rubella infection and cataract was first recognized in Australia in 1941. Since then additional congenital defects including deafness have been recognized. When the infection occurs before the 10th week of gestation spontaneous abortion may occur, and it is possible to grow the virus from the tissues of the affected fetus. After the 12th week the rate of abortion decreases, although if the pregnancy reaches term the baby may be stillborn, be born alive with congenital defects or may harbour the virus and exhibit the disease in infancy.

In clinically recognizable cases, the newborn is 'small for dates' and may have signs of early cataracts, micro-ophthalmia, deafness, micro-cephaly, chorioretinitis and malformations of the heart. Some neonates may also show signs and symptoms of meningoencephalitis, thrombo-cytopenia, hepatosplenomegaly with jaundice, pneumonitis and lymphadenopathy. Yet other neonates may appear normal at birth only to develop encephalitis or interstitial pneumonitis and a chronic rubelliform rash when several months of age. Congenital rubella is typically a multisystem disorder, although sensorineural deafness and pigmentary retinitis are the most common manifestations of the condition.

Once the virus has crossed the placenta, there is no method by which the infection can be cleared or its course modified. Immunity produced by the wild virus is more long-lasting than that produced by the vaccine virus. Because the virus crosses the placenta, immunization programmes require that the subject is not pregnant and does not become pregnant for several months afterwards.

Pathology

The brain may be small and have a simplified gyral pattern. There may be hydrocephalus. Histologically, there is a subacute/chronic meningoencephalitis and calcification. Foci of necrosis are seen, some of which appear to be due to a vasculitis possibly induced by immune mechanisms. Cyst formation results.

In addition to the obvious changes associated with inflammation, a wide variety of malformations have been described but it is not clear whether there is a definite relationship between these and maternal rubella.

Rarely, either in infancy or in adolescence, patients with recognizable stigmata of the congenital rubella syndrome may develop a slowly progressive panencephalitis, similar to the subacute sclerosing panencephalitis that may follow infection with measles (see Ch. 7).

Sudden infant death syndrome (cot death)

Children between the ages of 1 and 4 months are particularly at risk, death occurring quietly during sleep, due to a fatal apnoeic episode. The cause is not known, but pathological findings include changes in the lungs and evidence of hypoxic–ischaemic damage in the brain.

FURTHER READING

Crome L & Stern J (1972) *Pathology of Mental Retardation.* Edinburgh: Churchill Livingstone.
Friede R L (1989) *Developmental Neuropathology*, 2nd edn. Vienna: Springer-Verlag.
Johnson R T (1982) *Viral Infections of the Nervous System.* New York: Raven Press.
Larroche J C (1977) *Developmental Pathology of the Neonate.* Amsterdam: Excerpta Medica.
Hanshaw J B, Dudgeon J A & Marshall W C (1985) *Viral Diseases of the Fetus and Newborn*, 2nd edn. Philadelphia: Saunders.
Lenire R J, Loeser J D, Leech R W et al (1975) *Normal and Abnormal Development of the Human Nervous System.* Hagerstown, MD: Harper and Row.
McKusick V A (1988) *Mendelian Inheritance in Man: Catalogue of Autosomal Dominant, Autosomal Recessive, and X-Linked Phenotypes*, 8th edn. Baltimore: Johns Hopkins Press.

Norman M G (1978) Perinatal brain damage. In: *Perspectives in Perinatal Pathology*, Vol. 4. Edited by H S Rosenberg and R P Bolande. Chicago: Year Book Medical Publishers, pp. 41–92.
Pape K E & Wigglesworth J S (1979) *Haemorrhage, Ischaemia and the Perinatal Brain.* London: Heinemann Medical Books.
Remington J S & Klein J O (1976) *Infectious Disease of the Fetus and Newborn Infants.* Philadelphia: Saunders.
Rorke L B (1982) *Pathology of Perinatal Brain Injury.* New York: Raven Press.
Rorke L B & Younkin D (eds) (1992) Perinatal hypoxic–ischemic brain injury. *Brain Pathology* 2, 209–251.
Winter R M, Knowles S A S, Bieber F R & Baraitser M (1988) *The Malformed Fetus and Stillbirth: A Diagnostic Approach.* Chichester: John Wiley.

14. Ageing and the dementias

Ageing is a physiological process and although there may be structural alterations in the brain, there is not necessarily any intellectual impairment. Dementia, on the other hand, is 'an acquired global impairment of intellect, reason and personality but without impairment of consciousness'. Why these two subjects are dealt with together is because the commonest type of dementia is dementia of Alzheimer type, which is in many ways like an acceleration of the ageing process. In addition to the named types of dementia described in this chapter, and other named types of dementia referred to in other chapters, such as Creutzfeldt–Jakob disease (see Ch. 7), parkinsonism and the parkinsonian–dementia complex of Guam (see Ch. 12), and the multiple system atrophies (see Ch. 12), some degree of dementia is common in any disease process that causes widespread damage to the brain.

AGEING OF THE BRAIN

MACROSCOPIC APPEARANCES

At post mortem the dura, which is often very densely adherent to the calvaria, is slack because of a reduction in the size of the brain. With increasing years, and particularly over the age of 60, there is often thickening of the leptomeninges which, at the vertex, may acquire a distinctly gelatinous appearance often associated with prominence of the arachnoid granulations.

Atrophy of the brain is commonly present over the age of 60 years, but is not an invariable accompaniment of the ageing process. When present, however, there is narrowing of gyri and widening of sulci, particularly at the vertex in relation to the frontal and parietal lobes in which areas there is also an excessive amount of cerebrospinal fluid.

The weight and volume of the normal brain are maximum between the ages of 15 and 60 years; thereafter there is a slow atrophy, occurring earlier in women than in men. An assessment of the amount of atrophy can be gauged from the ratio of brain to skull volume, which remains constant at about 95 per cent up to the age of 60. Thereafter, even in intellectually normal subjects, although there is some variation, this ratio may fall to 80 per cent by the tenth decade.

The adult brain weighs between 1200 and 1600 g, with an average of 1400 g in men and 1250 g in women. The weight remains constant throughout middle age but after the age of 65 years it begins to decline, the mean loss being about 100 g. As the intracranial volume is not routinely measured post mortem, considerable reliance is placed upon the weight of the brain at autopsy as an index of cerebral atrophy. It should, however, be noted that both weight and volume increase by some 10 per cent during fixation in 10 per cent formol saline over a 2–3 week period. A useful index as to whether or not a brain is atrophied is to measure the ratio between the weight of the whole fixed brain and that of the whole fixed hindbrain, the former usually being between eight and ten times greater than the latter. In general, the cerebellum tends to be well preserved with increasing years.

Neuroimaging of the ageing brain has shown widening of sulci and some enlargement of the ventricular system. Hydrocephalus, however, is not a consistent finding. Sometimes in a small brain the ventricles maintain their normal relative proportions, whereas in other cases the brain is not much reduced in size, yet the ventricles are enlarged. This is one of the reasons why it is not possible to make a confident diagnosis of normal pressure hydrocephalus post mortem. In general, however, the volumes of the lateral and third ventricles increase progressively with age, starting from a mean of 15 ml in teenagers to 55 ml in individuals over the age of 60 years.

MICROSCOPIC APPEARANCES

Studies have suggested that there may be some diffuse loss of neurons from the cerebral cortex. Except in cases of marked atrophy the assessment of neuronal loss is difficult because it varies in the same region in different individuals. With the development of computerized image analysers, it has now been shown and generally accepted that normal ageing affects the frontal and temporal lobes more than the parietal lobes; there is considerable shrinkage of large neurons, with a consequent increase in the number of small neurons, and the constant neuronal density associated with diminished cortical volume indicates that some neuronal loss occurs with age, but the magnitude of this loss is much less than has been recorded previously. Particular attention has been devoted to the subcortical structures, one area of particular interest being the basal nucleus of Meynert, which is the main source of cholinergic fibres to the cortical mantle. Although some studies have shown a steady decline with age, others have shown that neuronal loss is minimal in adult life.

The hindbrain is not exempt from changes, there being some loss of Purkinje cells. In individuals over the age of 60 counts of motor neurons in the spinal cord and in most motor cranial nerve nuclei are normal, whereas in others, including the locus ceruleus, the main supply of cortical noradrenergic fibres, loss has been recorded. Loss of function may be due not only to neuronal loss but also to atrophy of the soma and the dendritic tree, as well as loss of synapses. Special staining techniques, including the use of the Golgi–Cox method, have shown that plasticity occurs in response to the normal ageing process and that, in particular, it is possible for pyramidal neurons of layer 2 of the parahippocampal gyrus to undergo considerable dendritic growth in response to loss of adjacent neurons.

Lipofuscin is a type of lysosome in which non-metabolizable substrates accumulate: it stains red with Sudan dyes and is PAS-positive. It is a normal organelle and is particularly conspicuous in certain neurons, such as those in the inferior olivary nuclei and in the ventral horns of the spinal cord. The amount of lipofuscin increases with advancing age in the hippocampus and in the various motor and basal nuclei of the brain stem, in the neocortex and in the cerebellum. There is no known relationship, however, between the amount of lipofuscin and neuronal loss, because loss of neurons with increasing age is also common in sites where lipofuscin is slight.

The amount of neuromelanin in the substantia nigra and in the pigmented nuclei of the pons decreases with advancing years, with up to a 50 per cent loss of pigmented neurons as part of the ageing process. The loss appears to be greatest in those neurons containing the most pigment, but whether or not the accumulation of pigment is directly associated with the changes that presage cell death is not clear.

Neuritic (senile) plaques

Known also as *dendritic or amyloid plaques*, these names emphasize the two most striking components of the many plaques found in the brain in ageing, since most consist principally of a central core of amyloid-like material enveloped by swollen abnormal neurites. Their appearances differ depending upon the staining method used. For example, there is difficulty in seeing them in H & E-stained preparations, but they are easily seen in either frozen or paraffin-embedded sections using silver impregnation techniques. The amyloid component of these plaques can be seen readily by Congo red or thioflavin S. More recently, immunohistochemical staining for βA4 amyloid protein has been used. The classic neuritic plaque measures between 5 and 20μm in diameter, and in a silver-stained preparation consists of a dark central core surrounded by an irregular clear halo composed of granular, filamentous or rod-like structures which, like the core, are argyrophilic (Fig. 14.1). The size and configuration vary

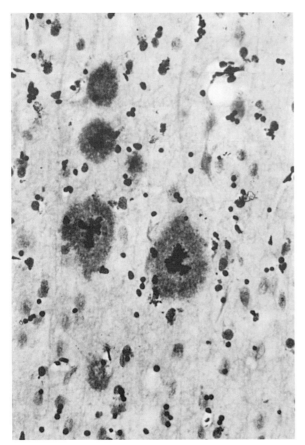

Fig. 14.1 Neuritic (senile) plaque. The plaques are granular and filamentous, and some have dense cores. (King's silver method for amyloid.)

depending on the state of development of the plaque and the plane of section. Plaques are commonly discrete, whereas in other areas they appear to fuse together into large irregular-shaped structures. Ultrastructural studies have shown that the central core is composed of amyloid fibrils which stain positively with Congo red, whereas the outer rim consists of a mixture of abnormal distended neuritic processes intermingled with astrocytes and microglia. Three stages in the light-microscopical appearances of neuritic plaques have been described. In the earliest stage, a *primitive plaque* consists of abnormal neurites intermingled with fibre-forming astrocytes and microglial cells. The second stage is the mature (*classic*) plaque, which shows all the typical features of the central core of amyloid, abnormal neurites, microglia and astrocytes. The last stage,

which is the *burnt-out plaque*, is composed mainly of amyloid. Recently another form of plaque has been described in which there is a diffuse deposition of amyloid unassociated with the central compacted amyloid or abnormal neurites. These lesions have been called *diffuse plaques*, (preamyloid deposits, senile plaque-like structures and diffuse senile plaques). This type of plaque is commonly found throughout the cortical mantle, occurring among other discrete classic plaques; they are also found, however, in areas of the brain where classic plaques are few, such as the brain stem and cerebellum. Such plaques have also been found in the 'punch drunk' syndrome following head injury. The relationship between this diffuse type of plaque and classic plaques is not clear.

Quantitative studies have demonstrated increasing numbers of neuritic plaques in the brains of normal individuals aged 50 years or more. In intellectually intact individuals plaques develop most often and in the largest numbers in the amygdala, but not all individuals accumulate plaques, even those living beyond their 90th birthday. From these and other studies has come the appreciation that the number of plaques found in individual brains of intellectually normal subjects also increases with increasing age. As a rule of thumb, it is unusual to find other than occasional plaques in a microscope field of 1.4 mm^2 in subjects up to the age of 60 years. Thereafter, counts of between four and five per field may be found, and between the ages of 70 and 80, counts of up to 10 per field may be found in some 10 per cent of normal subjects. Quantitative studies must, therefore, make allowance for the presence of an age-related number of neuritic plaques, and these should be taken into account when making a diagnosis of Alzheimer's disease.

Alzheimer's neurofibrillary degeneration

This change is difficult to see in H & E-stained sections, although various silver impregnation techniques will readily identify them and, more recently, antibodies to the various constituents of the tangle have been employed. Congo red stains tangles a deep pink colour and at the same time renders them birefringent under polarized light.

By light microscopy the configuration of the tangles is largely determined by the site and type of the neuron affected. Thus, in the small pyramidal neurons of the cerebral cortex, tangles are seen to extend from the base of the cell towards the apical dendrite (see Fig. 3.19). More complex forms develop in larger pyramidal cells, many resembling a skein of wool whereas tangles in the hippocampus may have a more complex configuration. Ultrastructural studies have shown that neurofibrillary tangles are made up of filaments that measure 20 nm across with a regular constriction of 10 nm occurring every 18 nm. Although originally thought to be twisted tubules, later studies have shown that these appearances are due to paired filaments wound in a double helix. Paired helical filaments are derived from components of the normal neuronal cytoskeleton, containing not only sequences from neurofilaments and microtubular associated proteins but also antigenic determinants which are unique to them. Current evidence suggests that the abnormal phosphorylation of the tau protein could play an important role in tangle formation.

In the normal ageing process neurofibrillary tangles are uncommon in non-demented subjects. They occur in the greatest numbers in the corticomedial portion of the amygdaloid nucleus and in the cortex of the anteromedial part of the temporal lobe; although their number increases with age, numerous tangles may be present in the anteromedial part of the temporal lobes in intellectually normal old people. It is unusual to find them to any great extent in the neocortex of normal old age.

The nature and origin of the tangles remains unclear, although it has been suggested that they contain the same proteins as the amyloid of blood vessels and plaques, despite the fact that ultrastructurally the neurofibrillary tangle does not resemble amyloid fibrils. Immunohistochemical studies, on the other hand, indicate that tangles share antigenic determinants with neurofilaments, with microtubules and tau protein. These studies tend to suggest that neurofibrillary tangles form as a result of a defective assembly of microtubules and/or neurofilaments which result from abnormal phosphorylation of tau or neurofilaments.

Granulovacuolar degeneration

This change is largely restricted to the pyramidal cells of the CA1 sector of the hippocampus. It consists of one or more intracytoplasmic vacuoles measuring some 3–5 μm in diameter, each containing a central granule between 1 and 2 μm in diameter (see Fig. 3.20). Multiple vacuoles are common, when they may displace the nucleus and normal cytoplasmic organelles; they occur occasionally in association with neurofibrillary tangles. They are easily seen in H & E-stained sections but are strikingly obvious in silver-stained preparations. Electron microscopy shows a dense granular core embedded in a translucent matrix, which appears to be separated from the rest of the cytoplasm.

Quantitative studies have shown that granulovacuolar degeneration is uncommon below the age of 65 years, but its frequency increases even in non-demented subjects to the extent that it is present in some 75 per cent by the ninth decade. The number of pyramidal cells showing this change increases to some 20 per cent in dements. Immunohistochemical techniques have shown that granulovacuolar degeneration contains phosphorylated epitopes, neurofibrillary tangles, neurofilaments and tau proteins, and variable staining for ubiquitin has been reported.

Hirano bodies

These ovoid eosinophilic structures measuring between 10 and 30 μm in length and 8 μm across may be seen easily in H & E-stained sections, although often they may be mistaken for columns of red cells (Fig. 3.21). They are present most commonly in the pyramidal cells of the hippocampus, where they are found with increasing prevalence in intellectually normal subjects: up to middle age only an occasional body is seen but late in life they are numerous. Ultrastructurally they are made up of parallel filaments 60–100 μm in length which alternate with longish sheet-like material. Immunohistochemistry has shown that Hirano bodies share epitopes with the actin-associated protein, and that a small proportion of the bodies also react with antibodies to tau protein and, therefore, probably derive from abnormal organization of neuronal cytoplasm.

VASCULAR CHANGES

Vascular changes are commonly found in the ageing brain. The incidence of stroke, for example, rises rapidly with increasing age: some 80 per cent occur in patients over the age of 65 years.

Atheroma

The amount of atheroma increases with increasing age but in the absence of hypertension does not usually affect blood vessels less than 2 mm in diameter, such as those supplying the basal ganglia and pons.

Hyaline arteriosclerosis

Although accelerated in hypertension similar changes occur in the elderly, comprising fibrous replacement of muscle whereas elastic tissue may break up and undergo partial absorption. The arterial walls are thickened and more rigid, lumina are dilated and the vessels become longer and tortuous. In blood vessels of 1 mm or less in diameter, in addition to hypertrophy of the media, the intima becomes thickened by a concentric increase in connective tissue. In the smallest arteries intimal change predominates and may result in narrowing of the lumen. In contrast to the dilatation seen in the larger arteries there may be hyaline thickening of arterioles (hyaline arteriosclerosis or lipohyalinosis), which gradually extends over the whole circumference and, when severe, replaces all structures except the endothelium.

Lacunae

These are cavities measuring from 3 to 20 mm in diameter, occurring principally within the diencephalon and the brain stem. Lacunae of small diameter are commonly seen in the basal ganglia in the ageing brain. Although some 90 per cent of lacunae are associated with hypertension, they may be found in some 9 per cent of normotensive subjects. They consist of expanded perivascular spaces with disintegration of the parenchyma and, around the blood vessel, the cavity contains very few cells and is limited by a narrow border of astrocytes. The term 'etat lacunaire' is used when the cavities are numerous in grey matter and 'etat crible' when similar cavities are numerous in the centrum semi-ovale and other richly myelinated regions. It has been suggested that 'lacunae are the result of spiralled elongations of small intracerebral arteries under the effects of raised blood pressure'. On the other hand, lacunae have been attributed to occlusive vascular disease: the smaller lesions appear to be due to lipohyalinosis and the larger to atheroma or emboli.

Microaneurysms

Miliary aneurysms have been demonstrated using radiological techniques following the injection of opaque material into the cerebral arteries in both hypertensive and normotensive patients post mortem. These microaneurysms occur on small arteries 100–300 μm in diameter and are seen as outpouchings of the vessel wall. Such aneurysms are uncommon under the age of 50 years, and they occur most commonly in the brains of hypertensive patients. Some miliary aneurysms have, however, been found in the brains of normotensive patients but not to the same extent as in elderly subjects.

Infarction and leukoaraiosis

Small infarcts are a common finding in the brains of elderly and non-demented subjects. In many instances they are found at autopsy as incidental findings and appear not to have been associated with clinical signs or symptoms, and particularly without any loss of or deterioration in higher mental functions. These lesions are small and are most commonly found in the basal ganglia and brain stem. If the infarcts are larger they may be the cause of the entity known as multi-infarct dementia, which is responsible for some 15 per cent of cases of dementia over the age of 65 years. They may also contribute to a further 10 per cent of cases of dementia in association with Alzheimer's disease.

The term leukoaraiosis is used to describe the changes in rarefied periventricular white matter seen on CT scans in both demented and elderly normal subjects. The changes are usually symmetrical and appear histologically as hyaline arteriosclerosis of blood vessels, astrocytosis and partial loss of myelinated axons and oligodendroglial cells. The appearances are thought to represent partial infarction confined to white matter, and vascular disease possible due to hypoperfusion because it occurs independently of grey matter and may be the only cerebral lesion in subjects without Alzheimer's disease.

Congophilic angiopathy

In this condition amyloid-like material is deposited in the small blood vessels of the meninges and cerebral cortex, and stains brightly and uniformly eosinphilic with H & E. If the complete circumference of the vessel is involved the arteriole appears as a thickened homogeneous tube which thus becomes congophilic when stained with Congo red: such staining also makes it birefringement in polarized light. Amyloid angiopathy is uncommon in normal individuals below the age of 60 years, the prevalence thereafter rising to about 30 per cent. The cortex of the parietal and occipital lobes is more comploy affected than that of the frontal or temporal regions. Rarely is there involvement of the brain stem. Although these vascular abnormalities are usually mild in normal old age, they are much more frequent in cases of Alzheimer's disease and in long-surviving cases of Down's syndrome.

Ultrastructurally the features are those of typical amyloid fibrils, which tend to accumulate first in the basal laminae and in the pericytes. The nature and origin of this vascular amyloid and its relationship to the amyloid found in the core of neuritic plaques remains uncertain.

In congophilic angiopathy, which may or may not be associated with Alzheimer's disease, many small blood vessels are affected. A not-infrequent complication is spontaneous intracerebral haemorrhage in any part of the brain. Thus in any elderly patient with an intracerebral haematoma

in an atypical site the possibility of congophilic angiopathy should be considered.

OTHER CHANGES

Other features are a subpial and subependymal astrocytosis and the occurrence of numerous corpora amylacea throughout the CNS, particularly immediately deep to the ependyma and throughout the spinal cord. Commonly, there are deposits of calcium in the walls of small blood vessels in the basal ganglia (Fig. 14.2), this material also staining positively with Perl's Prussian blue reaction.

THE DEMENTIAS

The generally accepted psychiatric definition of dementia is an acquired global impairment of intellect, memory and personality, without impairment of consciousness. There are many causes of

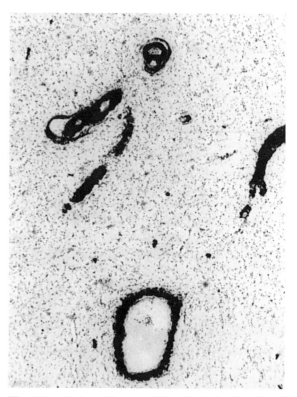

Fig. 14.2 Ageing of the brain. There is calcification of small blood vessels in deep grey matter. (Celloidin; cresyl violet.)

dementia but they must be distinguished from other causes of confusion and disorientation. In the elderly, dementia may be due to primary degeneration of either the cerebral cortex, such as in Alzheimer's disease, Pick's disease or diffuse cortical Lewy body disease, or of subcortical structures such as in Parkinson's disease, multisystem atrophy, Huntington's disease and progressive supranuclear palsy. Other causes are secondary to disease processes such as infection or inflammation, as in neurosyphilis, limbic encephalitis, multifocal leukoencephalopathy, Creutzfeldt–Jakob disease or AIDS (HIV infection), or to neurotoxins or metabolic disorders such as alcohol, hypothyroidism, hypoglycaemia, anticonvulsant drugs and barbiturates, neuroleptics or chronic uraemia associated with dialysis. Yet other causes are cerebral tumours and associated hydrocephalus, as occurs with gliomas or metastases, traumatic brain injury, e.g. diffuse axonal injury, subdural haematomas or dementia pugilistica, or vascular disease e.g. stroke, following subarachnoid haemorrhage.

It has been estimated that in developed countries some 10–15 per cent of the population over the age of 65 develop some degree of dementia, and that between 75 and 95 per cent of these cases are likely to be due to Alzheimer's disease or vascular disease, singly or in combination.

ALZHEIMER'S DISEASE

The term Alzheimer's disease was originally applied to presenile dementia occurring in patients under 60 years old, whereas the term senile dementia of Alzheimer type was applied to the over-60s. In pathological terms it is now realized that this is an artificial distinction, because the structural abnormalities are the same in all ages. Alzheimer's disease is by far the most common cause of dementia: it is an illness which usually lasts for an average of about 5 years, is more common in females than in males and the younger the age of onset the more aggressive seems to be the course of the illness.

STRUCTURAL ABNORMALITIES

On removing the calvaria the leptomeninges at the vertex are usually found to be rather thickened and opaque. The brain is atrophied, usually weighing 1000 g or less; the atrophy is accentuated in the frontal and temporal lobes. In the majority of cases there is little atheroma of the large cerebral blood vessels. Coronal sections of the brain show that the atrophy is global, although there tends to be relatively severe involvement of the insulae and the medial parts of the temporal lobes (Fig. 14.3). There is usually a reduction in the bulk of the white matter and generalized enlargement of the ventricular system. With the advent of *in vivo* techniques for brain morphometry, including MRI and CT scanning, it is now possible to define the distribution of the atrophy and to relate changes to functional mapping, as shown in SPECT and PET studies. The most characteristic pattern is reduced metabolic activity and blood flow in the temporal and frontal areas in which there is the greatest atrophy and the largest numbers of neuritic plaques and neurofibrillary tangles. Such studies have also provided evidence for involvement of the parietal lobe in cases of early onset of Alzheimer's disease.

Histological appearances

The most striking feature in the cortical ribbon in Alzheimer's disease is the presence of large numbers

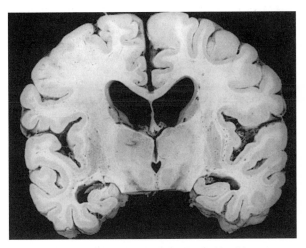

Fig. 14.3 Alzheimer's disease. There is considerable atrophy, particularly of the temporal lobes including the hippocampi, and enlargement of the lateral ventricles.

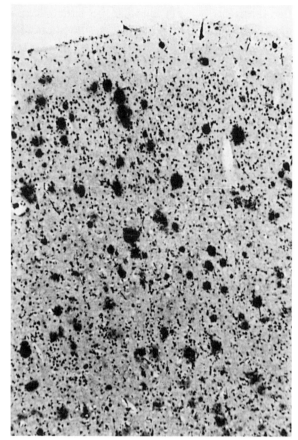

Fig. 14.4 Alzheimer's disease. There are many argyrophilic senile plaques in the cerebral cortex. (King's silver method for amyloid.)

of *neuritic plaques* (Fig. 14.4). As already discussed above, some neuritic plaques are frequently seen in the cortical ribbon in normal old age, but in cases of Alzheimer's disease their numbers far exceed those that would be expected for age- and sex-matched controls. Indeed, a number of studies have shown a significant relationship between the number of neuritic plaques and the severity of dementia. Neuritic plaques are found in greatest numbers in the medial parts of the temporal lobes, including the amygdaloid nuclei and their association areas, with relative sparing of the primary motor and sensory somatic cortical areas. Although neuritic plaques may be found in all layers of the cortex they are particularly common in the second and third layers; they are also present in subcortical grey matter, although not in the same numbers as in the

cortex, affected areas including the hypothalamus, the tegmentum of the upper brain stem and, to a lesser extent, the molecular layer of the cerebellar cortex.

A further feature is the presence of large numbers of *neurofibrillary tangles* throughout the neocortex, although again with relative sparing of the primary somatic and sensory areas. Large numbers of tangles are present in the hippocampi, in the amygdaloid nuclei, in the basal nucleus of Meynert and in the upper brain stem, the numbers being significantly different from age- and sex-matched controls. Quantitative studies have shown a closer relationship between the severity of the dementia and the numbers of neurofibrillary tangles than with neuritic plaques.

Granulovacuolar degeneration and *Hirano bodies* are also the rule. Another feature which is often quite marked is vacuolation of the subpial layers of the cortex, particularly in the temporal and parietal lobes. This spongy state is usually associated with neuronal loss, features that bear some resemblance to the status spongiosis of Creutzfeldt–Jakob disease.

The question of loss of neurons remains somewhat controversial, since many of the initial studies showed no statistical difference in cortical neuronal counts between age- and sex-matched controls and patients with Alzheimer's disease. However, subsequent studies which have addressed the issues of both cortical shrinkage and neuronal loss have shown that there is indeed loss of large pyramidal neurons in the frontal and temporal lobes, with much less involvement of the parietal and occipital lobes. Quantitative studies have also demonstrated considerable neuronal loss in the basal nucleus of Meynert and in the locus ceruleus. Although there are large variations in the overall counts between individual cases, it is now appreciated that between 40 and 70 per cent of the neuronal population of the basal nucleus of Meynert may be lost. This raises the possibility that degeneration of the neurons within this basal nucleus might be primary, the neocortical changes being secondary to the subcortical loss. It is, however, now accepted that the changes in the cortical mantle are far greater than can be accounted for by changes in the basal nucleus of Meynert, and that in all probability the latter are retrograde to what is otherwise a primary disease process of the cortical ribbon.

Other changes include loss of synapses, and various morphological changes in axons and dendrites that can be identified in Golgi-stained preparations. There is often an associated astrocytosis. Amyloid angiopathy occurs in over 80 per cent of patients with Alzheimer's disease. Amyloid is also deposited in the centre of neuritic plaques, and is made up of a polypeptide with a molecular weight of about 4000. It is termed A4 and is now known to be similar to if not identical to the amyloid deposited in the pia in cortical arteries in about 10 per cent of individuals over the age of 70 years. This amyloid lies external to the elastic lamina, stains pink with eosin and Congo red and is dichroic.

Pathogenesis

It has been suspected for many years that there are many and diverse factors of a both environmental and genetic nature that predispose to the onset of Alzheimer's disease.

Approximately 20 per cent of cases of Alzheimer's disease are thought to be familial, with almost 5 per cent exhibiting an autosomal dominant pattern of inheritance. Screening of the amyloid precursor protein (βAPP) gene and chromosome 21, which gives rise to the β amyloid protein found in neuritic plaques and in the amyloid of congophilic vessels, has revealed a single amino acid mutation in some families with Alzheimer's disease. However, not all families where the disease is of early onset have this mutation, and linkage analysis indicates that other genes, possibly on chromosomes other than 21, are also involved. Thus only a minor proportion of cases of Alzheimer's disease are thought to be related directly to gene abnormalities. Another genetically determined cause of Alzheimer's disease is that due to a partial duplication of chromosome 21.

Given that no more than about 20 per cent of all cases of Alzheimer's disease can be accounted for either by familial forms or Down's syndrome, it therefore follows that in by far the majority of cases of Alzheimer's disease the aetiology remains unknown. It is, however, now thought that a large proportion of the remaining cases are due to environmental factors, or to an interaction between genetic and environmental factors. Possible environmental factors include acute infections, alcoholism and intoxication with a number of agents such as aluminium and neurotoxic amino acids. Epidemiological studies have confirmed that there is a significant association between head injury and Alzheimer's disease, from the results of which it has been variously estimated that head injury plays a role in between 3 and 5 per cent of cases of Alzheimer's disease. The first indication that there is such an association came from detailed neuropathological studies of dementia pugilistica (see Ch. 8). Initial studies showed a cavum septum lucidum, neuronal loss, scarring of the cerebellum and marked neurofibrillary tangle formation, but an apparent absence of neuritic plaques as shown by conventional silver and Congo red stains. However, recent work has shown that, in dementia pugilistica, following treatment of tissue with formic acid using antibodies raised to βA4 amyloid protein, there are large numbers of diffuse plaques which are immunologically indistinguishable from those seen in cases of Alzheimer's disease. Further, cliniconeuropathological experience has confirmed that in up to 30 per cent of patients surviving severe head injury there are large numbers of diffuse βA4 protein plaques, and it would therefore seem that injury to the brain can trigger the deposition of βA4 protein in susceptible individuals which, under certain circumstances, may culminate in the development of the process of Alzheimer's disease. From these and experimental studies, including the use of transgenic mice, it would now seem that the induction of β amyloid precursor protein 751/770 in the brain is a normal response to neuronal stress, and is analagous to the induction of stress proteins (namely heat shock, ubiquitin). The basis of the susceptibility to the induction of Alzheimer's disease is, however, not known, although it seems reasonable to suppose that its molecular roots lie in some common polymorphism of the controlling elements of the β amyloid precursor protein gene which causes overexpression of the β amyloid precursor protein 751 transcript or its processing enzymes.

Relationship between neuritic plaques and neurofibrillary tangles

This remains of considerable interest, as a better understanding of the relationship between them might reveal clues as to whether they are causally related or are independent features of a common pathogenetic process. It has been known for many years that there are a number of diseases characterized by the presence of many neuro-fibrillary tangles in the absence of neuritic plaques, e.g. the parkinsonism–dementia syndrome of Guam, progressive supranuclear palsy and post-encephalitic parkinsonism. It has now, however, been established by immunohistochemical tech-niques using antibodies to βA4 amyloid protein, that plaques may be present in some of these conditions. The tangles are usually ubiquitinated and are now considered to be the means by which neurons try to remove abnormal phosphorylated proteins. There is, therefore, diminishing evi-dence that neuritic plaques are secondary to the formation of neurofibrillary tangles. Indeed, the emphasis has now changed with the recognition of the importance of βA4 amyloid protein and its precursor amyloid protein. Recent immunohisto-chemical studies, including those on transgenic mice, suggest that, whatever the cause of Alzheimer's disease, the abnormal metabolism of β amyloid precursor protein and the subsequent deposition of βA4 is the critical and central event in the pathogenesis and evolution of Alzheimer's disease. If this is indeed the sequence of events, then it would seem likely that neurofibrillary tangles are a consequence of the 'toxic' effects of the βA4 amyloid protein.

Changes in neurotransmitters and neuropeptides in Alzheimer's disease

Alzheimer's disease is associated with a distur-bance of many neurotransmitter systems, none of which in isolation satisfactorily accounts for either the symptomatology or the nature and distri-bution of the neuropathological changes. It is known, however, that a major biochemical abnormality in Alzheimer's disease is a 70–90 per cent deficiency of choline acetyltransferase, the synthesizing enzyme of acetylcholine, and that

acetylcholine in the neocortex, the hippocampal formation and the basal nucleus of Meynert is reduced. The degree of this reduction gives rise to the *cholinergic hypothesis*, the basis of which is that, since the cholinergic innervation of the neocortex originates mainly from the basal nucleus of Meynert, it is the atrophy of this subcortical structure that plays a crucial role in the genesis of Alzheimer's disease. Recent work, however, has challenged this rather simple concept, there now being good evidence that the abnormalities affect both pre- and postsynaptic sites and that the changes in the basal nucleus of Meynert are secondary to changes in the cortex. Furthermore, deficits have now been described in noradrenergic and serotinergic systems, and abnormalities have also been described in various neuropeptides, such as somatostatin. The increasing use of immunohistochemistry, however, has shown mul-tiple deficits none of which can fully account for the condition.

DOWN'S SYNDROME

Careful comparisons between age- and sex-matched controls and patients with Down's syndrome have clearly established that the patho-logical changes in the 45 per cent of cases of Down's syndrome that become demented in early middle age are identical to those found in cases of Alzheimer's disease (see Ch. 13). Fur-thermore, the distribution of the changes is similar, lesions starting in the medial parts of each temporal lobe before 'spreading out' into the asso-ciation neocortex and subcortical structures.

PICK'S DISEASE

The clinical separation of dementia of Alzheimer type and Pick's disease, a much less common disease, is difficult. Pick's disease is rare and may occur at any age from 21 to 90, although the peak incidence occurs at about the age of 60. The condition is slightly more common in women (5:4). Although most cases are sporadic, familial examples are known to occur, in which circumstances the disease is most likely to be transmitted by a dominant gene.

The presentation usually starts with changes of character and behaviour, which are attributable to damage to the frontal lobes. These are followed by insidious blunting of cognitive function and the patient may eventually become dysphasic, dyslexic and dyspraxic. The disease progresses slowly to severe dementia, death occurring usually between 5 and 10 years after onset. *In vivo* neuroimaging studies have confirmed the selective atrophy of the frontal and temporal lobes, with associated ventricular enlargement, and functional studies using PET have shown profound hypometabolism in the affected atrophic areas.

Pathology

There is selectively severe atrophy of the anterior parts of the temporal lobes (Fig. 14.5) and of the frontal lobes. The brain weighs 1000 g or less, and there are greatly narrowed gyri the crests of which are atrophied and yellowish-brown in colour, accounting for the so-called 'walnut' appearance. In the temporal lobes the poles are always affected, with the atrophy extending posteriorly towards the temporal gyri with relative sparing of the posterior two-thirds of the superior temporal gyri: this is in marked contrast to severe atrophy of the remaining temporal gyri and the medial parts of the temporal lobe, accounting for the gross description of the 'knife-blade' appearance. Often there is also involvement of the under aspects of the frontal lobes, including the medial orbital gyri and less commonly the convexity of the frontal lobes. There is associated ventricular enlargement and there may also be involvement of the caudate nucleus resembling that seen in Huntington's disease. In contrast, the hindbrain is normal.

The histological changes consist chiefly of neuronal loss in the outer layers of the affected cortex, accompanied by astrocytosis and pallor of staining of the subcortical myelin. In many, but not all cases there is a distinct type of change in neuronal perikarya, which become distended, the cytoplasm being eosinophilic and the nucleus eccentric. These are referred to as Pick's cells (Fig. 14.6). The most marked changes are in the large pyramidal cells of the neocortex, but they may also be quite striking in the basal ganglia, in the locus ceruleus and in the substantia nigra. Although these bodies may be identified by silver impregnation techniques, the advent of immuno-

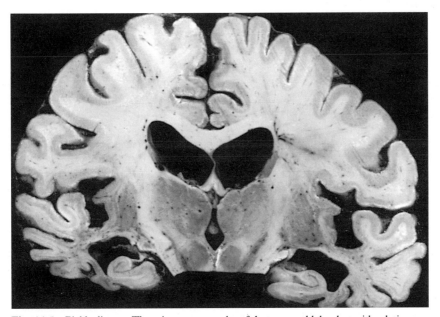

Fig. 14.5 Pick's disease. There is severe atrophy of the temporal lobes but with relative sparing of the superior temporal gyri. There is enlargement of the ventricles.

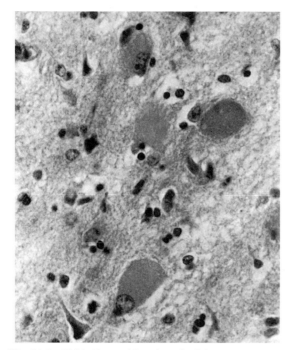

Fig. 14.6 Pick's disease. Note the pale globose neurons (Pick's cells). (H & E.)

histochemistry using antibodies to phosphorylated neurofilament epitopes makes their recognition easy. Ultrastructural studies have shown that Pick bodies are straight filaments, tubular profiles and paired helical filaments. The basis of the degenerative process is not known, but the similarities between Pick bodies and the tangles of Alzheimer's disease suggests that they may share a common molecular pathogenesis. Neuritic plaques are not prominent in Pick's disease, although occasional cases show the features of both Pick's and Alzheimer's disease. Neurochemical studies have not provided any clues to the pathogenesis of this disorder.

HUNTINGTON'S DISEASE

This is an autosomal dominant disorder in which the symptoms usually begin in the third or fourth decades. The incidence in Europe, North America and Australia is estimated at between 4 and 7 per 10 000 population. Recombinant DNA techniques have localized a genetic marker to the terminal band of the short arm of chromosome 4.

The disease typically starts as a tendency to fidget, which, over several months or years, develops into jerky choreic movements. During this time the patient may become truculent, irritable or apathetic. Where patients are aware of a family history suicide is common. The disease progresses with dementia, and death is usually from intercurrent infection.

Pathology

The brain is usually small and there may be some diffuse atrophy of the cerebral cortex. The most striking feature, however, is atrophy of the striatum. The head of the caudate nucleus, which normally bulges into the lateral ventricle, may shrink to a narrow brownish band of tissue and the putamen is also much reduced in size (Fig. 14.7). The head of the caudate nucleus, therefore, no longer bulges convexly into the lateral ventricle but becomes flattened or concave. The internal capsule may therefore appear prominent between the two atrophied parts of the striatum; the globus pallidus is also involved, but to a milder degree than in the putamen. Based on naked-eye and histological appearances, a grading system has been established, ranging in severity from 0 to 4, that correlates closely with the degree of clinical disability. In grade 0 the clinical abnormalities appear to precede morphological

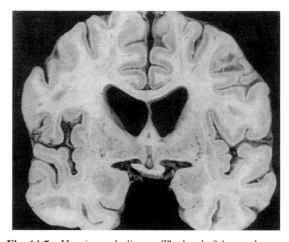

Fig. 14.7 Huntington's disease. The head of the caudate nucleus, instead of bulging into the floor of the ventricle, is reduced to a flattened narrow band of brownish tissue.

damage, in that there are no obvious neuropathological changes, whereas in grade 1 there may be loss of some 50 per cent of neurons in the caudate nucleus; in grade 4 this figure rises to 95 per cent. The earliest changes are seen in the medial paraventricular portion of the tail of the caudate nucleus and the dorsal part of the putamen, the most obvious histological changes being a preferential loss of small neurons in the striatum, with relative preservation of large neurons (Fig. 14.8a, b). The normal ratio of small to large neurons (160:1) is reduced to 40:1. The pattern of the abnormality suggests that there is involvement of a specific population of neurons. There is an apparent astrocytosis, although recent quantitative studies have suggested that this finding is spurious and that when the degree of atrophy is taken into account there is, in fact, a loss of astrocytes.

Morphometric studies have shown that the neocortex may be reduced in volume by about 15 per cent, neuronal loss being accentuated in layer 3. Such studies have shown that there appears to be some positive correlation between abnormal movements and striatal cell loss on the one hand, and between dementia and cortical cell loss on the other. Neuronal loss has been described in other subcortical structures, including the thalamus and hypothalamus.

Pathogenesis

Immunocytochemistry has revealed two principal types of neuron within the caudate nucleus and putamen – spiny and non-spiny. Spiny neurons comprise some 80 per cent of the total and account for most of the neuronal loss in Huntington's disease. These neurons contain γ-aminobutyric acid (GABA) and, together with the enzymes associated with it, such as glutamic acid decarboxylase, constitute the principal neurotransmitter system deficit in Huntington's disease.

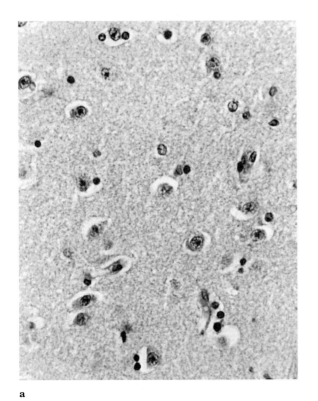

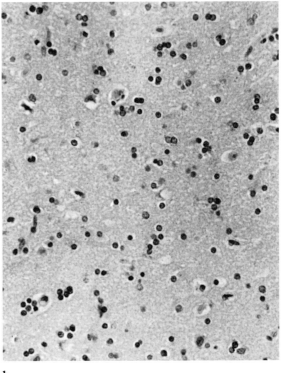

a   b

Fig. 14.8 Huntington's disease. (a) Normal caudate nucleus. (b) Caudate nucleus from a case of Huntington's disease. There is loss of neurons and an increase in astrocytes. (H & E (both same magnification).)

This is in contrast to the non-spiny neurons, which include the largest neurons of the caudate nucleus and putamen, which are relatively preserved, containing the neuropeptides somatostatin and neuropeptide Y. The vulnerability of spiny neurons in Huntington's disease may be related to the afferent glutamatergic innervation from the cortex. In support of this hypothesis is the observation that, when injected into the caudate nucleus and putamen of experimental animals, kainic acid, an analogue of glutamate, produces histological and biochemical abnormalities similar to those found in this disease.

DEMENTIA IN PARKINSON'S DISEASE

Although somewhat controversial, most recent studies have recorded that dementia occurs in between 30 and 40 per cent of patients with Parkinson's disease (see Ch. 12). Despite wide-ranging studies, any association between Parkinson's disease and Alzheimer's disease remains unproven, largely because of the use of different histological criteria for the diagnosis of Alzheimer's disease. Because of the prevalence of both disorders in the community, the occasional occurrence of Alzheimer's disease with Parkinson's disease is inevitable. The true incidence of the combined disorder will remain uncertain until such time as criteria for both diseases are agreed.

DEMENTIA IN PARKINSON'S DISEASE WITH CORTICAL LEWY BODIES

In the last 10 years an apparently new disorder, characterized by the finding of many Lewy bodies in the neocortex as well as in subcortical grey matter in dementing patients with Parkinson's disease, has been described.

Pathology

There may be some atrophy of the frontal and temporal lobes, with associated ventricular enlargement, and there is no obvious depigmentation of brain-stem nuclei. Histologically, there is neuronal loss and classic Lewy bodies are seen not only in subcortical structures but also throughout the neocortical ribbon. They can be difficult to distinguish from neurofibrillary tangles, even when using immunohistochemistry, as both are ubiquitin-positive.

DEMENTIA ASSOCIATED WITH PROGRESSIVE SUPRANUCLEAR PALSY

Starting usually between the 5th and 7th decades, this disease runs a progressive course over a 10-year period. The weight of the brain is usually normal, there being no evidence of frontal or temporal atrophy although there may be a degree of ventricular enlargement. Histologically the cortex of both the cerebral and cerebellar hemispheres is normal. The principal changes are neuronal loss and astrocytosis within the subthalamic nuclei and in the substantia nigra and superior colliculi. Residual neurons within these areas and elsewhere contain intracytoplasmic neurofibrillary tangles, which are usually made up of 15 nm straight filaments; occasionally, paired helical filaments are also seen.

OTHER PRIMARY CAUSES OF DEMENTIA

These include *progressive subcortical gliosis*, in which the most prominent histological feature is a pronounced subcortical gliosis without obvious involvement of the cerebral cortex and without any significant changes in myelin. Other causes include *thalamic dementia, dementia occurring in association with expressive dysphasia*, and *motor neuron disease*. A recently described syndrome is that of dementia of *frontal lobe type*, in which the symptoms suggest a frontal lobe disorder and yet there is a singular absence of the neuropathological changes of either Alzheimer's disease or Pick's disease.

DEMENTIA ASSOCIATED WITH VASCULAR DISEASE

For most practical purposes the term 'vascular dementia' implies *multi-infarct dementia*, but it is here extended to include dementias thought to be specifically associated with *chronic hypertension*, as well as entities such as *lacunar infarcts*. It may well be that these conditions are not separate, but represent a continuum based on a common vascular aetiology.

Infarcts are common in patients with dementia and may coexist with, say, Alzheimer's disease. For a number of reasons, however, chiefly based on the 'stepwise' progress of the illness, the presence of focal neurological signs and symptoms and the pattern of memory loss, the existence of 'multi-infarct' (arteriosclerotic) dementia is clinically recognizable. The presence of these features is often used to construct an 'ischaemic' score as a diagnostic aid to the differentiation of the vascular dementias. It is more common in men than in women, and is the second most common cause of dementia in the elderly, accounting for 10–20 per cent of cases aged over 65 years, and occurring in combined form with Alzheimer's disease in a further 10 per cent of cases.

Pathology

Multi-infarct dementia is essentially *ischaemic* in origin. Infarcts are numerous, although variable in size and site, and there may be compensatory ventricular enlargement. Both cerebral hemispheres are usually involved, but occasionally (fewer than 10 per cent of cases) there is only a single large infarct. In a minority of cases (about 20 per cent) there are small infarcts in the thalami and in the brain stem, especially in the pons. The cortex and basal ganglia in the distribution of the middle cerebral arteries are affected in nearly every case (Fig. 14.9a, b).

There appears to be an association between the dementia and the total volume of the infarcts rather than with their location. Thus, in most cases of multi-infarct dementia the volume of infarction is more than 50 ml, whereas if the volume is greater than 100 ml dementia is the rule. Dementia in cases with less than 50 ml infarction is probably due to a combination of infarction and Alzheimer's disease. Although hypertension is the most frequent cause, all the other principal causes of vascular disease may produce dementia (see Ch. 5).

Dementia in a patient with chronic hypertension may be associated with a peculiar pattern of ischaemic damage in the subcortical white matter. In such cases the cerebral cortex is relatively well preserved. This condition, which is often called *Binswanger's disease*, remains somewhat enigmatic since the relevant clinicopathological correlations are not always convincing. Post-mortem studies have shown a reduction in the volume of deep white matter, in which there are variably sized cysts and ventricular enlargement. Histologically there is patchy loss of myelin and axons, astrocytosis and widespread hyalinosis of small blood vessels. These changes probably represent

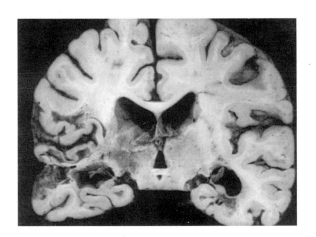

a

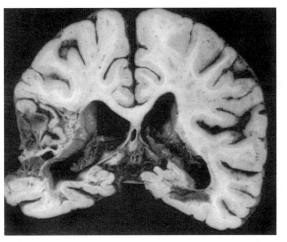

b

Fig. 14.9 Multi-infarct dementia. There are old infarcts in both cerebral hemispheres.

the severe end of a continuum in which the white matter changes occur in the presence of dementia. The other end of the spectrum is characterized by reduced density of periventricular white matter in elderly non-demented subjects. The latter has been referred to as *leukoaraiosis*, a term that is used to describe symmetrical incomplete ischaemia of deep white matter, and the histological features of which are similar to but less severe than those seen in Binswanger's disease.

The pathological basis of the periventricular changes is probably progressive narrowing of the lumina of arterioles, associated with hypertension. This would result in either a diminuation in blood flow to white matter or to loss of auto-regulatory capacity in that region.

OTHER DEMENTIAS

Transmissible encephalopathy

The archetype of the rare, unconventional transmissible dementias, which may occur at any age, especially in the 'presenile' period, is Creutzfeldt-Jakob disease (see Ch. 7). It is linked to a variety of other conditions, including *kuru*, *scrapie* in sheep, and *transmissible mink encephalopathy*.

Dementia and malignant disease

Psychiatric illness in the absence of metastases in the brain sometimes occurs in patients with malignant disease, especially those who have small-cell carcinoma of the bronchus. Some of these cases may be explained on the basis of re-active depression, adverse reactions to drugs, or some form of confusional state. Occasionally, how-ever, a true clinical dementia supervenes. Neuro-pathological examinations have been undertaken in only a few cases, and have shown perivascular cuffing with lymphocytes reminiscent of an encephalitis, mainly in the temporal lobe, hence the term 'limbic' encephalitis (see Ch. 10). The aetiology is obscure, but it may be due to some form of cancer-related immunosuppression, or possibly antigenic cross-reaction with a tumour product.

Alcoholic dementia

A long-term disability associated with chronic alcoholism is that of the Wernicke–Korsakoff syndrome (see Ch. 11). Being increasingly recognized is a diffuse form of brain damage in chronic alcoholics in which there are considerable and often severe neuropsychological deficits of a type that suggests a more global dementing process than occurs in the Wernicke–Korsakoff syndrome. Prolonged abstinence from alcohol may lead to improvement in both the clinical state and the *in vivo* evidence of structural brain damage of a type that may be identified on CT scanning. This comprises cerebral atrophy and associated ventricular enlargement, largely as a result of loss of white matter in the frontal lobes; the subcortical nuclei are unaffected. Morphometric studies have shown that these changes are due to reversible shrinkage of white matter following dehydration, although neuronal loss in the frontal cortex has been identified. The aetiology of this condition is probably multifactorial, including the direct neurotoxic affects of ethanol and vitamin deficiency.

Dementia in multiple sclerosis

There is an increasing awareness of cognitive impairment in patients with multiple sclerosis. In general, the severity of the cognitive impairment parallels the severity of demyelination in white matter, as detected by CT and MRI scanning. In the most severe cases there are extensive periventricular lesions, demyelination of the corpus callosum and considerable enlargement of the ventricular system.

Dementia pugilistica

Repeated blows to the head experienced by boxers – particularly professionals – are associated with the dementing syndrome known as dementia pugilistica (Ch. 8). As discussed above, it is now known that in the brains of patients with dementia pugilistica there are large numbers of diffuse plaques composed of βA4 amyloid protein that are immunologically indistinguishable from those seen in Alzheimer's disease (see p. 259).

Dementia associated with AIDS

Possibly the most common and most important cause of neurological illness in patients with AIDS results from the direct involvement of the brain by the virus. The resulting syndrome is the AIDS dementia complex, which develops in some 50 per cent of patients with the disease. CT scans may show some cortical atrophy and ventricular enlargement without focal lesions. Histologically, however, white matter abnormalities range from diffuse to extensive loss of myelin and axons, scattered microglial nodules and collections of macrophages. In 30 per cent of cases multinucleated giant cells (see Fig. 7.19), which are pathognomonic of HIV infection, are accompanied by macrophages, microglial cells and lymphocytes in the deep grey matter, white matter and cortex. This multifocal inflammatory process is referred to as HIV encephalitis. Involvement of the CNS by other infections is common, and so it is perhaps not surprising that there is not a clear relationship between HIV encephalitis and dementia.

Dementia of normal pressure hydrocephalus

Dementia of a disinhibited 'frontal lobe' type, together with urgency of micturition and a widely spaced ataxic gait, are often found to be due to normal pressure hydrocephalus, for which no cause can be found post mortem (see Ch. 4).

CSF pressure is usually normal at lumbar puncture, but continuous monitoring may record episodes of increased pressure, particularly during sleep. Thus the term intermittently raised pressure hydrocephalus may be more appropriate than normal pressure hydrocephalus. Underlying causes include previous subarachnoid haemorrhage, head injury or meningitis, and conditions which may lead to fibrous adhesion in the basal cisterns. CT scanning shows enlargement of the ventricles, whereas the sulci are normal or hardly discernible: this latter feature is in contrast to the widened sulci seen in cerebral atrophy and serves to distinguish this condition from the more common causes of dementia, namely Alzheimer's disease and multiple infarction.

PATHOLOGICAL CAUSES OF SEVERE MEMORY LOSS

There is an increasing awareness that bilateral involvement of the hippocampal formation is responsible for many amnesic states. The damage may involve the hippocampus, the fornix, the mamillary bodies, the mamillo-thalamic tracts, the dorsomedial thalamic nucleus or the various components of the amygdaloid or entorhinal cortex.

One of the best-known syndromes of profound memory disturbance is that of the Wernicke–Korsakoff syndrome often attributed to excessive alcohol consumption. Gross disorders of memory may also follow bilateral infarction of the medial parts of each temporal lobe, surgical removal of the temporal lobes, and in patients who survive acute necrotizing encephalitis due to herpes simplex virus and as a remote complication of malignant disease.

SCHIZOPHRENIA

This so-called functional psychosis has traditionally been considered not to have an organic basis. However, in the last 10 years neuroimaging, and particularly CT and MRI scan studies, have provided increasing evidence of a structural abnormality, particularly in the form of ventricular enlargement, observations that have been confirmed by morphometric studies post mortem. Structural changes are centred on the temporal lobe which has shown changes in its cytoarchitecture. The changes are not associated with degenerative, inflammatory or vascular processes, and are therefore thought to be developmental in origin. Current controversy revolves around whether these changes are present in all types of schizophrenia, but what appears to be increasingly certain is that the clinical symptoms predate the onset of ventricular enlargement, and that in many patients genetic factors play a role. It is yet to be determined how these structural abnormalities relate to particular neurochemical perturbations and the clinical signs and symptoms of the disease.

FURTHER READING

Davis P J M & Wright E A (1977) A new method for measuring cranial volume and its application to the assessment of cerebral atrophy at autopsy. *Neuropathology and Applied Neurobiology* **3**, 341–358.

Hubbard B M & Anderson J M (1985) Age-related variations in the neuron content of the cerebral cortex in senile dementia of Alzheimer type. *Neuropathology and Applied Neurobiology* **11**, 369–382.

Iversen L L, Iversen S D & Snyder S H (eds) (1988) *Handbook of Psychopharmacology*, Vol. 20. *Psychopharmacology of the Aging Nervous System*. New York: Plenum Press.

Kay D W K (1989) Genetics, Alzheimer's disease and senile dementia. *British Journal of Psychiatry* **154**, 311–320.

Khachaturian Z S (1985) Diagnosis of Alzheimer's disease. *Archives of Neurology* **42**, 1097–1105.

Lantos P L (1990) *Ageing and dementias*. In: *Systemic Pathology*, 3rd edn, Vol. 4. *Nervous System, Muscle & Eyes*. Edinburgh: Churchill Livingstone, pp. 360–396.

Masters C L & Beyreuther K (eds) (1991) Alzheimer's disease: molecular basis of structural lesions. *Brain Pathology* **1**, 226–296.

Reisberg B (ed) (1983) *Alzheimer's Disease: The Standard Reference*. New York: The Free Press.

Richardson E P (1990) Huntington's disease: some recent neuropathological studies. *Neuropathology and Applied Neurobiology* **16**, 451–460.

Stahl S M, Iversen S D & Goodman E C (1987) *Cognitive Neurochemistry*. London: Oxford University Press.

Tomlinson B E (1979) The ageing brain. In: *Recent Advances in Neuropathology*, 1. Edited by J B Cavanagh and W T Smith. Edinburgh: Churchill Livingstone, pp. 129–159.

15. Tumours

In many respects tumours of the nervous system have attracted greater attention than is justified by their incidence, several monographs having been written about them (see Further Reading). Only a very brief account therefore will be given here. There have also been numerous classifications, none completely satisfactory.

In the previous edition we incorporated a summary of the principal types of tumour of the nervous system, based on the WHO classification at that time. This year a new classification has been published (Table 15.1), and although this is not yet generally available it has been accepted by a panel of specialized neuropathologists. There are numerous minor changes but there are also some major ones. Perhaps the most important is that glioblastoma, previously classified as one of the poorly differentiated and embryonal tumours, now appears under the subheading of astrocytic tumours. As a result, tumours classified by experienced neuropathologists for many years as anaplastic astrocytoma based on the presence of necrosis and capillary endothelial hyperplasia, must now be classified as glioblastoma. The term glioblastoma multiforme has now been discarded; the definition of anaplastic astrocytoma is therefore rather vague. The common tumour of childhood, medulloblastoma, remains under the heading of embryonal tumours. This is quite understandable, but in the same subdivision we now have the concept of primitive neuro-ectodermal tumours (PNETs). There has been an increasing awareness of these poorly differentiated tumours in childhood for many years, and this has now been established. Another important point is that tumours of the cranial and spinal nerves are now referred to as schwannomas, which is preferable to the previous term of neurilemmoma because the neurilemma is the anatomical term for a nerve sheath and is not composed of potential tumour cells. Another commendable change is that haemangiopericytoma, which was previously classified as a type of meningioma, now appears as a malignant meningeal neoplasm. This is a very sensible decision because it is well known that these are very aggressive tumours of the meninges. Finally, it has been accepted that haemangioblastoma should *not* be classified as a tumour of blood vessel origin but rather as of uncertain origin.

As in other systems of the body, the name ascribed to any particular type of tumour is based on the similarity of the tumour cell to the appropriate developing or mature cell. Most of the tumours described in this chapter are restricted to the CNS, but tumours of nerve sheaths also affect cranial and peripheral nerves.

All intracranial tumours have essentially similar effects. They may produce *focal dysfunction*, e.g. hemiparesis or hemianopia, depending on their site; they may have an *irritant effect* on adjacent tissue and produce focal epilepsy; and they act as *intracranial expanding lesions*, leading ultimately to an increase in intracranial pressure (ICP) (see Ch. 4). With regard to the last of these, the effective size of the tumour is frequently contributed to by oedema in the adjacent brain. Furthermore, a high ICP is usually an early feature of any tumour in the posterior fossa because the frequently rapid occurrence of obstructive hydrocephalus (see Ch. 4). Spinal tumours, whether extradural or intradural, are characterized by signs of compression of, or focal damage to, the spinal cord.

Table 15.1   Histological classification of brain tumours

Tumours of neuroepithelial tissue

Astrocytic tumours
Astrocytoma
    Variants: Fibrillary
                    Protoplasmic
                    Gemistocytic
Anaplastic (malignant) astrocytoma
Glioblastoma
    Variants: Giant-cell glioblastoma
                    Gliosarcoma
Pilocytic astrocytoma
Subependymal giant-cell astrocytoma
(Tuberous sclerosis)

Oligodendroglial tumours
Oligodendroglioma
Anaplastic (malignant) oligodendroglioma

Ependymal tumours
Ependymoma
Anaplastic (malignant) ependymoma
Myxopapillary ependymoma
Subependymoma

Mixed gliomas
Mixed oligoastrocytoma
Anaplastic (malignant) oligoastrocytoma

Choroid plexus tumours
Choroid plexus papilloma
Choroid plexus carcinoma

Neuronal and mixed neuronal–glial tumours
Gangliocytoma
Ganglioglioma

Embryonal tumours
Medulloblastoma
    Variant: Desmoplastic medulloblastoma
Primitive neuroectodermal tumours (PNETs) with
multipotent differentiation: neuronal, astrocytic, ependymal,
muscle, melanotic etc.

Tumours of cranial and spinal nerves
Schwannoma (neurilemoma, neurinoma)
Neurofibroma
    Variants: Circumscribed (solitary)
                    Plexiform
Malignant peripheral nerve sheath tumour

Tumours of the meninges
Tumours of meningothelial cells
Meningioma
    Variants: Meningotheliomatous
                    Fibrous (fibroblastic)
                    Transitional (mixed)
                    Psammomatous
                    Angiomatous
Anaplastic (malignant) meningioma

Mesenchymal, non-meningothelial tumours
Benign neoplasms
Lipoma
Fibrous histiocytoma

Malignant neoplasms
Hemangiopericytoma
Malignant fibrous histiocytoma
Meningeal sarcomatosis

Primary melanocytic lesions
Malignant melanoma
    Variant: Meningeal melanomatosis

Tumours of uncertain histogenesis
Hemangioblastoma (capillary hemangioblastoma)

Haemopoetic neoplasms
Primary malignant lymphomas

Germ-cell tumours
Germinoma
Embryonal carcinoma
Yolk-sac tumour (endodermal sinus tumour)
Choriocarcinoma
Teratoma
Mixed germ-cell tumours

Cysts and tumour-like lesions
Rathke's cleft cyst
Epidermoid cyst
Dermoid cyst
Colloid cyst of the third ventricle
Enterogenous cyst
Neuroglial cyst
Other cysts
Lipoma
Granular-cell tumour (choristoma, pituicytoma)
Hypothalamic neuronal hamartoma
Nasal glial heterotopia
Plasma-cell granuloma

Tumours of the sellar region
Pituitary adenoma
Pituitary carcinoma
Craniopharyngioma

Local extensions from regional tumours
Paraganglioma
Chordoma
Chondroma
Chondrosarcoma
Adenoid cystic carcinoma (cylindroma)

Metastatic tumours
Meningeal carcinomatosis

INCIDENCE AND PREVALENCE

The precise incidence of tumours of the nervous system is difficult to establish since most surveys have been based on cases admitted to neuro-surgical units. In the previous edition our own experience over a 5-year period of nearly 12 000 tumours of the nervous system was presented. This is no longer valid because of the new WHO classification, and because many of the tumours classified as anaplastic astrocytoma would now be classified as glioblastoma. In general, in a neuro-surgical unit, tumours of neuroepithelial tissue account for some 40 per cent of cases, meningiomas for some 20 per cent, tumours of nerve sheath origin for some 20 per cent and metastatic carcinoma for a further 20 per cent. The figures should therefore give some idea of the incidence, at least of tumours within a particular region, but many patients thought to have cerebral metastases are not necessarily referred to a neurosurgical unit. The incidence of metastatic carcinoma therefore is probably higher than this, as many other surveys have found. Various reports have, however, suggested that the average annual incidence of neuroepithelial tumours is between 3 and 4 per 100 000 population. Others have suggested that about 1.5 per cent of all tumours affect the brain, and that almost half of these are of neuroepithelial origin.

The classification presented in Table 15.1 inevitably includes some very rare tumours. In this chapter many of these are catalogued in only a sentence or two, but it seemed appropriate that the pathologist faced with making a diagnosis of an unusual tumour should at least know of their existence, and their principal features.

The prognosis in patients with an astrocytic tumour – as indeed with any neuroepithelial tumour – is generally poor. There are certain exceptions, since astrocytomas of the optic nerve (if they have not spread into the hypothalamus) and pilocytic astrocytomas of the cerebellum in children, can be excised without subsequent recurrence. The same can be said about the rare subependymomas and choroid plexus papillomas. On the other hand, most neuroepithelial tumours progress inexorably, the duration of survival being in general related to the anaplasia of the tumour. Thus, the median survival for patients with glioblastomas is in the region of 4–6 months, whereas patients with astrocytomas, or other gliomas, that are well differentiated may survive for several years. These facts have led to considerable controversy about treatment: some clinicians are strong supporters of irradiation or chemotherapy, whereas others consider that survival is prolonged for such a short period by such regimens that it is inappropriate to subject the patient to such treatment. This has become a particularly difficult problem in the past decade, during which it has been established that steroids, by reducing or allaying cerebral oedema adjacent to a brain tumour and hence its effective volume, can have a dramatic effect on the clinical state of the patient. Should, therefore, a patient be subjected to what can be rather distressing treatment when he is neurologically normal and in full control of his mental faculties? These are rather philosophical arguments but are none the less practical considerations. On the other hand, medulloblastoma is being increasingly and successfully controlled by a combination of chemotherapy and irradiation of the neuraxis, some 35 per cent of patients so treated surviving for 5 years of longer.

In contrast, meningiomas and schwannomas can be eradicated surgically, hence the importance of early diagnosis. Only too often, however, they have attained such a large size by the time the diagnosis is made that surgery is not as successful as it might be. The treatment of metastases in the CNS can, at best, only be palliative but treatment with steroids and, on occasion, the excision of an accessible metastasis can dramatically improve the clinical state of the patient.

DIAGNOSIS

Despite the increasing sophistication of non-invasive neuroradiological techniques such as CT (Figs 15.1, 15.2) and MRI (Fig. 15.3) in establishing the most likely diagnosis, a good case can be made for always obtaining a precise tissue diagnosis of the nature of an expanding lesion within the brain or the vertebral canal. Even if the tumour is deeply seated, stereotactic techniques are increasingly being used to obtain an appropriate biopsy. With brain tumours, the biopsy can be obtained through a burr hole or in the course of an open craniotomy. For spinal tumours, either percutaneous biopsy or laminectomy are required. Conventions vary in different countries, but the simplest technique with most intracranial tumours is burr-hole biopsy. In our experience, the best method for examining the small, soft pieces of tissue so obtained is the smear technique (Figs 15.4, 15.5; see Ch. 3), although frozen sections or touch preparations may be more applicable to larger biopsies or to tough tissue. Some laboratories, however, prefer frozen sections for the examination of even small, soft pieces of tissue. In our hands, provided the biopsy has come from the appropriate site, the correct diagnosis has been

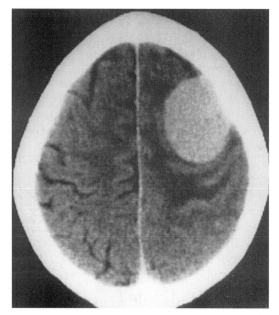

Fig. 15.1 Contrast enhanced CT scan. This sharply defined uniformly enhancing tumour is a meningioma with its base against the vault of the skull. There is some associated oedema. (Courtesy of Dr Peter Macpherson, Department of Neuroradiology, Institute of Neurological Sciences, Glasgow.)

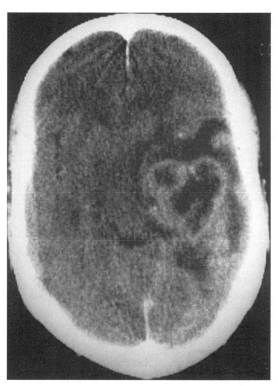

Fig. 15.2 Contrast CT scan. There is an ill-defined lesion in a cerebral hemisphere with irregular peripheral enhancement and low central enhancement. This is an anaplastic astrocytoma with surrounding oedema. (Courtesy of Dr Peter Macpherson, Department of Neuroradiology, Institute of Neurological Sciences, Glasgow.)

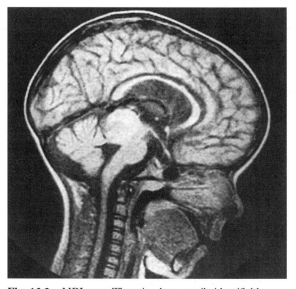

Fig. 15.3 MRI scan. There is a large, easily identifiable mass in the pineal region. (Courtesy of Dr Donald M. Hadley, Department of Neuroradiology, Institute of Neurological Sciences, Glasgow.)

made on the basis of examination of smears in some 93 per cent of biopsies, and in another 5 per cent it was possible to make a positive diagnosis of a malignant tumour although its precise type could not be identified. The technique is not restricted to the identification of tumours, since the smear technique can help in the diagnosis of cerebral infarction, cerebral abscess and viral encephalitis. The smear technique is not incorporated in this chapter but we have already published a monograph on it (see Further Reading). Nevertheless, it is probably better to defer the definitive diagnosis until paraffin sections have been examined.

The examination of a small biopsy from the CNS is an important and sometimes difficult task. The logic of the diagnostic process rests on an understanding of the likely nature of the tumour, this being based predominantly on the site of the tumour and the age of the patient. If the immediate diagnosis on smears or on frozen sections is not readily apparent, the pathologist has to bear in mind the possibility that the biopsy has been derived from a rare tumour, when some

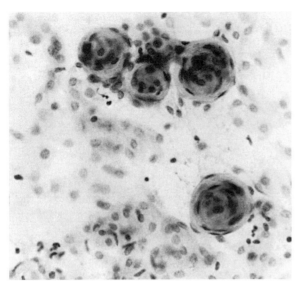

Fig. 15.4   The brain smear technique. In this smear from a meningloma there are numerous cell whorls. (cf. Fig. 15.47). (Toluidine blue.)

material must be preserved for special diagnostic techniques such as immunohistochemistry and electron microscopy. A major problem for a pathologist relatively inexperienced in the examination of brain biopsies is the distinction of intense reactive changes from a neuroepithelial tumour. There is no easy answer to this problem, apart from practical experience. Another particular problem in which the implications of an incorrect diagnosis may be important is the recognition of the less common variants of meningioma. There are also occasions when it is difficult to differentiate astrocytoma from schwannoma.

Neuropathologists have traditionally used three principal stains in the examination of biopsies from suspected tumours: H & E as a general stain, HVG to distinguish between glial and collagen fibrils, and PTAH to identify astrocytic fibrils. The last of these is not always reliable in biopsy material and has been superseded by immuno-histochemical techniques. Occasionally selective silver impregnations are of value, but this is a field for the expert.

Immunohistochemistry

Various markers are helpful in elucidating the diagnosis of tumours of the nervous system. They

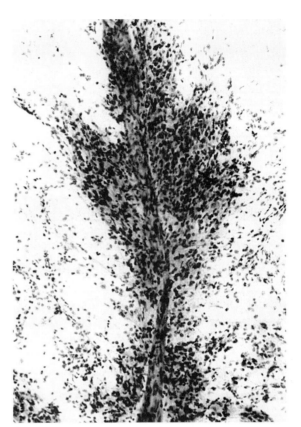

Fig. 15.5   The brain smear technique. There is a pseudopapillary appearance with tumour cells tending to be concentrated around blood vessels. This is the appearance of anaplastic astrocytoma. (Toluidine blue.)

include glial fibrillary acidic protein (GFAP), subunits of neurofilaments (NF), neuron-specific enolase (NSE), S-100 protein and prealbumin. Other markers that are not specific for neuroepithelial structures but are helpful in the diagnosis of other tumours that affect the nervous system are vimentin, cytokeratin, immuno-globulins, Factor VIII/von Willebrand-related antigen and pituitary hormones. Although immunofluorescence is still widely used, the horseradish peroxidase–anti horseradish peroxidase (PAP) procedure remains the method of choice.

Although there is considerable heterogeneity of microscopical appearances, and therefore of staining by immunohistochemistry, in gliomas, a panel that includes several antibodies is often of use in diagnostic neuro-oncology (Table 15.2). Patterns of staining may vary depending upon

Table 15.2   Immunoreactivity of selected brain tumours

	GFAP	EMA/CK	LCA	NF	VIM	S 100	NSE
Astrocytoma	+	–	–	–	+/–	+/–	+/–
Glioblastoma	+	+/–	–	–	+	+	+
Oligodendroglioma	+/–	–	–	–	+/–	+	+
Ependymoma	+	+/–	–	–	+	+/–	+/–
Choroid plexus tumour	+/–	+	–	–	+	+	+
Ganglioglioma	+	–	–	+/–	+/–	+/–	+/–
Medulloblastoma	+/–	–	–	+/–	+	+	+
Schwanomma	–	–	–	–	+	+	–
Neurofibroma	–	–	–	–	+	+	–
Meningioma	–	+/–	–	–	+	+	+
Haemangioblastoma	+/–	–	–	–	+	+/–	+/–
Lymphoma	–	–	+	–	–	–	–
Metatastasis	–	+	–	–	–	+/–	–

GFAP   = Glial fibrillary acidic protein; EMA = Epithelial membrane antigen; CK = Cytokeratin;
LCA   = Leucocyte common antigen; NF = Neurofilament; VIM = Vimentin;
NSE   = Neuron-specific enolase
+   = Positive; ± = Variably positive; – = Negative

fixation, the type of antibody and the degree of differentiation within any category of tumour, and even under optimal conditions staining may be either focal or diffuse.

Glial fibrillary acidic protein (GFAP)

Antibody to GFAP is one of the most reliable and widely used agents because of its specificity for cells of the astrocytic series. There is a positive reaction with astrocytoma but also with some other tumours, including certain ependymomas, subependymomas, gliosarcomas, gangliogliomas and in the better differentiated areas of glioblastoma. A number of non-glial tumours contain GFAP-positive cells, namely choroid plexus papilloma, pituitary adenoma, pineoblastoma and medulloblastoma. The presence of GFAP-positive cells in the last of these is usually taken as evidence of astrocytic differentiation in the primitive cells. However, reactive astrocytes within tumours also give a positive reaction.

S-100 protein

Despite initial hopes that it might be a specific marker for tumours of neuroepithelial origin, S-100 protein has not established itself as such because a wide range of tumours of different ontogeny are positive for the protein. It is present not only in glial and non-glial cells, but also in some tumours of non-neuroepithelial origin, e.g. meningioma and melanoma.

Neurofilaments

Neurofilaments (NF) are exclusive to neurons and do not cross-react with other intermediate filaments, e.g. GFAP, vimentin or cytokeratin. This makes NF a reliable marker for ganglion cells and their precursors, e.g. in a ganglioglioma, but they may not be present in primitive neuroepithelial tumours thought to be of neuroblastic derivation, such as neuroblastoma and medulloblastoma.

Neuron-specific enolase

Enolase has three distinct subunits, α, β and γ. The homodimer $\gamma\gamma$ or neuron-specific enolase (NSE) is essentially confined to neurons and cells of the neuroendocrine cell system. Antisera against NSE help to identify peripheral neuroblastoma, melanoma and tumours of the APUD system. Lymphomas and various carcinomas are also occasionally positive for NSE. $\alpha\alpha$ enolase (the non-specific enolase) is present in some astrocytomas, ependymomas, oligodendrogliomas and meningiomas.

Vimentin

This is a protein subunit of the intermediate

filaments that occur in endothelial cells, fibroblasts, macrophages and lymphoid cells, but it is not specific for any particular mesenchymal tissue because positive staining also occurs in melanomas, lymphomas and in some ependymomas. Strongly positive staining has been reported in meningiomas, but this may not be helpful as similar staining occurs in sarcomas and fibrous histiocytomas.

Cytokeratin

All carcinomas are said to contain cytokeratins, irrespective of their degree of differentiation. Specific antisera are therefore useful in differentiating between metastatic carcinoma and other anaplastic tumours of the nervous system.

Immunoglobulins

Although the role of various histochemical techniques in the diagnosis of lymphomas is now well established, their application to tumours of the nervous system is often unsatisfactory, as the diagnosis may not be suspected preoperatively and therefore appropriate samples are not taken for study.

Other diagnostic antisera

Factor VIII/von Willebrand-related antigen is synthesized by endothelium and has been used to label normal and hyperplastic endothelial cells in malignant gliomas. α-fetoprotein is helpful in the diagnosis of certain gonadal germ-cell tumours and in the identification of extragonadal-cell tumours occurring in the pineal and suprasellar regions. Germinomas do not stain, whereas embryonal carcinoma and endodermal sinus tumours are strongly positive. Mature teratomas are negative, so that positive staining tends to be associated with a poorer outcome. Human chorionic gonadotrophin is secreted by the trophoblastic epithelium of the placenta. Positive staining may be found in primary intracranial choriocarcinoma and mixed malignant germ-cell tumours in which some trophoblastic elements are intermingled with germinoma, embryonal carcinoma and in yolk-sac tumours. Prealbumin is of value in identifying cells of choroid plexus origin.

TUMOURS OF NEUROEPITHELIAL TISSUE

The great majority of tumours of neuroepithelial tissue (Table 15.1) are derived from the neuroglia, i.e. *astrocytes*, *oligodendrocytes* and *ependymal* cells, or their precursors. The corresponding tumours, *astrocytomatous tumours*, *oligodendrogliomas* and *ependymomas* are often referred to collectively as the *gliomas*. Medulloblastoma is conventionally not included among the gliomas since its cell of origin is thought to be an embryonal precursor of the neuronal series. There are many variants of these tumours, but the name applied often has to be based on the predominant cell type since many neuroepithelial tumours contain more than one type of neoplastic cell. Thus, astrocytes can be identified within many tumours classed as oligodendrogliomas or ependymomas.

The *gliomas* as a group share many common features. Some are composed of cells that are very similar to mature neuroglial cells, whereas others are anaplastic (malignant). The term 'anaplasia' includes features like cellular pleomorphism, loss of cellular differentiation, the presence of mitotic figures, the occurrence of vascular endothelial hyperplasia and the presence of necrosis. The terms 'benign' and 'malignant' have a different connotation than they have with most tumours in other systems of the body: no matter how well differentiated or benign a glioma appears, it almost invariably infiltrates and cannot be successfully removed surgically; and no matter how poorly differentiated or malignant the glioma appears, they very rarely metastasize. Any type of glioma, however, may occasionally spread diffusely throughout the subarachnoid space, this being termed '*meningeal gliomatosis*'. Often the site of the tumour is more important than its type: thus very little can be achieved for a patient with a deeply seated, well differentiated glioma, whereas there may be temporary benefit from the debulking of a highly anaplastic tumour in an accessible site, such as the frontal, the temporal or the occipital pole of the non-dominant hemisphere. The precise classification of a glioma rarely, if ever, influences neurosurgical management.

There was a tendency in the past to grade gliomas numerically on the basis of their degree of differentiation, Grade 1 being a tumour composed essentially of mature cells and Grade 4 being a highly anaplastic tumour. Because of the great variation of individual features in gliomas, this approach has tended to fall into disrepute. Furthermore, precise classification cannot be based on the appearance of a small biopsy since, in many gliomas, various grades are present within the one tumour. There is, however, a tendency to think of gliomas as being well differentiated or showing varying degrees of anaplasia. This may well influence therapy once the diagnosis has been established, because of the aggressive behaviour of highly anaplastic gliomas.

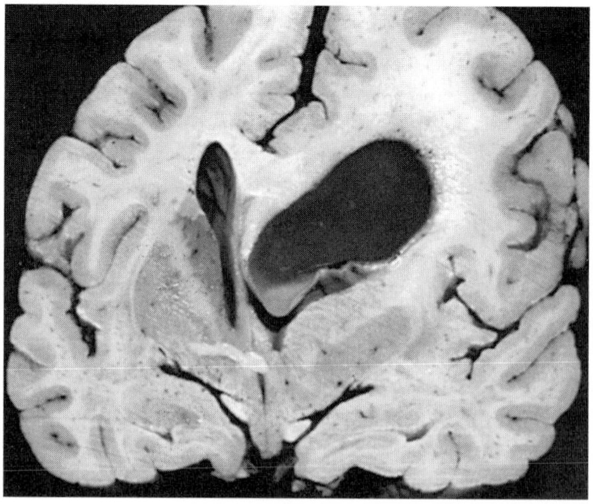

Fig. 15.7   Astrocytoma. Most of the lesion consists of a cyst, there only being a narrow rim of tumour around it.

ASTROCYTIC TUMOURS

The majority of gliomas are astrocytic in origin. Astrocytomas occur principally in the white matter, and they vary greatly in appearance. Some are reasonably well demarcated from the adjacent tissue, but others mainly cause expansion of the affected region and are very poorly demarcated (Fig. 15.6). Affected grey matter tends to be pale and expanded, and there is a loss of differentiation between grey and white matter. Many are firmer than normal brain, but some are softer and some are cystic (Fig. 15.7). Anaplastic astrocytoma is grossly similar to astrocytoma, the diagnosis of

anaplasia being based on the microscopical appearances (see below). Glioblastomas, in contrast, are characterized by the presence of foci of haemorrhage and necrosis (Fig. 15.8): they often appear better circumscribed than astrocytomas. As indicated above, the effective size of any astrocytoma may be increased by oedema of the adjacent white matter. Very occasionally astrocytomas may be multicentric, but such an occurrence can only be accepted if histological studies have established that there has been no

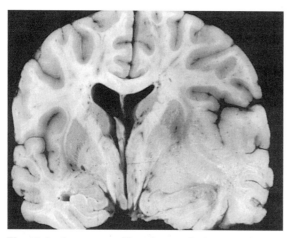

Fig. 15.6   Astrocytoma. There is a poorly demarcated mass causing expansion of the right temporal lobe.

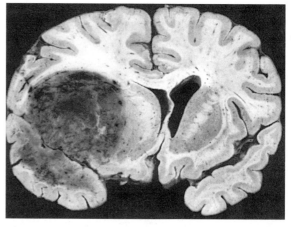

Fig. 15.8   Glioblastoma. There is a sharply defined haemorrhagic tumour in the inferior part of the left frontal lobe and in the adjacent temporal lobe.

spread of the astrocytoma via the subarachnoid space to another site within the brain.

A particular type of astrocytoma is the cystic astrocytoma of the cerebellum: this is a pilocytic astrocytoma (see below) that occurs in children. It is one of the few astrocytomas that can occasionally be successfully excised surgically. Pilocytic astrocytoma also occurs in the hypothalamus (Fig. 15.9). Another type of astrocytoma is the optic nerve glioma: if this is restricted to the optic nerve it also may not recur after resection, but extension into the hypothalamus is common. Gliomatosis cerebri – often referred to in the past as diffuse astrocytoma – is now classified (WHO) as a neuropithelial tumour of uncertain origin. The affected area is expanded and firm (Fig. 15.10) and the tumour is very poorly demarcated from the adjacent brain tissue. This type of tumour frequently occurs in the brain stem – the so-called pontine astrocytoma (Fig. 15.11) – and in the spinal cord.

A rare variant of astrocytic tumours is the subependymal giant-cell astrocytoma, which is associated with tuberous sclerosis (see Ch. 13),

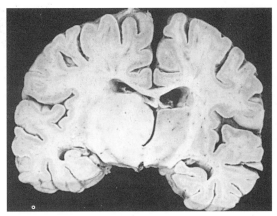

Fig. 15.10 Gliomatosis cerebri. The left thalamus is expanded by tumour.

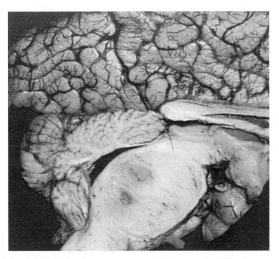

Fig. 15.11 Pontine astrocytoma. The pons is diffusely enlarged by poorly demarcated tumour.

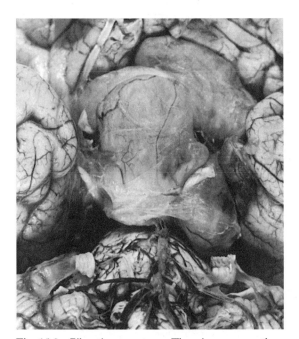

Fig. 15.9 Pilocytic astrocytoma. There is an apparently encapsulated mass in the region of the hypothalamus.

and takes the form of a firm, pale subependymal nodule. They are often multiple.

Histological appearances

More than one histological type may be present in the same tumour. *Fibrillary* astrocytoma is composed of unevenly distributed, often loosely arranged, elongated cells (Fig. 15.12), among which there is a characteristic fibrillary eosinophilic matrix and varying numbers of fine and coarse glial fibrils that stain with PTAH and GFAP and can be seen by electron microscopy (Fig. 15.13a, b and c). Microcystic spaces and small foci of

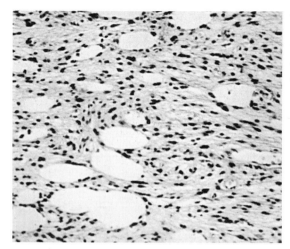

Fig. 15.12   Fibrillary astrocytoma. The tumour is composed of elongated cells with some microcysts. (H & E.)

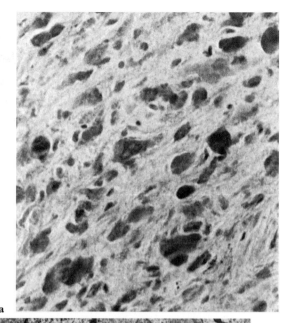

a

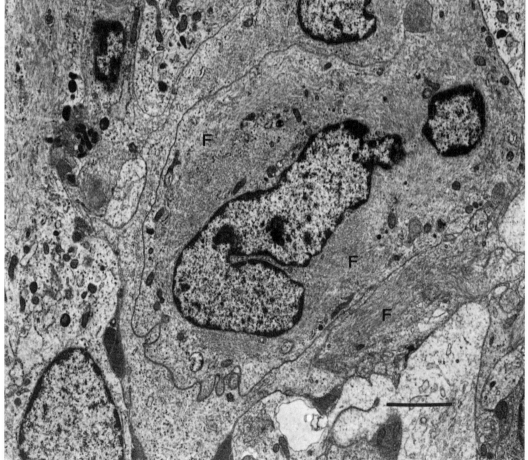

b

Fig. 15.13   Fibrillary astrocytoma. (a) The tumour cells are positive with antibody of GFAP. (b) and (c) On electron microscopy there are intracytoplasmic glial fibrils (F). ((a) PAP; (b) bar = 2.5 μm; (c) bar = 0.5 μm)

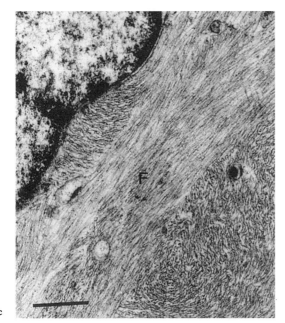

c

Fig. 15.13 (contd.)

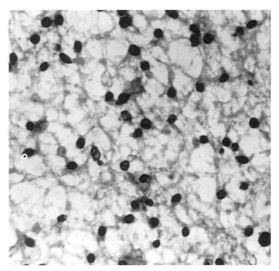

Fig. 15.15 Protoplasmic astrocytoma. The tumour cells have short processes and there is obvious microcystic change. (H & E.)

calcification (calcospherites) are often present. Where a fibrillary astrocytoma affects grey matter, residual neurons are often recognizable. Fibrillary astrocytes tend to predominate in cases of gliomatosis cerebri, and in such tumours there is remarkable preservation of neurons (Fig. 15.14). *Protoplasmic* astrocytoma occurs mainly in grey matter and is composed of rather stellate cells with short processes and swollen cytoplasm, separated by an eosinophilic matrix within which glial fibrils are very scanty (Fig. 15.15).

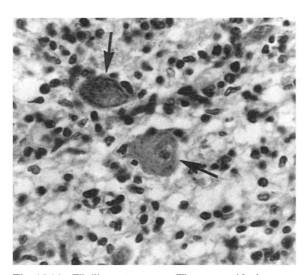

Fig. 15.14 Fibrillary astrocytoma. There are residual neurons (arrows) within the tumour. (H & E.)

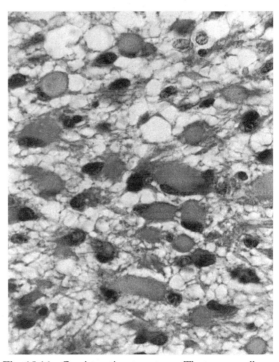

Fig. 15.16 Gemistocytic astrocytoma. The tumour cells have abundant cytoplasm. (H & E.)

Microcystic change is usually very prominent. *Gemistocytic* astrocytoma is composed of large globoid or polygonal cells which have abundant homogeneous cytoplasm separated by glial fibrils (Fig. 15.16).

Anaplastic astrocytoma is one of increased cellularity with atypical nuclei and some mitotic activity (Fig. 15.17). There is no necrosis or endothelial proliferation. *Glioblastoma* is a highly cellular tumour composed of poorly differentiated rounder pleomorphic cells. Multinucleate giant cells are not infrequent (Fig. 15.18). There is great variation in the degree of mitotic activity. Essential for the diagnosis of glioblastoma is the presence of foci of necrosis and endothelial proliferation (Figs 15.19, 15.20). A particularly characteristic feature is the so-called pseudo-palisading of tumour cells around areas of necrosis.

Variants of glioblastoma are the *giant-cell glioblastoma* and *gliosarcoma*. Giant-cell glioblastoma is indistinguishable from glioblastoma macro-

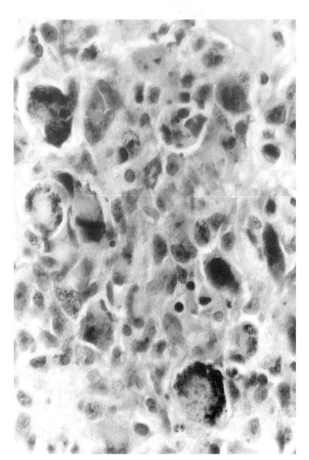

Fig. 15.18 Glioblastoma. There are multinucleate giant cells in the tumour. (H & E.)

scopically. The characteristic features on histological examination are the presence of large numbers of multinucleate giant cells (Fig. 15.21). There is usually also a considerable amount of reticulin. In gliosarcoma there is a distinctive sarcomatous element, presumably arising from the vascular endothelial hyperplasia that is common in glioblastoma (Fig. 15.22). The sarcomatous areas are composed of spindle cells and vast amounts of reticulin. These cells are negative for GFAP.

Pilocytic astrocytoma is composed predominantly of elongated cells which have long fibrillary processes. The latter tend to form parallel bundles among which there are loosely structured microcystic areas (Fig. 15.23). The term 'compact-spongy', which was previously used for this type of astrocytoma in the cerebellum, is

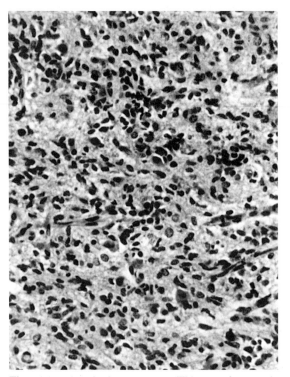

Fig. 15.17 Anaplastic astrocytoma. This type of tumour is highly cellular.

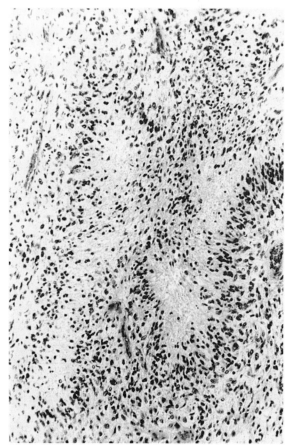

Fig. 15.19 Glioblastoma. Tumour cells form a palisade around foci of necrosis. (H & E.)

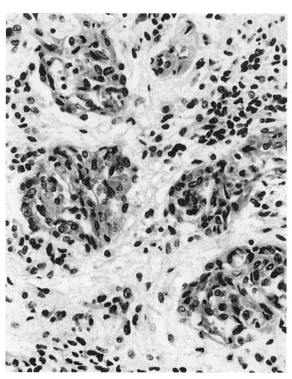

Fig. 15.20 Glioblastoma. Capillary endothelial hyperplasia leads to the formation of glomeruloid structures. (H & E.)

particularly descriptive. Optic nerve gliomas are usually of pilocytic type, but the loosely structured 'spongy' areas are less conspicuous than in the cerebellum or in the hypothalamus.

Subependymal giant-cell astrocytoma consists of large astrocytes surrounded by glial fibrils. Focal calcification is frequent.

In *gliomatosis cerebri*, a tumour now classified as of uncertain origin, the affected region is diffusely permeated by neoplastic astrocytes and there is remarkable preservation of neurons. The tumour cells are usually well differentiated, but anaplastic change may supervene.

Two other features are commonly seen in astrocytomas. If the cerebral cortex is involved there is almost invariably a subpial band of tumour astrocytes extending some distance from the main tumour, and if the tumour invades the

subarachnoid space it often evokes a desmoplastic reaction, with the result that there may be a considerable amount of collagen in this part of the tumour.

OLIGODENDROGLIAL TUMOURS

Oligodendrogliomas occur principally in the cerebral hemispheres and tend to be more sharply defined than astrocytomas, and slightly gelatinous. Calcification may be such that it can be seen in X-rays of the skull.

Histological appearances

Oligodendroglioma is composed of compact masses of uniform round cells that tend to have well defined boundaries. The cytoplasm is typically clear, thus giving a 'honeycomb' appearance (Fig. 15.24). The scanty stroma contains many small thin-walled blood vessels, often with a 'chicken-wire' appearance. There are usually some

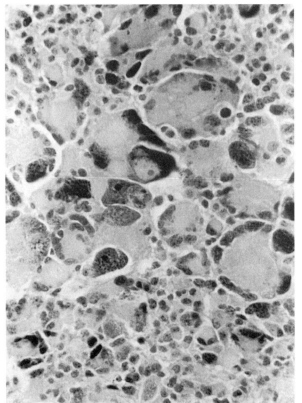

Fig. 15.21 Giant-cell glioblastoma. Within the tumour there are multinucleate giant cells. (H & E.)

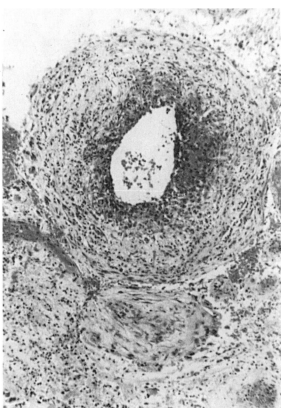

Fig. 15.22 Glioblastoma. Within the tumour there may be hyperplasia of the mesenchymal elements in the walls of blood vessels. (H & E.)

astrocytes within an oligodendroglioma, but when they are numerous or when part of the tumour has the appearances of astrocytoma, the term *oligoastrocytoma* is used (Table 15.1). In anaplastic oligodendroglioma the characteristic vascular pattern tends to be retained, and some areas of the tumour are clearly composed of cells of oligodendroglial type. There is, however, also cellular pleomorphism, vascular endothelial hyperplasia, necrosis and haemorrhage.

EPENDYMAL TUMOURS

Ependymoma

This type of tumour occurs more commonly in childhood and adolescence than in adult life. Because of their cell of origin, they occur in relation to any part of the ventricular system but they have a particular predilection for the fourth

ventricle (Fig. 15.25). They also are a relatively frequent tumour of the spinal cord, since ependymal cells run the entire length of the cord in relation to the central canal and are present in the filum terminale. Ependymomas tend to grow into the ventricles, but they also infiltrate into adjacent tissue. If the tumour is in the third or the fourth ventricle, hydrocephalus develops rapidly. Ependymomas tend to be friable and rather papillary, but when they infiltrate into the paraventricular tissue they are usually firm and solid. Cyst formation also occurs. Because of the relative ease by which tumour cells can be desquamated into the CSF pathways, ependymomas are a relatively common cause of meningeal gliomatosis. As with other gliomas, *anaplasia* in an ependymoma is shown by the presence of haemorrhage and necrosis.

Ependymomas arising in the region of cauda

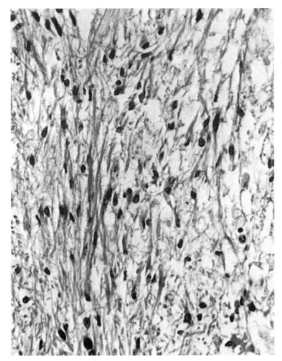

Fig. 15.23 Pilocytic astrocytoma. Many of the tumour cells are elongated and have conspicuous fibrillary processes. (H & E.)

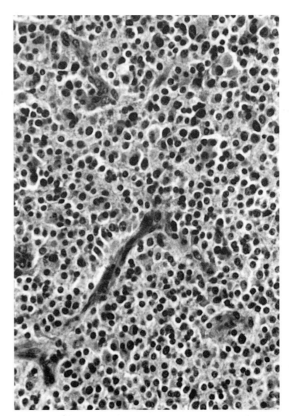

Fig. 15.24 Oligodendroglioma. The cells are uniformly small and capillaries are conspicuous. (H & E.)

equina tend to be of the *myxopapillary* variety. This is a slowly growing, rather gelatinous tumour which frequently spreads in the subarachnoid space to ensheathe the nerve roots of the cauda equina, and it often also extends rostrally in the subarachnoid space around the spinal cord. This type of ependymoma may erode through the dura into the adjacent bone. Ependymomas of the filum, however, are occasionally encapsulated, when they can sometimes be successfully removed surgically.

As the name implies, *subependymomas* arise deep to the ependyma, usually in the lateral or fourth ventricles, and then protrude as smooth firm nodules into the ventricle. They often appear to behave as hamartomas rather than invasive tumours, and small ones are an occasional incidental finding post mortem.

Histological appearances

The cells in *ependymomas* frequently have a distinctly epithelial appearance, but the most

characteristic feature is the perivascular pseudorosette, which takes the form of a perivascular fibrillary eosinophilic cuff between blood vessels

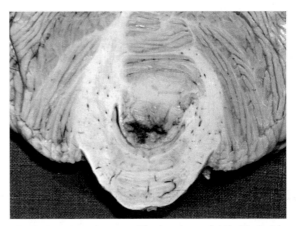

Fig. 15.25 Ependymoma. The fourth ventricle is filled with tumour.

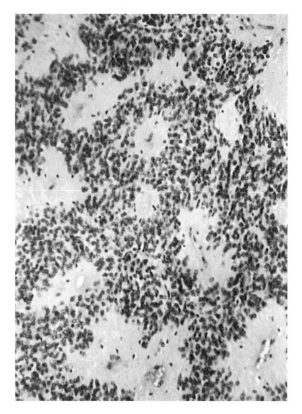

Fig. 15.26 Ependymoma. Blood vessels are separated from tumour cells by a perivascular fibrillary halo. (H & E.)

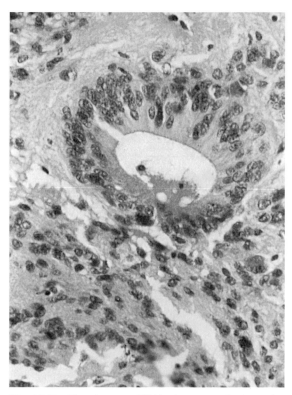

Fig. 15.27 Ependymoma. Within the tumour there may be canaliculi lined by the columnar cells. (H & E.)

and tumour cells (Fig. 15.26). Less frequently, there are canaliculi (Fig. 15.27). PTAH-positive, rather elongated bodies may be identifiable along the luminal margin of the cells lining the canaliculi. These are part of the ciliary apparatus and are known as *blepharoplasts*. Occasionally, ependymomas have a distinctly papillary architecture, when the term *papillary ependymoma* is appropriate. The latter have similarities to choroid plexus papillomas but there is usually less collagen in their stroma, and they are negative with prealbumin. Astrocytes often figure prominently within ependymomas, particularly where they infiltrate into brain tissue. *Anaplastic* features in an ependymoma consists of cellular pleomorphism, mitotic figures, capillary endothelial hyperplasia, necrosis and haemorrhage.

In myxopapillary ependymoma, ependymal cells are arranged in a papillary fashion around blood vessels that frequently have rather thick hyaline walls (Fig. 15.28). The tumour cells tend to be

large and contain clear spaces that may stain for mucopolysaccharide. The principal feature of *subependymoma* is the presence of closely packed trabeculae of astrocytic fibres, among which there are small and fairly compact groups of ependymal cells (Fig. 15.29).

MIXED GLIOMAS

With the increasing use of immunocytochemical techniques there has been an increased recognition of mixed gliomas composed of oligodendroglial and astrocytic elements.

CHOROID PLEXUS TUMOURS

Choroid plexus papilloma

These tumours occur most frequently in childhood and adolescence, and form bulky papillary masses of friable tumour within the ventricular system

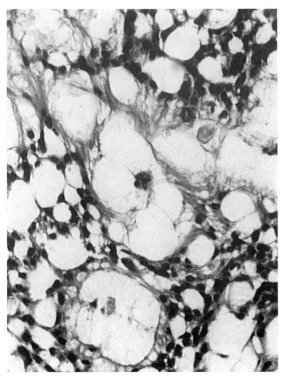

Fig. 15.28 Myxopapillary ependymona. The tumour cells are large and contain clear vacuoles. (H & E.)

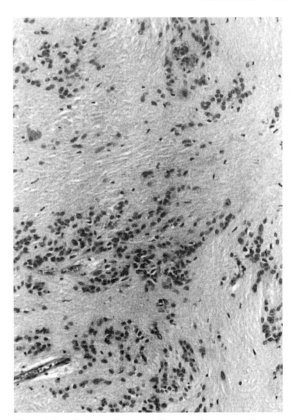

Fig. 15.29 Subependymoma. Groups of tumour cells are separated by bands of astrocytic fibres. (H & E.)

(Fig. 15.30). Hydrocephalus is an almost invariable accompaniment. This may be contributed to by excessive secretion of CSF by the tumour, but a second cause of hydrocephalus is desquamation of tumour cells into the CSF pathways, which has an irritant effect leading to obliteration of the CSF pathways.

Histological appearances

The appearances are those of a papillary tumour composed of cuboidal cells on a delicate stroma of fibrovascular tissue, and almost indistinguishable from normal choroid plexus (Fig. 15.31). These tumours rarely become anaplastic (choroid plexus carcinoma).

NEURONAL AND MIXED NEURONAL–GLIAL TUMOURS

These are rare. *Gangliocytoma* is a very slowly growing tumour composed predominantly of mature ganglion cells. They often seem to behave more as hamartomas than true tumours. *Ganglioglioma* is commoner and its macroscopic appearances are the same as astrocytoma. Histological examination, however, discloses the presence of bizarre cells of ganglionic type, as shown by the presence of large vesicular nuclei with prominent nucleoli and typical Nissl substance, in addition to tumour astrocytes (Fig. 15.32). Many of the ganglion cells are binucleate, and throughout the tumour there are frequently groups of small dark cells that are usually interpreted as being neuroblasts. The bizarre and atypical features of the ganglion cells usually allow this type of tumour to be distinguished quite easily from astrocytomas invading grey matter, within which there are residual neurons. The ganglionic nature of these bizarre cells can usually be demonstrated by silver staining, immunohistochemistry for neurofilaments and

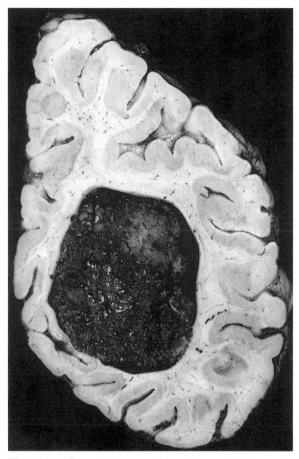

Fig. 15.30 Choroid plexus papilloma. The occipital horn of the ventricle is filled with a papillary tumour.

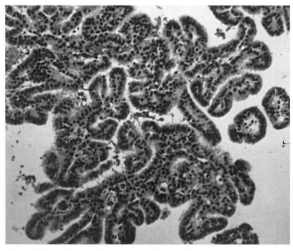

Fig. 15.31 Choroid plexus papilloma. The tumour is composed of cuboidal cells on a fibrovascular papillary stroma.

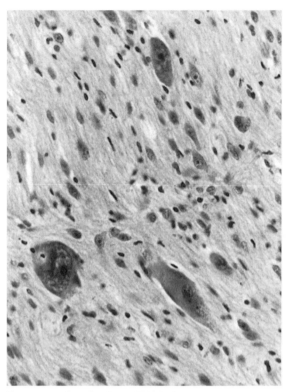

Fig. 15.32 Ganglioglioma. Within the tumour there are aberrant cells of ganglionic type. (H & E.)

the ultrastructural demonstration of putative synapses. When anaplastic change occurs within a ganglioglioma it is usually in the astrocytic element. Primitive tumours composed of cells resembling neuroblasts are dealt with below.

EMBRYONAL TUMOURS

Medulloblastoma

Medulloblastoma is a tumour of the cerebellum and probably arises from nests of cells originating in the external granular layer. It is seen most commonly in children, but it does occur in adolescence and occasionally in early adult life. Most frequently it arises in the midline and presents as a mass of soft, rather grey tumour that frequently fills the fourth ventricle (Fig. 15.33). Hydrocephalus then occurs rapidly. Medulloblastomas, however, can also arise laterally in one of the cerebellar hemispheres. Medulloblastoma has a particular propensity to spread

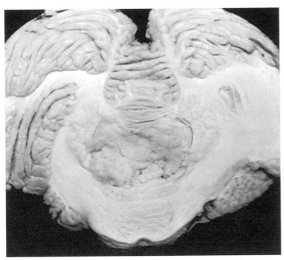

Fig. 15.33 Medulloblastoma. The fourth ventricle is filled with tumour.

within the subarachnoid space as a continuous or discontinuous sheet of tumour (Fig. 15.34), or as seedlings into the lateral ventricles or into the spinal subarachnoid space. There are often small nodules of tumour on spinal nerve roots.

When a medulloblastoma extends into the subarachnoid space it usually provokes an intense desmoplastic reaction. Sometimes such a reaction is seen throughout the greater part of the

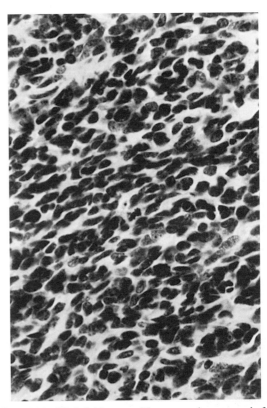

Fig. 15.35 Medulloblastoma. The tumour is composed of closely packed, rather elongated cells. (H & E.)

tumour, when it is referred to as a desmoplastic medulloblastoma.

Histological appearances

Medulloblastoma consists essentially of sheets of closely packed, often slightly elongated, cells that have scanty cytoplasm (Fig. 15.35). The classic feature is the presence of neuroblastic rosettes (Fig. 15.36), but they are not present in every medulloblastoma. The tumour cells in the ventricles and in the subarachnoid space are of similar appearance to those in the main tumour.

In *desmoplastic medulloblastoma* there is a rich network of reticulin and collagen fibrils. A particularly striking feature is the presence of 'islands' of slightly larger and paler cells that are devoid of reticulin (Fig. 15.37). In some medulloblastomas parts of the tumour have the classic appearances, whereas in other areas the features are those of desmoplastic medulloblastoma.

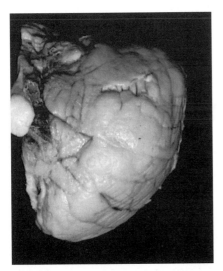

Fig. 15.34 Medulloblastoma. There are plaques of tumour within the subarachnoid space on the inferior surface of the cerebellum.

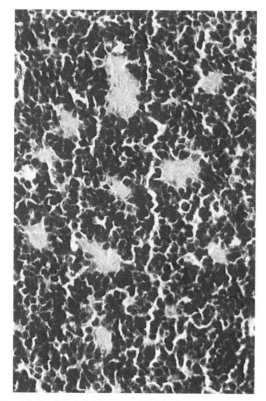

Fig. 15.36 Medulloblastoma. Within the tumour there may be neuroblastic rosettes. (H & E.)

Primitive neuroectodermal tumours (PNETs)

Tumours with the histological features of medulloblastoma occur occasionally elsewhere in the CNS, usually in a cerebral hemisphere in a young child. There is an increasing awareness of this type of tumour and they are now referred to as *primitive neuroectodermal tumours*. Immunocytochemical studies suggest that the cells are related to neuroblasts, but there is often evidence suggestive of astrocytic, ependymal or neuroblastic differentiation.

TUMOURS OF CRANIAL AND SPINAL NERVES

Schwannoma (Neurilemoma)

This is the commonest type of nerve sheath tumour and is composed basically of Schwann cells. They are slowly growing encapsulated tumours that do not infiltrate but can cause considerable distortion of adjacent tissue, such as the brain stem or the spinal cord. On section they are frequently cystic, and there may also be distinctly yellow areas. The commonest cranial nerve affected is the VIIIth ('acoustic neuroma'), where the tumour causes considerable distortion of the cerebellopontine angle (Fig. 15.38; see also Fig. 13.17). It also causes enlargement of the internal auditory meatus, and this may be a

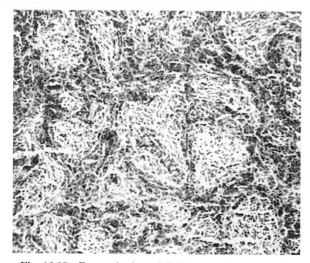

Fig. 15.37 Desmoplastic medulloblastoma. There are groups of rather pale cells between closely packed darker cells. (H & E.)

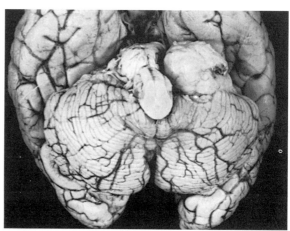

Fig. 15.38 Acoustic schwannoma. There is an encapsulated tumour in the cerebellopontine angle.

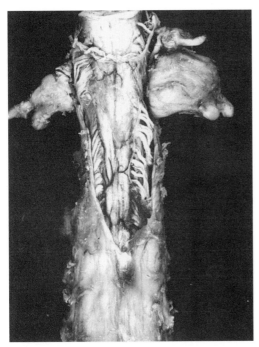

Fig. 15.39 Spinal schwannoma. Bilateral tumours are present on cervical nerve roots.

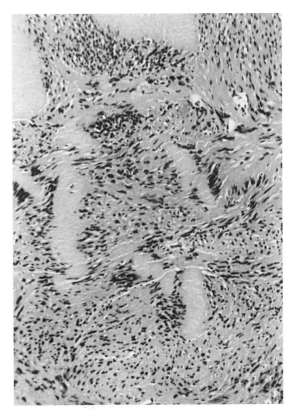

Fig. 15.40 Schwannoma. There is palisading of the nuclei of elongated cells. (H & E.)

helpful radiological sign. A schwannoma occasionally develops from the Vth cranial nerve. Spinal schwannomas almost invariably arise on posterior nerve roots, the tumour distorting and compressing the adjacent cord (Fig. 15.39). There is occasionally continuity through an intervertebral foramen between the spinal tumour and a paravertebral extension, but this is more commonly seen with neurofibroma (see below). Schwannomas may also arise on peripheral nerves.

Histological appearances

Schwannomas are essentially paraneural tumours and it is often possible to identify remnants of the affected nerve in the capsule of the tumour. The tumour itself is of variegated appearance, two features being particularly common, namely the occurrence of interlacing bundles of greatly elongated cells whose nuclei often show some palisading (Antoni A, Fig. 15.40), and tissue of a much looser texture containing large, often pleomorphic, polygonal cells (Antoni B, Fig. 15.41).

Small cysts and evidence of previous haemorrhage are common. The electron microscopic appearances are characteristic (Fig. 15.42).

Neurofibroma

These tumours are composed of Schwann cells and fibroblasts, and lead in the first instance to fusiform enlargement of the affected segment of nerve. They may be circumscribed, i.e. solitary, but frequently several adjacent nerves are affected, the ensuing condition being known as a *plexiform neurofibroma*. Neurofibromas rarely, if ever, affect cranial nerves, but do affect spinal nerve roots, when they are frequently in continuity with a paravertebral mass. Any peripheral nerve may be affected. They may attain a very large size and, on section, the tissue has a pale, rather mucoid appearance.

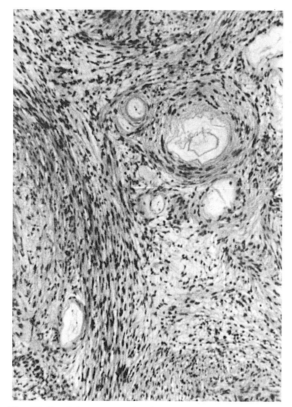

Fig. 15.41   Schwannoma. In addition to closely packed elongated cells, there are more loosely arranged cells. (H & E.)

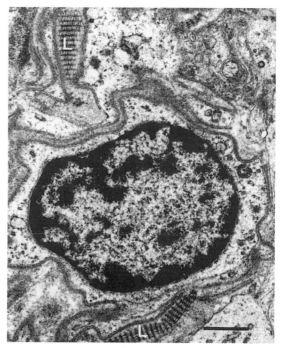

Fig. 15.42   Schwannoma. On electron microscopy there are multiple cytoplasmic processes coated by electron-dense basement membrane. Luse (L) bodies are seen in the matrix. (Bar = 1 μm.)

Histological appearances

The affected nerve is expanded and, because of the presence of a considerable amount of pale inter-cellular matrix, often appears of low cellularity. Throughout the nerve there are varying numbers of elongated, rather twisted cells and some collagen fibrils (Fig. 15.43). Residual axons can usually be recognized.

In many respects the classic types of schwannoma and neurofibroma should be thought of as the ends of a spectrum, since many tumours arising from nerve sheath cells have features suggestive of both schwannoma and neurofibroma. Any nerve sheath tumour may occasionally become malignant but, in our experience, malignant changes and local recurrence occur more frequently in tumours with the appearances of neurofibroma rather than of schwannoma, and in association with von Recklinghausen's neurofibromatosis.

VON RECKLINGHAUSEN'S NEUROFIBROMATOSIS

This genetically determined autosomal dominant disease is characterized by the presence of multiple tumours of nerve sheath cells and multiple pigmented lesions in the skin (see Ch. 13). Many of the nerve sheath tumours are subcutaneous, but they may occur on any nerve, including those supplying the viscera. Bilateral acoustic schwannoma are not uncommon (see Fig. 13.17). It has also been stated that there is an increased incidence of other tumours of the CNS, such as neuroepithelial tumours and meningiomas.

TUMOURS OF THE MENINGES

TUMOURS OF MENINGOTHELIAL CELLS

Meningioma

This is a common tumour and the majority originate in arachnoidal cells, it being generally accepted that many arise in arachnoidal granu-

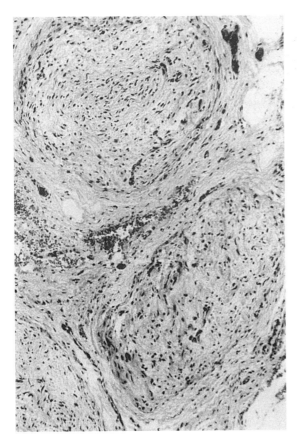

Fig. 15.43   Neurofibroma. Small nerves are expanded by tumour. (H & E.)

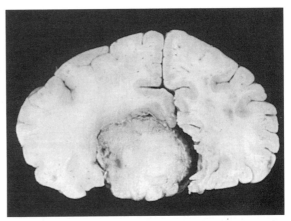

Fig. 15.44   Meningioma. The tumour is sharply defined and has excavated a cavity for itself in the frontal lobe.

lations. They occur mainly above the tentorium cerebelli in relation to venous sinuses. About 10 per cent occur in the posterior fossa or in the vertebral canal. Most spinal meningiomas occur in women. Occasionally meningiomas occur within a lateral ventricle or in the orbit.

Because of their slow rate of growth, meningiomas may attain a quite remarkable size before giving rise to symptoms. They are solid, lobulated tumours, often attached by a broad base to the dura. As they enlarge they excavate a cavity for themselves in the adjacent brain (Fig. 15.44), from which they are usually sharply demarcated. There is often some loss of cortex. Meningiomas vary greatly in appearance, some being soft and fleshly whereas others are hard and gritty. Sometimes the tumour grows as a thick sheet on the surface of the brain, this being referred to as *meningioma-en-plaque* (Fig. 15.45). Meningiomas often evoke reactive changes in the adjacent bone to produce hyperostosis.

Histological appearances

There are several named types of meningioma (Table 15.1), based on the histological appearances, but there is little correlation between these and the site of the tumour or its gross appearance. *Meningotheliomatous* meningioma is composed of polygonal cells with poorly-defined cell boundries (Fig. 15.46). There is frequently considerable pleomorphism of these cells and

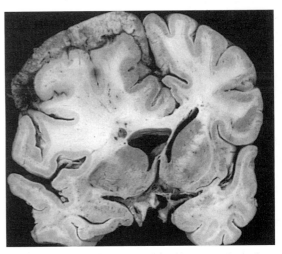

Fig. 15.45   Meningioma-en-plaque. There is a sheet of tumour on the surface of the left cerebral hemisphere.

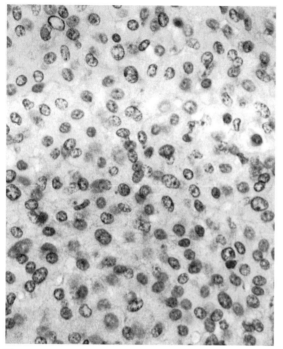

Fig. 15.46 Meningotheliomatous meningioma. This is composed of sheets of cells of arachnoidal type. (H & E.)

there are often compact groups of closely packed smaller cells within the tumour. The cells in a *fibrous* meningioma are characteristically elongated, and reticulin is conspicuous throughout the tumour. The classic feature of a *transitional* meningioma, which is probably the commonest type, is the presence of whorls composed of concentrically arranged cells (Fig. 15.47), often with small blood vessels in their centre. Cell whorls are very similar in appearance to normal arachnoidal granulations. There is a tendency to believe that cell whorls are always present in a meningioma. This is not so, and if the diagnosis is in doubt electron microscopy is helpful (Fig. 15.48). The whorls often become calcified, when they are referred to as psammoma bodies and, if they are numerous, the tumour is distinctly gritty on section and it is then referred to as a *psammomatous* meningioma (Fig. 15.49). In an *angiomatous* meningioma there are many vascular channels of varying size, usually with thick hyaline

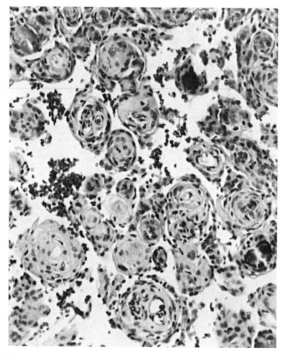

Fig. 15.47 Transitional meningioma. Within the tumour there are numerous cell whorls (cf. Fig. 15.4). (H & E.)

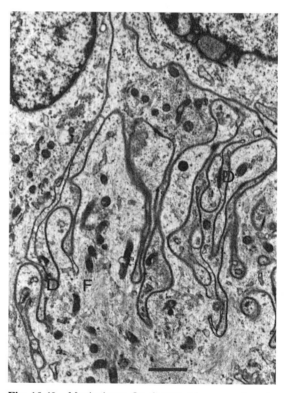

Fig. 15.48 Meningioma. On electron microscopy there is marked interdigitation of adjacent cells. There are also some desmosomes (D) and cytoplasmic filaments (F). (Bar = 1 μm.)

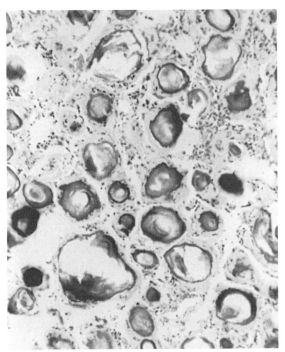

Fig. 15.49 Psammomatous meningioma. Within the tumour there are numerous foci of calcification. (H & E.)

MESENCHYMAL NON-MENINGOTHELIAL TUMOURS

Benign neoplasms

Tumours such as *lipomas* and *fibrous histiocytomas* may affect the menginges. Their appearances are similar to those elsewhere in the body.

Malignant neoplasms

Haemangiopericytoma

Because of certain macroscopic similarities to meningioma, this tumour was known in the past as the haemangiopericytic type of meningioma. Its behaviour, however, was rather different and its appearances are identical to those of haeman-giopericytoma elsewhere in the body. It is composed of sheets of plump polygonal cells with poorly defined cell boundries (Fig. 15.50). There are many thin-walled vascular channels of varying size and there is a dense network of reticulin throughout the tumour. Foci of necrosis, accu-

walls. Among the blood vessels the cells tend to be similar to those seen in meningotheliomatous meningioma.

Although meningiomas are essentially benign, any type may occasionally metastasize, usually to the lungs. This is usually attributed to invasion of a venous sinus by the tumour, or to the shedding of tumour cells into the circulation at the time of operation. Nevertheless, meningiomas can, and often do, infiltrate through the dura into the adjacent bone and, in relation to hyperostosis, groups of tumour cells are seen within the bone. Many meningiomas recur; this may be because of incomplete removal for technical reasons, or it may sometimes be due to the growth of a small satellite meningioma adjacent to the main tumour. Various studies have established how difficult it is to predict when a meningioma is likely to recur, but numerous mitotic figures and foci of necrosis are not good prognostic factors. A pitfall for the unwary is necrosis due to embolization prior to surgery. Anaplastic meningioma is very rare.

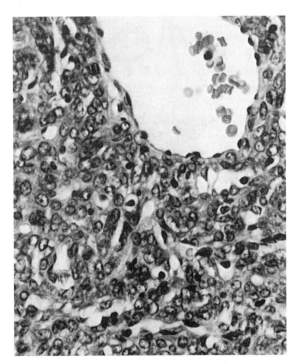

Fig. 15.50 Haemangiopericytoma. Closely packed cells with poorly defined cell margins are in direct continuity with a vascular channel. (H & E.)

mulations of lipid and mitotic figures are usual. The tumour cells are separated from the thin-walled vascular channels simply by a basement membrane.

Meningeal sarcomatosis

This is a very rare type of tumour that takes three principal forms – *fibrosarcoma*, resembling similar tumours elsewhere in the body; *polymorphic cell sarcoma*, which is composed of small, poorly differentiated mesenchymal cells showing some cellular pleomorphism; and *primary meningeal sarcomatosis*, which is a diffuse proliferation of mesenchymal elements in the subarachnoid space. It is often difficult to identify these types of tumour precisely, particularly when they are spreading within the subarachnoid space, but the situation can often be clarified by appropriate immunocytochemical staining.

Primary melanocytic lesions

Primary malignant melanoma can arise from melanocytes in the pia-arachnoid. Most commonly this takes the form of diffuse meningeal melanomatosis (Fig. 15.51) with varying degrees of infiltration into the brain. Rarely, the tumour is a solid greyish haemorrhagic mass growing into the adjacent neural tissue from the meninges. Meningeal melanomatosis is particularly common in patients who have one or more benign pigmented naevi on the skin. This syndrome is known as *neurocutaneous melanosis* (see Ch. 13).

TUMOURS OF UNCERTAIN HISTOGENESIS

Haemangioblastoma (capillary haemangioblastoma), previously considered to be a tumour of blood vessel origin, occurs almost exclusively within the cerebellum in adult life. Occasionally they arise in relation to the caudal brain stem or the cervical cord. The classic type of cerebellar haemangioblastoma consists of a large cyst containing xanthochromic fluid (Fig. 15.52), with a mural nodule of tumour. Sometimes, however, the tumour is a solid mass. The solid areas usually have a distinct yellow colour. They are basically benign tumours but recurrence is not

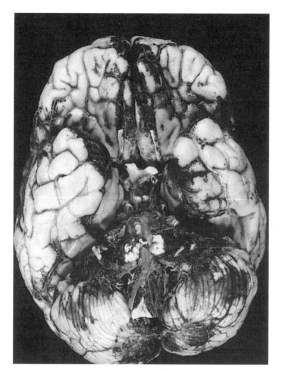

Fig. 15.51 Meningeal melanomatosis. There is extensive infiltration of the subarachnoid space by melanoma.

uncommon, and some recurrent tumours become more aggressive and infiltrate through the craniectomy into the tissues of the scalp. Some patients with a haemangioblastoma also have polycythaemia.

Cerebellar haemangioblastomas may exist as solitary lesions, but they may also be a component of *Lindau's syndrome*, when there may be multiple

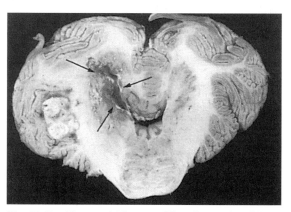

Fig. 15.52 Haemangioblastoma. There is a partly solid and cystic (arrows) tumour within the cerebellum.

haemangioblastomas, similar tumours in the retinae, congenital cysts in the pancreas and the kidneys, and clear-cell tumours in the kidney.

Histological appearances

The tumour consists of a closely packed network of vascular channels of varying size, and a stroma composed of large polygonal cells that are usually distended with lipid (Fig. 15.53). There is a dense reticulin network throughout the tumour.

HAEMOPOIETIC NEOPLASMS

Lymphomas may affect the CNS in several ways, the commonest being compression of the spinal cord by an extradural deposit. Lymphoma can also occur in the extradural and subdural spaces within the skull, and is one of the causes of non-

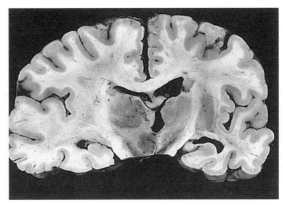

Fig. 15.54 Cerebral lymphoma. There are two masses of tumour within the left thalamus.

metastatic complications of malignant disease (see Ch. 10). Lymphoma, however, also occurs intrinsically within the brain and spinal cord, and in the past was often referred to as micro-gliomatosis; there may be no evidence of systemic lymphoma but in some the brain appears to be affected as part of a generalized process. Intrinsic *cerebral lymphomas* vary greatly in appearance. Some are fairly well defined, rather fleshy masses (Fig. 15.54), whereas others are ill-defined, sometimes rather granular lesions. Occasionally the appearances are very similar to those of astrocytoma, including cyst formation. Multi-centric deposits are not uncommon. Deposits of lymphoma often seem to replace brain tissue rather than to act as expanding lesions; there is therefore often no evidence of a high intracranial pressure.

Histological appearances

The main part of the tumour is usually richly cellular, being composed of round or oval cells with a distinctly lymphoid appearance and usually containing oval or slightly twisted nuclei (Fig. 15.55). Mitotic figures and varying degrees of pleomorphism may be present, and there are sometimes foci of necrosis. Even within the main tumour, tumour cells are particularly dense adjacent to blood vessels. Enlarged astrocytes and hypertrophied microglia are often conspicuous throughout the tumour. The edge of the tumour is very poorly defined, and in the

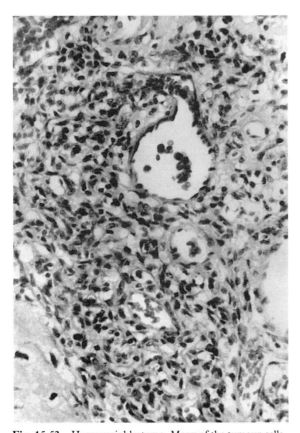

Fig. 15.53 Haemangioblastoma. Many of the tumour cells have clear spaces because of the presence of lipid. (H & E.)

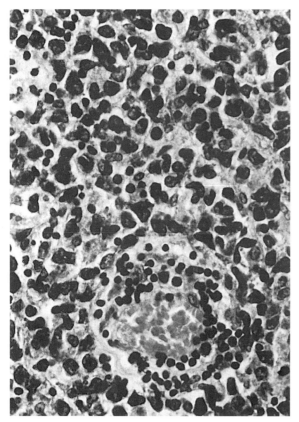

Fig. 15.55   Cerebral lymphoma. The cells are closely packed and many of the nuclei have a distinctly convoluted appearance. (H & E.)

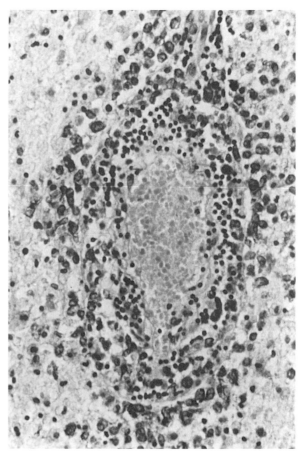

Fig. 15.56   Cerebral lymphoma. Adjacent to the main tumour there are many tumour cells around blood vessels. (H & E.)

immediately adjacent brain blood vessels are surrounded by cells similar to those in the main tumour (Fig. 15.56). A particularly characteristic feature is concentric reduplication of reticulin around the blood vessels within the tumour, and in the blood vessels surrounded by tumour cells in the adjacent brain (Fig. 15.57). Extension into the subarachnoid space is common. Even when macroscopic examination suggests there is only a solitary mass of tumour, histological examination will often show collections of tumour cells around blood vessels in the immediately adjacent tissue and in other parts of the CNS.

In the past considerable emphasis was placed on the fact that a proportion of the tumour cells in an intrinsic cerebral lymphoma would, with silver impregnation, show the staining properties of microglia. It now appears, however, that these cells are reactive and not an intrinsic component

of the tumour. This has been established by immunocytochemical studies, which have indicated that nearly all intrinsic cerebral lymphomas are of diffuse, non-Hodgkin type composed of B lymphocytes. Hodgkin's disease is very rarely seen within the brain.

Meningeal leukaemia

The meninges may be affected in acute leukaemia, in children. There is diffuse infiltration of the meninges by leukaemic cells. The latter are readily identifiable in cytospin preparations (see Ch. 1), hence the importance of routinely monitoring CSF cytology in patients with acute leukaemia.

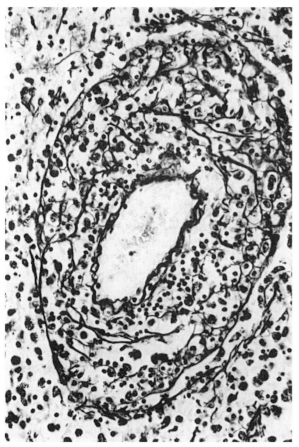

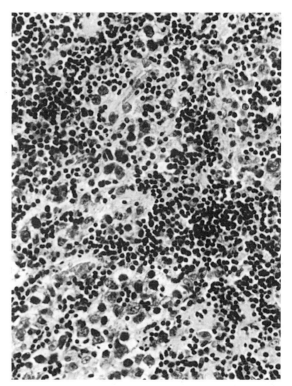

Fig. 15.58   Germinoma. Two cell types are apparent – large round cells and groups of small cells. (H & E.)

Fig. 15.57   Cerebral lymphoma. There is reduplication of reticulin around blood vessels within and adjacent to the tumour. (Reticulin.)

GERM-CELL TUMOURS

The commonest germ-cell tumour is the *germinoma*, a tumour that is virtually restricted to the pineal and hypothalamic regions, where it appears as a grey, rather friable, sometimes focally haemorrhagic mass.

Histological appearances

This tumour is composed of two cell types – large round cells with clearly defined cell margins and relatively large nuclei, and small cells with the appearances of lymphocytes (Fig. 15.58) – and is basically indistinguishable from seminoma and ovarian dysgerminoma. There is often a granulomatous reaction within the tumour.

Other rare germ-cell tumours encountered, almost always in the pineal region, are *embryonal carcinoma*, *choriocarcinoma* and *teratoma*. Immunocytochemistry is of value in defining their hisotogenesis (see p. 274).

CYSTS AND TUMOUR-LIKE LESIONS

A *Rathke's cleft cyst* is a lesion arising within the pituitary gland and often bulging upwards through the diaphragma sella. It is lined by low cuboidal epithelium and is basically an enlargement of the cleft that is normally found in the pituitary gland in lower primates and vertebrates between the anterior and intermediate lobes.

Epidermoid and *dermoid* cysts are the same as similar cysts that occur elsewhere in the body. They occur particularly in the posterior fossa and in the vertebral canal, when there may be a fistula connecting the cyst with the overlying skin. They also occur within the diploe of the skull. They are encapsulated lesions and sharply defined from

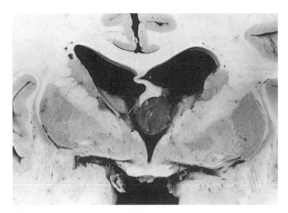

Fig. 15.59   Colloid cyst. There is an encapsulated cyst within the third ventricle.

the adjacent tissue, which they compress. On section they contain grey or white cholesteatomatous material, as a result of which they are sometimes referred to as 'pearly' tumours. The cyst is lined by rather flattened stratified squamous epithelium, with or without skin appendages. There is usually some reactive astrocytosis in the adjacent neural tissue.

Not all epidermoid cysts are developmental, since they also occur in the region of the cauda equina as a result of small pieces of squamous epithelium being implanted there in the course of lumbar puncture, particularly when several lumbar punctures have been undertaken in young children.

Colloid cysts occur in the third ventricle and there is considerable doubt as to their precise cell of origin, since some lie in the lower part of the third ventricle and others near its roof. The cyst is encapsulated (Fig. 15.59) and usually contains green, rather gelatinous fluid. The lining epithelium may be flat, cuboidal or pseudo-stratified, with or without cilia. Sometimes the cells are PAS-positive. A colloid cyst may have an intermittent ball-valve effect on the interventricular foramina, leading to episodes of raised ICP. Not infrequently, however, a patient with a colloid cyst may die within hours as a result of acute hydrocephalus and a high ICP.

Enterogenous cysts are developmental abnormalities that occur within the vertebral canal. If a sinus develops in the midline between endoderm and ectoderm early in gestation, some ectopic endodermal cells may remain within the vertebral canal. The cysts are most frequently lined by epithelium of respiratory type, but cysts of gastrointestinal type are also encountered.

Arachnoid cysts are collections of CSF enclosed within the pia-arachnoid. Their pathogenesis is not clear, but they may attain a considerable size without producing any increase in ICP. The commonest site is adjacent to a Sylvian fissure,

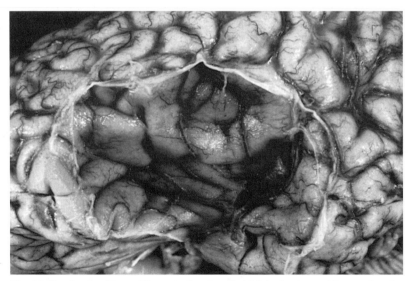

Fig. 15.60   Arachnoid cyst. The cyst, the edge of which is clearly seen, has produced considerable widening of the Sylvian fissure to expose the insula.

when the typical features post mortem are a collection of fluid on the surface of the brain and considerable displacement of the insular opercula, such that the insula may be clearly seen (Fig. 15.60).

Other rare lesions in this group of tumours include *lipomas*, which occur particularly in the hypothalamus and above the corpus callosum; *choristomas*, which are composed of oncocytic or granular cells in the posterior lobe of the pituitary gland; *hypothalamic neuronal hamartomas*, which are nodules protruding from the base of the brain in the region of the mamillary bodies, and composed of a mixture of ganglion cells and astrocytes; and *nasal glial heterotopia* ('nasal glioma'), which is a nodule of ectopic neural tissue in the roof of the nose. The ectopic tissue may be in continuity with the cranial cavity and, if it is thought to be a nasal polyp and removed, there is a danger of post-operative meningitis.

TUMOURS OF THE SELLAR REGION

PITUITARY ADENOMAS

The previous classification of pituitary adenomas was based on the types of cell identified in the anterior lobe of the pituitary gland with conventional staining, namely acidophil, basophil and chromophobe. Acidophil cells account for about 40 per cent of the total cell complement, basophils for about 10 per cent and chromophobes for the remainder. As a result of developments in immunocytochemistry, however, it is now possible to identify specific cells (Fig. 15.61) related to a particular hormone (see Tables 15.3 and 15.4). Electron microscopy has also made a major contribution, in that the numbers and size of secretory granules can be assessed and related to the functional activity of the cell (Fig. 15.62). A particular impetus to these developments in the assessment of pituitary adenomas is the increasing interest in microsurgical techniques for the excision of microadenomas. A full description of the various types of adenoma is beyond the scope of this chapter (see Further Reading).

Pituitary adenomas are benign tumours composed of secretory cells of the anterior lobe of the pituitary gland. These vary greatly in size

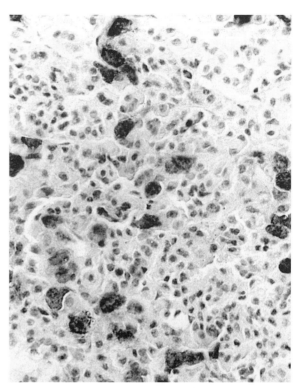

Fig. 15.61 Normal anterior pituitary. The darkly stained cells have reacted with antibody to ACTH. (cf. Fig. 15.63) (PAP.) (Courtesy of Dr Anne Marie McNicol, Department of Pathology, University of Glasgow.)

and appearance, from microadenomas no more than 1–2 mm in diameter (such adenomas occur as an incidental finding in some 10–15 per cent of pituitary glands if they are examined routinely post mortem) to lesions several centimetres in diameter.

The adenomas have two principal effects – hormonal and/or compressive. The former may take the form of increased production of hormone, as in acromegaly or Cushing's disease, or of a reduced secretion of hormones brought about by a non-functioning adenoma replacing the greater part of the anterior lobe. Compressive signs are usually secondary to a suprasellar expansion of the tumour, leading to compression of the optic chiasma (hence the high incidence of defects in the visual fields) and the hypothalamus. The tumour may also extend laterally into the cavernous sinuses.

Table 15.3   Normal anterior pituitary: morphological and functional features

Cell	Hormone	Location	Percentage of cells	Histological staining[a] (H & E; PAS/Orange G)	Immunoperoxidase staining
Somatotroph[b]	Growth (GH)	Lateral wing	50	Acidophilic; PAS (–)	GH
Lactotroph[b]	Prolactin (Prl)	Generalized	15–20	Acidophilic; PAS (–)	Prl
Corticotroph	Adrenocorticotrophic (ACTH)	Mucoid wedge	15–20	Basophilic; PAS (+)	ACTH, β-LPH, α -endorphin
Gonadotroph	Follicle-stimulating and luteinizing (FSH/LH)	Generalized	10	Basophilic; PAS (+)	FSH and LH[c]
Thyrotroph	Thyrotrophic (TSH)	Anterior mucoid wedge	about 5	Basophilic; PAS (+)	TSH

Non-secretory: follicular or stellate cells, primitive precursor cells

[a] The tinctorial characteristics of normal pituitary cells depend upon sufficient cytoplasmic granule storage. If sparsely granulated, cells otherwise functional may appear non-reactive or 'chromophobic'.
[b] Rare acidophilic stem cells (presumed somatotroph- and lactotroph-precursor cells producing both GH and Prl) are present in the normal pituitary.
[c] Many gonadotrophs are capable of producing both FSH and LH, although immunohistochemical and ultrastructural evidence suggests that some gonadotrophs may produce only one hormone.

(Reproduced in modified form with permission from Scheithauer B, Surgical pathology of the pituitary: the adenomas, Part 1. In: *Pathology Annual*, Vol. 19, Part 1. Appleton-Century-Crofts, Conn. USA, 1984, pp. 317–374.)

Table 15.4   Pituitary adenomas: histochemical and immunocytological staining characteristics

Adenoma type	H & E	Orange G	PAS	Immunochemistry
Prolactin cell	C, A[a]	+/–	–	Prl
Growth-hormone cell	A, C[a]	+	–	GH
Mixed growth hormone cell–prolactin cell	A, C	+ or –	–	GH and Prl
Mammosomatotroph[c] cell	A	+	–	GH, strong +; Prl weak +
Acidophil stem cell	C	–	–	Prl +, GH variably +
Corticotroph cell	B, C	–	+	ACTH[b]
Gonadotroph cell	B, C	–	+	Either FSH or LH or both
Thyrotroph cell[c]	B, C	–	+	TSH ±
Null cell	C or A	–	–	None

[a] Sparsely granulated variants appear chromophobic.
[b] b -lipotropin and endorphins also demonstrated.
[c] Rare.
A = acidophilic; B = basophilic; C = chromophobe

(Reproduced in modified form with permission from Scheithauer B.
Surgical pathology of the pituitary: the adenomas, part 1. In: *Pathology Annual*, Vol 19, part 1. Appleton-Century-Crofts, Conn. USA, 1984, pp. 317–374.)

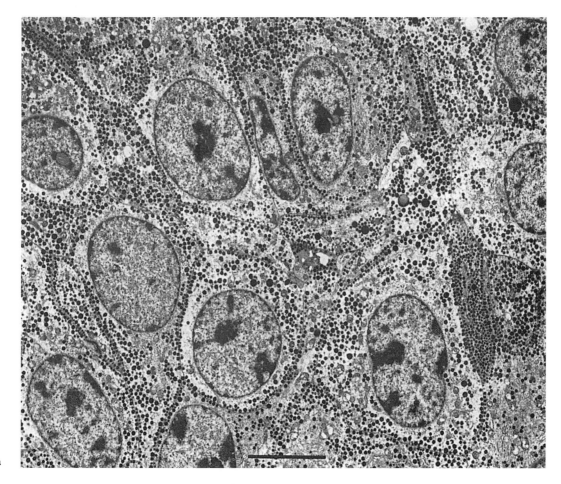

a

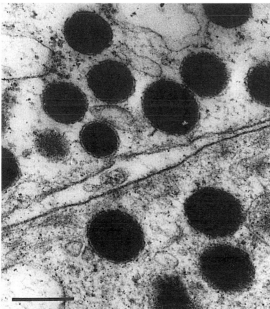

b

Fig. 15.62 Pituitary adenoma. There are numerous intracytoplasmic membrane-bound secretory granules. (a) Bar = 5 μm; (b) bar = 0.25 μm.

Types of adenoma

Depending on the type of cell present, adenomas were in the past classified as acidophil, basophil, mixed or chromophobe. Sometimes there is a good correlation between the histological findings and the clinical syndrome, i.e. the presence of numerous acidophil cells in a patient with acromegaly, and an adenoma composed of chromophobe cells in a patient with panhypo-pituitarism. Immunocytochemical studies, however, have established that many cells that are chromo-phobe by conventional staining stain positively for a specific hormone by immunocytochemical techniques (Table 15.4). Hence the current ability to recognize, for example, prolactin-cell adenomas (a common cause of infertility and galactorrhoea in young women), growth hormone-cell adenomas, mixed growth hormone-cell–prolactin-cell adenomas, corticotrophic adenomas (Fig. 15.63), gonadotroph-cell adenomas and thyrotroph-cell adenomas.

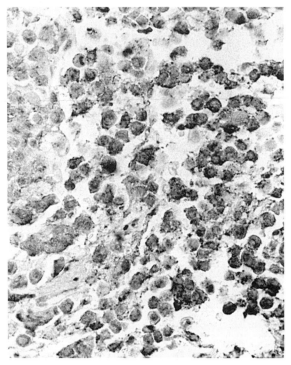

Fig. 15.63 Pituitary adenoma. The great majority of cells have reacted with antibody to ACTH. (PAP.) (Courtesy of Dr Anne Marie McNicol, Department of Pathology, University of Glasgow.)

In some 20–30 per cent of surgically resected pituitary adenomas there is no clinical or biochemical evidence of hypofunction, nor is there any immunocytochemical evidence of functional differentiation. This type of tumour tends to be aggressive, the patient usually presenting either with hypopituitarism or compressive effects. These are often referred to as null-cell adenomas, but some 25 per cent are strikingly acidophilic because of an intense accumulation of mitochondria. This type of adenoma is often referred to as a pituitary oncocytoma.

Histological appearances

These vary greatly. The great majority of adenomas are composed of trabeculae of oval or polygonal cells with single nuclei. In tumours devoid of any evidence of endocrine activity the cytoplasm is often scanty, but in other adenomas there may be a considerable amount of cytoplasm. In active adenomas binucleate cells are frequently present. It is not uncommon, particularly for a non-secreting tumour, to have a distinctly papillary appearance. The stroma varies considerably in amount, but in prolactinomas it often contains amyloid.

Pituitary apoplexy

This is brought about by haemorrhage into, or infarction of, a pre-existing adenoma, and the pathogenesis is not known. The classic clinical presentation is the sudden onset of acute deterioration of vision and headache.

Pituitary carcinoma

This is a rather controversial issue but there are occasional reports of pituitary tumours metastasizing elsewhere in the CNS. On the other hand, there is no doubt that tumours of the anterior lobe of the pituitary can infiltrate into the cavernous sinuses and the base of the skull. Such tumours are probably better referred to as invasive pituitary adenomas.

CRANIOPHARYNGIOMA

This is a tumour arising in the region of the pituitary stalk from ectopic nests of squamous epithelial cells derived from Rathke's pouch, or from cells in the pars tuberalis of the pituitary gland that have undergone squamous metaplasia. It characteristically occurs as a suprasellar mass projecting upwards into the hypothalamus and the third ventricle, and sometimes downwards into the pituitary fossa. It is encapsulated and sharply circumscribed from the adjacent brain tissue. Much of the tumour is usually cystic (Fig. 15.64), the fluid having the colour and consistency of dark engine oil. The solid areas are rather grey or white, and there is usually considerable calcification that can be seen in straight X-rays of the skull.

The solid parts of the tumour are composed of keratinizing stratified squamous epithelium and, despite the apparent encapsulation of the tumour macroscopically, small cell nests are often seen infiltrating for 1 or 2 mm into the adjacent brain. The stratified squamous epithelium undergoes a peculiar change where the individual cells become separated by clear spaces, thus producing appearances similar to adamantinoma (Fig. 15.65). The fibrous tissue stroma is also rather rarefied. Throughout the tumour there are deposits of keratin, cholesteatomatous masses with multinucleated giant cells around cholesterol clefts, and calcification. There can be a quite remarkable degree of reactive astrocytosis in the adjacent brain, such that the appearances of a biopsy taken immediately adjacent to a craniopharyngioma may be very similar to fibrillary astrocytoma.

LOCAL EXTENSIONS FROM REGIONAL TUMOURS

These are summarized in Table 15.1. *Glomus jugulare* tumours present as extradural masses in the cerebellopontine angle. *Chordomas* arising in

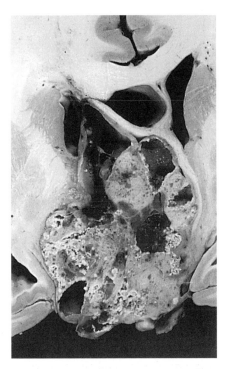

Fig. 15.64 Craniopharyngioma. There is a focally cystic tumour within the hypothalamus.

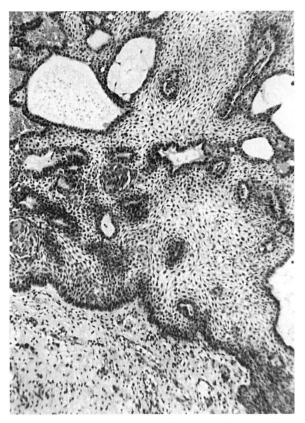

Fig. 15.65 Craniopharyngioma. The tumour is composed of rather dissociated stratified squamous epithelium within which there are cystic spaces. (H & E.)

the clivus produce compression of the brain stem and usually pareses of cranial nerves where they are affected by the tumour as it infiltrates the base of the skull. Sacral chordomas compress the lower spinal cord and cauda equina. *Chondromas* and *chondrosarcomas* can affect any part of the CNS. *Olfactory neuroblastomas* arise in the olfactory bulbs, where they can ultimately act as expanding lesions. *Adenoid cystic carcinoma* occasionally presents as a tumour affecting the temporal lobe, having extended upwards from the middle ear and sinuses. Any nasopharyngeal tumour may spread upwards into the skull.

METASTATIC TUMOURS

As indicated at the start of this chapter, the incidence of metastatic carcinoma in the CNS is difficult to establish. It is, however, common and may be as common or even commoner than neuroepithelial tumours. The primary tumour may be of any type, but there is a particular predilection for small-cell carcinoma of the bronchus to metastasize to the CNS. Metastases occur most frequently in the posterior frontal and parietal regions and in the cerebellum. They are characteristically multiple, but not infrequently a patient presents with what appears to be a large solitary metastasis. Comprehensive histological examination of the brain in such cases, however, will usually disclose the presence of other metastases.

Deposits of metastatic carcinoma are characteristically sharply defined from the adjacent brain tissue (Fig. 15.66). They vary greatly in appearance, some being granular, others gelatinous and others – particularly malignant melanomas– being haemorrhagic. Oedema in the adjacent brain tissue is often very severe, with the result that the effective size of even a small metastasis can be such that there is severe distortion and herniation of the brain and a high intracranial pressure. In contrast, in some patients with multiple metastases, a corresponding amount of brain appears to be destroyed and there is no evidence of a high intracranial pressure.

Another common site for metastatic carcinoma is the extradural spinal space.

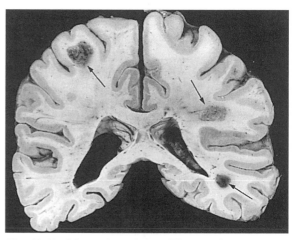

Fig. 15.66   Metastatic carcinoma. There are three metastases (arrows) in this brain slice.

Meningeal carcinomatosis

Neuroepithelial tumours – particularly medulloblastoma – and lymphomas may spread throughout the subarachnoid space, but meningeal carcinomatosis is the commonest type of diffuse meningeal tumour. In the majority of cases there is no other evidence of metastatic carcinoma in the brain. In some cases the tumour cells reach the subarachnoid space by spreading centripetally along cranial or spinal nerve roots, but carcinoma cells usually reach the subarachnoid space by haematogenous spread, possibly via the choroid plexus. It is often possible to identify some thickening and opalescence of the pia-arachnoid, particularly on the superior surface of the cerebellum, such that surface markings on the brain are obscured. There are often small nodules of tumour on the nerve roots of the cauda equina (Fig. 15.67), which also tend to be rather matted together and difficult to separate. Not infrequently, however, the layer of carcinoma cells is so thin that there are no macroscopic abnormalities. Hence the importance of post-mortem screening of the brain from any patient with carcinoma who also has some neurological dysfunction. The great majority of tumours that cause meningeal carcinomatosis are adenocarcinomas.

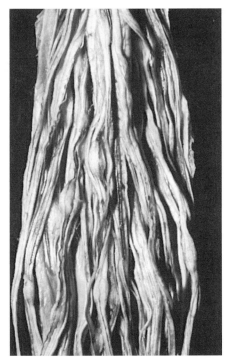

Fig. 15.67 Meningeal carcinomatosis. There are small nodules of tumour on the cauda equina.

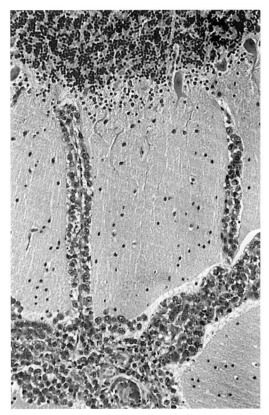

Fig. 15.68 Meningeal carcinomatosis. There are tumour cells within the subarachnoid space and around blood vessels in the molecular layer of the cerebellum. (H & E.)

Histological appearances

Carcinoma cells are seen diffusely throughout the subarachnoid space. They are particularly conspicuous on the surface of the cerebellum, where they often show a tendency to extend into the adjacent cortex along perivascular spaces (Fig. 15.68). It is not uncommon to see a monolayer of cells growing on the pia-arachnoid (Fig. 15.69). The fact that the CSF protein is usually elevated and the glucose is reduced means that the abnormalities in the CSF are similar to those encountered in tuberculous meningitis, but in patients with diffuse meningeal carcinomatosis tumour cells can usually be identified in the CSF, although several specimens may have to be examined.

TUMOURS IN PARTICULAR ANATOMICAL SITES

There are several sites where tumours, whose type can usually only be established histologically, produce particular clinical syndromes.

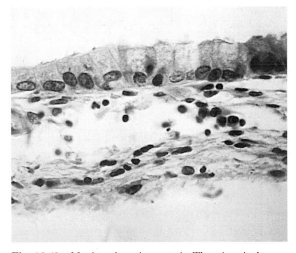

Fig. 15.69 Meningeal carcinomatosis. There is a single layer of columnar cells on the pia. (H & E.)

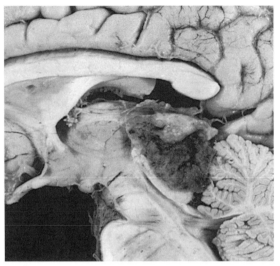

Fig. 15.70   Pineal region tumour. The tectal plate adjacent to the pineal is replaced by metastatic carcinoma (cf. Fig. 15.3).

Pineal region

Some of these arise within the pineal gland and include the germ-cell tumours referred to above (see p. 297). Pineal-cell tumours are rare: they include pineocytomas, which are composed of small, slightly elongated cells with processes often radiating towards blood vessels, and pineoblastoma, which is a highly cellular tumour similar in many respects to medulloblastoma (see p. 286). Other tumours that occur in this region are neuroepithelial tumours, particularly astrocytomas affecting the tectal plate, ependymomas and metastatic carcinoma (Fig. 15.70).

Cerebellopontine angle

Acoustic schwannoma (neurinoma) is by far the commonest tumour encountered in this situation, but meningiomas and metastatic carcinoma may have very similar macroscopic features. Other tumours that may fill the angle include ependymomas, astrocytomas, a haemangioblastoma originating in the cerebellum, epidermoid cysts, and intracranial extension of a glomus jugulare tumour.

Spinal

These may be extradural, intradural and extramedullary, or intramedullary. All produce essentially similar clinical features. The commonest extradural tumours are metastatic carcinoma and lymphoma, including plasmacytoma. Rarer lesions include simple or malignant mesenchymal tumours and angiomas. Intradural extramedullary tumours are usually tumours of nerve sheath cells or meningiomas. Most intramedullary tumours are neuroepithelial (astrocytoma or ependymoma), but metastases also occur.

Suprasellar

Perhaps the commonest suprasellar tumour is the upward extension of a pituitary adenoma. Other tumours that occur in this region include suprasellar meningioma, gliomas in the hypothalamus, craniopharyngiomas, carcinoma of the nasal sinuses, metastatic carcinoma and lymphoma, and chordoma.

Orbital

A wide range of neuroepithelial and non-neuroepithelial tumours may occur in the orbit (see Ch. 16). The former include glioma of the optic nerve and tumours of nerve sheaths, whereas the latter include meningioma, metastatic carcinoma and lymphoma. In some patients the fibro-fatty constituents of the orbit react in an unusual manner to produce the condition known as *pseudotumour*: in some cases the changes are akin to a hypersensitivity reaction, whereas in others there is a sclerosing fibroblastic response.

Intraventricular

Almost any neuroepithelial tumour may protrude into the ventricular system and appear as an intraventricular lesion on CT scanning. Rarely, meningiomas arise in a lateral ventricle. Tumours that can protrude into the third ventricle include pituitary adenoma, craniopharyngioma and germinoma.

FURTHER READING

Adams J H, Graham D I & Doyle D (1981) *Brain Biopsy: the Smear Technique for Neurosurgical Biopsies*. London: Chapman & Hall.

Burger P C, Scheithauer B W & Vogel F S (1991) *Surgical Pathology of the Nervous System and its Coverings*, 3rd edn. New York: Churchill Livingstone.

Franks A J (1988) *Diagnostic Manual of Tumours of the Central Nervous System*. Edinburgh: Churchill Livingstone.

Hovath E & Kovacs K (1986) Identification and classification of pituitary tumours. In: *Recent Advances in Neuropathology*, Vol 3. Edited by J B Cavanagh. Edinburgh: Churchill Livingstone, pp. 75–93.

Rubinstein L J (1972) *Tumours of the Central Nervous System*. Washington, DC: Armed Forces Institute of Pathology.

Rubinstein L J (1986) Immunohistochemical signposts – not markers – in neural tumour differentiation. *Neuropathology and Applied Neurobiology* **12**, 523–537.

Russell D S & Rubinstein L J (1989) *Pathology of Tumours of the Nervous System*, 5th edn. London: Edward Arnold.

Scheithauer B W (1984) Surgical pathology of the pituitary: parts 1 and 2. In: *Pathology Annual*, Vol 19, parts 1 and 2. Edited by S C Sommers and P P Rosen. Conn. USA, Appleton-Century-Crofts, pp. 317–374 and pp 269–316.

Thomas D G T (ed) (1990) *Neuro-Oncology. Primary Malignant Brain Tumours*. London: Edward Arnold.

Vanden Berg S R (1992) Current diagnostic concepts of astrocytic tumours. *Journal of Neuropathology and Experimental Neurology* 51, 644–657.

Weller R O (1990) Tumours of the nervous system. In: *Systemic Pathology*, 3rd edn, Vol. 4. *Nervous System, Muscle and Eyes*. Edinburgh: Churchill-Livingstone pp 427–503.

16. Diseases of the orbit

W. R. Lee

Neoplasms and other mass lesions can be accurately localized in the orbit by modern imaging techniques, but the ultimate diagnosis depends on a surgical exploration and an adequate biopsy. In general, the use of biopsy is restricted to tumours or inflammatory processes in the orbit (pseudotumour) that simulate neoplasia, but it should be appreciated that the biopsy may not be representative. This is due to the difficulties encountered in the exploration of the narrow confines of the apical part of the bony orbit, and the risk of damage to vision by interruption of nerves or division of the ophthalmic artery or vein. If the disease is not successfully cured by wide excision or radiotherapy, the contents of the orbit, with the attached eyelids, will be removed *in toto*. This procedure of orbital *exenteration* (see p. 334) will be required not only for neoplastic diseases, but also for inflammatory processes which have led to exposure and ulceration of the cornea and blindness.

CLINICOPATHOLOGICAL BACKGROUND

Proptosis, visual loss and double vision are the most significant symptoms of orbital disease. The investigation and preoperative assessment of the precise size, shape and location of a space-occupying mass in the orbit have been greatly improved by the application of ultrasonography, computerized tomography and MRI scanning. Although there are many conditions that will not require intervention, those which are encountered most commonly in a diagnostic service are chronic idiopathic orbital inflammatory disease with fibrosis (so-called sclerosing pseudotumours),

vascular tumours, non-Hodgkin's lymphomas, lacrimal gland tumours, and tumours of the optic nerve. Occasionally inflammatory infiltrations such as Wegener's granulomatosis and orbital myositis, either associated with endocrine exophthalmos or an idiopathic non-granulomatous reaction, can simulate a neoplasm. The effects of a space-occupying lesion within the rigid confines of the bony orbital wall may be rapid and serious in terms of visual function. Massive transudation into the conjunctiva and eyelids follows compression of the orbital veins, and irreversible ischaemic damage to the optic nerve or retina causes blindness when the ophthalmic artery or its branches are occluded. Any retro-ocular mass will displace the globe and cause proptosis, and if unalleviated, results in corneal exposure, ulceration and endophthalmitis.

ANATOMY OF THE ORBIT

The following are features of importance in the pathological processes that occur in the orbit.

BONY ORBIT

The superior wall is separated from the frontal lobes of the brain by a thin bony plate, which can easily be penetrated by a sharp object passing into the orbit. Anteriorly the frontal sinus may be the source of an inflammatory process extending into the orbit. The lacrimal fossa is located in the anterolateral bony orbit, and erosion of the bone indicates a potentially malignant extension of a tumour of the lacrimal gland. The inferior orbital wall is easily penetrated by neoplasms arising in the maxillary sinus, and the medial wall, formed by the thin ethmoid bones, is similarly affected when a tumour arises in the nasal cavity or the paranasal sinuses. The lower aspect of the medial wall contains the lacrimal fossa, which surrounds the lacrimal sac and is therefore eroded by extension of inflammatory or neoplastic processes. At the apex of the orbit the optic nerve and the ophthalmic artery pass through the narrow optic foramen. The sensory nerves (V) and the motor nerves (III, IV and VI) to the extraocular muscles enter the orbit in close relation with the ophthalmic vein through the superior orbital fissure. It is in this region that a space-occupying lesion can cause most damage to the blood vessels and nerves.

THE EXTRAOCULAR MUSCLES

The four rectus muscles arise from the connective tissue which lines the optic foramen (annulus of Zinn), and insert into the episclera anterior to the equator of the globe. The aponeuroses of the four muscles unite to form a conical capsule (Tenon's) which ensheathes the globe and the fat which surrounds the optic nerve and the closely related nerves and blood vessels. The superior oblique muscle has an origin from the annulus, but passes through the trochlear at the upper medial orbital rim before turning back to attach to the posterolateral episclera of the globe. The inferior oblique muscle is attached to the anterior part of the inferior wall of the orbit, and the insertion is to the back of the globe on the lateral (or temporal) side just below the midline.

ORBITAL APONEUROSES

Tenon's capsule is surrounded by orbital fat, and this allows smooth movement of the globe within the orbit. Anteriorly, the capsule fuses with a septum derived from the periosteum of the orbital rim and the orbital septum separates the stroma of the conjunctiva from the orbital fat. The septum is condensed in the horizontal plane to form the medial and lateral orbital ligaments. If the septum or ligaments are divided, the eye and extraocular muscles are no longer stabilized and ocular movement is abnormal.

EYELIDS

The eyelids form the anterior boundary of the orbit and serve to protect the anterior surface of the eye.

INFLAMMATORY DISEASE IN THE ORBIT

IDIOPATHIC INFLAMMATION

This is one of the most difficult areas in diagnostic orbital pathology, and in the majority of cases a definitive diagnosis cannot be provided. The disease resembles retroperitoneal fibrosis in terms of the histological features and clinical progression. The clinical presentation usually includes proptosis, pain, chemosis and restriction in movement of the extraocular muscles; the onset can be acute or slowly progressive. The condition may be unilateral or bilateral, and appears to be self-propagating, with dense fibrosis at the end-stage causing total restriction of ocular movements. The term 'pseudotumour' has long been used to describe the chronic non-granulomatous inflammatory process that is observed on histological examination. Predictably, special stains for fungi and bacteria are negative and it has not been possible to identify viral particles using modern technology. In the past, the term 'pseudotumour' was used as an umbrella to include a variety of entities, such as lymphoid pseudotumour, plasma-cell pseudotumour, orbital myositis, lipo-granulomatous pseudotumour and 'sclerosing' pseudotumour. With immunohistochemistry lymphocytic infiltrates can now be classified as reactive or neoplastic, and tumours consisting of plasma cells are either benign solitary plasma-cytomas or orbital manifestations of multiple myeloma. Destruction of orbital fat at the edge of a lesion leads to the formation of a lipogranulomatous reaction, and this almost always represents a secondary response (Fig. 16.1) overlying the primary pathology. If the biopsy is adequate and representative – a mixed inflammatory reaction associated with fibrosis – the conventional diagnosis is 'sclerosing pseudotumour'. There is good reason for the adoption of the term 'multifocal fibrosclerosis' to bring this condition into line with general pathology.

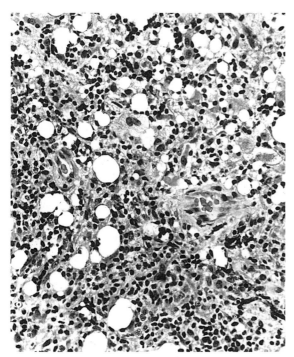

Fig. 16.1 Reactive changes. Foamy macrophages and fat spaces are prominent in a non-specific lipogranulomatous pseudotumour. This reactive change may be seen at the periphery of a primary tumour. (H & E.)

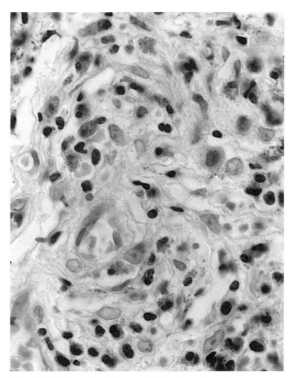

Fig. 16.2 Reactive changes. A lymphocytic and lipomacropyhagic reaction consisting of lipid-containing macrophages adjacent to prominent fat spaces. This histology was seen at the edge of an orbital tumour which was probably a lymphoma, since this disease appeared elsewhere shortly after the orbital biopsy. (H & E.)

Multifocal fibrosclerosis (sclerosing pseudotumour)

This condition is encountered in a biopsy of the orbital soft tissues or in an exenteration specimen at the end stage. The histological pattern consists simply of a mixed inflammatory reaction, which includes focal lymphocytic and plasma-cell infiltration and neutrophil (often eosinophil) polymorphonuclear leucocytes. The banal nature of this cellular change (Fig. 16.2) contrasts with the sinister and sometimes relentlessly progressive clinical course, which can end with bilateral blindness and exposure keratitis. As the disease progresses, the fibroblastic response becomes more prominent and the sclerosing process is accompanied by a peripheral lipogranulomatous reaction in the orbital fat. The extraocular muscle fibres are destroyed by inflammatory cell infiltration and interstitial fibrosis. Progressive orbital fibrosis (Fig. 16.3) interferes with the function of the sensory and motor nerves in the orbit, and can occasionally cause impairment of blood flow to the eye. However, it is important to establish the absence of a necrotizing vasculitis: the identification of this abnormality would indicate Wegener's granulomatosis.

INFLAMMATION IN EXTRAOCULAR MUSCLE

Endocrine exophthalmos

On very rare occasions in a patient with proptosis, the laboratory tests for hyperthyroidism are negative, and the ophthalmologist may elect to biopsy an extraocular muscle which is swollen on CT scan. The presence of clusters of lymphocytes between the muscle bundles (lymphorrhages) (Fig. 16.4) is strongly suggestive of endocrine

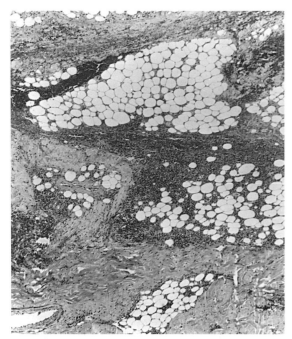

Fig. 16.3   Orbital pseudotumour. At the end-stage of progression in an orbital pseudotumour there is dense fibrous tissue containing clumps of lymphocytes around orbital fat. (H & E.)

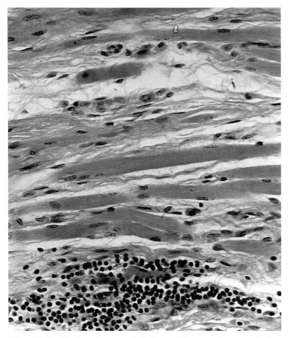

Fig. 16.4   Endocrine exophthalmos. Extraocular muscle in endocrine exophthalmos contains lymphorrhages and an accumulation of alcianophilic connective tissue between the fibres. The muscle fibres are in part atrophic. (H & E.)

exophthalmos. The spaces between the muscle fibres are enlarged by deposition of Alcian blue-positive mucopolysaccharide initially, but later in the disease there is replacement fibrosis.

Biopsy of extraocular muscle is rarely, if ever, considered ethical in patients with unilateral (15 per cent) or bilateral exophthalmos. Diagnosis is usually made by abnormally high values for triiodothyronine and thyroxine, and low values for thyroid-stimulating hormone. It should be noted, however, that patients with exophthalmos and ophthalmoplegia may be euthyroid according to biochemical tests. The demonstration of uniform swelling of the extraocular muscles on CT scanning is probably the most valuable confirmation of endocrine exophthalmos.

The pathologist will also encounter this disease in autopsy material. The orbital tissues should be removed *in toto* and dissection of the fat will demonstrate swollen extracular muscles. Histology of the extraocular muscles demonstrates perivascular lymphocytic infiltration with mast cells and mucopolysaccharide accumulation within and around muscle fibres. As the disease progresses there is replacement fibrosis between the muscle fibres. Study of the nerves at the orbital apex will reveal loss of larger axons in the motor nerves: this is attributed to compression by the swollen muscle.

The pathogenesis of the disease remains poorly understood, but it is accepted that genetic factors are important (HLA antigens BW35 and DR-3 are related) and that the disease is autoimmune in nature.

Acute orbital myositis

In children this condition may be bilateral and may involve more than one muscle, but commonly in adults only one extraocular muscle is affected. Proptosis can be accompanied by congestion of the conjunctiva, when the inflammation extends along, the tendinous insertion of the extraocular muscles and ocular movements are painful or limited. CT scanning reveals localized swelling of the muscle and the diagnosis is confirmed by a rapid and sustained response to steroids. A diagnostic biopsy is usually unnecessary but a persistent

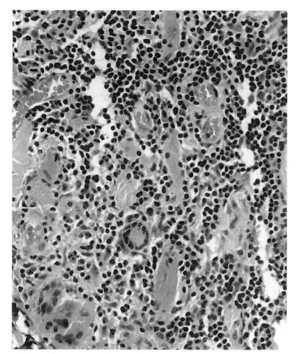

Fig. 16.5   Orbital myositis. Massive lymphocytic infiltration between the muscle fibres is characteristic of acute orbital myositis. The multinucleate giant cells are probably derived from the muscle fibres. (H & E.)

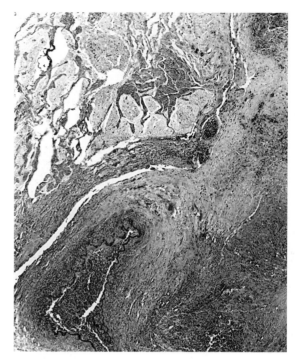

Fig. 16.6   Orbital apical syndrome. The bundles of axons in the optic nerve have undergone infarction and there is chronic inflammation in the wall of the ophthalmic artery. The adjacent fibro-fatty tissue is infiltrated by inflammatory cells. (H & E.)

squint may require correction, and in tissue from this source there is an intense inflammatory reaction between the muscle fibres (Fig. 16.5). Without treatment the disease progresses to fibrous replacement of the muscle.

Orbital apical syndrome (Tolosa Hunt syndrome)

On rare occasions, and without any preceding or related disease, a non-granulomatous inflammatory reaction occurs in the apex of the orbit and in the nerve sheath, and in this location the effects of compression on blood vessels and nerves are serious. Retro-ocular pain and visual loss are the principal symptoms. Pathological examination reveals a non-specific chronic inflammation in the tissues and a vasculitis that is accompanied by infarction of the optic nerve (Fig. 16.6).

SPECIFIC INFLAMMATORY DISEASE

Bacterial infection: orbital cellulitis

Acute bacterial infection of the orbit is a well recognized clinical event, but it is unlikely that the disease will be encountered in routine histopathology. Such infections may be blood-borne or may spread from adjacent sinuses. In current practice granulomatous infection due to syphilis, tuberculosis or *Klebsiella rhinoscleromatosis* (rhinoscleroma) is virtually unknown.

Fungal infection

Aspergillosis

Infection by *Aspergillus* sp. was in the past a recognized complication of infection via the nasal cavity or the paranasal sinuses, presenting as proptosis and visual loss. The giant-cell granulomatous reaction to large branching septate hyphae of uniform diameter (identifiable even in H & E preparations) is diagnostic.

Mucormycosis

Mucor sp. acts as an opportunistic infection in patients who coincidentally suffer from poorly controlled diabetes mellitus or are immuno-compromised. In the past, the disease was well recognized as a cause of necrosis of the nose in undernourished children. In adults there is a unilateral proptosis which progresses to affect both orbits and involves the nasal cavity. Biopsy reveals a dense non-granulomatous reaction around the hyphae, which are most easily identified in the walls and lumina of thrombosed blood vessels. The PAS stain will demonstrate widespread hyphae in the orbital tissues, many of

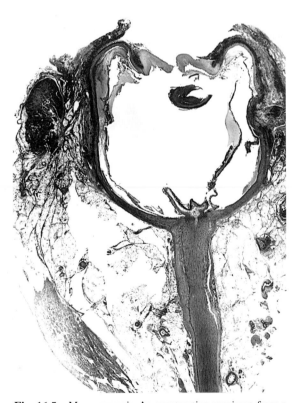

Fig. 16.7 Mucormycosis. An exenteration specimen from a patient who ultimately died of mucormycosis. The branches of the posterior ciliary arteries are filled with fungal hyphae and the cornea is ulcerated as a consequence of ischaemic infarction of the anterior segment with secondary infection. (H & E.) (Section by courtesy of Professor F. Stefani.)

which show the changes of infarction (Fig. 16.7). The organism is larger than *Aspergillus* and *Candida* spp. and can be identified with certainty by marked variation in the dimensions of the hyphae. The only available treatment in the past was radical surgery, and the outlook was poor. Treatment with antifungal agents has been encouraging, and better responses have been described in recent reports.

Parasitic infections

Infestation by intestinal nematodes (*Ascaris* and *Strongyloides*) and hookworms (*Ancylostoma Necator*) is a rare affection of the eye, and even more rarely the orbit. *Taenia échinococcus* infestation leads to the growth of a hydatid cyst (containing scolices) in the orbit and the cyst can sometimes be as large as the globe, so that proptosis may be severe.

Inflammatory reactions due to ruptured cysts

Haematic cyst

A haematoma in the orbit (spontaneous or post-traumatic) may progress to the formation of an expanding tumour-like mass with erosion of bone. In some cases the diploic bones are the source of bleeding. Histology from the curetted tissue reveals a haemogranuloma with prominent iron deposition and a giant-cell granulomatous reaction to cholesterol crystals (Fig. 16.8).

Mucocoele

A cystic evagination of the mucosa of a paraorbital sinus may pouch into the orbit and present as an orbital tumour. On macroscopic examination an excised mucocoele will show, cystic tissue with a thickened wall. On histological examination the cystic space (Fig. 16.9) is lined by flattened, but sometimes recognizable, stratified upper respiratory tract epithelium. Haemorrhage and fibrosis may complicate the histology of the wall of the mucocoele. This is usually a condition of elderly patients with a history of sinusitis, but it has been reported in younger patients with an allergic diathesis.

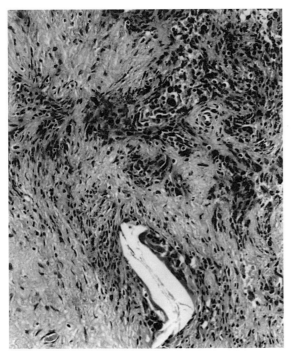

Fig. 16.8 Haematic cyst. The wall of a haematic cyst contains cholesterol clefts within a fibrous and chronic inflammatory reaction in which iron-containing macrophages are prominent. (H & E.)

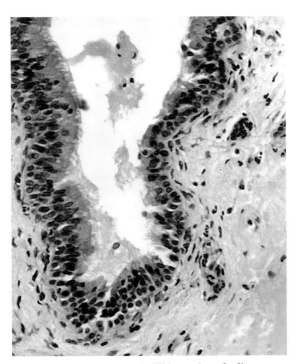

Fig. 16.9 Orbital mucocoele. This consists of a fibrous capsule lined internally by columnar epithelial cells which are atrophic in parts. (H & E.)

Dermoid cysts

These are encountered in the deeper tissues of the eyelid and, in children, excision may be necessary to exclude the possibility of a more sinister orbital neoplasm, particularly if there is spontaneous rupture and an inflammatory process leads to a rapid increase in size. The intact cyst is lined by stratified squamous epithelium with pilosebaceous follicles in the wall. Rupture of the cyst gives rise to a giant-cell granulomatous reaction to keratin (Fig. 16.10). The cysts may also occur in the bony wall of the orbit.

Sarcoidosis

This condition may present as an inflammatory mass in the orbit, and the lesion is usually located in the region of the lacrimal gland. Histological demonstration of non-caseating granulomas within the orbital fat (Fig. 16.11) is adequate for a firm diagnosis. A biopsy is rendered unnecessary by a positive gallium scan, a positive Kveim test and a raised level of angiotensin-converting enzyme in the serum.

Amyloidosis

So-called amyloid tumours occur as a rarity in the orbit. Middle-aged or elderly patients are

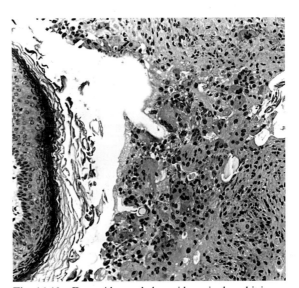

Fig. 16.10 Dermoid cyst. A dermoid cyst in the orbit is lined by stratified squamous epithelium: the cyst wall is broken down in one part to release keratin, with a resultant giant-cell granulomatous reaction. (H & E.)

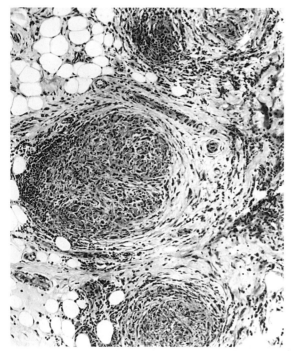

Fig. 16.11   Sarcoidosis. Sarcoid granulomas in the orbital tissues may be surrounded by fibrous tissue or clusters of lymphocytes. (H & E.)

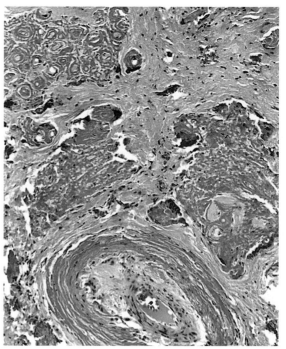

Fig. 16.12   Amyloidosis. In amyloidosis involving the orbit, fat spaces are surrounded by a ring-like deposit and there is a giant-cell reaction to the amyloid protein. The lumen of the vessel is narrowed by the deposition of amyloid. (Sirius red.)

affected. Clinically the mass causes a slowly progressive proptosis. After bisection, the cut surface of the mass has the characteristic waxy texture of amyloidosis. The histological appearance of the nodules of acellular eosinophilic material may be characteristic, but variants include deposition of amyloid in the form of rings around fat cells, in addition to deposition in the walls of blood vessels. Multinucleate giant cells and calcification may also be found (Fig. 16.12). Lymphocytes and plasma cells occur in clusters in the surrounding tissues.

Wegener's granulomatosis

Although the lungs, the orbitonasal tissues and the kidneys are involved in this destructive granulomatous inflammatory disease, ulceration of the anterior sclera and cornea presents a serious management problem for ophthalmologists, as does an orbital pseudotumour which may be a further complication. Necrotizing arteritis and venulitis with fibrinoid necrosis are essential

features for the histological diagnosis of Wegener's granulomatosis. This is accompanied by areas of smudgy necrosis containing nuclear dust in the orbital fat and fibrous tissue. The areas of necrosis may be surrounded by palisaded (epithelioid) macrophages with multinucleate giant cells, which can have a triangular appearance (Fig. 16.13). The demonstration of anti-neutrophil cytoplasmic antibodies in the serum can be a useful additional diagnostic tool in this condition.

Idiopathic midline destructive disease (IMDD)

Previously termed lethal midline granuloma, this condition resembles Wegener's granulomatosis without renal and pulmonary involvement. Formerly the clinical and pathological features in the orbit were regarded as being essentially the same as in classic Wegener's granulomatosis. As information has accumulated, it now appears that in many cases the idiopathic midline destructive

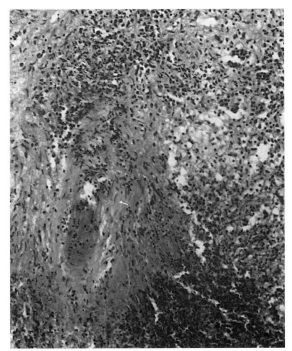

Fig. 16.13 Wegener's granulomatosis. The muscular arteries are blocked by fibrin thrombi and there is smudgy necrosis within the blood vessel wall and the surrounding tissue. The macrophages are arranged in palisades. (H & E.)

disease precedes the development of a histiocytic lymphoma or a diffuse T-cell lymphoma which involves skin, lymph nodes, liver and spleen. The feature which should give rise to suspicion of a malignant lymphoma is the nuclear architecture of the infiltrating histiocytes, which is markedly abnormal in terms of infolding and chromatin distribution. Biopsies may be superficial to the primary orbital disease, and anterior orbital inflammatory reactions should be interpreted with caution.

LYMPHOHISTIOPROLIFERATIVE DISORDERS

GENERAL

Jakobiec and his colleagues have made a major contribution to the classification and pathogenesis of benign and malignant lymphoid proliferation in the orbit. It is important to appreciate that, if the lacrimal gland is disregarded, the tissues behind the orbital septum do not normally contain either lymphatics or lymphoid elements. Thus any lymphoid proliferation within the retroseptal part of the orbit could be regarded as primary or metastatic neoplasia. It is not surprising, therefore, that in practice the majority of retroseptal orbital lymphohistiocytic lesions ultimately transpire to be neoplastic, and that the prognosis for survival is worse when the tumour occurs in this location. Conversely, 'preseptal' lymphoid tissue is normally present in the conjunctival stroma, the lacrimal gland and the lacrimal drainage system, and since this is exposed to antigenic stimulation these locations are the site of reactive lymphoid proliferations and can be equated with extranodal lymphohistiocytic proliferations arising in other 'mucosa-associated lymphoid tissues' (MALT).

When systemic disease occurs coincidentally or soon after the presentation of an orbital lymphoma, the process is obviously part of a generalized disease and the treatment and prognosis are those of the primary disease. The most interesting features of lymphomas confined to the orbit(s) are that the disease remains confined to the orbit(s) in many cases, and that the prognosis for all lymphocytic proliferations is relatively good, with a better than 80 per cent survival.

The lymphoid proliferations that are encountered in orbital biopsies can be classified into three broad groups: those in which the characteristics suggest a benign or a reactive proliferation; those in which the proliferation consists of uniform immature lymphocytes; and those that exhibit all the characteristic histological features of small- or large-cell lymphoid malignancy. The diagnosis may be suggested by the relatively slow onset of painless proptosis in an elderly patient and the demonstration of a mass which appears to spread like putty on CT scan. The tumours can occur within orbital fat or within orbital muscle.

In practice, Hodgkin's disease and myeloma only rarely present as isolated orbital tumours, and orbital involvement usually occurs during the course of a systemic disease. Involvement of the orbit in mycosis fungoides is rare, and can be recognized by the presence of hyperchromatic crenated nuclei, which are said to have a cerebriform appearance in this T-cell lymphoma.

Plasmacytomas are encountered from time to time and are usually solitary benign tumours. Presentation in the form of an orbital cellulitis is a rare event.

In multiple myeloma the B-lymphocyte tumour cells are IgM-positive as a rule, but sometimes IgA λ staining is observed.

BENIGN LYMPHOCYTIC PROLIFERATIONS

Lymphocytic proliferations, which are obviously benign to the experienced eye, occur in two patterns. In one there is a predominance of the lymphocytic and plasma-cell component of an inflammatory pseudotumour. In this group, the cellular infiltrate includes macrophages and polymorphonuclear leucocytes of both neutrophil and eosinophil type, and the lymphoid cells are mature without evidence of atypia. In the second group there is a lymphoid proliferation, which may be of follicular type (Fig. 16.14). This is characterized by sheets of uniform small lymphocytes within which follicles containing larger, less mature cells, are easily found. The cells in the follicles may exhibit mitotic activity to a degree exhibited in a reactive lymph node, but the mitotic activity is confined to this region. It is highly likely that tumours with this histological pattern will be anterior in the orbit or will be close to the lacrimal gland. These tumours are polytypic, with T- and B-cell markers, and T-helper cells predominate over T-suppressor cells. With steroid therapy, this disease has a good prognosis.

Kimura's disease

Although presentation in the eyelid is common in angiolymphoid hyperplasia with eosinophilia (Kimura's disease) this benign condition has been included in the differential diagnosis of inflammatory pseudotumour in the orbit. The histology is characterized by a follicular lymphoid reaction, conspicuous infiltration by eosinophil polymorphonuclear leucocytes, and thin-walled blood vessels with swollen endothelial cells (Fig. 16.15).

'Grey zone' lymphoma

It has been traditional in ophthalmic pathology to use the term 'grey zone' lymphoma for lymphocytic proliferations which consist of uniform small cells with a low mitotic rate. The difficulty in assessing the degree of malignancy in such banal proliferations should not be underestimated. The tumours, which are often anterior in location, consist of sheets of small lymphocytes which exhibit little variation in nuclear size and chromatin pattern, and the immunohistochemical studies do not point convincingly to either tumour (the presence of light chains) or a reactive process (polyclonality) (Fig. 16.16). The majority of these tumours, however, are monotypic and will respond permanently to a relatively low dose of irradiation. Jakobiec and Knowles have widened the histological criteria to include a group of tumours in which there is a scattered subpopulation of cells with large hyperchromatic nuclei, and they recommend the term 'atypical lymphoid hyperplasia' as an alternative to 'grey

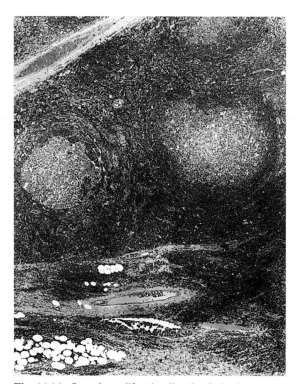

Fig. 16.14 Lymphoproliferative disorder. In benign lymphoid hyperplasia, follicles are obvious at low magnification: the cytological architecture is that of a normal follicular reactive response. (H & E.)

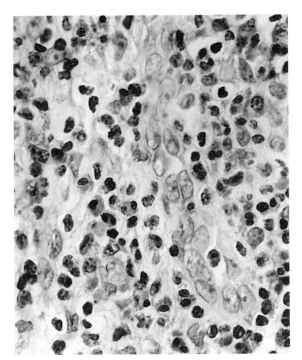

Fig. 16.15 Kimura's disease. Bilobed eosinophils are prominent and the endothelial cells lining the vessels are hyperplastic. (H & E.)

zone' lymphoma. Whatever the name, predictions must be cautious as to the outcome in terms of cure, recurrence or progression to systemic disease in an individual case.

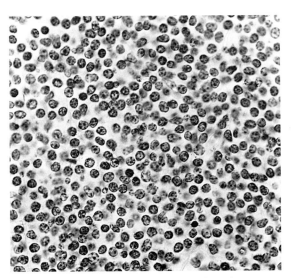

Fig. 16.16 Lymphoma. 'Grey zone' lymphocytic tumours consist of monotonous small lymphocytes of uniform size. (H & E.)

MALIGNANT LYMPHOID TUMOURS

Since there is as yet no agreement among pathologists for the classification of nodal malignant lymphoma, the classifications in ophthalmic pathology for orbital tumours are usually simplified into follicular or diffuse proliferations of atypical lymphoid cells which have a high mitotic rate, and which are either of small, medium or large cell type (Fig. 16.17); and histiocytic large-cell lymphomas (Fig. 16.18), which were previously classified as reticulum-cell sarcoma.

It is not uncommon for retroseptal lymphomas to be predominantly of B-cell type but to have a significant T-cell component. The most recent studies have shown that the majority of the cytologically malignant tumours are monotypic. It should be stressed that malignant lymphomas in the orbit can herald a generalized disease, and this should be excluded by careful systemic screening. The presental tumours contain masses of neoplastic lymphocytes which have a mixed population of polyclonal cells at the periphery. The majority of posterior orbital lymphomas will respond to irradiation at moderate levels (35 Gy),

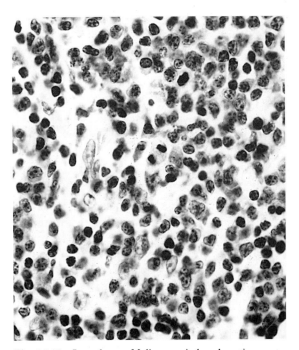

Fig. 16.17 Lymphoma. Malignancy in lymphocytic tumours is recognized by variations in size and shape of the lymphocytes and by mitotic figures. (H & E.)

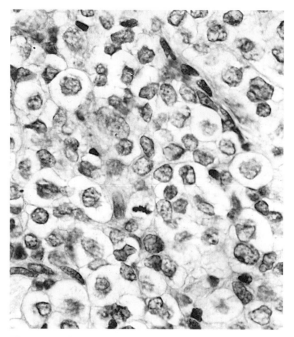

Fig. 16.18 Lymphoma. This is a large-cell lymphoma with a high mitotic rate located in an extraocular muscle. (H & E.)

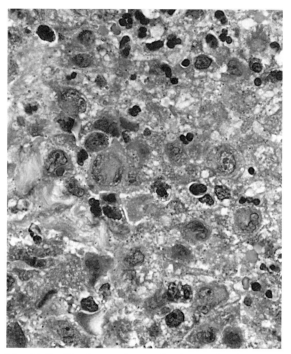

Fig. 16.19 Xanthogranuloma. The characteristic features of juvenile xanthogranuloma include eosinophil leucocytes and multinucleate (Touton) giant cells within a population of lymphohistiocytic cells. (H & E.)

but there are serious complications and the monotypic cytologically malignant tumours have a 50 per cent risk of progression to systemic disease within the subsequent 15 years.

The current explanation for the unpredictable behaviour of lymphoproliferative disorders in the orbit is that some of the tumours which appear to be reactive may harbour clones of neoplastic lymphocytes.

Juvenile xanthogranuloma

Juvenile xanthogranuloma only very rarely occurs in the orbit and the disease usually affects the skin, the iris or the eyelid. The predominantly histiocytic proliferation contains diagnostic multinucleate giant cells with peripheral nuclei (Touton) and foamy cytoplasm. Histology will also reveal an admixture of eosinophil polymorphonuclear leucocytes (Fig. 16.19).

Eosinophilic granuloma

This tumour can be unifocal or multifocal, and it

forms part of a spectrum with histiocytosis X at the malignant end. The histology is that of a histiocytic neoplasm with a scattered infiltrate of eosinophils.

TERATOMAS, HAMARTOMAS AND VASCULAR NEOPLASMS

ORBITAL TERATOMA

Teratomatous cysts in the orbit are lined by epithelia of various embryological origin – intestinal, keratinizing or respiratory etc., and the stroma contains a variety of mesodermal tissues, fat, cartilage and fibrous tissue (Fig. 16.20). Such teratomas are usually massive and unilateral, occurring in the newborn and causing the eye to prolapse between the lids. These tumours are encountered in the form of an exenteration specimen. Abnormalities in the formation of the cranial bones can lead to defects through which heterotopic brain may project.

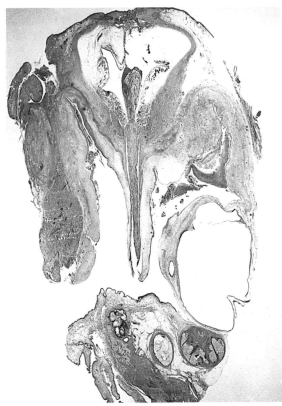

Fig. 16.20   Teratoma. An orbital teratoma which prolapsed the eye and caused exposure keratitis and corneal ulceration. The cystic spaces are lined by squamous epithelium and intestinal villi. (H & E.)

increase in size in later years as a consequence of haemorrhage into the tumour. Haemorrhage into the walls leads to deposition of haemosiderin and a response by macrophages to plasma lipid (Fig. 16.21). Fibrosis may be pronounced and clusters of lymphocytes may be prominent. Channels containing pink-staining lymph indicate a lymphangiomatous component, and there is logic in classifying the large compound tumours as *vascular choristomas*. Lymphangiomas are a well recognized entity in orbital pathology, and cystic hygromas can also occur in the orbit: treatment of the latter with a CO_2 laser is successful.

Capillary haemangiomas are more often located in the eyelid in childhood and tend to regress with time, but the process may be speeded by treatment with steroids, laser therapy or irradiation. The distinction between spontaneous regression and treatment-induced regression is difficult on histological examination, although the request for such an assessment may be made by the clinician managing the case.

Vascular malformations consist of dilated and enlarged orbital veins – 'orbital varix' – or are shown to be 'arteriovenous malformations with shunts'. These masses tend to bleed heavily during surgery, so that intervention is avoided if

VASCULAR HAMARTOMAS

Cavernous haemangiomas are diagnosed with confidence in adults by MRI, and in many cases are not treated. The malformations are relatively common and may be totally or partially excised for cosmetic reasons, or 'debulked' because the physical compression is causing secondary tissue damage to important structures, e.g. the optic nerve or nerves to the extraocular muscles.

Vascular spaces are evident on the cut surface on macroscopic examination of a cavernous haemangioma. Histologically the origin of the tumour from dilated vascular channels is obvious. The walls of the vascular spaces outline with the reticulin stain.

A cavernous haemangioma may occupy the whole or a major part of the orbit and may

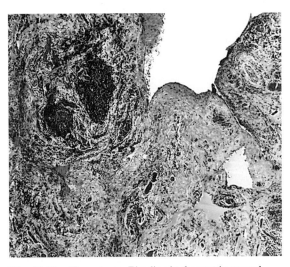

Fig. 16.21   Hamartoma. Bleeding in the matrix around large vascular channels leads to the formation of dense masses of fibrous tissue containing macrophages and other inflammatory cells. (H & E.)

not essential. Histological examination of the excised tissue reveals large venous channels and muscular arteries.

VASCULAR NEOPLASMS

A *haemangioendothelioma* is characterized by proliferation of endothelial cells (Factor VIII-positive) within the spaces surrounded by thin blood vessel walls which are demonstrated by the reticulin stain (Fig. 16.22). The stain is also essential for the diagnosis of a haemangiopericytoma, which is formed by the proliferation of pericytes around normal endothelial cells.

NEURAL TUMOURS

NEUROFIBROMA

A neurofibroma can occur as a solitary tumour within the orbit. Multiple tumours with *café au lait* spots form the major part of the von Recklinghausen's syndrome of diffuse neurofibromatosis (see Ch. 15). As the name implies, this is a tumour of Schwann cells and the fibrocytes of the perineurium. Myelinated nerve fibres are present within the tumour, and these are best demonstrated with stains for axons and myelin or with antibodies against S-100 protein.

The fibromatous component of the tumour may predominate, but myxomatous degeneration can occur within the fibrous matrix. Total excision may be difficult and specimens should be examined carefully for clearance: recurrence of inadequately excised tumours is not uncommon.

There is a very rare variant of neurofibroma, in which the spindle cells transform into rhabdomyoblasts – the *Triton tumour* (Fig. 16.23). This term is derived from the observation that an amphibian, *Trituris*, is capable of regenerating a whole limb from a stump of sciatic nerve. Rhabdomyosarcomas arising in plexiform neurofibromas have a better prognosis than the spontaneous tumours.

Malignant peripheral nerve sheath tumours are rare, but those which arise in the orbit tend to spread to the middle cranial fossa.

SCHWANNOMA

These benign neural tumours grow slowly and are more commonly present in orbital fat rather

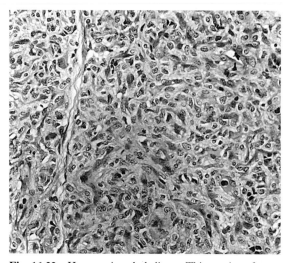

Fig. 16.22 Haemangioendothelioma. This consists of a mass of proliferating endothelial cells around slit-like vascular channels. (H & E.)

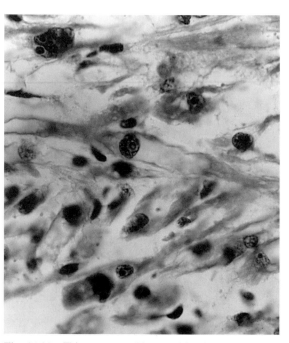

Fig. 16.23 Triton tumour. Pleomorphism is pronounced in this example of rhabdomyosarcomatous differentiation in a Triton tumour. (H & E.)

than in extraocular muscle. The characteristic patterns include spindle cells arranged in a dense palisade around acellular areas or loosely arranged cells in a myxoid matrix. Schwannomas may occur in neurofibromatosis or may be the presenting feature of this disease. Structures resembling a Meissnerian body may be found as a rare variant (Fig. 16.24), although these are more likely to be found in neurofibromas.

PIGMENTED NERVE SHEATH TUMOURS

If a spindle-cell orbital tumour contains melanin, the first assumption is that this represents spread from an intraocular melanoma. Isolated well circumscribed pigmented tumours have, however, been described within the retro-ocular soft tissues, and the prognosis is good after excision. Such tumours can be included with the group of melanocytic nerve sheath tumours. The cells may possess malignant characteristics (Fig. 16.25) and contain melanosomes, but there is a marked tendency for the cell nuclei to form palisades. Further study and documentation is required for a better understanding of the behaviour of this very rare form of tumour in the orbit.

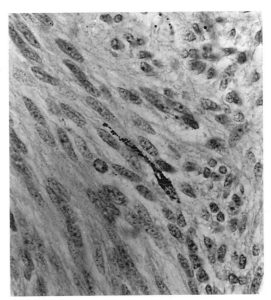

Fig. 16.25   Pigmented nerve sheath tumour. In this melanocytic nerve sheath tumour the spindle cells contain melanin granules. (Masson Fontana.)

ESTHESIONEUROBLASTOMA

The differential diagnosis of a small round-cell tumour in the orbit of a patient of any age should include this diagnosis. This is a primitive neuro-ectodermal tumour of the olfactory bulb.

SOFT TISSUE TUMOURS

RHABDOMYOSARCOMA

This tumour is high on the clinical differential diagnostic list of orbital and eyelid tumours in a child presenting with proptosis. On macroscopic examination the tumour is homogeneously tan-coloured (unless there had been treatment by irradiation). Rhabdomyosarcomas are subclassified into *differentiated*, *undifferentiated* (or *embryonal*) and *alveolar*. The differentiated variant is rarer than the undifferentiated, and the diagnosis is obvious – the pleomorphic malignant rhabdomyo-blasts have eosinophilic cytoplasm which exhibits cross-striations (Fig. 16.26). Some of the cells are elongated to form an obvious strap shape, whereas others have been likened to tadpoles or tennis rackets. Multinucleate cells are a common feature.

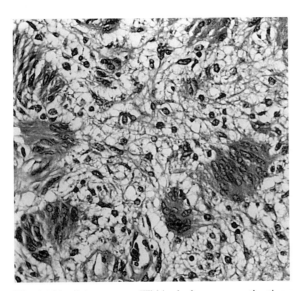

Fig. 16.24   Schwannoma. Within the loose connective tissue (Antoni type B) of a schwannoma there are Meissnerian corpuscles. (H & E.)

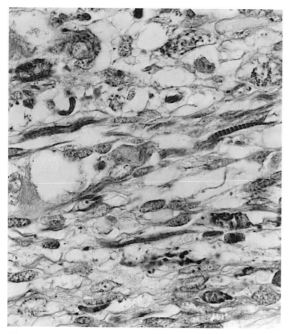

Fig. 16.26 Rhabdomyosarcoma. The characteristic appearances of a well differentiated rhabdomyosarcoma include strap cells with cross-striations and large oval (tadpole) cells. (PTAH.)

Undifferentiated tumours consist of spindle cells in a loose myxoid matrix and the tissue has an embryonal appearance. Rhabdomyoblasts are desmin-positive and on electron microscopy there are clumps of intracytoplasmic myofilaments which often require a long search for identification. Apoptosis is seen as phagocytosis of dead cells by living cells, and the former resemble polymorphonuclear leucocytes.

In an alveolar rhabdomyosarcoma the individual tumour cells have the cytological features of malignant mesenchymal tumours, but the cells tend to line spaces in the connective tissue and these approximate in size and pattern to pulmonary alveoli.

This tumour can be mistaken clinically for an inflammatory process in the orbit, and the diagnosis may be delayed. In the past the prognosis was very poor, even with early recognition, but with pulsed chemotherapy a 50 per cent survival can now be anticipated. Irradiation and/or chemotherapy results in large areas of necrosis within the tumour, but evidence of viability will be found easily as the surviving unaffected cells continue to grow.

MALIGNANT 'RHABDOID' TUMOURS

This group of malignant tumours must be distinguished from rhabdomyosarcoma, with which there is a superficial resemblance. The tumour cells have eosinophilic cytoplasm which contains hyaline bodies (Fig. 16.27) and the staining reaction is positive with cytokeratin and vimentin, but not with desmin. The characteristic ultrastructural feature is the presence of whorls of intermediate filaments in the cytoplasm.

OTHER SOFT-TISSUE TUMOURS

Alveolar soft-part sarcoma bears some resemblance to an alveolar rhabdomyosarcoma, but a confident diagnosis can be made when diastase-resistant PAS-positive crystals are identified in the cytoplasm of the tumour cells (Fig. 16.28).

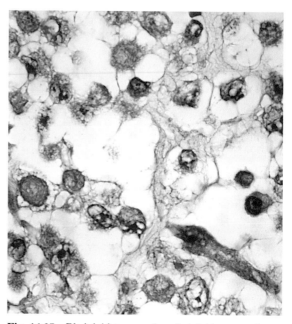

Fig. 16.27 Rhabdoid tumour. In a rhabdoid tumour the cells resemble rhabdomyoblasts and there are filamentous whorls in the cytoplasm. (H & E.) (Section by courtesy of Dr F. A. Jakobiec.)

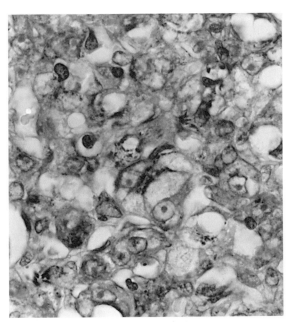

Fig. 16.28 Sarcoma. In an alveolar soft-part sarcoma a diagnosis is aided by the recognition of PAS-positive rod-shaped structures in the cytoplasm of the cells. (PAS.) (Section by courtesy of Professor A. Garner.)

TUMOURS DERIVED FROM BONE-FORMING TISSUE

ORBITAL OSTEOMA

Proptosis may be due to an ovoid mass of compact bone arising in the bony wall of the orbit and projecting into it. This slowly growing benign tumour does not present clinical or pathological diagnostic problems. The difficulty arises on macroscopic examination (Fig. 16.29), when a band saw is required to divide the specimen. The cut surface often reveals an outer layer of compact bone around a central cancellous component. Although in parts histology shows active osteoblastic and osteoclastic activity, with prominent pagetoid cement lines, the cells retain benign characteristics. There is a tendency to recurrence and wide primary excision is to be recommended. An orbital osteoma has been described in Gardner's syndrome (intestinal polyposis, soft-tissue and skeletal osteomas).

RARE BENIGN BONE-FORMING TUMOURS IN THE ORBIT

Reports of benign osteoblastoma, aneurysmal bone cyst and brown tumour appear occasionally in the literature. Accurate diagnosis of these benign tumours of osteoblasts and osteoclasts requires specialist knowledge of orthopaedic pathology.

OSTEOSARCOMA AND FIBROSARCOMA

Highly malignant spindle-cell tumours, with or without bone formation (Fig. 16.30), can occur spontaneously in the orbit. The association of orbital and extraorbital fibrosarcomas and osteogenic sarcomas with the retinoblastoma gene has aroused considerable interest in the genetics of malignancy. In a small percentage of cases of retinoblastoma it is possible to detect a deletion of a gene located on the long arm of chromosome 13 at the q14 locus. The current view is that the gene behaves as a suppressor for malignancy in the neuroblasts in the retina. This concept can be extended to explain the high incidence of fibrosarcoma and osteosarcoma occurring in the second and third decades at sites which have not been irradiated. Children suffering from bilateral retinoblastomas are also at risk of developing a pinealoblastoma (trilateral retinoblastoma syndrome).

TUMOURS DERIVED FROM LIPOCYTES

LIPOMAS

Lipomatous hamartomas may arise from lipocytes in the orbit and can project forwards into the eyelid. The distinction from native or prolapsed orbital fat is far from easy, but infiltration of muscle, for example, can be a helpful sign of the hamartomatous nature of the lesion.

PLEOMORPHIC LIPOSARCOMAS

Primary liposarcomas are usually located behind the globe and are well demarcated on CT scan. Such malignant tumours derived essentially from lipocytes are rare, and can occur at any age. Local

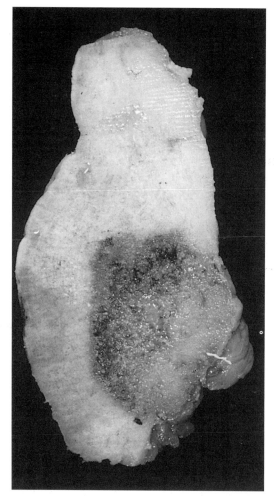

Fig. 16.29 Osteoma. The macroscopic appearances of the cut surface of an osteoma of the orbit.

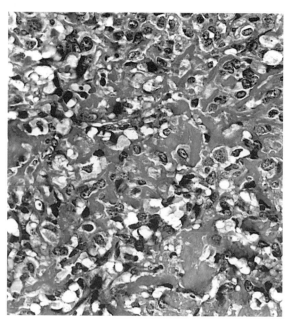

Fig. 16.30 Osteosarcoma. An osteogenic sarcoma is characterized by the presence of pink-staining osteoid between malignant spindle cells. (H & E.)

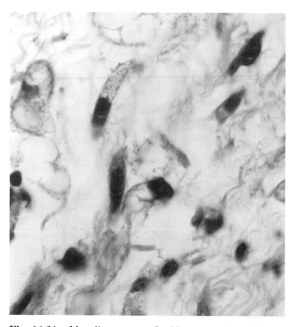

Fig. 16.31 Myxoliposarcoma. In this tumour the malignant lipoblasts with foamy cytoplasm lie within the myxoid matrix. (H & E.)

recurrence is common and the death rate from metastases is about 50 per cent. Microscopic examination reveals a pleomorphic tumour cell with vacuolated lipid-containing intracytoplasmic spaces. The mitotic rate is low, but haemorrhage and necrosis are common features.

PRIMARY MYXOLIPOSARCOMA

This orbital tumour occurs in the fourth to sixth decades. The gelatinous mass invades the para-orbital tissues and the cranial cavity, and the limits are poorly defined on imaging. On macroscopic examination there is no obvious capsule. Local spread is the major problem, and metastatic disease is a late event. On histological examination the tumour cells are of lipoblastic type with small or large intracytoplasmic fat globules and markedly pleomorphic nuclei, and the surrounding matrix is myxoid and Alcian blue-positive (Fig. 16.31). Mitotic figures are sparse and a characteristic vascular pattern in the tumour – so-called chicken-wire appearance – has been described.

TUMOURS DERIVED FROM FIBROBLASTS

NODULAR FASCIITIS

In this tumour the fibroblastic proliferation occurs in a storiform pattern, and the corresponding deposition of a collagenous matrix is particularly well demonstrated with the reticulin stain (Fig. 16.32). The mitotic rate is very low and the uniform appearance of the cells, in addition to the radiating arrangement, is sufficient for a histological diagnosis in this well circumscribed tumour.

FIBROUS HISTIOCYTOMA

Tumours formed by proliferating fibroblasts and foamy histiocytes can be classified as benign or malignant fibrous histiocytomas, according to the degree of cellular dedifferentiation and the mitotic rate. The contribution of the histiocytic cells to the neoplasia has been questioned, so that the diagnosis of malignant fibrous histiocytoma is contentious. Enzinger and Weiss (1988) have used this term as an umbrella for a variety of morphological variants.

A fibrous histiocytoma is similar to nodular fasciitis, however, in that the proliferating fibroblasts tend to grow in a storiform pattern. The presence of large round foamy histiocytes (Fig. 16.33) merits separate classification. The histiocytic component can be predominant in the fibroxanthogranulomatous infiltrate in Erdheim–

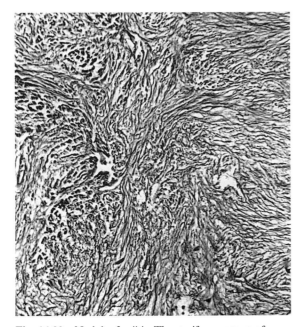

Fig. 16.32 Nodular fasciitis. The storiform pattern of collagen deposition is an important feature of nodular fasciitis. (Reticulin stain.)

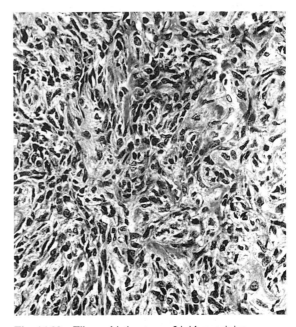

Fig. 16.33 Fibrous histiocytoma. Lipid-containing macrophages are seen between fibroblasts arranged in a radiating (storiform) pattern. (H & E.)

Chester disease, in which the lungs, heart, bones and retroperitoneum are involved, in addition to the eyelids and orbit.

Malignant fibrous histiocytoma is characterized by cytological features of malignancy in the fibroblastic population. The cells vary markedly in size and shape and the nuclear chromatin is irregular. The mitotic rate is high and multi-nucleate cells are prominent (Fig. 16.34). Recurrence is common when this tumour occurs in the orbit and the prognosis is poor.

TUMOURS OF THE OPTIC NERVE

In practice it is important to appreciate that there are only two forms of tumour in the optic nerve: a low-grade pilocytic astrocytoma that occurs in children, and meningioma, which is the common form of neoplasia in adults.

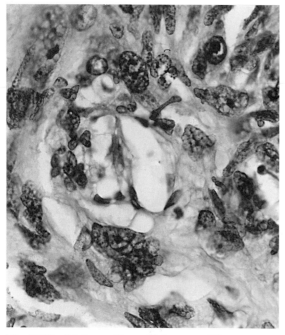

Fig. 16.34 Malignant fibrous histiocytoma. Bizarre multinucleate cells arising from neoplastic fibroblasts are distinctive in this type of tumour. (H & E.)

GLIOMA

Although both juvenile and adult forms of this tumour are recognized, the latter are very rare and invariably lethal. The adult tumour has the pattern of a glioblastoma (see Ch. 15) and is complicated by extensive intracranial spread.

Juvenile gliomas cause visual loss and proptosis, with downward and lateral displacement of the eye; upward movement is markedly limited. The tumour is easily identified by CT scan (which may show a pronounced kink in the nerve) and is usually unilateral, except in individuals suffering from neurofibromatosis. The slow increase in size of intraorbital gliomas is attributed by some authors to water uptake in areas of myxomatous degeneration within the tumour. Although the prognosis is good in the majority of cases, in a small group there has been spread of the glioma to the chiasma and blindness in the opposite eye has followed.

The benign behaviour of the tumour in the majority of cases has led to the practice of excising the affected region of the nerve, leaving the blind eye *in situ*. If the tumour is too extensive, or if there are secondary complications such as exposure keratitis, it is more likely that the eye will be excised with the affected segment of the optic nerve (Fig. 16.35). The cut surface of the fusiform tumour is white and homogeneous, and it is desirable to make the macroscopic dissection so that the sections pass through the centre of the eye and the centre of the tumour. In a localized resection it is important to provide histological evidence of clearance of the nerve at the proximal end, and an orientation suture is to be recommended.

The proliferation of neoplastic astrocytes within the nerve bundles destroys the myelinated axons, but spares the pial septae. The tumour cells are of pilocytic type and have uniform nuclei, but the cytoplasmic extensions form a disorderly array; mitoses are rare. The filaments in the extended processes can be demonstrated with a PTAH stain. The application of immunocytochemistry reveals a positive staining reaction for GFAP, S-100 and vimentin, and with HNK-1 (a marker for type 1 astrocytes). At the ultrastructural level, 10 nm filaments are

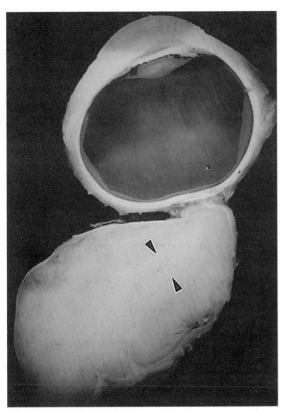

Fig. 16.35   Optic nerve glioma. Macroscopic appearance of an optic nerve glioma. The outline of the optic nerve is barely visible (arrowheads) (× 2).

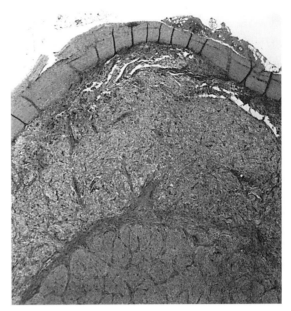

Fig. 16.36   Optic nerve glioma. A glioma causes diffuse thickening of the nerve and reactive arachnoidal proliferation between the pia mater and the dura mater. (H & E.)

present in the cytoplasm of the astrocytes, and the cytoplasm is lined by a basement membrane.

In the matrix, Rosenthal fibres – small irregular glial eosinophilic masses – are an uncommon finding, but areas of myxoid (Alcian blue/PAS-positive) degeneration are frequently seen.

The glioma rarely perforates the dura mater and it is important to appreciate that the tumour induces proliferation in the cells in the arachnoid of the optic nerve. This presents a major problem in the diagnosis of optic nerve gliomas if the surgeon takes a biopsy from the anterior or posterior periphery of the tumour (Fig. 16.36).

The development of mathematical models led to the conclusion that these tumours, generally regarded as low-grade astrocytomas, actually have a very wide but continuous range of growth rate. Some grow rapidly enough to be explained by simple exponential doubling, but most behave as though their growth rate decelerates, a feature that makes comparison of various groups of patients difficult. No support is currently given for the classic hypothesis that these gliomatous tumours are hamartomas.

Tumours of the optic nerve (intracranial as well as intraorbital), however, have an excellent prognosis following complete surgical excision, and only a slightly poorer prognosis following irradiation. About 5 per cent of optic nerve gliomas recur in the chiasma following 'complete' intraorbital excision. Patients with neurofibromatosis have about twice the recurrence rate following an apparently complete excision of an intraorbital glioma. Gliomas of the optic chiasma will respond to irradiation.

MENINGIOMAS OF THE OPTIC NERVE

This tumour may occur within the meninges of

the optic nerve or may arise in the intracranial meninges and spread into the orbit around the nerve. Growth of an optic nerve meningioma is slow in adults, but children may be affected by a more aggressive form. The symptomatology includes visual loss and proptosis, with infero-lateral displacement of the globe. The tumour is identified *in vivo* by CT or MRI, and high-density calcified psammoma bodies within the tumour may be demonstrated. Surgical excision is the treatment of choice and, depending on the location of the tumour, the involved optic nerve may be submitted separately or with the globe attached.

A meningioma may form a tube-like sheath around the optic nerve and the mass can achieve a diameter of 2–3 cm. It may be difficult to find the compressed and atrophic nerve within the tumour if longitudinal sections are taken on macroscopic examination. The nerve is easily found in transverse blocks, but this plane is not optimal if the globe is attached. The histological pattern in the majority of cases is that of a transitional (syncytial) type of tumour, with prominent psammoma bodies (see Ch. 15). Indeed, if the diagnosis of fibroblastic, meningo-thelial or angioblastic meningioma is under con-sideration, then the differential diagnosis should include primary haemangioendothelioma, hae-mangiopericytoma or malignant fibrous histio-cytoma (of angiomatoid type).

LACRIMAL GLAND TUMOURS

NORMAL STRUCTURE

The gland is located in the lacrimal fossa in the upper outer orbit, and is pale brown in colour and ovoid in shape (1.5 cm). It is divided into two parts, orbital and palpebral, by an extension of the levator palpebrae superiores, and the ducts lead into the superolateral conjunctival fornix. The tarsal plate and the stroma of the fornix contain accessory lacrimal glands. The secretory component of the lacrimal gland is formed by lobules containing acini and draining tubules. The acini are formed by cuboidal cells which

secrete the solutes and glycosaminoglycans which are found in the tears. The antibacterial sub-stances lysozyme and lactoferrin are also produced by the acinar cells. Immunoglobulins (IgA and IgM) are formed in the plasma cells lying in the interstitium, and are transferred across the epithelium into the ductular system. The secretions from the acini drain into ductules which are formed by epithelial cells surrounded by a myoepithelium. The large drainage ducts (10–12 in number) are accompanied by blood vessels and lymphatics during their course to the superior fornix. The function of the gland is controlled by sympathetic and parasympathetic nerve fibres, and the blood supply is via the ophthalmic artery.

PLEOMORPHIC ADENOMA

This tumour grows slowly over a period of more than 2 years, and is painless. Enlargement of the lacrimal fossa is by bone erosion rather than destruction, and the clinical features provide strong evidence for the diagnosis. The tumour is surrounded by a fibrous pseudocapsule which contains micronodular extensions of tumour, and it is essential that the tumour is excised widely at the first intervention and not shelled out of the pseudocapsule, since recurrent tumour within the pseudocapsule is in many cases less well differentiated and more aggressive in behaviour.

The cut surface of the excised tumour, which may be 2–3 cm in diameter, often reveals cystic spaces containing mucoid material and areas of haemorrhage. Good sampling of the periphery of the tumour is an important responsibility of the pathologist, and numerous blocks should be taken to assess clearance.

Histological examination reveals duct-like cords and acini of uniform cuboidal cells (Fig. 16.37), which are lined externally by spindle-shaped myoepithelial cells. The acinar lumen usually contains eosinophilic proteinaceous material and the stroma is predominantly fibrous, with alcianophilic myxoid areas, although fat and cartilage may be present; release of material from

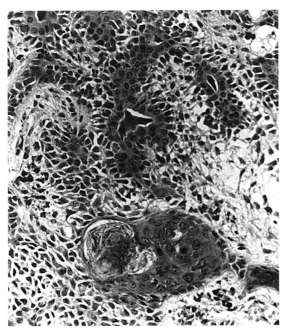

Fig. 16.37   Adenoma of lacrimal gland. In a pleomorphic adenoma the epithelial component is either glandular or squamous, and the myoepithelial cells proliferate to form a loose myxoid stroma. (H & E.)

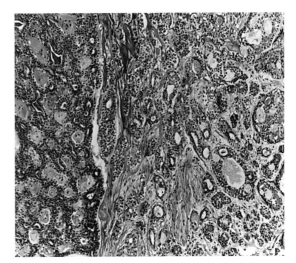

Fig. 16.38   Adenocarcinoma of lacrimal gland. Malignant transformation in a pleomorphic adenoma with loss of glandular architecture and epithelial cell cohesion. (H & E.)

the cysts can stimulate an inflammatory reaction. The stroma is formed by myoepithelial cells which stream out from the edge of the epithelial clusters.

ADENOCARCINOMA

When an adenocarcinoma arises in an adenoma (Fig. 16.38) the event can be recognized by areas of poorly differentiated pleomorphic glandular tissue with a high mitotic rate. The clinical progression of adenocarcinoma of the lacrimal gland is more rapid than that of a pleomorphic adenoma, and pain is a characteristic feature in some cases because the adenoid cystic variant infiltrates sensory nerves. The mass is located in the upper outer orbit and the globe is displaced medially. Adenocarcinomas are radioresistant, so that radical surgery (exenteration) will be required because of involvement of the periosteum and

orbital wall. Thus it is likely that the exenteration specimen will include the superolateral wall of the bony orbit.

Histologically the malignant epithelial cells exhibit a considerable degree of pleomorphism and mitotic activity, although the acinar or tubular characteristics are retained.

ADENOID CYSTIC CARCINOMA

Separate consideration of this variant is justified because the tumour is commoner and growth is faster than that of an adenocarcinoma. Pain and ptosis are a manifestation of the proclivity to invade nerves, and individuals in the first three decades are affected. Various histological patterns are encountered, and the basaloid pattern carries a worse prognosis than the cribriform pattern (Fig. 16.39). Perineural spread and invasion of orbital bone should be features sought in histological examination of the exenteration specimen.

Immunohistochemical studies of the epithelial cells in the benign and malignant tumours of the lacrimal gland have demonstrated a positive

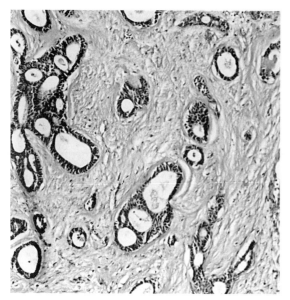

Fig. 16.39   Adenocarcinoma of lacrimal gland. An adenocarcinoma of the lacrimal gland with adenoid cystic transformation. (H & E.)

reaction for keratin. The myoepithelial cells label actin, but not for vimentin.

LYMPHOMAS AND SJØGREN'S SYNDROME

The gland normally contains a significant population of lymphoid cells and is frequently the primary location of a reactive or neoplastic proliferation, which does not differ from those described previously. The term Mikulicz's syndrome is applied when the lacrimal and the parotid glands are involved bilaterally and are enlarged by an inflammatory or neoplastic process. The term Mikulicz's disease is preferred if the patient is suffering from the dry eyes and dry mouth of Sjøgren's syndrome and this is complicated by enlargement of the lacrimal and salivary glands. By accepted definition the lymphoid infiltrate in Mikulicz's disease must be benign, and be accompanied by reactive hyperplasia of the acinar and tubular cells (i.e. benign lymphoepithelial hyperplasia).

LACRIMAL SAC

FUNCTIONAL ANATOMY

Tear fluid drains through the punctae at the medial end of the eyelids and through the canaliculi into the lacrimal sac. The sac is located in the lacrimal fossa in the inferomedial part of the orbit, and the duct leads into the nasal cavity. The canaliculi are lined by stratified epithelium, and the lacrimal sacs by a stratified columnar epithelium.

INFLAMMATORY DISEASE

Dacryocystitis occurs in an acute or chronic form. The latter is of relevance to the histopathologist because the procedure of dacryocystectomy is used for removal of the chronically inflamed sac in the treatment of pain, swelling and epiphora. Excessive watering of the eyes is treated by probing an obstructed sac, and this can lead to the presence of a pyogenic granuloma in the lumen when the mucosa is traumatized. Persistent obstruction is treated by forming a passage between the sac and the nasal cavity (*dacryocystorhinostomy*).

The excised lacrimal sac will be thickened by fibrosis of the wall and mucus in the lumen (mucocoele). Histological examination reveals a variable pattern of lymphoplasmacytoid infiltration and fibrosis. The inflammatory reaction is densest in the submucosa, which is often ulcerated and the epithelium undergoes metaplasia from columnar ciliated with goblet cells to stratified cell type.

Inspissated mucus and polymorphonuclear leucocytes will be found in the lumen, which infrequently contains fungal elements or bacteria or both. The surrounding tissue may contain some fibres from the orbicularis muscle, and these may show a wide variety of reactive non-specific changes.

DACRYOLITH

On most occasions the material within a lacrimal sac is soft, mucoid or mucopurulent. If the contents becomes inspissated and a foreign body such as an eyelash acts as a nidus, a dacryolith is formed and this can be expressed by the ophthalmologist and submitted for pathology. Histology of a dacryolith will reveal a mixed bacterial and fungal infection around an eyelash swathed in layers of mucus.

A solid mass of yellow granular tissue (formed by clumps of actinomyces) may be expressed from the sac in some cases and this is sufficient to effect a cure. Such mycetomas are of interest and the actinomyces are best demonstrated by a Gram stain. These fine, beaded elongated rods are said to branch, but this feature is not easily demonstrable. Usually clusters of large and eosinophilic bar-like crystals are present within the fungal masses, which may also contain bacteria. The nature of the crystalline eosinophilic material is uncertain.

LACRIMAL SAC TUMOURS

Benign tumours of the lacrimal sac epithelium are *unusual*. Malignant tumours are also very rare, and most commonly of poorly differentiated squamous-cell type, although transitional-cell carcinomas are encountered more frequently than squamous carcinomas. The tumour is resected with the lacrimal sac *in toto*, or more widely if there is spread into the orbit. Lymphomas occuring in the region of the lacrimal sac are usually of a reactive type.

METASTATIC TUMOURS

Metastases from carcinomas arising in the breast or the thoracic and abdominal viscera are rarer than those spreading directly from the maxillary or ethmoidal nasal sinuses. Nevertheless, the possibility of a metastasis should always be entertained in a patient who presents with proptosis due to an adenocarcinoma, a squamous carcinoma or an anaplastic orbital tumour, even although at the time of orbital surgery a primary tumour had not been identified. The commonest locations for a 'silent' primary are the oesophagogastric junction, the kidney and prostate or a skin melanoma.

Rather surprisingly, metastatic carcinoid tumours to the orbit have been reported frequently by ophthalmic pathologists. Seminoma of the testis has a tendency to metastasize to the facial bones and the orbit.

In children, metastatic neuroblastoma should always be a consideration and leukaemia (which may be aleukaemic) can elude immediate diagnosis. Granulocytic sarcoma can present in an otherwise healthy child, and with symptoms resembling an inflammatory pseudotumour: the diagnosis is made by the greenish appearance of the tumour at biopsy and histologically by the presence of myeloblastic cells with a high nuclear/cytoplasmic ratio and positive staining for esterase activity.

INTRACRANIAL REMOVAL OF THE ORBITAL CONTENTS POST MORTEM

The eye can be made firm by intravitreal injection of fixative (glutaraldehyde is preferred). The roof of the orbit is removed with a saw and bone forceps. The levator palpebrae is identified, divided and elevated to reveal the superior rectus, which is divided and removed. This exposes the fat within the conus and dissection will identify the optic nerve, which can be isolated as far as the orbital apex where it is divided. The lateral and medial rectus and the oblique muscles can now be identified and dissected, and divided at the apex of the orbit. The eye is separated from the eyelids by cutting through the conjunctiva at the limbus and the fornix from the front with curved scissors. The medial and lateral ligaments are divided and the eye is now mobile and can be pushed back into the orbit. The orbit is packed with cotton wool to prevent collapse of the lids, which can be sutured from the internal surface. An artificial eye can be inserted to provide the best cosmetic result.

If it is necessary to leave the cornea and conjunctiva for cosmetic reasons, the globe can be cut across the equatorial plane, initially with a sharp blade and subsequently with scissors. It will also be necessary to divide the inferior rectus to free the inferior part of the globe. If the anterior part of the eye is left *in situ*, the cavity in the orbit must be filled with cotton wool which is dyed with black ink. With this method it is impossible to tell from the exterior that there has been any interference.

The eye and the attached muscles and fatty tissue should be fixed in formol saline or glutaraldehyde prior to further dissection. Penetration of the orbital fat by the fixative is slow and it is advisable to make a loose dissection of the extraocular muscle to facilitate fluid movement.

THE EXENTERATION SPECIMEN

An exenteration procedure entails surgical removal of the eyelids, the globe, the optic nerve, the extraocular muscles, the orbital fat and the periosteum. The indications for this procedure are most commonly malignant tumours of the eyelid, such as basal-cell carcinoma and squamous or sebaceous-cell carcinomas. If the procedure is a radical excision of an adenocarcinoma of the lacrimal gland, the superolateral bony wall of the orbit will be attached to the orbital tissue. Similarly, if an excision of an ethmoidal tumour is required, or if a (sclerosing) basal-cell carcinoma extends down the medial wall of the orbit, the ethmoidal bones will be included. Radical resections of the maxilla may be extended to incorporate the orbit, but in this case the orbital component will be transferred to the ophthalmic pathologist and another specialist pathologist (dental or ENT) will deal with the maxilla and the main bulk of the tumour.

Orientation of exenteration specimens is easy if a careful description is provided with the request form, but if not, it is useful to remember that the lashes on the upper lid are longer than those on the lower and that the upper lid has a fold. The medial canthus is identified by the caruncle and the punctae.

Frequently the normal anatomy is distorted by the primary pathology and secondary swelling due to inflammation, and a certain amount of intuition is required for proper orientation. The first step is to remove the bony tissues, which may subsequently require several days in a decalcifying fluid. Tumours can be palpated within the soft fibrofatty tissue and the overall dimensions measured approximately. At this stage removal of the fat and superior rectus from the upper part of the orbit will allow the identification of the superior oblique muscle by the tendinous insertion, and dissection of the optic nerve gives a landmark for the first cut. The aim is to get one block which passes just off the centre of the principal lesion and just off the edge of the optic nerve and the pupil. The block thus obtained can be quite large, and there is much to be said for a 24-hour period of secondary fixation for penetration of the orbital fat. It is also advisable to prolong the processing cycle to improve the impregnation of the orbital fat with wax.

For the study of clearance in eyelid tumours, radial blocks should be taken through the eyelids in a systematic manner, going, for example, from lateral to medial along the upper lid, round the inner canthus and then medial to lateral along the lower lid. In the case of an orbital tumour the blocks can be taken in a horizontal or vertical plane to search for tumour extension through the orbital periosteum. The purpose of the exercise is to advise the surgeon or the radiotherapist of the possible sites where there may be a recurrence.

FURTHER READING

Alford E C Jr & Lofton S (1988) Gliomas of the optic nerve or chiasm. Outcome by patients' age, site and treatment. *Journal of Neurosurgery* **68**, 85–98.

Bray W H, Giangiacoma J & Ide C H (1988) Orbital apex syndrome. *Surgery of Ophthalmology* **32**, 136–140.

Bullen C L, Liesegang T J, McDonald T H & DeRemee R A (1983) Ocular complications of Wegener's granulomatosis. *Ophthalmology* **90**, 279–290.

Enzinger F M & Weiss F W (1988) soft tissue tumors. St Louis: Mosby.

Goldberg R A, Rootman J & Cline R A (1990) Tumours metastatic to the orbit: a changing picture. *Survey of Ophthalmology* **35**, 1–24.

Grossniklaus H E, Abbuhl M F & McLean I W (1990)

Immunohistologic properties of benign and malignant mixed tumor of the lacrimal gland. *American Journal of Ophthalmology* **110**, 540–549.

Knowles D M, Jakobiec F A, McNally L & Burke S J (1990) Lymphoid hyperplasia and malignant lymphoma occurring in the ocular adnexa (orbit, conjunctiva and eyelids): a prospective multiparametric analysis of 108 cases during 1977 to 1987. *Human Pathology* **21**, 959–973.

Lee W R (1993) *Ophthalmic Histopathology*. London: Springer-Verlag.

Lee W R & McGhee C N J (1989) Pseudotumours in the Orbit. In: *Recent Advances in Pathology*. Edited by P P Anthony and R N M MacSween. Edinburgh: Churchill Livingstone, pp. 123–137.

Mansour A M, Barber J C, Reinecke R D & Wang F M (1989) Ocular choristomas. *Survey of Ophthalmology* **33**, 339–358.

Marquardt M D & Zimmerman L E (1982) Histopathology of meningiomas and gliomas of the optic nerve. *Human Pathology* **13**, 226–235.

Mauriello J A & Flanagan J C (1989) Pseudotumour and lymphoid tumour: distinct clinicopathologic entities. *Survey of Ophthalmology* **34**, 142–148.

Satorre J, Antle C M, O'Sullivan R *et al.* (1991) Orbital lesions with granulomatous inflammation. *Canadian Journal of Ophthalmology* **26**, 174–195.

17. Diseases of muscle

Janice R. Anderson

Skeletal muscle fibres are highly specialized cells subject to tissue-specific and often hereditary diseases, but muscle is also a large, richly vascular, widely distributed tissue, with high metabolic activity that is adversely affected in many systemic disorders. Secondary changes induced by diseases of the peripheral nervous system underline the essential role of continued neural stimulation to preserve muscle function and integrity.

The interpretation of skeletal muscle histopathology was revolutionized by the advent of muscle enzyme histochemistry supplemented by electron microscopy. However, its description can be baffling and uninformative and muscle pathology often seems shrouded in mystery. This chapter aims to rectify the situation. It attempts not only to describe morphological changes observed in skeletal muscle, but to elucidate pathogenetic mechanisms. It is certainly not encyclopaedic and many rare disorders have been omitted, although others are included where they illustrate a pathological principle.

All cells of the body show only a limited reaction to injury as discerned by light microscopy. Nevertheless, in skeletal muscle cells, the pathological changes frequently distinguish between two broad categories of muscle disease: *myopathic*, where the muscle cell is the primary target of pathological insult, and *neurogenic*, secondary to disease of the nervous system, principally the lower motor neuron. This division is useful, although undoubtedly an oversimplified basic concept. The myopathic category shows a far greater spectrum of morphological change, and encompasses four major clinicopathological categories: relatively static congenital myopathies; progressive genetically determined wasting diseases or dystrophies; inflammatory myopathies; and metabolic disorders.

The new era of muscle histochemistry was followed by the explosion of molecular biology applied to muscle disease. The identification and cloning of genes responsible for several common diseases has already shed new light on their pathogenesis, provided definitive diagnostic tests and accurate antenatal diagnosis. Nevertheless, there is still a major role for an initial diagnosis on muscle histopathology. There is no doubt that in a large proportion of cases the pathologist can quickly provide useful diagnostic information on the basis of routine H&E frozen sections combined with a small number of histochemical stains.

GENERAL COMMENTS

BIOPSY TECHNIQUE

Muscle biopsy, obtained by either needle or open biopsy, is a minor procedure that can be performed under local anaesthesia in most patients, but the specimen can be rendered worthless unless it is rapidly and carefully frozen. Frozen sections are mandatory for enzyme histochemistry, but routine H&E staining is also vastly superior in frozen sections and the measurement of fibre diameter is more reliable. Slow freezing invariably causes ice-crystal artefact, which can obscure genuine pathological changes and mimic a vacuolar myopathy. For diagnostic purposes transverse sections generally yield the most information. Fibre atrophy is one of the commoner pathological changes and fibre size can be accurately assessed from fibre diameter,

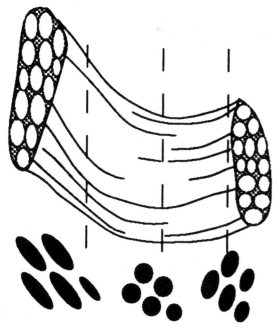

Fig. 17.1   Elongated profiles in oblique sections. True transverse sections are required for accurate comparison of fibre size.

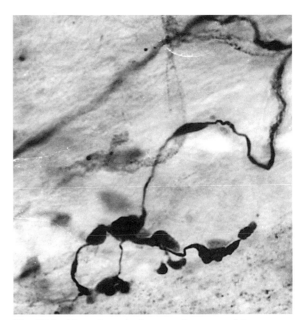

Fig. 17.2   Normal terminal axon and motor endplate. (Methylene blue vital stain.)

but only in genuine transverse sections (Fig. 17.1). A tiny strip should be fixed in glutaraldehyde for electron microscopy and the reserve kept frozen, so that genetic and biochemical investigations can be performed if necessary.

BIOPSY SITE

The site of biopsy is best determined by the clinical picture. A severely wasted muscle in a patient with a chronic disorder should be avoided. A tender muscle may yield a positive result in inflammatory disorders, and electromyographic abnormalities on one side in symmetrical disease may assist localization of an appropriate muscle to biopsy in the opposite limb. CT and MRI scanning are being used increasingly to map the distribution of atrophic muscles and to monitor the progression of wasting. MRI signal intensity also indicates disease activity and may prove valuable in directing the biopsy.

Motor end-point biopsy

The terminal innervation can be demonstrated by methylene blue vital staining (Fig. 17.2) or silver impregnation. Significant abnormalities occur in denervating disease and myasthenic disorders, but unless by chance, axon terminals and motor endplates will only be obtained in a specifically directed motor end-point biopsy.

MUSCLE FIBRE TYPES AND STAINING REACTIONS

A wide variety of enzyme histochemical and tinctorial stains are available, but only a few are necessary for initial screening (Table 17.1). Differences in physiological properties, i.e. differences

Table 17.1

Myosin ATPase*	Fibre typing
Oxidative enzyme e.g. NADH-TR*	Intermyofibrillar network Mitochondria
Gomori trichrome	Ragged red fibres Nemaline rods
Acid-phosphatase*	Lysosomes, macrophages
Periodic acid–Schiff	Glycogen
Oil red O	Lipid

*Histochemical reaction

in twitch speed and fatiguability correlate with differences in enzyme profile of individual muscle fibres. One fibre category may be selectively involved in diseases, and therefore identification of fibre types and variation from the normal pattern are important diagnostic criteria. The myosin adenosine triphosphatase (ATPase) histochemical reaction is the best and most readily reproducible method by which three fibre types can be distinguished in all human limb muscles: slow twitch, fatigue-resistant type 1, and fast twitch type 2 fibres, which are subdivided into 2A with intermediate fatiguability and 2B that fatigue rapidly (Figs 17.3, 17.4 and 17.5). The muscle fibres within a motor unit are of uniform type but fibres from adjacent units are intermingled, creating a normal mosaic pattern in all normal human limb muscles. A fourth type, 2C fibres, are immature fibres found only in fetal, neonatal or regenerating muscle. Other stains give additional information about sarcoplasmic contents, the arrangement of myofibrils and other organelles (Fig. 17.6). Immunocytochemistry to demonstrate dystrophin normally gives uniform linear staining of the cell membrane of every fibre. Immunocytochemical techniques may also be used to identify and type infiltrating lymphocytes and macrophages in inflammatory disease. Electron microscopy is unlikely to detect significant abnormalities if none is evident by light microscopy, but is of particular value in revealing the structure of various cytoplasmic inclusions and confirming the presence of abnormal mitochondria.

Extraocular muscles

Extraocular muscles are richly innervated and have

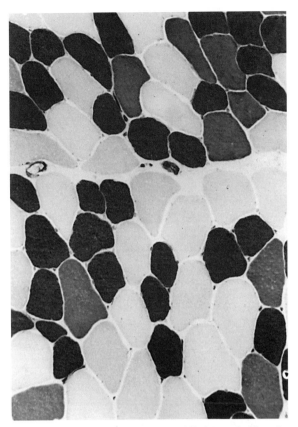

Fig. 17.4 Three fibre types in normal limb muscle. Type 1 fibres dark, type 2A fibres pale, type 2B fibres grey. Type 2 fibres are frequently larger than type 1 fibres in young men. Myosin ATPase reaction at pH 4.6

unique physiological properties which may explain their selective disease involvement and different enzyme profiles from limb muscle. A proportion combine characteristics of type 1 and type 2 fibres and there is a wide normal size variation. Understandably, they are rarely examined in life.

NORMAL PARAMETERS AND BASIC PATHOLOGICAL REACTIONS

Normal human limb muscles show roughly equal proportions of the three fibre types, creating the normal mosaic histochemical pattern (Fig. 17.5). Cross-sections of whole muscle examined at autopsy may show a predominance of one or other fibre in superficial and deep zones, but this is rarely evident in a small biopsy. Fibres are collected into *fascicles* bounded by a thin collagenous *perimysium*. Within

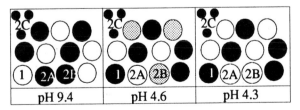

Fig. 17.3 Myosin ATPase reaction distinguishes the major fibre types. At pH 9.4 type 1 fibres are pale and type 2 fibres are dark, whereas this reactivity is reversed at pH 4.3. The type 1 fibres are also dark at intermediate pH 4.6, but at this pH type 2 fibre subtypes can be distinguished: 2A pale, 2B grey. Regenerating 2c fibres are dark at all pHs.

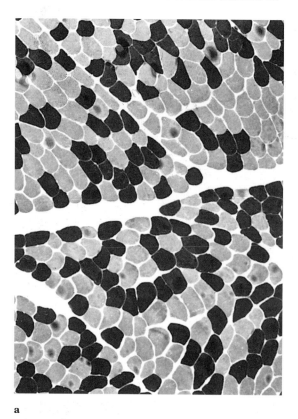

a

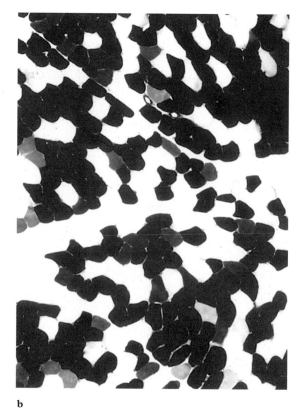

b

c

Fig. 17.5   Myosin ATPase reaction. Serial sections demonstrate the different intensities of staining of the three fibre types after preincubation of the tissue at different pHs. (a) pH. 9.4 (b) pH 4.6. (c) pH 4.3.

the fascicles, although individual muscle fibres are encased by a basement membrane and there is a very fine collagenous scaffold and capillary network, these are inconspicuous and fibres appear closely packed in a frozen section. There are only minor variations in fibre size in normal muscle. The type 2 fibre population is generally larger in athletic males (Fig. 17.4) and the reverse may be seen in sedentary females. Fibres obviously increase in diameter in the growing child and may become smaller with inactivity in old age, but there is a wide normal variation, and size is also affected by freezing. Although accurate measurement has aided the recognition of patterns of atrophy in disease, in diagnostic work obvious disparity in fibre size is usually equally informative.

The multiple nuclei of normal muscle fibres are inconspicuous and peripheral. Oxidative enzyme

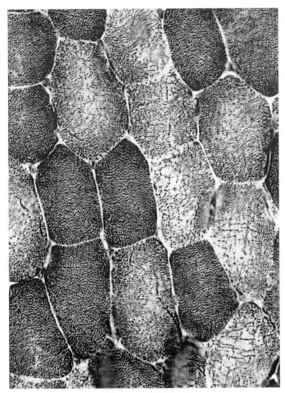

Fig. 17.6 The orderly intermyofibrillar network shown by an oxidative enzyme reaction. Type 1 fibres with higher oxidative enzyme concentration are more darkly stained. (NADH-TR.)

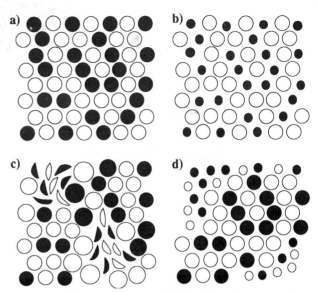

Fig. 17.7 Patterns of atrophy. (a) Normal mosaic pattern: for simplicity, only two fibre types are shown. (b) Selective fibre type atrophy, e.g. type 1 atrophy in myotonic dystrophy. (c) Small group atrophy and compensatory hypertrophy in denervation. (d) Perifascicular atrophy at the periphery of the vascular field in dermatomyositis.

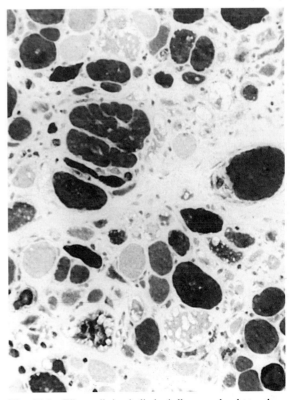

Fig. 17.8 Fibre splitting in limb girdle muscular dystrophy. Two large type 1 fibres appear separated into several tiny fragments. (Myosin ATPase pH 4.6.)

reactions, such as NADH-TR, which stain mitochondria and the intermyofibrillar cytoplasm, highlight normal orderly cytoarchitecture and display disturbances in disease. Fibre atrophy and hypertrophy are common abnormalities in disease and various patterns of atrophy within a fascicle may give a clue to pathogenesis (Fig. 17.7). Hypertrophied fibres frequently show some degree of myofibrillar disarray and may contain central nuclei, often a prelude to fibre splitting. Longitudinal clefts separate the sarcoplasm into small fragments. In transverse section these fit together like pieces of a jigsaw, and are of uniform histochemical type (Fig. 17.8). Increased interstitial fibrous tissue, central nuclei, variation in fibre size and disturbances in fibre architecture are all indicative of disease, except at the site of insertion into a tendon or fibrous septum. Although probably due to repetitive minor injuries at this site, they are a normal finding (Fig. 17.9). Such biopsies are often obtained from corrective orthopaedic procedures

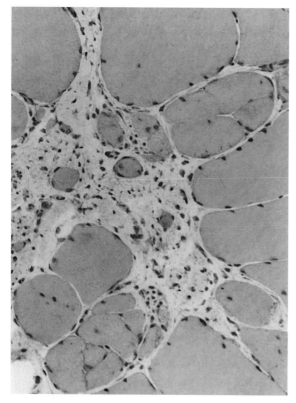

Fig. 17.9   Muscle close to the tendon insertion, showing variation in fibre size, fibre splitting and interstitial fibrosis. Such changes are normal at this site and should not be interpreted as muscular dystrophy.

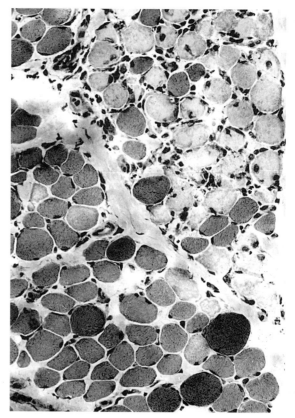

Fig. 17.10   Necrosis in Duchenne muscular dystrophy. Group of pale-staining necrotic fibres. Scattered deeply stained fibres are hyaline hypercontracted fibres. (H & E.)

and should not be interpreted as evidence of a muscular dystrophy. A variety of cytoplasmic inclusions occur in disease, and these are described in relation to individual disorders.

Necrosis and *regeneration* represent the final common pathway of injury in many disorders, including dystrophies (Fig. 17.10) and inflammatory myopathies. Limb muscle fibres are several centimetres long and focal injury generally causes segmental necrosis, followed by segmental regeneration. Hypercontraction, recognized by deeply eosinophilic cytoplasm due to clumped myofibrils, may precipitate necrosis. Striations are lost in the necrotic segment and the cytoplasm appears pale and structureless. Mononuclear phagocytic cells, which rapidly invade and ingest the cytoplasmic debris, are well demonstrated with an acid-phosphatase reaction. The stumps of the undamaged portion of the fibre are sealed by the formation of new

plasma membrane. Undifferentiated mononuclear satellite cells that lie between the basement membrane and sarcolemma are normally impossible to identify by light microscopy, but injury stimulates their proliferation and migration. Regeneration retraces the steps of embryogenesis. The mononuclear cells line up and fuse to form thin basophilic myotubes with large vesicular nuclei, initially at the periphery of the disintegrating segment. As the necrotic debris is removed, so the myotubes fuse together and with the parent fibre to restore normal structure. Until they mature, tiny regenerating fibres show a type 2C histochemical reaction and stain strongly for desmin.

CLINICOPATHOLOGICAL CORRELATION

Morphological changes in skeletal muscle, including fine structural abnormalities, however distinctive, are rarely pathognomonic of a single disorder, and the need for close clinicopathological correlation cannot be overemphasized. Diagnosis of muscle disease based on morphology alone will frequently be wrong and, furthermore, may be responsible for failure to instigate appropriate further investigations.

MUSCULAR DYSTROPHIES

Muscular dystrophies are genetically determined, progressive wasting diseases of skeletal muscle which show different clinical patterns of selective fibre atrophy and rates of progression, but considerable overlap in histology. The slowly progressive dystrophies show many common histological features, but the rapid evolution of the most severe form, Duchenne dystrophy, is reflected in distinctive histology.

DUCHENNE AND BECKER MUSCULAR DYSTROPHY

Duchenne (DMD) and Becker (BMD) muscular dystrophy are sex-linked recessive disorders resulting from different mutations of the same gene on band p21 of the short arm of the X chromosome. Cloning of the DMD/BMD gene and identification of the gene product, dystrophin, was a triumph of molecular biology that elucidated the pathogenesis of these diseases and provided an explanation for the histopathological abnormalities.

Clinical aspects

DMD is a relentlessly progressive wasting disease of muscle, with onset in childhood and an inevitable downhill course. Affected boys become chairbound before 12 years of age and rarely survive beyond 20 years. In contrast, the clinical manifestations of BMD are milder, the progression slower and there is far greater phenotypic variation. Patients with BMD are usually not confined to a wheelchair until at least 15 years of age, and a minority with exceptionally mild myopathy remain ambulant into the fourth decade.

DMD is usually detected clinically between 4 and 6 years of age, when it is appreciated that the apparently clumsy little boy has a genuine physical disability. Clinical examination reveals proximal muscle weakness and mild wasting, but usually hypertrophy of the calves. The latter sign disappears with progression of the disease. The serum creatine kinase is grossly elevated throughout childhood, gradually declining in the teens as the total muscle mass becomes severely diminished. Two-thirds of cases are sporadic, due to new mutations, but where there is a family history and the mother is a carrier, much greater awareness leads to earlier diagnosis. The characteristic histological changes can be recognized in the first year.

Histology

The key histological features are segmental muscle fibre necrosis and regeneration (Figs 17.10 and 17.11). Necrotic and subsequently regenerating

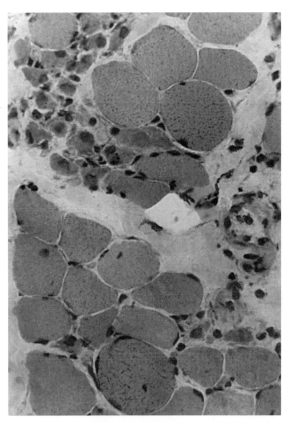

Fig. 17.11 Regeneration in Duchenne muscular dystrophy. Groups of small fibres with large nuclei are regenerating fibres that have basophilic cytoplasm and show type 2C fibre staining reactions with myosin ATPase. The large rounded fibre with a central nucleus is a hyaline hypercontracted fibre. (H & E.)

muscle fibres frequently occur in small clusters. The necrotic fibres frequently contain macrophages phagocytosing cytoplasmic debris, and a careful search also reveals a few isolated, non-necrotic fibres invaded by lymphocytes. The latter are shown by immunocytochemistry to be CD8+ cytotoxic T cells. Apart from occasional small foci of perimysial lymphocytes, inflammatory cells in the interstitium are generally sparse. Uninvolved fibres show a normal internal architecture and a few may be hypertrophied, adding to the low-power impression of excessive variation in fibre size. The calf hypertrophy in childhood is at least partly due to genuine compensatory hypertrophy preceding muscle fibre necrosis. Regeneration fails to keep pace with fibre breakdown and thus progression of the disease is associated with loss of muscle fibres. Endomysial and perimysial fibrosis appear early in the course of the disease, and in advanced disease there is striking fibrofatty replacement of muscle (Fig. 17.12). In addition to pale-staining necrotic fibres throughout the course of the disease,

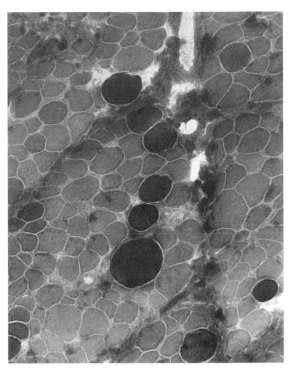

Fig. 17.13 Hyaline hypercontracted fibres stain darkly with Gomori's trichrome.

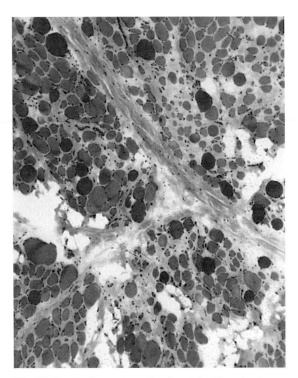

Fig. 17.12 Duchenne muscular dystrophy. Variation in fibre size, hyaline fibres, interstitial fibrosis and fatty replacement. (H & E.)

the biopsy also reveals scattered large, rounded fibres with homogeneous deeply eosinophilic cytoplasm, which also stain darkly with Gomori's trichrome (Fig. 17.13). Fibre typing with the ATPase reaction shows involvement of all fibre types, but the normal clear distinction between types 1, 2A and 2B fibres is blurred by the presence of many regenerating fibres showing a type 2C reaction.

The histopathological changes in BMD are more diverse. The picture may be very similar to DMD, although generally less florid. It is frequently indistinguishable from other mild dystrophies (Fig. 17.14), with variation in fibre size, atrophic and hypertrophic fibres, increased central nuclei, non-specific disturbances of myofibrillar arrangement and mild endomysial fibrosis. A proportion may show only mild atrophy, with small angular fibres suggestive of denervation.

Pathogenesis

The so-called 'hyaline fibres' are in fact hyper-

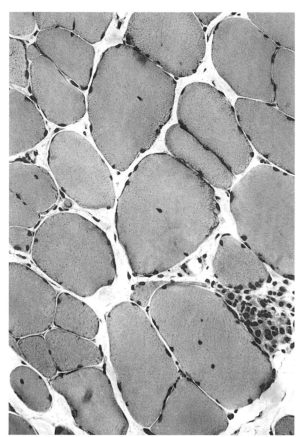

Fig. 17.14   Becker muscular dystrophy. Non-specific myopathic changes: variation in fibre size including hypertrophied fibres with central nuclei, a solitary necrotic fibre invaded by inflammatory cells and a mild increase in endomysial connective tissue. (H & E.)

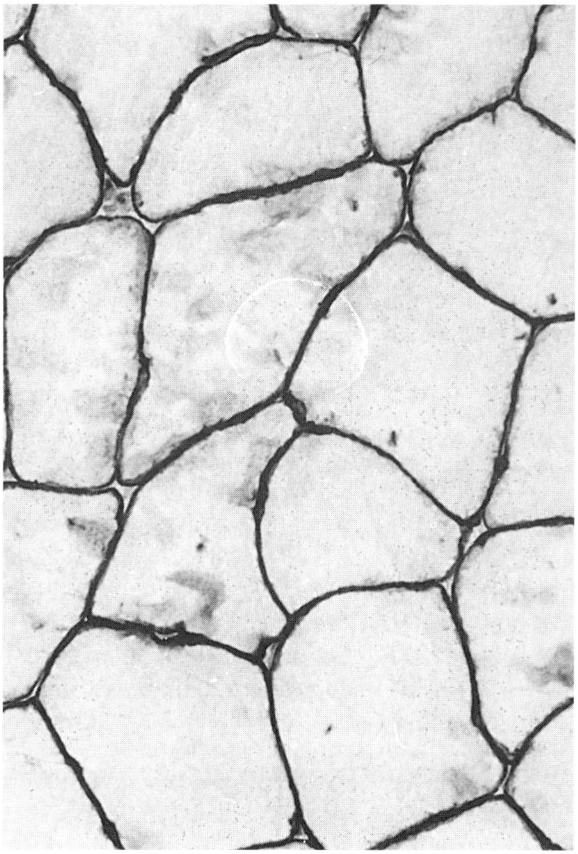

Fig. 17.15   Immunocytochemical reaction for dystrophin. Normal uniform staining of the sarcolemma of every muscle fibre. (Immunoperoxidase method.)

contracted fibres, shown to have an increased calcium ion content. These fibres reflect the fundamental pathological defect in DMD and BMD. Dystrophin is a large rod-shaped protein, localized to the inner surface of the sarcolemma (Fig. 17.15). Its function appears to be to connect the cell membrane internally to the contractile machinery, the actin and myosin filaments, and externally to the basement membrane (Fig. 17.16). Dystrophin is linked to a large glycoprotein complex that spans the sarcolemma and binds to laminin in the extracellular matrix. The arrangement and hinge-like properties of the dystrophin molecules convey a degree of elasticity to the cell membrane and protect its integrity during the contraction and relaxation process. In the absence of dystrophin

small defects may be produced in the cell membrane during contraction. The lesions have long been recognized by electron microscopy in DMD. Focal membrane defects permit an influx of calcium ions which activate myosin ATPase and trigger segmental hypercontraction. Cell membrane injury is exacerbated and the continued influx of calcium ions activates proteases and initiates coagulative necrosis. The complete absence of dystrophin in DMD is readily confirmed by immunoperoxidase staining. Deficiency of dystrophin also causes loss of the dystrophin-associated membrane glycoproteins, thereby weakening the links between the basal lamina and the sarcolemma, such that separation occurs. Loss of basal lamina support may further enhance membrane fragility.

Western blotting shows that in DMD dystrophin

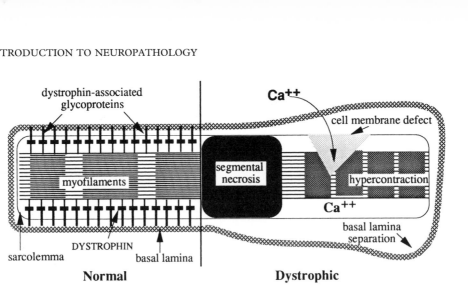

Fig. 17.16 Dystrophin rods in the normal subsarcolemmal location link sarcolemma to myofilaments, and to basement membrane via the dystrophin-associated glycoproteins. Absence of dystrophin reduces flexibility of the sarcolemma, predisposing to breaks during contraction and separation from basal lamina. Sarcolemmal defects allow influx of calcium ions and trigger events leading to segmental necrosis.

is absent or barely measurable (less than 3 per cent of normal levels). Two-thirds of these patients have a deletion or duplication in the very large (2 kb) dystrophin gene, readily detected with the gene probes now available. The remainder may have a point mutation. Dystrophin levels are less drastically reduced in BMD and the majority, including those least affected, show qualitative abnormalities, usually a truncated protein. A plausible explanation for these differences is that DMD is the result of a frame-shift deletion, such that a nonsense sequence is created distal to the mutation, whereas in BMD, despite a deletion, the distal reading frame is maintained and a partially functional protein is translated. This attractive hypothesis of genotype– phenotype correlation explains many, but not all cases, and other mechanisms, such as alternative splicing of exons, may operate. Immunostaining of the muscle biopsy for dystrophin is an important diagnostic aid to the histopathologist. There is no sarcolemmal staining in DMD, but a variable picture is obtained in BMD and in female carriers of DMD/BMD. In the majority of patients with BMD staining is either weak or patchy and a proportion of fibres are negative. As histological changes are far less specific than in DMD, the muscle biopsy of any male with an undiagnosed proximal myopathy should be stained for dystrophin. However, BMD patients with only a small

in-frame deletion or duplication may show normal sarcolemmal immunostaining, and the diagnosis cannot be refuted until Western blotting for dystrophin and gene probing have also been performed.

Several clinical trials have clearly established that steroids improve muscle strength in DMD, although side effects may limit their long-term use. The mechanism of action is still unclear. Although there is no reduction in the numbers of necrotic fibres, the number of cytotoxic T lymphocytes is reduced. Therefore, a possible explanation is that cytotoxic T-cell activity perpetuates the initial fibre injury, and reduction in cytotoxic T cells allows damaged fibres to undergo regeneration.

Female carriers

A minority of female carriers are symptomatic. Any girl with a mild unexplained myopathy should be evaluated as a possible sporadic DMD carrier. Carriers may show minor non-specific abnormalities on biopsy, and most will show a mosaic pattern of immunostaining for dystrophin, attributed to random inactivation of the normal X chromosome in somatic cells. In asymptomatic carriers a small number of negative fibres may be observed, but others may show entirely normal staining. Thus, as with BMD, a single investigation is not reliable. Amplification of lymphocyte RNA by the polymerase chain reaction is a rapid method of detection of deletion and duplication mutations, requiring only venous blood samples and likely to gain widespread use for carrier detection in the future.

Females with a DMD phenotype

A very small number of females have been identified with typical DMD clinical and biopsy abnormalities. These girls all have a karyotypic abnormality involving the X chromosome, in some a translocation with breakpoint in band Xp21. All show absence of dystrophin by Western blotting and immunostaining of the biopsy.

OTHER MUSCULAR DYSTROPHIES

SEVERE CHILDHOOD AUTOSOMAL RECESSIVE MUSCULAR DYSTROPHY

In a comparatively rare autosomal recessive muscular dystrophy, with onset in childhood and DMD-like phenotype and histology, dystrophin is present, but there is a deficiency of a 50kDa protein of the dystrophin-associated glycoprotein complex.

FACIOSCAPULOHUMERAL DYSTROPHY

Facioscapulohumeral dystrophy (FSHD) is a dominantly inherited disorder characterized by progressive weakness of these named muscle groups. However, this clinical distribution is not exclusive to the hereditary disease and, as biopsy shows no pathognomonic features and the genetic abnormality has yet to be identified, the diagnosis is not straightforward. The gene locus has been mapped to the distal long arm of chromosome 4. Diagnostic criteria for FSHD have been defined as: onset of the disease in facial or shoulder girdle muscles, with sparing of the extraocular, pharyngeal, lingual muscles and myocardium; facial weakness in more than 50 per cent of affected family members; autosomal dominant inheritance; and evidence of myopathic disease in muscle biopsy in at least one affected member, without features specific to alternative diagnoses. Obviously, if all these criteria are fulfilled diagnosis is relatively easy, but the information may not be forthcoming. The criteria rely heavily on family data, but it is well known

that patients may not disclose or even be aware of a family history. Minimally affected family members, who may comprise 30 per cent of cases, are unlikely to be detected without thorough neurological examination. Sporadic cases also occur. The age of presentation varies: it is usually in early adult life, but may be in childhood. Facial and shoulder girdle weakness are usually in early adult life, but may be in childhood. Facial and shoulder girdle weakness are usually asymmetrical. The myopathy is associated with progressive deafness, and thus audiometry is a useful adjunct to diagnosis. A retinal vasculopathy has been reported in some families. In the absence of a family history, the diagnosis must rely upon attention to clinical detail and clinicopathological correlation. Biopsy serves to exclude other disorders and can only provide confirmation in an appropriate clinical setting.

Muscle biopsy should obviously be taken from an affected muscle and, despite shoulder girdle weakness, deltoid may be preserved. Thus biceps or triceps may be preferable. The histological abnormalities may be minimal. Variation in fibre size is usually mild. Scattered, angular atrophic fibres frequently occur, which hints at denervation, but they are rarely grouped. Definite grouped atrophy challenges the diagnosis. Necrotic or regenerating fibres are usually isolated and are not numerous. The oxidative enzyme reactions sometimes reveal a lobulate pattern in type 1 fibres, due to focal accumulation of mitochondria and sarcoplasmic reticulum. Large interstitial chronic inflammatory cell infiltrates are an occasional confusing finding which resembles an inflammatory myopathy (Fig. 17.17). Distinction may be difficult without a family history, but the absence of MHC Class 1 expression, except on regenerating fibres, may be helpful. The significance of lymphocytic infiltration is uncertain, but it seems likely that, as in DMD, it is a response to muscle cell degeneration, rather than a cause.

LIMB GIRDLE DYSTROPHY

For many years now it has been acknowledged that limb girdle syndromes are heterogeneous. In the past, cases labelled as limb girdle dystrophy have undoubtedly included many cases of chronic

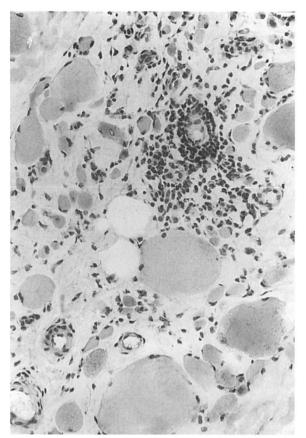

Fig. 17.17 Facioscapulohumeral muscular dystrophy. Excessive variation in fibre size, interstitial fibrosis and an aggregate of chronic inflammatory cells. Inflammation may mimic polymyositis. The dystrophic changes are often far less severe than shown here. (H & E.)

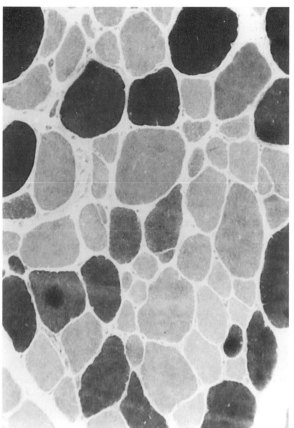

Fig. 17.18 Emery–Dreifuss muscular dystrophy. Excessive variation in fibre size and a suggestion of fibre splitting. (Myosin ATPase pH 4.6.)

spinal muscular atrophy (SMA) and Becker dystrophy. Today, histology alone is an inadequate investigation. Immunocytochemistry, dystrophin assay and genetic analysis are essential for accurate diagnosis. Only when Becker dystrophy and SMA are excluded can the diagnosis of limb girdle dystrophy be entertained.

Familial cases of limb girdle dystrophy are easier to define than sporadic, and both autosomal dominant and recessive genotypes are described. Clinically these patients most often show early adult onset of symmetrical slowly progressive weakness and wasting of pelvifemoral and scapulohumeral muscles. Muscle biopsy can usually be described as 'myopathic', but quite non-specific. There is excessive variation in fibre size, disturbances of

myofibrillar arrangement, but no distinctive cytoplasmic inclusions. Occasional necrotic fibres occur. In the more chronic cases, fibre hypertrophy may be accompanied by fibre splitting (see Fig. 17.8). Fibre atrophy and loss is accompanied by endomysial fibrosis. The tiny fibres derived from splitting may mimic the grouped atrophy of denervation. There is normal sarcolemmal staining for dystrophin. Fine structural abnormalities are equally non-specific.

EMERY–DREIFUSS MUSCULAR DYSTROPHY

This is an X-linked recessive disorder of childhood characterized by the three main features of selective weakness of the proximal arm and distal leg muscles, early contractures and a cardiomyopathy. It has been clearly separated from DMD and BMD by mapping of the gene to a separate locus on the X chromosome. The clinical picture is more specific than the muscle histology, which shows only mild myopathic changes (Fig. 17.18). The cardiac abnormalities are the most sinister, as cardiac arrhythmias may cause sudden death. Recognition of the phenotype may avert early death through cardiac pacing.

OCULOPHARYNGEAL DYSTROPHY

For many years chronic myopathies associated with ptosis and progressive external ophthalmoplegia (PEO) were under a general umbrella of ocular myopathy. It is now clear that there are two entirely separate categories that can be distinguished by histology. PEO is a manifestation of a mitochondrial myopathy, with ragged red fibres. Oculopharyngeal muscular dystrophy (OPMD) is an autosomal dominant disorder of late onset, particularly prevalent in French and French-Canadian families, where PEO is associated with dysphagia and limb weakness. Although limb involvement is generally mild, biopsy is likely to reveal characteristic cytoplasmic rimmed vacuoles. These are large lysosomal structures which, with an H&E stain, show an irregular small vacuole surrounded by a rim of coarse basophilic granules. The granules stain strongly for the lysosomal enzyme acid-phosphatase. The periphery is eosinophilic with Gomori's trichrome. Electron microscopy shows a collection of large membranous whorls, typical of muscle lysosomes, derived from the sarcoplasmic reticulum. The whorls are associated with masses of cytoplasmic filaments (approximately 16–18 nm diameter) that have been shown to be ubiquitinated. In addition, aggregates of finer filaments (8.5 nm diameter) are found in muscle cell nuclei. The nature and origin of both filamentous inclusions are unknown. Apart from variations in fibre size, including scattered angular atrophic fibres, there are no other significant abnormalities. Although the histology is unusual and diagnostically informative, rimmed vacuoles and the cytoplasmic filaments are not pathognomonic of OPMD. They occur in other chronic neuromuscular diseases, particularly inclusion body myositis (see p. 364), emphasizing once again the importance of clinico-pathological correlation.

CONGENITAL MUSCULAR DYSTROPHY

This label is given to muscle disease in infancy showing histological changes that characterize muscular dystrophies in older patients. The disease presents with neonatal hypotonia, weakness and contractures, and often congenital dislocation of the hips. Neuroradiological surveys have disclosed a high frequency of unsuspected CNS abnormalities. Fukuyama dystrophy is a similar condition associated with severe CNS anomalies that is prevalent in Japan. It has been shown to be a separate autosomal recessive disorder by the discovery of abnormally low expression of the dystrophin-associated glycoproteins, (DAGs) although staining for dystrophin is normal. No deficiencies of DAGs or dystrophin have been detected in other forms of congenital muscular dystrophy.

Unlike the congenital myopathies, congenital muscular dystrophy shows endomysial fibrosis and fatty replacement in early infancy (Fig. 17.20). There is usually normal fibre type differentiation but excessive variation in fibre size, due to a combination of atrophy and hypertrophy. The non-Fukuyama form is probably heterogeneous and despite an alarming biopsy the muscle disease may be static and even improve. The contractures may respond to physiotherapy. Autosomal recessive inheritance is suggested by involvement of siblings, but intrauterine infection is postulated as a causative factor. The severity at birth and lack of progression in some cases could be explained by a single intrauterine insult.

MYOTONIA

MYOTONIC DYSTROPHY

Clinical aspects

Myotonic dystrophy (MyD) is a dominantly inherited, progressive disease that is clinically and pathologically quite distinct from the other dystrophies. Myotonia and progressive weakness of the facial muscles are hallmarks of the disorder. They are associated with a variety of systemic abnormalities, including cataracts, premature balding, cardiac arrhythmias and endocrine disturbances.

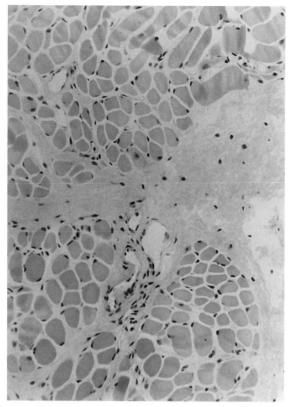

Fig. 17.19 Congenital muscular dystrophy. Endomysial and perimysial fibrosis in muscle biopsy from a 2-year-old child. (H & E.)

The onset of clinical symptoms is usually between 20 and 30 years, although myotonia may cause little inconvenience and is often disregarded by patients until muscular weakness becomes disabling in middle age. Patients with MyD may have cardiac abnormalities – usually conduction defects, and also mitral valve prolapse – and there is a peculiar association with multiple pilomatricomas. The combination of myotonia and clinical weakness is diagnostic, but one or other may be difficult to discern in the early stages. Biopsy from a clinically affected muscle in a typical case shows characteristic histology, but there is wide phenotypic variation, and mild histological abnormalities in minimally affected patients are difficult to assess. This difficulty has been completely resolved by cloning of the MyD gene on chromosome 19q13.3. The mutation responsible for MyD is an expansion of a trinucleotide (CTG) repeat DNA sequence in a gene encoding a protein kinase. The larger the expanded sequence in this unstable DNA the greater is the clinical severity.

Histology

The earliest change in a muscle biopsy is a selective atrophy of type 1 fibres. This is accompanied by type 2 fibre hypertrophy, although there may be a relative paucity of type 2B fibres. Central nuclei are another early feature, initially present in only a small proportion of atrophic type 1 fibres, but later in the majority of type 1 fibres and in many hypertrophied type 2 fibres. In advanced disease, longitudinal sections show very thin, atrophic fibres containing long chains of nuclei. Cytoarchitectural abnormalities, best demonstrated by an oxidative enzyme reaction, also become more pronounced. Motheaten and targetoid fibres may be found, but ring fibres are especially common (Fig. 17.20) and are due to malalignment of myofibrils. Peripheral myofibrils run circumferentially, creating the ring, whereas there is a normal longitudinal arrangement of the innermost myofibrils (Fig. 17.21). Possibly these are an *in vitro* artefact of handling irritable muscle, but nevertheless they are a useful diagnostic finding. Sarcoplasmic masses are another common disturbance in cell architecture. These are sarcolemmal blebs of homogeneous eosinophilic cyto-

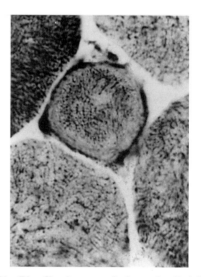

Fig. 17.20 Ring fibre in myotonic dystrophy. Peripheral myofibrils are orientated circumferentially, whereas inner myofibrils show normal longitudinal arrangement.

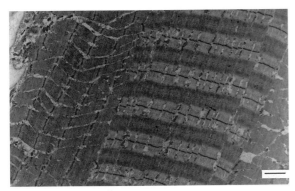

Fig. 17.21   Ring fibre displaying the malaligned peripheral myofibrils. (Bar = 1 μm.)

plasm devoid of myofibrils (Fig. 17.22) that are PAS-positive and show variable oxidative enzyme activity. In advanced disease all myopathic abnormalities become more obvious. There is greater variation in fibre size, greater disturbance in fibre architecture and fibrofatty replacement. Apart from occasional fibres, necrosis is unusual. Wasting in MyD is due to progressive atrophy.

CONGENITAL MYOTONIC DYSTROPHY

Myotonic dystrophy may present at birth in infants born to affected mothers. Although it is an autosomal dominant disorder, the congenital form is transmitted exclusively by the mother, who may herself be only mildly affected or even unaware of her disease. By no means all children born to affected mothers show this early onset. The maternally derived factor modifying the MyD genome is unknown, but the expanded nucleotide sequence is always very large. Pregnancy may be complicated by polyhydramnios. Affected neonates show generalized hypotonia and severe respiratory problems. Those who survive show delay in motor development and are often mentally retarded. Although there is a myopathic facies, clinical myotonia is not detected in early childhood. Moreover, its presence strongly suggests the rarer condition of myotonia congenita. Muscle histology in the neonate is quite different from the adult, and the classic changes evolve during childhood. The neonatal biopsy conveys a picture of immaturity and may resemble myotubular

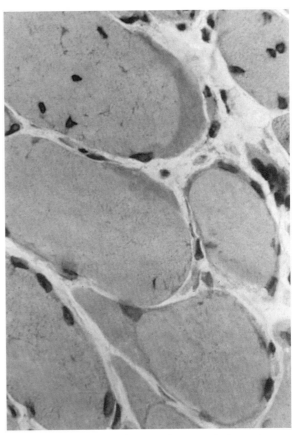

Fig. 17.22   Sarcoplasmic masses in myotonic dystrophy. Peripheral blebs of cytoplasm devoid of myofibrils. (H & E.)

myopathy, as many fibres contain large central nuclei (Fig. 17.23). The majority of fibres have a halo of peripheral cytoplasm, devoid of organelles and therefore unstained by the oxidative enzyme reaction. Although there is variation in fibre size, a situation which is always abnormal in the neonate, selective type 1 atrophy is not present at this stage. Immaturity is described in other organs, including nesidioblastosis and persistence of fetal glomeruli.

OTHER MYOTONIC DISORDERS

Myotonia congenita and paramyotonia congenita are also familial disorders in which patients exhibit clinical myotonia, but are extremely rare in comparison with MyD. Unlike MyD, there is no muscle wasting and myotonia is the dominant clinical

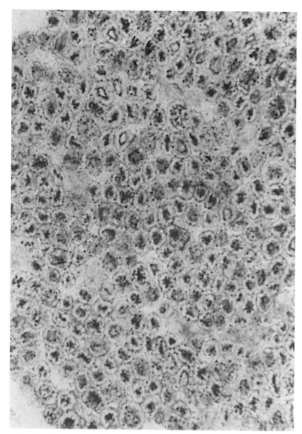

Fig. 17.23 Myotubular myopathy. Peripheral rim of sarcoplasm devoid of myofibrils. Many fibres contain central nuclei and also show absence of myofibrils in the central zone. A similar appearance may be seen in congenital myotonic dystrophy (NADH-TR).

attack contains large cytoplasmic vacuoles, but between times is normal or shows only minor abnormalities. The vacuoles may be present in a large proportion of fibres and appear to be derived from the sarcoplasmic reticulum, as are tubular aggregates, which have a very distinctive electron microscopical picture (Fig. 17.24) and frequently occur in the periodic paralyses.

CONGENITAL MYOPATHIES

The congenital myopathies are a group of disorders that are often familial and present in early childhood. The main features are delayed motor development, hypotonia, proximal muscle weakness and, often, facial weakness. In contrast to progressive muscular dystrophies and the early-onset

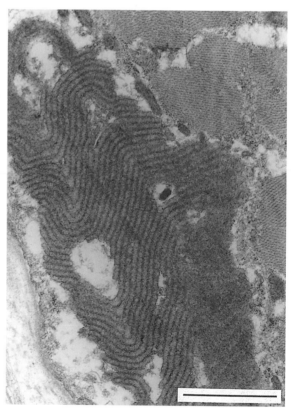

Fig. 17.24 Tubular aggregates. Subsarcolemmal array of closely packed tubules derived from the sarcoplasmic reticulum. Large aggregates are visible by light microscopy and are intensely stained by the NADH-TR reaction. (Bar = 10 μm.)

feature, often severe and sometimes precipitated by cold. Muscle histology is usually normal, or shows only minor abnormalities. Sodium channel abnormalities are incriminated in the pathogenesis.

Disorders characterized by transient episodic weakness, i.e. periodic paralysis, are likely to present in a very different manner. Myotonia may be detected in some, and paramyotonia congenita and hyperkalemic periodic paralysis appear to be allelic mutations of the same gene on chromosome 17. Different categories of hyper-, hypo- or normokalemic periodic paralysis are equated with changes in serum potassium levels during attacks. Muscle biopsy taken during or shortly after an spinal atrophies, the congenital myopathies are frequently static or only slowly progressive. Type 1 fibre predominance and/or small type 1 fibres are common histological features, together with a variety of cytoarchitectural abnormalities upon which diagnosis and nomenclature are based. The pathological changes originally suggested a pathogenesis of maturation arrest, and the recent discovery of retention of fetal or embryonic myosins have given support to this hypothesis in some cases. Whereas in single families there is clear evidence of phenotypic variation and histological overlap, there is also evidence of genetic heterogeneity in disorders with similar histological features. Currently these disorders are perhaps best considered as different disturbances of myogenesis that adversely influence maturation, growth and function, but do not predispose to necrosis. However, long survival is often associated with slow progression, and repeat biopsies may reveal fibre loss and fibrofatty replacement. The diagnosis may be suspected clinically, but can only be proven by biopsy. It is very probable that identification of the genetic abnormalities will soon justify the lumping or splitting of these disorders.

CENTRONUCLEAR MYOPATHIES

As the name implies, central nuclei are the key histological feature of this myopathy. However, wide variation in age of onset, clinical picture and modes of inheritance indicate that different entities exhibit the same abnormality.

Myotubular myopathy

The best-defined entity is an X-linked recessive disorder presenting with profound neonatal hypotonia that frequently causes death from respiratory failure in the first few months. These male infants show a very distinctive biopsy picture, likened to fetal myotubes. In transverse section many fibres contain central sarcolemmal nuclei, (Fig. 17.25) and in the majority the myosin ATPase reaction demonstrates a large central or perinuclear unstained zone. The oxidative enzyme reaction shows a reversed pattern, with a thin pale-staining peripheral rim and a dark centre (Fig. 17.23). There may be normal differentiation of type 1 and 2 fibres, or type 1 predominance. Type 1 fibres are usually smaller than type 2. Electron microscopy confirms the absence of myofibrils from the centre of the fibre, which contains glycogen, normal mitochondria and, sometimes, lysosomes. Although the the myotube analogy may be an oversimplification, recent studies have demonstrated the persistence of fetal cytoskeletal distribution of vimentin and desmin and fetal myosins. The gene for this X-linked myopathy has recently been mapped to the Xq28 region. Congenital myotonic dystrophy may look very similar in the neonatal muscle biopsy, and should always be excluded by examination of the mother.

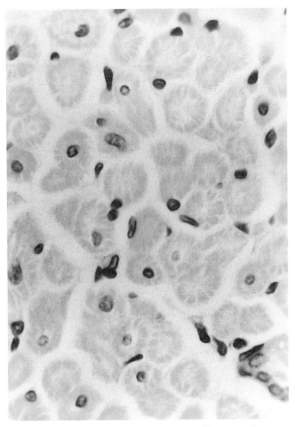

Fig. 17.25   Myotubular myopathy. Many fibres contain central nuclei and most show a large pale central zone devoid of myofibrils. (H & E.)

Other centronuclear myopathies

Multiple central nuclei also characterize a milder, autosomal dominant disorder with variable onset in infancy, later childhood or even in adult life. Sporadic cases occur and a small number of patients with identical histology have presented in the fifth or sixth decades. Central nuclei are found in a large proportion of fibres, both type 1 and type 2. The nuclei form long chains in longitudinal sections. There is a small perinuclear halo (Fig. 17.26), but not the large central clear area of the X-linked form. Type 1 predominance is common and type 1 fibres are usually small, but degenerative changes are absent. Histological variation discovered within families has led to the inclusion of cases with type 1 predominance and small type 1 fibres without central nuclei. The difficulties of

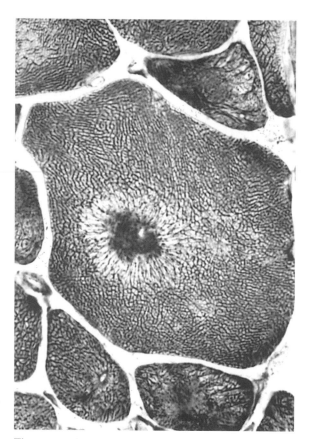

Fig. 17.26 Centronuclear myopathy. Central nucleus and perinuclear clear zone of radiating myofibrils. (NADH-TR.)

classification and counselling posed by sporadic cases with these changes are obvious.

NEMALINE MYOPATHY

Congenital nemaline myopathy provides one of the most eyecatching muscle biopsy appearances. The disorder shows a clinical spectrum. The most severely affected present with generalized neonatal hypotonia and often succumb to respiratory insufficiency in early life. Hypotonia, diminished muscle bulk and facioskeletal abnormalities, including a high arched palate and kyphoscoliosis, draw clinical attention in childhood. A minority present with a limb girdle syndrome in adult life. Inheritance is usually autosomal recessive.

Nemaline rods (a misnomer because nema means worm) are the key diagnostic feature and unmistakable, provided the appropriate special stains are employed. Although perfectly visible they are easily overlooked with H&E staining, but with Gomori's trichrome tiny purple rod-shaped cytoplasmic bodies stand out against the bright green background (Fig. 17.27). Rods are present in a high percentage of fibres, forming large subsarcolemmal aggregates or dispersed among the myofibrils and imparting a speckled appearance. The numerous rods are often found in the setting of type 1 predominance and type 1 atrophy or hypoplasia. Electron microscopy shows that the rods are composed of parallel cross-linked filaments, occasionally in continuity with a Z band (Fig. 17.28). γ-actinin, a normal Z-band component that binds actin filaments, is the major rod constituent, suggesting that rod formation results from aberrant development of the normal cytoskeleton. Nemaline rods are not unique to congenital nemaline myopathy. A few rods may be found in other disorders, particularly neurogenic disease, thus their significance, particularly in adults, must be interpreted with caution. γ-actinin is a component of intercalated disks in cardiac muscle, and a rare nemaline rod cardiomyopathy has been reported, usually in adults with only a mild skeletal myopathy.

CENTRAL CORE DISEASE

This disorder has comparatively mild manifestations, and weakness is usually not detected before

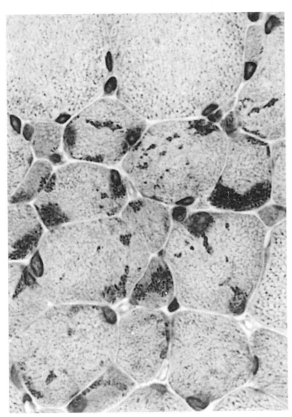

Fig. 17.27 Nemaline myopathy. Rod bodies in peripheral clumps and scattered within the fibre. Rods are more numerous in atrophic fibres. (Gomori's trichrome.)

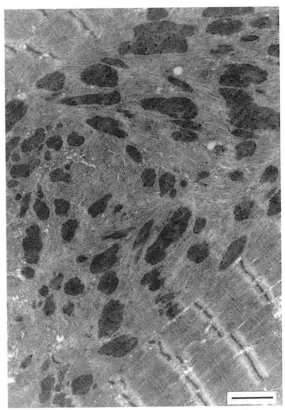

Fig. 17.28 Nemaline rods. Arrays of electron-dense parallel filaments. (Bar = 1 μm.)

the child has started walking, and sometimes not until adulthood. It is usually dominantly inherited. The myopathy of central core disease may be mild, but an unknown proportion of patients also have the potentially fatal malignant hyperpyrexia trait. The name describes the key morphological feature. A central core is a well demarcated zone in the centre of a muscle fibre that extends for the greater part of its length and is devoid of normal histochemical reactivity. Cores are not easy to see with H&E or myosin ATPase, and are best demonstrated with an oxidative enzyme stain (Fig. 17.29). They are also clearly visible under fluorescent or polarized light (Fig. 17.30). Cores only occur in type 1 fibres, and typical central core disease shows type 1 predominance or uniformity and type 1 fibres are frequently small. A high percentage, and in some cases all fibres, contain cores. Although cores are often central and

single, there may be several eccentric cores in a single fibre. The diameter varies, a proportion of up to 30 μm occupying a large part of the cross-sectional area; others are far smaller. Electron microscopy reveals variable disorganization of fibre architecture in the core (Fig. 17.31). The myofibrils may be completely disrupted or preserved, with abnormally short sarcomeres and malalignment of the Z bands creating a zigzag pattern. Mitochondria and triads formed by T-tubules and sarcoplasmic reticulum are absent. Central cores and the target fibres of neurogenic disease have a similar appearance and structure, but the latter are far shorter and only temporary.

MINICORE DISEASE

This is yet another early-onset and generally mild myopathy, in which the diagnosis is based on a

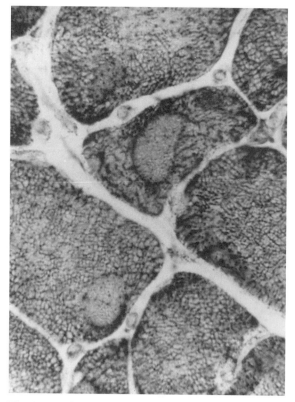

Fig. 17.29   Central cores. Well circumscribed, roughly circular pale-staining zones in sarcoplasm. (NADH-TR.)

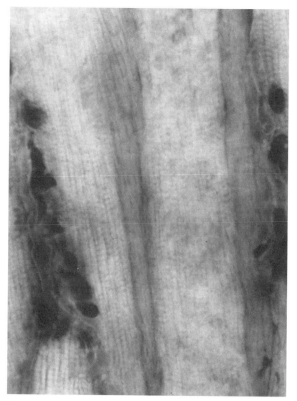

Fig. 17.30   Central cores. Longitudinal section in fibres viewed by fluorescent light.

structural peculiarity. Minicores are numerous tiny areas of loss of oxidative enzyme activity due to focal myofilament disruption involving only a few sarcomeres, with Z-band streaming and absence of mitochondria. Multiple minicores in individual fibres impart a smudgy appearance in cross-section. They occur in all fibre types, although again type 1 fibres may be predominant and atrophic.

CONGENITAL FIBRE TYPE DISPROPORTION

Congenital fibre type disproportion describes a benign myopathy of early onset in which small type 1 fibres are the only histopathological abnormality (Fig. 17.32). This is by no means a disease-specific abnormality: it is a characteristic not only of almost all congenital myopathies, but also of myotonic dystrophy. It is therefore a diagnosis of exclusion, but does seem to be a genuine entity in a small

proportion of cases. Although accurate measurement can be used to confirm the diagnosis, the disparity in fibre size should be at least 18 per cent, and thus easily discernible by eye.

METABOLIC MYOPATHIES

All muscle diseases affect some aspect of muscle cell metabolism, but this category refers particularly to disorders in which there are specific enzyme defects in the pathways of energy production. The functional effects depend on the nature and severity of the defect. Defective energy production may cause exercise intolerance, but when severe, cell integrity is threatened and massive cell death may result in frank myoglobinuria. Enzyme deficiency frequently causes morphological changes because the enzyme substrate accumulates and distorts cell architecture. The major energy sources of muscle are glycogen, glucose and free fatty acids. Enzyme

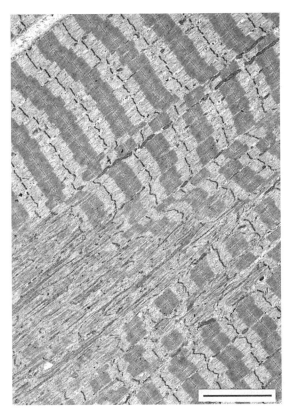

Fig. 17.31 Central core. Disorganization of myofilaments in the centre of the fibre, with smearing and loss of Z bands. Normal myofibrils at the edge of the core. (Bar = 5 µm.)

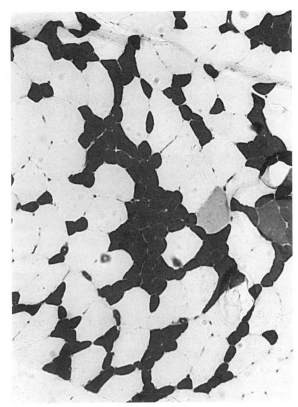

Fig. 17.32 Congenital fibre type disproportion. Uniformly small type 1 fibres contrast with mildly hypertrophied type 2 fibres. Fourteen-year-old girl, hypotonic with poor muscle bulk since birth, but no progressive weakness. (Myosin ATPase.)

defects have been identified at many points in their biochemical pathways.

DISORDERS OF GLYCOGEN METABOLISM

Glycogen is normally stored in resting muscle cells and utilized in the initial stage of exercise, after which fuel stores are replenished by blood-borne glucose and fatty acids. Glycogen is the obligate substrate in high-intensity exercise, such as weight lifting, when muscle contraction occurs under anaerobic conditions. Defects of glycolysis prevent the rise of venous lactate that normally occurs in ischaemic exercise. Myophosphorylase deficiency (McArdle's disease) and phospho-fructokinase deficiency are both autosomal recessive conditions responsible for cramps on exercise and myoglobinuria. Muscle histology shows glycogen storage, in the form of large clear subsarcolemmal blebs that are positive with PAS. Histochemical reactions for both enzymes are available, and give a negative result. A muscle biopsy taken shortly after an episode of myoglobinuria may reveal spotty fibre necrosis and regeneration. In McArdle's disease, the presence of the fetal isoenzyme in regenerating fibres gives a misleading positive histochemical reaction. Other defects of glycolysis that affect muscle metabolism do not always show obvious glycogen storage.

Acid-maltase deficiency

Acid-maltase deficiency is a lysosomal storage disease and, although a defect in glycogen metabolism, it does not directly interfere with energy production. The disease is autosomal recessive and may present in infancy (Pompe's disease), childhood or adult life. A generalized enzyme defect in the infantile form causes hepatosplenomegaly, macroglossia and early death due to cardiac muscle involvement. Disease of later onset affects only skeletal muscle, causing progressive limb girdle and truncal weakness, that may resemble a muscular dystrophy.

Lysosomal glycogen storage causes a vacuolar myopathy. In infantile cases, vacuoles fill the cytoplasm of every cell, so that at lower magnification, in transverse section, muscle resembles adipose tissue. There are fewer vacuoles in older cases. The vacuoles, which appear empty with H&E (Fig. 17.33), show PAS positivity due to their glycogen content and are positive for the lysosomal enzyme acid-phosphatase. Electron microscopy shows numerous membrane-bound lysosomal vacuoles filled with glycogen granules, and also an excess of free cytoplasmic glycogen. The diagnosis can be confirmed by biochemical analysis of muscle or lymphocytes. Antenatal diagnosis is possible using cells obtained by amniocentesis.

MITOCHONDRIAL ENCEPHALOMYOPATHIES

Clinical syndromes and pathogenesis

In recent years inborn errors of mitochondrial metabolism have emerged from obscurity and been recognized as the cause of a group of multisystem disorders with diverse clinical manifestations but in which muscle and/or cerebral disorders predominate. Over the same period the mitochondrial genome has been sequenced and its role established. Respiratory chain defects are the commonest of the many specific biochemical errors detected at different stages of mitochondrial metabolism. The five enzyme–protein complexes of the respiratory chain are assembled within the mitochondria from precursor proteins derived from two sources (Fig. 17.34). The majority of precursor proteins are encoded by nuclear DNA and transported across the mitochondrial membrane, but the mitochondrion also contains its own unique circular DNA (mtDNA), which encodes the remainder and directs synthesis within the mitochondrion.

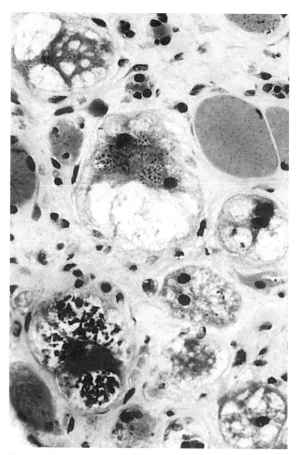

Fig. 17.33 Acid-maltase deficiency, adult form. Vacuolated fibres contain stored glycogen. Large lysosomes appear as dark, basophilic granules. (H & E.)

Mitochondrial DNA has a different genetic code from that of nuclear DNA, and it also shows a strictly maternal pattern of inheritance. Mitochondria within the fertilized egg are almost exclusively derived from the ovum. Thus, mitochondrial encephalomyopathies due to genetic defects of the respiratory chain may be transmitted either by mendelian or maternal inheritance.

Within a wide spectrum, from neonatal onset of severe and rapidly fatal encephalomyopathy to late adult onset of ptosis and mild myopathy, several clinical syndromes are particularly associated with mitochondrial defects. These are CPEO (chronic progressive external ophthalmoplegia), MELAS (myopathy, encephalopathy lactic acidosis and stroke) and MERRF (myoclonic epilepsy and

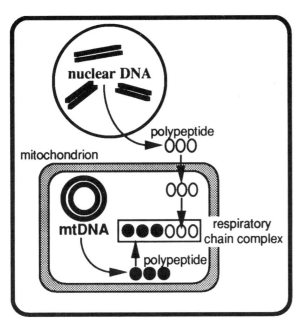

Fig. 17.34 Dual genetic control of mitochondrial enzyme synthesis – enzyme complexes contain polypeptides encoded by both nuclear DNA and mtDNA and assembled in the mitochondrion.

chain polypeptides, and also genes encoding ribosomal and transfer RNAs. The clinical features depend not only upon the molecular lesion but also the severity of the biochemical defect and the tissues involved. The preferential involvement of muscle, both skeletal and cardiac, and the nervous system may reflect the permanence of their mature cells. Continued cell turnover may serve to eliminate cells with large numbers of abnormal mitochondria. All cells contain thousands of mitochondria; thus phenotypic expression of a mitochondrially encoded defect will depend on the proportion of mitochondria containing mutant mtDNA. Age is also a relevant factor. Mitochondrial energy production declines with age; thus the presence of a proportion of abnormal mitochondria may not be manifest until middle or even old age. Point mutations of the mitochondrial genome are usually maternally transmitted, whereas large deletions occur sporadically. Large deletions may not be transmitted because they affect the viability of the ovum.

Histology

Skeletal muscle frequently contains distinctive and diagnostically significant abnormal 'ragged red fibres' (Fig. 17.36). 'Ragged red' refers to the appearance of an irregular red rim of peripheral

ragged red fibres). Although there is overlap between these syndromes, probing the mitochondrial genome has disclosed a definite correlation between clinical phenotypes and specific mtDNA defects (Fig. 17.35). Point mutations in different mitochondrial genes have been identified in MELAS and MERRF, and large deletions in cases with CPEO. Human mtDNA contains genes encoding messenger RNAs specifying respiratory

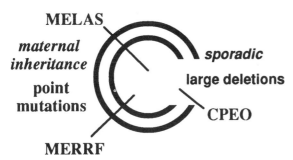

Fig. 17.35 MtDNA mutations. Point mutations responsible for syndromes such as MELAS and MERRF are usually maternally inherited. Large gene defects, as in CPEO, are sporadic and not transmitted because ova are non-viable.

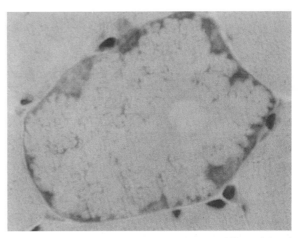

Fig. 17.36 Ragged red fibres. Irregular basophilic peripheral rim and faintly granular appearance of sarcoplasm. (H & E.)

cytoplasm with Gomori's trichrome stain. However, the fibres are evident with H&E and show a basophilic border and granular cytoplasm that are very well demonstrated by the oxidative enzyme reactions, where the border is dark. These staining reactions are due to large subsarcolemmal aggregates of mitochondria, in which electron microscopy reveals an abnormal structure, either excessive and whorled cristae or crystalline inclusions (Fig. 17.37). Ragged red fibres are not exclusive to mitochondrial enzyme defects. As an occasional finding in a wide variety of muscle diseases they are attributed to secondary disturbances in mitochondrial metabolism. Nevertheless, when numerous, they provide strong evidence of a mitochondrial myopathy. Ragged red fibres are indicators of a generalized reduction in mitochondrial protein synthesis, but there is no correlation between fine structural abnormalities and specific biochemical defects. The latter must be determined by biochemical analysis. An acquired mitochondrial myopathy, with ragged red fibres, may develop in AIDS patients on long term zidovudine (AZT) therapy because the drug is an inhibitor of a mitochondrion-specific DNA polymerase.

Severe myopathies of early onset are described in which tissue specific mtDNA depletion are attributed to a defect of nuclear directed mtDNA replication. A histochemical stain for complex 1, cytochrome C oxidase, is available and even in the absence of ragged red fibres enzyme deficiency can be detected by lack of staining of a variable proportion of fibres.

Lipid storage

In normal muscle neutral lipid is inconspicuous, seen as tiny faint red dots with an Oil red O stain and mostly in type 1 fibres. Mitochondrial oxidative metabolism depends on transportation of fatty acid substrates into the mitochondrial matrix, performed by specific carrier molecules. Carrier deficiency limits transport and impairs mitochondrial respiration and leads to the accumulation of fatty acids in the cytoplasm. Carnitine and carnitine palmitoyl transferases (CPT) are involved in the transfer process. Primary carnitine deficiency may be systemic or limited to skeletal muscle, and in both cause a dramatic increase in diffuse large cytoplasmic lipid droplets. Systemic carnitine deficiency is usually fatal in early childhood, due to cardiac muscle involvement. Secondary carnitine deficiency is not uncommon in a variety of totally unrelated muscle diseases, including cachexia, but the lipid accumulation is less (Fig. 17.38). CPT deficiencies are a cause of exercise intolerance and myoglobinuria, but not progressive disease. Although muscle biopsy may show lipid accumulation immediately after an attack, at other times it is likely to be deceptively normal.

Normal histology

Mitochondrial biochemical defects may not produce any histological abnormalities. Despite a negative biopsy, exercise-induced serum lactate elevation is strong evidence of defective mitochondrial metabolism and warrants biochemical analysis of the muscle. Part of the biopsy should always be frozen and preserved for this purpose. Genetic analysis may be performed on muscle, but also on peripheral lymphocytes, if mutant mtDNA is amplified by PCR.

INFLAMMATORY MYOPATHIES

Inflammatory myopathies are disorders in which muscle cell injury is directly or indirectly attributable to the inflammatory reaction. Mononuclear

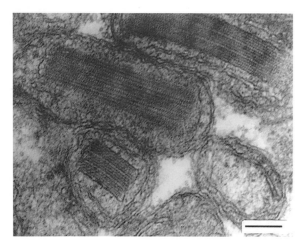

Fig. 17.37 Mitochondrial myopathy. Mitochondria are enlarged and contain crystalline inclusions. (Bar = 1 μm.)

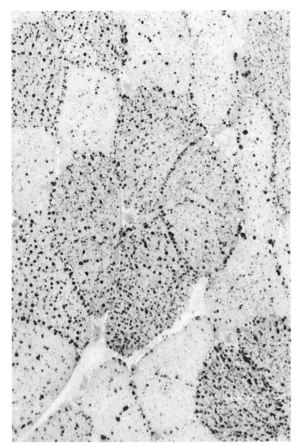

Fig. 17.38 Lipid droplets. Moderate increase in cytoplasmic lipid droplets, particularly in type 1 fibres. This change arouses suspicion of a mitochondrial metabolic disorder, but an increase of this degree is not specific and may reflect an acquired metabolic disturbance, including the effects of steroid therapy, high alcohol intake and, paradoxically, starvation. (Oil red O.)

chronic inflammatory cells are usually present in the muscle.

INFECTIOUS AGENTS

Infective myositis due to active proliferation of bacterial, fungal or parasitic organisms in muscle may elicit a vigorous inflammatory response, but is rare except in the tropics, and unlikely to be confused with the immunological disorders. Acute viral myositis is attributable to viral invasion of muscle cells, for example by influenza or enteroviruses, but is a self-limiting disorder. Infectious agents have long been incriminated as trigger factors

of the immunologically mediated destruction of muscle in polymyositis (PM) and dermatomyositis (DM), but micro-organisms are consistently absent in muscle examined by light and electron microscopy or tissue culture. However, recent *in situ* hybridization detection of enteroviral RNA in macrophages in muscle biopsies has strengthened the viral hypothesis. In addition, a steroid-responsive inflammatory myopathy, indistinguishable from idiopathic PM, occurs in patients infected with human immunodeficiency virus, and retroviral antigens have been identified in sparse macrophages in muscle biopsies.

POLYMYOSITIS AND DERMATOMYOSITIS

Polymyositis and dermatomyositis are the commonest clinically important inflammatory myopathies and are responsible for both chronic and debilitating diseases, showing both clinical and pathological overlap. Polymyositis is a disease of adult life, commonest in women over 40 years. Patients exhibit symmetrical proximal muscle weakness, usually of insidious onset. These muscles may be tender to palpation. The CK is usually at least moderately elevated and there are EMG abnormalities in affected muscles. In DM there is similar muscle weakness, but it is associated with a characteristic faint erythematous scaly rash. Dermatomyositis occurs at all ages, including childhood and, when severe, chronic cases may develop contractures and subcutaneous calcinosis over the heels and elbows. PM or DM may occur in association with other connective-tissue diseases. A minority of older adults with dermatomyositis have an underlying systemic malignancy.

Histology and immunopathogenesis

In both PM and DM there is mononuclear cell infiltration of muscle and fibre necrosis, and in chronic disease there is likely to be a degree of replacement fibrosis. In small biopsies the disorders may be indistinguishable, but in larger samples there may be differences in the distribution and character of the inflammatory cells which probably reflect different immune effector mechanisms (Fig. 17.39). In both disorders the cellular infiltrate

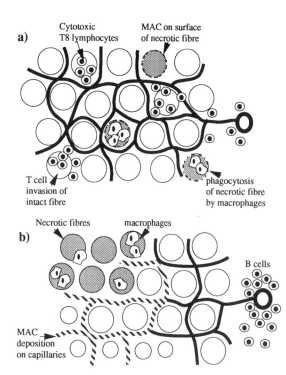

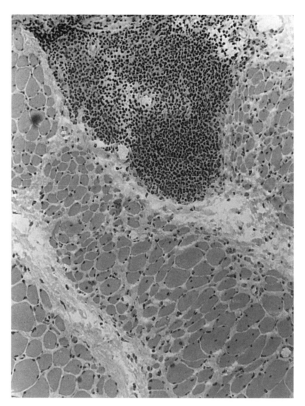

Fig. 17.39 Different pathogenetic mechanisms in inflammatory myopathies. (a) Polymyositis: inflammation mainly endomysial where T cells predominate. Spotty fibre necrosis and cytotoxic T-cell invasion of intact muscle fibres. Normal capillary vasculature. (b) Dermatomyositis: MCA deposition leads to capillary loss. Perifascicular atrophy due to ischaemia and peripheral group of necrotic fibres, indicating a microinfarct. Inflammation mainly perimysial where B cells predominate.

Fig. 17.40 Dermatomyositis. Large perivascular lymphocytic aggregate in the perimysium and perifascicular fibre atrophy. (H & E.)

is predominantly lymphocytic, but in PM it is chiefly endomysial and focal. Individual, apparently healthy, muscle fibres are surrounded and invaded by lymphocytes (Fig. 17.40), shown by immunocytochemistry to be cytotoxic T cells accompanied by macrophages. This invasion of non-necrotic muscle fibres implicates cell-mediated cytotoxicity in PM. In contrast, in DM the infiltrate is dispersed in the perimysial connective tissue surrounding fascicles, and frequently forms perivascular aggregates (Fig. 17.41). Endomysial inflammation is less conspicuous. B cells are more numerous in DM than in PM, but the character of the infiltrate changes from B-cell dominance in the perivascular location to increasing numbers of T cells, mainly T4, approaching the endomysium. The relative abundance of B cells suggests that local humoral immune mechanisms have a more important role in DM. PM and DM are the archetypal disorders, but the same patterns of inflammation may occur in any of the connective-tissue disorders.

All stages of necrosis and regeneration may be seen in a single biopsy in the active phase of PM and DM, but different patterns of fibre necrosis are observed (Fig. 17.40). In PM, in addition to invasion by cytoxic T cells, the fibres are damaged by a second immunological mechanism. There is frequently spotty, single fibre necrosis. These necrotic fibres are not surrounded by T lymphocytes, but react for membrane attack complex (MAC). MAC deposition implicates the humoral antibody-dependent mechanism of cell death that is mediated by complement. In a minority of patients with an idiopathic inflammatory myopathy clinically compatible with polymyositis, and with

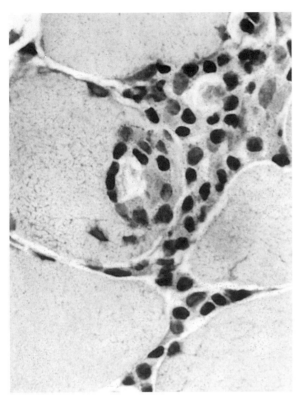

Fig. 17.41 Polymyositis. Endomysial lymphocytic infiltration and invasion of non-necrotic muscle fibre.

seen in arterioles and venules in DM, particularly the juvenile form.

Fibre atrophy is also common in PM and DM. Perifascicular atrophy, involving type 1 and type 2 fibres, is particularly characteristic of DM (Fig. 17.40) and is also attributed to ischaemia, secondary to the microangiopathy but insufficient to cause necrosis. The distribution coincides with the periphery of the vascular field, where the effects of a reduced blood supply are most severe. Selective type 2 fibre atrophy may occur in association with an inflammatory cell infiltrate, but sometimes is the only histological abnormality (Fig. 17.43), particularly in patients whose inflammatory responses have been suppressed by steroids

no drug exposure, the muscle biopsy is completely devoid of inflammatory cell infiltration and shows only segmental necrosis. The same picture is seen in a proportion of patients with AIDS-related myopathy, and is recorded in Lyme disease.

In DM necrotic fibres frequently occur in small clumps, with the appearance of microinfarcts (Fig. 17.42). Primary immunological attack upon the vasculature may be responsible for these ischaemic foci. Capillary vessels positive for the complement membrane attack complex and decreased capillary density are consistent findings, and present early in the disease. Microtubular inclusions of uncertain nature, revealed by electron microscopy in endothelium in DM, and also in systemic lupus erythematosus, may be a cellular response to injury. In addition to microangiopathy, fibrinoid necrosis, attributable to immune complex deposition in blood vessel walls, is occasionally

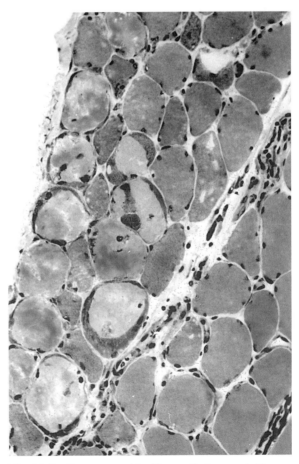

Fig. 17.42 Dermatomyositis. Cluster of pale necrotic fibres suggesting a microinfarct at the periphery of a fascicle. Several show regenerating myotubes surrounding the necrotic centre. (H & E.)

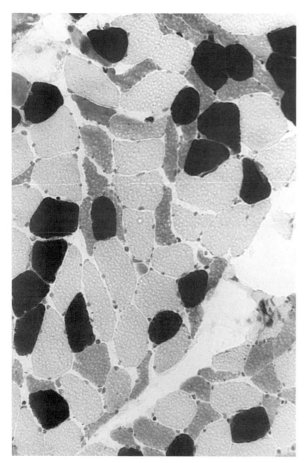

Fig. 17.43   Selective type 2B fibre atrophy. (ATPase pH 4.6.)

before biopsy. However, as there are many possible causes of type 2 atrophy, including disuse atrophy and immobility associated with joint pain, malignancy, cachexia and steroid therapy, a firm diagnosis of PM or DM cannot be based on this sole histological criterion. Muscle biopsy is often employed in an attempt to distinguish between steroid-induced myopathy and an exacerbation of myositis. If the only abnormality is type 2 atrophy, the many possible contributory factors and the patchy nature of the inflammatory process make distinction impossible.

Granulomatous inflammation

The 'tuberculoid' granuloma, a histological marker of cell-mediated immunity, is a tight focus of epithelioid histiocytes and multinucleate Langhans' giant cells. Granulomas are rare, inconspicuous components of the predominantly lymphocytic inflammation of muscle fascicles in PM. In contrast, sarcoidosis involving skeletal muscle shows discrete non-caseating tuberculoid granulomas, chiefly in the interstitium, but without accompanying endomysial inflammation or muscle fibre necrosis.

Vasculitis

Acute necrotizing arteriolitis and arteritis are not uncommon in juvenile DM, and may on occasion be seen in skeletal muscle in systemic lupus erythematosus and rheumatoid arthritis. In polyarteritis nodosa (PAN), fibrinoid necrosis of medium-sized arteries is the essential diagnostic feature. In PAN, muscle fascicles in the territory of an affected vessel may show ischaemic atrophy, or a pattern of denervation atrophy because the motor nerve is ischaemic, but there is no endomysial inflammation. Muscle infarcts due to arteritis in the absence of associated microangiopathy are very unusual, probably because there is a good collateral blood supply and the full capacity of the capillary network is only required during strenuous exercise.

Eosinophilic fasciitis

Skeletal muscle may be involved in the spectrum of hypereosinophilic disorders in which eosinophil-derived toxins probably contribute to tissue damage. In eosinophilic fasciitis, a mixed chronic inflammatory infiltrate containing many eosinophils is present in an oedematous and sclerotic fascia, often spreading deeply into the perimysium. In some cases the infiltrate involves the endomysium and is associated with spotty muscle fibre necrosis, i.e. an eosinophilic polymyositis. Indistinguishable eosinophilic inflammation of fascia and muscle may be found in the eosinophilia – myalgia syndrome attributable to tryptophan ingestion.

INCLUSION BODY MYOSITIS

Inclusion body myositis (IBM), an insidious inflammatory myopathy of elderly patients, was originally distinguished from PM and DM by the presence of rimmed vacuoles and failure to respond to steroids. Although cytotoxic T-cell invasion and destruction of non-necrotic muscle cells occurs in IBM, autophagy may be the more important mechanism of muscle degradation. The numerous cytoplasmic vacuoles, rimmed by basophilic material, are large acid-phosphatase-positive lysosomes, identical to those described in oculopharyngeal dystrophy (Fig. 17.44). Failure to demonstrate acid-phosphatase activity is probably because lysosomal bodies are dislodged in preparation of the sections. Small pale eosinophilic inclusions, found within or closely associated with the vacuoles, are shown by electron microscopy to be composed of masses of electron-dense filaments, 16–18 nm in diameter (Fig. 17.45). These should not be confused with cytoplasmic spheroid bodies, which are more strongly eosinophilic, composed of desmin filaments and often present but separate from the vacuoles. Spheroid bodies are probably Z-line abnormalities and occur in association with myofibril degeneration in a wide variety of myopathies. The origin and composition of the

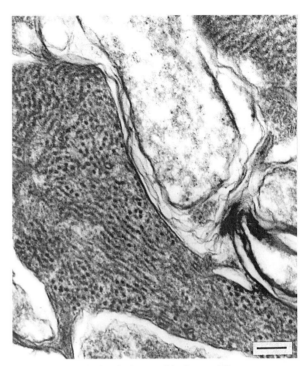

Fig. 17.45 Inclusion body myositis. Array of filaments (16–18 nm) in the cytoplasm adjacent to lysosomal membranous whorls. In IBM identical filaments are occasionally found in sarcolemmal nuclei. (Bar = 0.1 μm.)

larger filaments is unknown. Despite resemblance to paramyxoviral nucleocapsids, negative viral DNA *in situ* hybridization studies refute a mumps virus aetiology. The filaments are ubiquitinated and are reported to contain βA4 amyloid, but are are not disease-specific. In addition to IBM and OPMD, they are found in rare distal myopathies and other chronic wasting neuromuscular disorders, and may only represent proteins resistant to degradation in cells undergoing slow degeneration. The autophagic lysosomal system plays a central role in these conditions, but the trigger factors are unknown.

IBM has been divided into inflammatory and non-inflammatory forms and the term inclusion body myopathy is preferred. However, this may not be the fundamental issue. If inflammation is a secondary phenomenon, as in muscular dystrophies, it is important to look for other changes, such as clear evidence of denervation, and to pay careful attention to the clinical picture. Sporadic IBM in the elderly patient with inflammation and autophagy

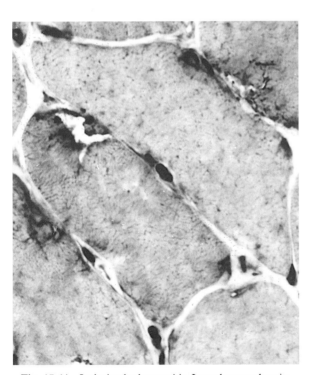

Fig. 17.44 Inclusion body myositis. Irregular cytoplasmic vacuoles rimmed by darker basophilic material. (H & E.)

may be a distinct entity, but the undisputed presence of abnormal mitochondria with crystalline inclusions in occasional patients suggests heterogeneity.

NEUROGENIC DISEASE

Myopathies are characterized by a wide variety of different histopathological changes that reflect different pathogenetic mechanisms. In contrast, the histopathological changes of denervating diseases are stereotyped. The major changes are those due to disease of the lower motor neuron, essentially atrophy following denervation and compensatory hypertrophy of surviving fibres. This picture may be complicated by reinnervation, which not only reverses fibre atrophy but may rearrange the normal distribution of fibre types.

DENERVATION ATROPHY

Pathological insult of the lower motor neuron may primarily be directed towards the anterior horn cells, the axon, the myelin sheath and the motor end plate. The composition and architecture of the motor unit is fundamental to interpretation of changes in muscle induced by denervation. One anterior horn cell innervates a large number of muscle fibres: over 1000 in a large limb muscle but only a fraction of that in a small hand muscle. The muscle fibres within a motor unit have uniform physiological and thus enzyme histochemical properties. Within the body of the muscle, although the fibres of a single motor unit are in close proximity they are intermingled with those of adjacent units, creating the normal mosaic pattern of fibre type distribution (Fig. 17.46a). Impulses from the motor neuron trigger simultaneous contraction of all the fibres within the motor unit. Denervated fibres cease to contract and gradually shrink (Figs 17.46b and 17.47). It follows, therefore, that disease of the anterior horn cell and proximal axon will simultaneously affect all

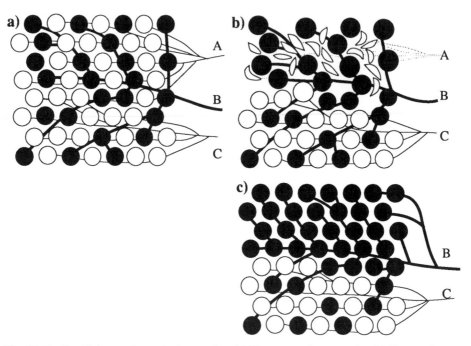

Fig. 17.46 Partial denervation and reinnervation. (a) Three normal motor units. (b) Denervation atrophy in motor unit A. Muscle fibres within a single unit are in close proximity, giving a pattern of type grouping. (c) Reinnervation of motor unit A from subterminal axons of adjacent motor unit B has created giant motor units and reversed atrophy. A change in fibre type has created a pattern of type grouping.

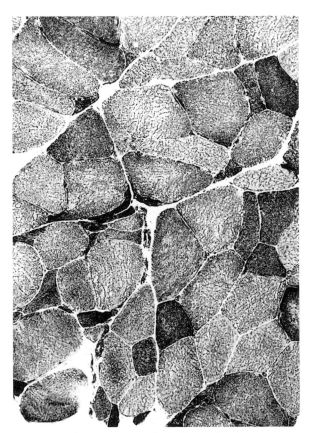

Fig. 17.47 Small group atrophy in denervation due to motor neuron disease. Atrophic fibres are thin and angular, easily overlooked with H & E, but stain darkly for oxidative enzyme. (NADH-TR.)

the muscle fibres in that motor unit, whereas patchy involvement of the myelin sheath will have far less effect. Motor end plates (MEP) have a large reserve capacity and, although the MEP may itself be damaged, most MEP disorders cause transitory physiological disturbance, i.e. myasthenia, as opposed to permanent structural changes in muscle. Hence, routine muscle biopsy is not the most appropriate diagnostic test for the myasthenic disorders, but in doubtful cases serves to eliminate other diseases, and a precise motor end-plate biopsy could reveal specific fine structural abnormalities.

REINNERVATION

Denervation is always followed by some attempt at reinnervation. In traumatic nerve trunk injuries, it is well recognized that suturing the severed ends enables axons sprouting from the proximal stump to follow their original path guided by Schwann cell tubes to reinnervate the muscles and restore function. In disease, denervated muscle fibres provide a stimulus to sprouting from the preterminal region of adjacent healthy axons. In human muscle the axons of the motor neuron lie in tight bundles that branch repeatedly until they reach the innervation zone, where a spray of short myelinated preterminal axons emerges, and each supplies a single motor end plate to one muscle fibre. Only a very small proportion of human preterminal axons are branched, giving rise to two end plates on the same or adjacent fibres. After partial denervation of a muscle, frequent branching of the remaining fine preterminal axons may be detected, such that three or more muscle fibres are innervated. Reinnervation not only restores the structure and function of the muscle fibre but it creates giant motor units, with greater action potential that can be detected by EMG. In addition, reinnervation may transform the normal mosaic pattern. The physiological properties, and hence the enzyme profile of muscle fibres are not intrinsic but dictated by the electrical stimulus of the motor nerve. Reinnervation can induce fibre type conversion, reflected in a biopsy by the occurrence of large clumps of uniform fibre type, referred to as type grouping (Fig. 17.46c). Reinnervation may convert type 1 to type 2 fibres or the reverse, but type 2 fibre grouping is usually only seen in the most chronic slowly progressive denervating disease, whereas type 1 grouping predominates in more rapidly progressive disease and may be a reflection of earlier sprouting from type 1 axons. Following a single insult, as in poliomyelitis or nerve injury, reinnervation may be complete, and only the disturbance of the pattern testifies to its occurrence. In chronic progressive denervating disease there is a balance between denervation and reinnervation. In the more rapidly progressive, such as most cases of motor neuron disease and the severe infantile form of spinal muscular atrophy, the scales are tipped towards denervation and thus atrophy. In slowly progressive disorders, such as milder late-onset forms of spinal muscular atrophy and hereditary peripheral neuropathies, evidence of reinnervation and compensatory hypertrophy are more conspicuous. Furthermore, uniform atrophic fibres may also show type grouping, as reinnervated motor units are subsequently denervated.

HISTOLOGY

Small angular denervated fibres tend to stain deeply with the oxidative enzyme reaction (Fig. 17.47) irrespective of fibre type, a consequence of comparatively greater loss of myofibrils than the cytoplasmic constituents which bind the reaction product. Other disturbances of the cytoskeleton are not seen in denervation, with two exceptions, namely target fibres and fibres damaged by functional overloading. Target fibres are a striking, aptly named abnormality, well demonstrated by the NADH-TR reaction in which a small, circular zone devoid of enzyme activity is bounded by a rim of increased activity (Fig. 17.48). The central zone shows myofibrillar disarray and depletion of mitochondria, whereas the dark rim is rich in mitochondria. The disturbance of cell architecture appears to be a temporary phenomenon, perhaps related to abnormal contractions. Numerous target fibres are almost pathognomonic of neurogenic disease, and probably appear during early reinnervation. In the most chronic denervating diseases, increased functional stresses on surviving fibres causes a remarkable degree of fibre hypertrophy, but this functional overloading may also cause segmental necrosis and fibre splitting. Rarely, these secondary myopathic changes may mask the basic pathology.

LOSS OF ANTERIOR HORN CELLS

Anterior horn cell loss occurs in poliomyelitis, in spinal muscular atrophy and in motor neuron disease. All these diseases are characterized by grouped atrophy of muscle fibres, the pattern created by simultaneous atrophy of all the fibres within affected motor units. Initially there are only small groups of atrophic fibres, typically showing an angular contour as though moulded by the contractions of healthy innervated fibres in overlapping motor units. The contrast is further heightened as innervated fibres undergo compensatory hypertrophy. In progressive disease, as more

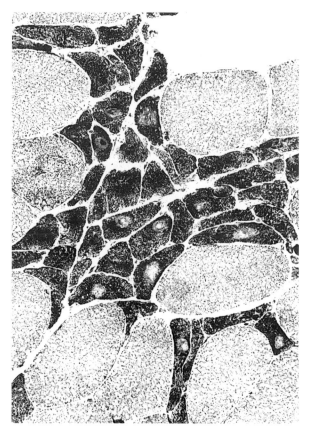

Fig. 17.48   Target and targetoid fibres due to chronic partial denervation in chronic spinal muscular atrophy. Grouped type 1 atrophic fibres show pale circular central zones. (NADH-TR.)

motor units are affected, larger groups of atrophic fibres appear. None of the anterior horn cell diseases shows motor unit selectivity, so that all fibre types are randomly affected.

Motor neuron disease (MND)

MND is a progressive disease of middle to old age characterized by widespread degeneration of motor neurons. The anterior horn cells, brain-stem nuclei and Betz cells of the cerebral cortex are all involved, giving the combined upper and lower motor neuron signs of wasting associated with spasticity and brisk reflexes. Different clinical patterns depend on the maximal site of neuron loss. Bulbar involvement has a particularly poor prognosis because dysphagia leads to death from aspiration pneumonia. Sensory neurons and the autonomic nervous system are spared. Extraocular and cardiac muscles are not affected. The great majority of cases are sporadic, but the rare familial form shows earlier onset and slower progression. The aetiology is still obscure, but is probably multifactorial. The increasing incidence and geographical variation in the western world incriminate environmental factors. Summation of the effects of a variety of environmental neurotoxins may eventually cause death of ageing neurons.

The majority of patients with sporadic MND have a rapidly progressive course and, whereas there may be type 1 grouping and mild compensatory hypertrophy, small group atrophy is the principal abnormality (Fig. 17.49).

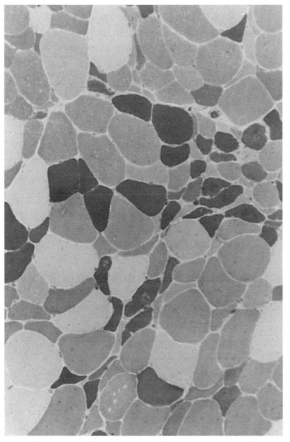

Fig. 17.49   Small group atrophy in motor neuron disease. Atrophic fibres include both type 1 and type 2 fibres. (Myosin ATPase pH 4.6.)

Spinal muscular atrophy (SMA)

The spinal muscular atrophies are inherited disorders showing progressive loss of anterior horn cells. Three grades of severity of childhood SMA have been distinguished on the basis of age of onset and clinical course. Severe acute infantile (SMA type 1: Werdnig–Hoffmann disease) is characterized by profound global weakness, evident at birth or shortly thereafter and inevitably progressing to death from respiratory failure before 3 years, and often before 1 year. Intermediate, chronic (type 2 SMA) is also associated with early onset (before 3 years), but a slower progression and longer survival, although most patients are severely incapacitated and many never manage to walk. The mildest form, juvenile (type 3 SMA: Kugelberg–Welander disease) presents later in childhood and patients retain mobility for many years. These are all autosomal recessive disorders that map to chromosome 5, and are thus probably due to different mutations of the same gene.

A separate X-linked disorder affecting bulbar and spinal muscles presents in adult life and is associated with gynaecomastia. There is a rare, genetically heterogeneous, distal form.

Both severe and intermediate childhood SMA show florid large group denervation atrophy (Figs 17.50 and 17.51), and cannot be distinguished by biopsy alone. Evidence of reinnervation (Fig. 17.52) and secondary myopathic changes dominate mild childhood and adult-onset disease.

Hereditary motor and sensory peripheral neuropathies

These disorders differ from MND and SMA in that there is also involvement of sensory neurons. Although there is a complex clinicopathological classification, there are two major categories: HMSN 1, or hypertrophic neuropathy of Charcot–Marie–Tooth, and HMSN 2, or the neuronal type of peroneal muscular atrophy. The term peripheral neuropathy is confusing because these are also anterior horn cell disorders, characterized by dysfunction, gradual dying back of the axon and eventual cell death. Neuronal degeneration and therefore muscle wasting in the lower limbs is more severe in type 2. Sensory involvement distinguishes HMSN type 2 from distal SMA. In type 1,

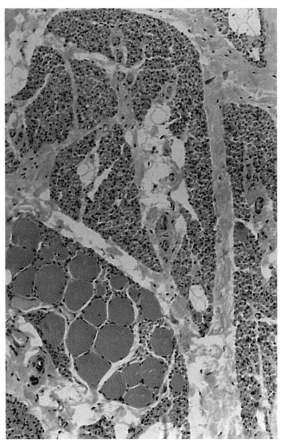

Fig. 17.50   Large group atrophy in severe infantile spinal muscular atrophy and a single group of greatly hypertrophied, residual innervated fibres. (H & E.)

repetitive demyelination and remyelination is the cardinal pathology responsible for reduced nerve conduction velocity and clinically palpable nerves. HMSN 1 is an autosomal dominant disorder in which a gene mutation has been identified on chromosome 17. The muscle biopsy typically shows all the features of chronicity, and thus compensatory hypertrophy and type grouping are well developed.

MYASTHENIA

Myasthenia gravis

Myasthenia gravis (MG) is an autoimmune disease in which the motor end plate is damaged by antibodies – usually IgG class – to the acetylcholine receptor. The deposition of these complement-fixing antibodies leads to degeneration of junctional folds and simplification of the postsynaptic membrane, which thereby impairs neuromuscular transmission. These changes can only be recognized by electron microscopy. Methylene blue vital staining or silver impregnation shows fine terminal sprouts and elongation of the end plates. Routine muscle biopsy shows no significant abnormalities in MG or other myasthenic syndromes, and it is not an appropriate diagnostic test. Patients with chronic myasthenia gravis may eventually develop some permanent muscle weakness and show corresponding changes of mild denervation atrophy.

Neonatal myasthenia

Neonatal myasthenia gravis is a transient disorder, mediated by the transplacental passage of AChR antibody in 10–15 per cent of babies born to affected mothers. High maternal antibody levels during pregnancy are a major determining factor. Rare congenital myasthenic syndromes are due to various non-autoimmune defects of the motor end plate, including acetylcholinesterase deficiency and defective AChR resynthesis.

The Eaton-Lambert myasthenic syndrome

This myasthenic syndrome is a rare non-metastatic manifestation of malignancy, usually oat-cell carcinoma of the bronchus. Occasionally it occurs in association with other autoimmune diseases, without malignancy. The syndrome may resemble MG clinically but it has a different pathogenesis and shows different fine structural disturbances of the motor end plate. The myasthenia is due to diminished release of acetylcholine from the nerve terminals affected by antibody bound to the presynaptic membrane. The axon terminals may be filled with synaptic vesicles and the postsynaptic membrane shows increased folding and complexity.

SYSTEMIC DISEASE

Muscle weakness and wasting are not uncommon manifestations of a wide variety of systemic disorders, including endocrine disturbances (par-

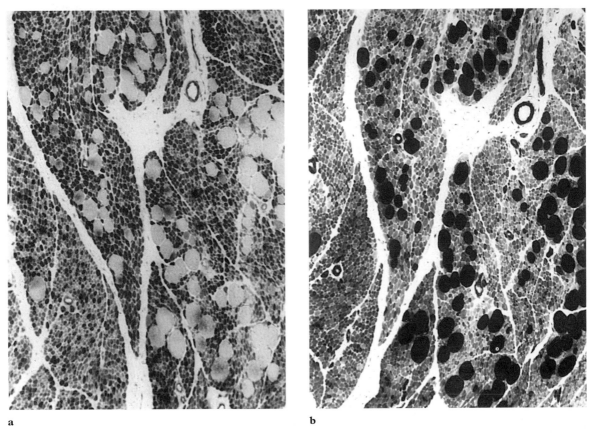

Fig. 17.51 Large group atrophy in severe infantile spinal muscular atrophy. Atrophic fibres are both type 1 and type 2, indicative of involvement of many motor units. Hypertrophied fibres are all type 1 and probably reinnervated fibres. (Myosin ATPase serial sections (a) pH 9.4, (b) pH 4.6.)

ticularly Cushing's syndrome), hyper- and hypo-thyroidism, chronic renal failure, systemic infection, malignancy, and cachexia from any cause. In general, the large proximal muscles are affected and the histological changes are non-specific. Diminished muscle mass in cachectic patients is first reflected by selective type 2B fibre atrophy and is common in any debilitated and immobilized patient. Occasional degenerate and necrotic fibres occur. The pathogenetic mechanisms are diverse. Endocrine dysfunction may interfere with muscle metabolism, powerful cytokines may damage muscle cells and immunological mechanisms may be invoked. Antiganglioside antibodies have been detected in a rare motor neuron syndrome associated with neoplasia. The association of inflammatory myopathy and neoplasia has been mentioned.

DRUG-INDUCED MYOPATHIES

Although steroid-induced myopathy is probably the commonest iatrogenic cause of muscle wasting, many unrelated drugs can cause myopathies. Adverse reactions may be idiosyncratic and unpredictable or due to toxicity. Clinical and pathological changes can resemble other neuromuscular diseases, and medication is easily overlooked. Steroid myopathy is most often a consequence of prolonged high dosage with fluorinated steroids. The steroidal effect on muscle metabolism results in generalized type 2 fibre atrophy, and sometimes an increase in lipid droplets. The most severe drug reaction is an acute necrotizing myopathy, which can cause rhabdomyolysis, myoglobinuria and renal failure. Drugs of addiction, such as heroin and the new designer drug Ecstasy (3, 4-methylenedioxy-

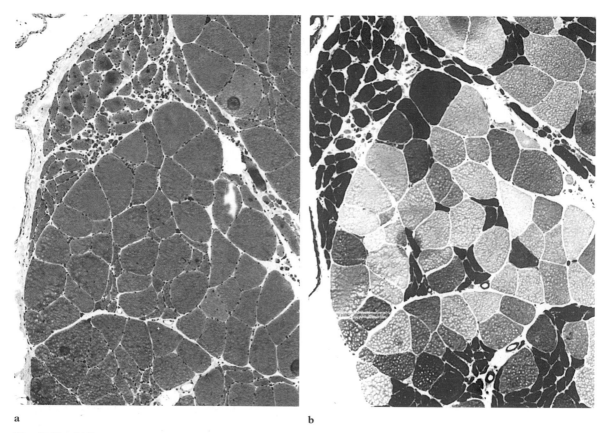

a   b

Fig. 17.52   (a) Large group atrophy and compensatory hypertrophy in an adult with chronic spinal muscular atrophy. (b) Type grouping. All the atrophic type 1 fibres are type 1 fibres. This uniform grouping, which contrasts with the surrounding mosaic pattern, is strong evidence of reinnervation. Large uniform groups also suggests repeated episodes of denervation and reinnervation.

methamphetamine) are important causes to be aware of, as the patient may be comatose on admission.

MALIGNANT HYPERPYREXIA

Malignant hyperpyrexia is due to an abnormal susceptibility to certain inhalational anaesthetic agents and muscle relaxants that trigger an acute prolonged rise in intracellular calcium ions, leading to sustained rigid contractions and arise in body temperature. The abnormal response is occasionally seen in patients with a recognized myopathy, particularly central core disease, but others with an autosomal dominant trait may have no overt physical disability, hence the first indication is an adverse reaction to anaesthesia. Following such an incident, muscle biopsy is indicated but should only be performed in a specialized centre where *in vitro* testing is available. Any histological abnormalities are usually minor and non-diagnostic.

FURTHER READING

Engel A G, Banker B Q (1986) *Myology, Basic and Clinical,* Vols. 1 & 2. New York: McGraw-Hill.
Rowland L P, Wood D S, Schon E A & DiMauro S (1989) *Molecular Genetics in Diseases of Brain, Nerve, and Muscle.* New York: Oxford University Press.

DiMauro S (1992) Symposium. Mitochondrial Encephalopathies. *Brain Pathology* 2, 111–162.
Dubowitz V (1985) *Muscle Biopsy. A Practical Approach,* 2nd edn. London: Bailliére Tindall.

18. Diseases of peripheral nerves

R. H. M. King

The study of peripheral nerves began in the middle of the 19th century and depended, until recently, largely on silver staining and paraffin embedding. The development of electron microscopy and resin embedding over the last 30 years has enormously improved our knowledge of the details of the normal and abnormal structure. More recently, immunohistochemistry and cytochemistry have made further advances possible. Despite this, most neuropathies cannot be diagnosed simply by examining a sample of nerve, but this may be needed to confirm the results of clinical and other investigations.

STRUCTURE OF PERIPHERAL NERVES

NORMAL STRUCTURE

Peripheral *nerve trunks* consist of bundles of axons connecting neuronal cell bodies in the central nervous system (CNS), or in dorsal root or sensory ganglia, to their target organs. The myelin sheath of axons in the peripheral nervous system (PNS) is derived from Schwann cells; in the CNS it is produced by oligodendroglial cells. The glial cells between the axons in the CNS are replaced in the PNS by an extensive collagenous matrix, hence its totally different mechanical properties.

Nerve trunks are composed of varying numbers of *fascicles*. Each of these consists of an intrafascicular component containing axons and their associated Schwann cells, embedded in collagenous endoneurial connective tissue and surrounded by a sheath of perineurial cells and collagen (Fig. 18.1). This *perineurium* consists (in the sural nerve) of about 6–11 concentric layers

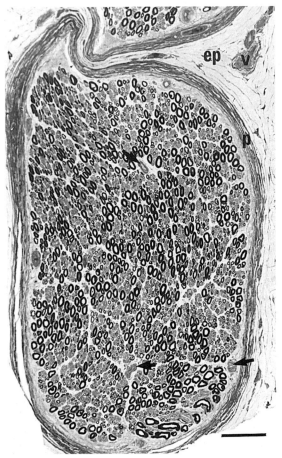

Fig. 18.1 Light micrograph of normal peripheral nerve: one fascicle. p = perineurium, ep = epineurium, arrows = capillaries, v = venule. (Araldite section, thionin and acridine orange. Bar = 50 μm.)

of flattened cells connected by tight junctions and separated from each other by organized sheets of collagen fibrils. This cylindrical sheath provides support and protection, both mechanically and because of its function as a diffusion barrier.

Fibrous long-spacing collagen, with a longitudinal periodicity of 125 nm instead of 67 nm, may be found in the perineurium, usually in abnormal nerves (see, for example Fig. 18.30b), and in the endoneurium in neurofibromatosis.

Fascicles are bound together by an *epineurium*, consisting mainly of collagen fibrils and varying amounts of fat and elastic fibres. The cross-sectional diameter of collagen fibrils in the epineurium is larger than that in the endoneurium or perineurium. The *blood supply* of the nerve is provided by a longitudinal anastomotic network of arterioles and venules in the epineurium, via blood vessels that penetrate the perineurium, to a capillary network running longitudinally in the endoneurium.

Pacinian corpuscles (encapsulated nerve endings) may be closely associated with the nerve trunk. In these a single myelinated nerve fibre is encircled by multiple layers of flattened cells and collagen and enclosed by a capsule of perineurial-type cells (Fig.18.2); these act as pressure sensors.

Axons in the PNS vary in diameter from 0.2 μm to 12 μm; those larger than 2.5 μm are normally surrounded by a myelin sheath (Fig. 18.3). The plasma membrane of axons is called the *axolemma*. The axoplasm contains 25 nm diameter microtubules, 10 nm neurofilaments, mitochondria, vesicles of smooth endoplasmic reticulum, multivesicular bodies and, occasionally, free or membrane-bound glycogen granules (see Fig. 18.5) and polyglucosan bodies. Cytoplasmic components associated with protein synthesis, such as rough endoplasmic reticulum and ribosomes, do not occur away from the neuronal perikaryon.

There is continuous movement of the various components of the axon from the neuronal cell body to (anterograde transport) and from (retrograde transport) the axon terminal. This transport occurs at several different rates, roughly separable into slow and fast types. Fast axonal transport, both anterograde and retrograde, carries vesicles and mitochondria at a speed of 400 mm/ day along the microtubules. The proteins of the axoplasmic cytoskeleton are also transported along

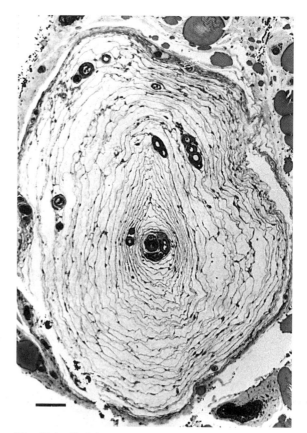

Fig. 18.2   Pacinian corpuscle on sural nerve. (Bar = 100 μm.)

the axon at 0.25–4 mm/day. This slow transport system has two components, 'a' and 'b'. Microtubules and neurofilaments move at the slowest rate (component a), and actin and other proteins move slightly faster (component b). Actin filaments perform an important structural function at the growing tip in developing and regenerating axons, but they are difficult to identify in mature, stable axons.

Unlike oligodendroglia in the CNS that myelinate several axons simultaneously, one Schwann cell myelinates only one segment of an axon. This arrangement develops in the fetus, starting at about 17 weeks' gestation. Initially, large numbers of very small axons lie in groups surrounded by processes of Schwann-cell cytoplasm. The Schwann cells multiply and some axons grow in size to about 2 μm diameter. These become separated, to lie singly in individual Schwann cells

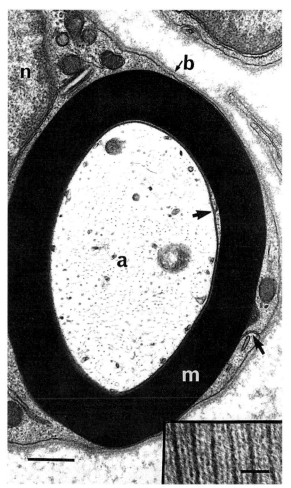

Fig. 18.3 Electron micrograph of myelinated nerve fibre. m = myelin, a = axon, n = Schwann-cell nucleus, and b = basal lamina, arrows = inner and outer mesaxons. Bar = 0.5 μm. Inset shows details of myelin structure, major dense line and intraperiod lines. (Lead citrate and methanolic uranyl acetate (collagen unstained)). (Bar = 20 nm.)

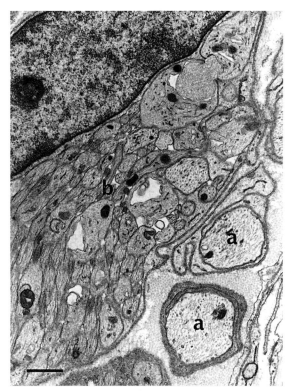

Fig. 18.4 Fetal nerve (21 weeks), with a large bundle of small unmyelinated axons (b) and two larger separate axons ready to be myelinated (a). (Bar = 1 μm.)

(Fig. 18.4). Some remain small and unmyelinated, but become individually wrapped by Schwann-cell processes. All the Schwann cells are the same; the signal for myelinogenesis comes from the axon. When an axon becomes deeply indented into a Schwann cell the adjacent Schwann-cell plasma membranes come together to form a mesaxon. This lengthens and spirals around the axon. The elimination of cytoplasm from the spirals produces the myelin sheath. The major dense line of myelin is formed from the cytoplasmic surfaces of the Schwann cell, and the

intermediate line from the outer surfaces. Fresh, unfixed myelin is a white, runny, glistening substance. The periodicity of PNS myelin is approximately 17 nm in fresh tissue. Shrinkage during fixation reduces the periodicity seen in electron micrographs to about 14 nm (Fig. 18.3 inset). Chemically, myelin consists of lipid bilayers in which intra- and transmembrane proteins are embedded.

The mature myelin sheath remains connected to the outer surface of the Schwann cell by the outer mesaxon, and to the inner surface by the inner mesaxon (Fig. 18.3). There is a positive correlation between the thickness of the myelin sheath and the length of the myelinated segment, and both are normally related to the diameter of the axon. The length of one internode in the largest diameter fibres is greater than 1 mm, whereas in the smallest fibres it is only 100 μm. In a normal nerve all the internodes along any one fibre are the same length. The myelin sheaths of the whole nerve fibre population do not reach their full thickness until late childhood. In the sural nerve the final adult ratio of myelinated/unmyelinated axons is approximately 1:4.

The external surface of the Schwann-cell plasma membrane is covered by a basal laminal sheath composed of collagens IV and V, glycosaminoglycans, fibronectin, laminin and other connective-tissue components. This basal laminal sheath is continuous along the axon from one Schwann cell to the next. Basal laminae only occur around Schwann cells, perineurial cells and capillary endothelial cells, thus differentiating them from fibroblasts, mast cells, macrophages and infiltrating lymphocytes.

The *node of Ranvier* is a break in the continuity of the myelin sheath where two adjacent Schwann cells abut. The basal lamina is continuous from one Schwann cell to the next. Nodes may be seen by light microscopy of longitudinal sections (see Fig. 18.9) and on teased fibre preparations. Electron microscopy shows that, in the unmyelinated region between the termination of the myelin lamellae, the axon is surrounded by Schwann-cell *nodal microvilli*, embedded in a specialized extracellular gap substance rich in ferric ions. In large fibres these form a halo of radially arranged interdigitating processes ending very close to the axolemma (Fig. 18.5). There are fewer and less regularly organized processes in the nodes of small fibres. The axoplasm in the nodal region contains a higher density of microtubules and large organelles and fewer neurofilaments, a reversal of the proportions in the internodal axoplasm. The nodal gap axolemma has an electron-dense undercoating. Sodium channels are concentrated in this area; in unmyelinated axons sodium channels are evenly distributed along the axon. The presence of an insulating layer of myelin and the localization of sodium channels at the nodes forms the structural basis for saltatory conduction. This greatly increases the speed of nerve impulse transmission in myelinated axons compared to unmyelinated ones. Abnormalities in this region may therefore have a deleterious effect on the function of the axon.

In a normal fibre, myelin lamellae produced by adjoining Schwann cells terminate on the

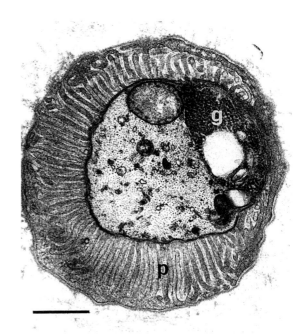

Fig. 18.5   Transverse section through a node of Ranvier. Schwann-cell nodal processes (p) surround the axon. There are glycogen granules in the axon (g). (Bar = 1 μm.)

axolemma, where they open up to contain small pockets of cytoplasm containing occasional organelles. In small fibres all the lamellae terminate consecutively on the axon; however, in large fibres some of the lamellae do not reach the axolemma but end in an organized, stepwise fashion against other lamellae. These can be seen in suitable preparations by light microscopy and are sometimes called the 'spiny bracelets of Nageotte', after their original observer.

The continuity of the myelin lamellae may be interrupted along the internode by Schmidt–Lanterman incisures (Figs 18.6 and 18.9). These are regions of non-compaction where the lamellae open at the major dense line to form a helical cytoplasmic pathway between the Schwann cell exterior to the myelin sheath and that inside it, adjacent to the axon (Fig. 18.6). The cytoplasm contained within the incisure often contains microtubules.

The bulk of Schwann-cell cytoplasm occurs either in the nuclear region or near the node. It contains the usual intracellular organelles, such as microtubules, centrioles, intermediate filaments,

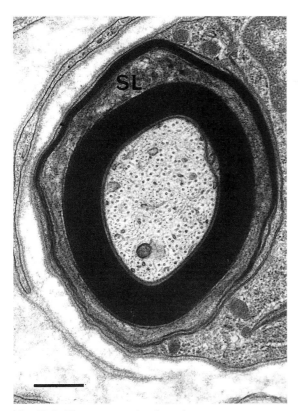

Fig. 18.6 Transverse section through a Schmidt–Lanterman incisure (SL). (Bar = 0.5 μm.)

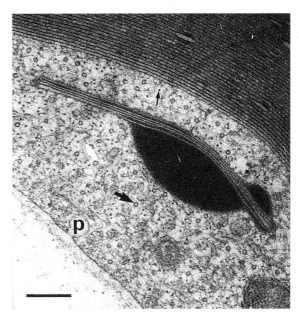

Fig. 18.7 Reich granule in Schwann-cell cytoplasm; also visible are microtubules (large arrow), intermediate filaments (small arrow) and a pinocytotic vesicle (p). (Bar = 0.2 μm.)

granular and agranular endoplasmic reticulum and mitochondria. In addition, a normal Schwann cell may contain lamellar lipid bodies called Reich or π granules (Fig. 18.7). Their numbers may be increased in old age and in some neuropathies, and they do not usually occur in Schwann cells associated with unmyelinated axons. Another dense inclusion, again more common in abnormal situations, is the Marchi-positive Elzholz or μ granule. These are globular bodies of unsaturated lipid with a myelin-like structure but a smaller periodicity; one can be seen close to the myelin sheath in Fig. 18.16b. A normal myelinated fibre is approximately circular in cross-section along most of the internode, except in the nuclear region of small fibres and near the node in large ones. In the paranodal region the myelin is crenated to form longitudinal grooves containing cytoplasm and large collections of mitochondria.

The relationship between Schwann cell and axon is different when the axons are not my-elinated. During development, those destined to remain unmyelinated remain small but become more intimately associated with the enveloping Schwann cells. Seen in cross-section, there are usually several unmyelinated axons associated with one Schwann-cell profile. The term 'Remak fibre' is often used for a Schwann cell plus its associated axons. The axons may either be completely invaginated into the Schwann cell, or merely indent the surface under the basal lamina. They may be difficult to distinguish, even with the electron microscope, from small Schwann-cell processes (see Fig. 18.4).

There is no equivalent of a node of Ranvier where two Remak fibres join, as the Schwann cells form longitudinal chains of cells with branching anastomosing processes connected by small tight junctions; unmyelinated axons pass through these processes.

ABNORMAL STRUCTURE

Demyelination

Primary segmental demyelination is the loss of one or more segments of myelin from the axon in the absence of axonal pathology. Demyelination may sometimes be restricted to the paranodal region. Loss of myelin disrupts the saltatory conduction mechanism, resulting in a conduction block, and hence the occurrence of clinical signs and symptoms. In primary Schwann-cell disorders or myelinopathies, myelin debris may be seen in the Schwann cells before invasion and removal by macrophages. *Autoimmune demyelination* (EAN – see p. 388) is characterized by the presence of macrophages that insert processes through the Schwann-cell membrane and strip the myelin sheath from the axon (Fig. 18.8). Myelin is only lost from axons where they pass through auto-immune inflammatory lesions, and is normal elsewhere.

Secondary demyelination is the loss of myelin due to alteration in axonal calibre, usually from atrophy. If the change in axonal size is transient or very slow, remyelination of the demyelinated segments can occur (see below).

After demyelination, there may be a brief period when the demyelinated internode is covered only by Schwann-cell basal lamina. This stage is very short-lived, and the bare axon is rapidly ensheathed by the cytoplasmic processes of Schwann cells. The differential effect of demyelination on adjacent internodes is best seen by the examination of individual teased fibres that will typically show both normal and demyelinated internodes along the length of the same axon.

Remyelination

After removal of the myelin debris, the Schwann cells divide and move along the denuded axon. New nodes of Ranvier form where adjacent cells abut, so once these have lined up along the axon new internodes are effectively defined before remyelination begins. The resultant remyelinated segments are of varying lengths, but all will usually be shorter than the original unless only paranodal widening has occurred (Fig. 18.9). The myelin sheath will initially be inappropriately thin, compared with the axonal diameter and, even if Schwann-cell function is normal, may take some considerable time to return to normal. In cross-section the thinly remyelinated fibres often show considerable deviations from the usual circular cross-section; as the myelin sheath becomes thicker it tends to resume a normal circular shape.

Repeated episodes of demyelination and remyelination may result in the production of excess Schwann cells that move away from the axon to form hypertrophic whorls, often called '*onion bulbs*', around it. These can so thicken the nerve trunk that it may be enlarged to palpation (Fig. 18.10). Axonal loss may result from prolonged or recurrent demyelination.

The changes seen in hereditary demyelinating diseases (HMSN I and III; Refsum's disease) could be expected to affect all fascicles equally, and thus may help to distinguish this from chronic inflammatory demyelinating polyneuropathy (CIDP) (see p. 389), where the disease process is more likely to be patchy (Fig. 18.11a and b).

Abnormalities of myelin sheath thickness in the

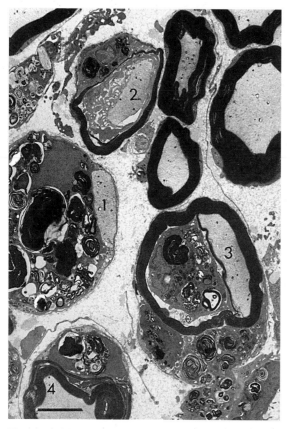

Fig. 18.8 EAN: guinea pig ventral root. Macrophages are stripping myelin from axons. (1) is completely bare, (2) (3) and (4) are under attack. (Bar = 5 μm.)

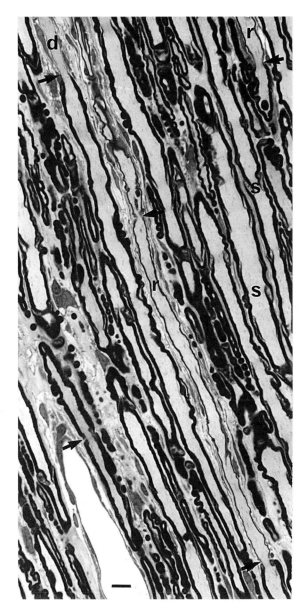

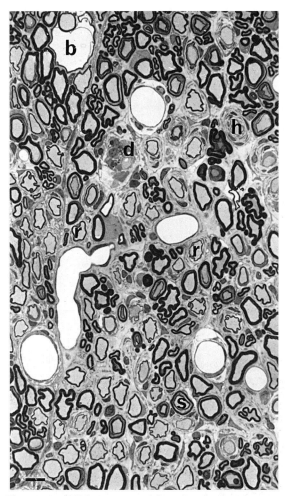

Fig. 18.10 EAN: transverse section of same specmen as Fig. 18.9. There are numerous thinly remyelinated axons (r), whorls of excess Schwann cells (h), intramyelinic oedema (b) and demyelinated axons (d). Schmidt–Lanterman incisures appear as two concentric circles (s). The holes are capillaries distended due to perfusion fixation. (Bar = 10 μm.)

Fig. 18.9 EAN: longitudinal section: lumbar ventral root; nodes (arrows) include one normal, a demyelinated segment (d) and remyelinated segments (r). Several Schmidt–Lanterman incisures are clearly visible (s). (Bar = 10 μm.)

form of an excess of lamellae for a particular size of axon, or the formation of reduplicated folds of myelin lamellae, such as is seen in hereditary liability to pressure palsy (see p. 398), also occur in hereditary motor and sensorimotor neuropathies and in neuropathies associated with abnormal serum paraproteins. In some instances of simple hypermyelination the axon may be so small that atrophy is suggested, but redundant folds and loops seem more related to overproduction of myelin than axonal atrophy.

Axonal degeneration

In this situation, the primary event is axonal damage. When a myelinated axon disintegrates, the myelin sheath also collapses to form ovoids of myelin around axonal debris. When axonal transport ceases organelles collect locally, particularly

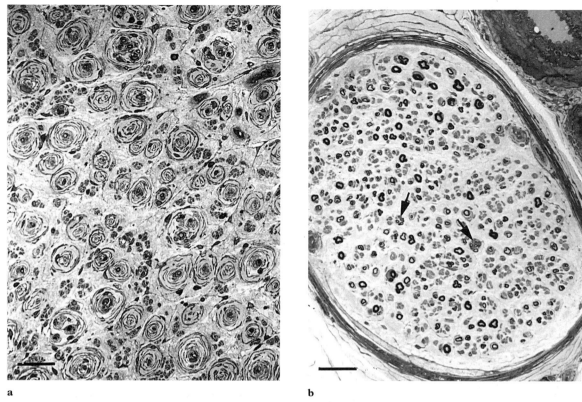

a   b

Fig. 18.11   CIDP. (a) Part of a large fascicle with hypertrophic clusters of Schwann cells around central myelinated axons. (b) Adjacent smaller fascicle with axonal loss and some regenerative clusters (arrows) but no hypertrophic changes. (Bar = 50 μm in both.)

at nodes in large fibres, as these are regions of axonal constriction. The fibre then breaks at the nodes of Ranvier and the Schmidt–Lanterman incisures. Longitudinal sections show various stages of this disruption (Fig.18.12). If individual fibres are teased out, the appearance of the myelinated fibre can be seen to change from a smooth cylinder broken at regular intervals by the nodes to a series of myelin ovoids like a string of beads. These further degenerate into simpler lipids and eventually neutral fats, and are removed by macrophages that enter the nerve fascicle from the endoneurial capillaries.

Persisting excess Schwann cells may remain scattered in the endoneurium, often rounding up and resembling small lymphocytes in size and shape. They may be differentiated by immunological staining or electron microscopy, which will show their basal laminal ensheathment (Fig. 18.13). When axonal damage results from a decrease in neuronal function, degeneration typically progresses in a distal–proximal direction in what is often described as a *dying-back neuropathy*. The neuronal cell body reacts to axonal injury with chromatolytic changes, and the cell may die if the site of damage is close to the perikaryon.

Bands of Büngner are the longitudinally continuous columns of Schwann cells resulting from proliferation after the loss of myelinated fibres. These remain within the basal laminal sheath that had surrounded the original fibre. The cell profiles are rounded in cross-section (as in Fig. 18.16b). These may contain the Reich granules associated with the original myelin sheath. If the Büngner band is only invaded by unmyelinated axon sprouts, the Reich granules serve as a marker to differentiate the result of myelinated fibre degeneration from a normal Remak fibre.

Degeneration of unmyelinated axons is less

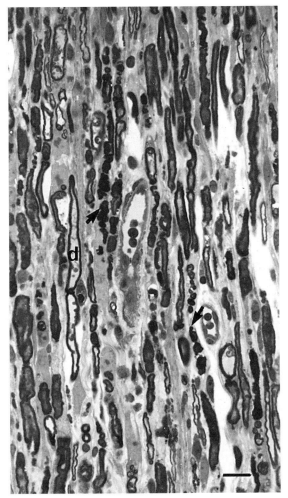

Fig. 18.12 Experimental Wallerian degeneration, 4 days after nerve section. In some fibres the myelin is still normal although the axon has gone (d); others have been replaced by chains of densely staining myelin ovoids (arrows). (Bar = 20 μm.)

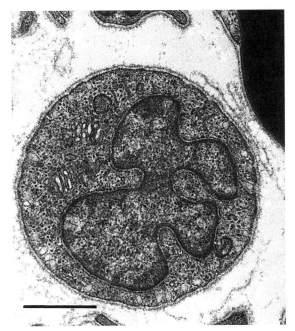

Fig. 18.13 Schwann cell unassociated with an axon. (Bar = 1 μm.)

conspicuous due to the lack of degenerating myelin. The cessation of axonal transport results in the formation of large aggregates of organelles in localized regions of the axon. These may be much larger than similar accumulations occurring during the degeneration of myelinated axons. Both organelles and axoplasm rapidly disappear, leaving Schwann-cell processes around an empty space. This collapses after a short time and the Schwann-cell processes form flattened cytoplasmic processes. Macrophages invade the tissue, but the lack of degenerating myelin renders them

relatively inconspicuous. Schwann-cell multiplication after unmyelinated axonal loss is much less prolific than after myelinated fibre loss.

Axonal regeneration

Regenerating axonal sprouts arise from interrupted axons, either from their tips or from preterminal nodes of Ranvier. They grow along the Büngner bands and may become myelinated when they attain an appropriate size. If these axon sprouts fail to contact a suitable end-organ, they will eventually degenerate. Examination of teased regenerated fibres shows a sequence of internodes of equal length, but shorter than in a normal fibre of the same calibre. If several sprouts from one fibre become myelinated they remain closely associated, forming a regenerative cluster as is just visible in Figure 18.11b. This persists and provides a marker for recovered axonal damage. Some clusters form a concentric arrangement of Schwann cells and unmyelinated axons around a central myelinated fibre. These may superficially resemble onion bulbs, but the circles are incomplete and fewer than those produced by repeated episodes of remyelination. There may be unmyelinated axons in the rings of Schwann cells in both cases. A band of Büngner or axonal sprouts may occur in the centre of a hypertrophic whorl as a result of axonal degeneration secondary to demyelination. If the concentric arrangement is limited, electrophysiological investigations should also be helpful in differentiating demyelination and degeneration. Teasing apart both regenerated clusters and hypertrophic nerves for individual examination is rendered very difficult by the firmly attached excess collagen and cellular processes.

There are particular problems associated with regeneration of unmyelinated axons. They arise from the inability of the resultant sheets of flattened Schwann-cell processes to act as guides. The regenerating sprouts may track along regenerating myelinated axons instead, and be misrouted to the wrong end-organ.

If traumatic damage to a nerve trunk has resulted in the separation of proximal and distal stumps, the growing sprouts may be unable to enter the distal stump. In this situation, they may turn back along the proximal stump and form a tangle of small fibres around it called a *traumatic neuroma*. This structure may be the source of unpleasant and anomalous nerve impulses. Removal of the neuroma and, if possible, apposition of the two ends of the nerve may result in improved regeneration.

NERVE BIOPSY

The sural nerve at the ankle or the superficial peroneal nerve in the lower leg are the most commonly biopsied nerves. A fascicular biopsy should be performed if possible, so that any resultant sensory deficit is minimized. The radial nerve or the dorsal ulnar nerve at the wrist are also accessible, and may be taken if clinically indicated. Biopsy of motor nerves such as the deep peroneal is only rarely performed, in cases where the neuropathy appears only to involve these nerves. Where a disease affects the entire nervous system, peripheral nerve biopsy is a convenient diagnostic test.

BIOPSY TECHNIQUES

As myelin is a semi-liquid material, fresh nerves must be handled with the utmost care and all stretching, pressure and bending avoided. It is also important to fix or freeze the nerve as soon as possible after removal, as post-mortem changes rapidly occur.

Fixation problems and handling artefacts

The nerve specimen should be fixed without delay for at least 1 hour before being cut into smaller pieces: it is still quite common to see the result of mishandling or poor processing interpreted as pathological changes. Figure 18.14 illustrates the result of damage caused in this

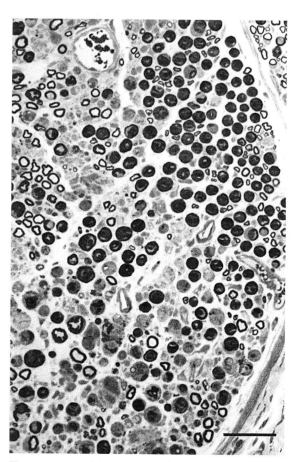

Fig. 18.14 Dark filled-in fibres resulting from trauma at the time of biopsy. (Bar = 50 μm.)

way. Large fibres are more readily damaged than small ones, and the resultant artefacts superficially resemble early Wallerian degeneration (see Fig. 18.24).

Traditional formaldehyde-based fixatives followed by paraffin embedding are unsatisfactory for specimens of peripheral nerves, because of the resultant poor myelin preservation. Glutaraldehyde is a better fixative than formaldehyde, but penetrates more slowly. The most generally satisfactory buffer so far seems to be 0.1 M PIPES (piperazine-N,N'-bis-2-ethanesulfonic acid) at pH 7.4.

The perineurium around the fascicles hinders penetration by solutions, so that processing times need to be much longer than those employed for more homogeneous and permeable tissues. Osmium tetroxide is usually used as a secondary fixative after aldehyde fixation and before resin embedding, and also as a component of Fleming's fixative for paraffin embedding. Semithin (1 μm) sections from resin blocks give simultaneous staining of axons and myelin, and greatly superior resolution compared with paraffin processing (see Figs 18.1 and 18.32). The former system also permits the cutting of ultrathin sections for electron microscopy from the same block.

A common result of poor fixation is the disruption of the Schmidt–Lanterman incisures, so that the light microscopic appearance is of two concentric circles (see Fig. 18.10). The myelin lamellae in the paranodal region also are very susceptible to artefactual distortion. Suboptimal preservation or delays in fixation may easily produce vacuolar changes in mitochondria, particularly those in the axons. Vesicular structures in myelin need careful interpretation, as they may result from the movement of lipids either during post-mortem delays or during aldehyde fixation. The different compositions of PNS and CNS myelin means that fixatives producing good results in CNS may not do so in the PNS.

Immunocytochemistry has recently become increasingly useful in diagnosis, and can usually be performed on formalin-fixed material. Unfortunately glutaraldehyde and osmium tetroxide are efficient protein cross-linkers, and so inactivate many antigen–antibody reactions that are the basis of these stains.

Frozen sections for light microscopy may be useful for the quick diagnosis of inflammatory lesions, for the localization of soluble lipids or the identification of particularly fixation-sensitive antigens. Cryoimmunocytochemistry for electron microscopy is a useful research technique, but it is doubtful if it has a place in routine diagnosis.

Morphometric techniques, both at the light and the electron microscopic level, can provide further useful information. In particular, histograms of the sizes of myelinated fibres and unmyelinated axons can be helpful in identifying fibre size changes and the loss of particular calibres of fibres or axons. Measurements of myelin thickness or g ratio (axon diameter/fibre diameter) also assist in identifying abnormal thickening or thinning of the myelin sheath. The latter can of course suggest remyelination, but axonal sprouts with short internodes also have inappropriately thin myelin. The myelin of regenerated axons remains thin due to the short internodal length. Regenerated sprouts usually have a smaller diameter than the parent axon. When assessing the significance of inappropriately thin myelin, the examination of teased fibre preparations will probably also be necessary. Segmental demyelination can then be distinguished by the presence of varying internodal lengths, contrasting with the short, regularly spaced nodes found on regenerated axons. Even on teased preparations, very small calibre fibres that normally have rather short internodes can still present interpretation problems.

DISORDERS OF PERIPHERAL NERVES

NERVE INJURY

Mechanical injury

Neurapraxia

This is the mildest degree of mechanical nerve injury and may result, for example, from acute compression injury such as tourniquet paralysis and 'Saturday-night palsy'. Clinically, there is a focal conduction block due to mechanical alteration of the paranodal structures. Recovery may take several weeks, but demyelination is not a persistent problem.

It has been suggested that mild crush or percussion injury may cause myelin to move away from the site of injury and flow back once pressure is removed, but there is little direct evidence for this. Slightly more severe injury causes local paranodal myelin retraction or segmental demyelination of the whole internode. In this situation the original Schwann cell may produce an extension of the remaining myelin sheath to cover the defect, or repair may be by insertion of a short intercalated internode. After demyelination of a whole internode, Schwann-cell multiplication leads to the formation of several shorter remyelinated internodes within a few weeks. Only a thin myelin sheath is necessary to re-establish saltatory conduction and abolish the dysfunction.

Axonotmesis

This term is used to describe a more severe injury, resulting in axonal as well as myelin disruption while leaving the Schwann-cell basal laminal sheath intact. The distal part of the nerve fibre then undergoes Wallerian degeneration and the muscles or end-organs atrophy. Recovery by sprouting from the undamaged region is aided by the presence of the basal laminal tubes, which guide the sprouts. New axons may appear even before macrophages have removed the debris. Individual sprouts will then be myelinated by new Schwann cells, which form another basal laminal sheath. The original redundant basal laminal sheath around the regenerated axon or cluster of axons eventually disappears. When the basal laminal tubes are left intact by the injury there is a good possibility of axons reinnervating their original end-organ, thus leading to total functional recovery. Axonal sprouts grow at a rate of approximately 2 mm/day, so the delay before recovery depends on the site of injury. If reinnervation is delayed for longer than 1 year, muscle fibres start to disappear and few will survive 3 years' denervation. Permanent muscle weakness will therefore result.

Persistent nerve compression or entrapment produces a region of narrowing with endoneurial expansion, particularly on the proximal side and, to a lesser extent, on the distal side. The axons on the proximal sides of these regions show abnormal bulbous swellings related to impaired axonal transport, with axonal atrophy distally. At the site of compression there may be demyelination and axonal degeneration. Morphologically, there is fibrosis of the whole nerve fascicle, proliferation of endoneurial Schwann cells and fibroblasts, and axonal loss. Mucopolysaccharide deposits and Renaut bodies may be seen, although the latter, which are ovoid hyaline structures, also occur in the endoneurium of normal nerves (Fig. 18.15).

Neurotmesis

If continuity of a nerve is interrupted by

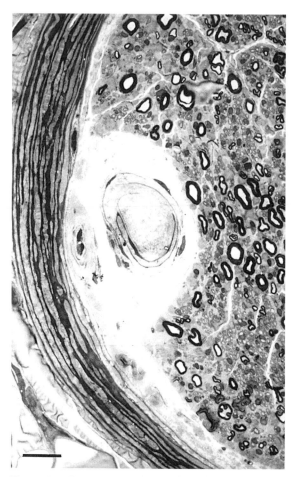

Fig. 18.15 Renaut body in a radial nerve at the wrist. (Bar = 20 μm.)

a penetrating wound or a severe stretch injury, the basal laminal sheaths no longer form continuous tubes to guide the regenerating sprouts. Recovery is much more limited after this type of injury, even if the two ends are sutured together. In addition, fibroblasts rapidly produce a collagenous barrier to axonal outgrowth. Even if the sprouts penetrate into the distal stump, misrouting of the regenerating axons impairs the chances of successful reinnervation of end-organs; this problem is reduced by the development of multiple regenerating sprouts from each axon. Aberrant regeneration and neuroma formation may further complicate recovery.

Neuroma

A traumatic neuroma forms when a nerve trunk is damaged and continuity is lost between the proximal and distal stumps, or when the perineurium is damaged and regrowing axons leave the nerve trunk through the defect. When endoneurial components are unprotected by perineurium, many small circles of perineurial cells or fibroblasts enclose small numbers of myelinated or unmyelinated axons, leading to the formation of minifascicles (Fig. 18.16a). The perineurial cells around these originate as fibroblasts that encircle the fibres. When the circle is complete, tight junctions and a basal laminal sheath form (Fig. 18.16b). The collagenous

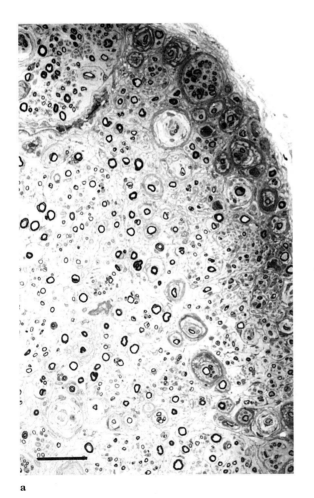

a

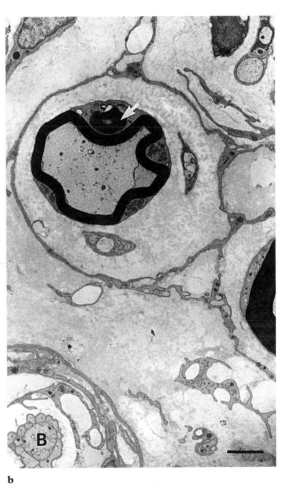

b

Fig. 18.16   (a) Minifascicles at the edge of a traumatic neuroma. (Bar = 50 μm.) (b) Detail showing a circle of perineurial cell around an axon sectioned through the paranodal region. The Schwann-cell cytoplasm contains an Elzholz body (arrow). There is a band of Büngner in the lower minifascicle (B). (Bar = 2 μm.)

components may also be of abnormal size or periodicity. At the centre of the neuroma, the axonal sprouts may form a twisted undirected mass that can develop to a considerable size.

Cold injury

Peripheral nerves seem particularly vulnerable in non-freezing ('trench foot') cold injury. Experimental studies have shown that the blood–nerve barrier is damaged, and extensive progressive endoneurial oedema occurs. This progression possibly explains why the early rapid recovery from initial conduction block and failure of axonal transport is followed in a few days by axonal degeneration of the large myelinated fibres.

Radiation damage

The neuropathy associated with radiation injury has an unusually long development time. There is a delay of at least 6 months, with a peak latency of 3–4 years. The nerves show axonal loss and extensive fibrosis. The mechanism is uncertain, but may be due to ischaemia related to changes in blood vessels. Alternatively, it has been suggested that the long-term effects seen after radiation therapy may be related to an inability of the Schwann cells to repair injury. Normally, adult Schwann cells only multiply after damage, and cell division is impaired by irradiation. Although necrosis is the result of large doses, both benign and malignant nerve sheath tumours have been reported in man and experimental animals as late sequelae of lower (20 Gy) doses of irradiation.

ACQUIRED NEUROPATHIES

Nutritional deficiency

Neuropathic beriberi

The nerves most commonly involved in beriberi are the distal limb, vagus and phrenic nerves, in which there is degeneration and loss of axons. Proximally there is secondary segmental demyelination and chromatolysis in the neurons of the dorsal root ganglia and anterior horns in the spinal cord. There is also a rostral degeneration in the posterior columns of the spinal cord. Thus the picture is of a central–peripheral distal axonopathy.

It is probable that the nerve damage is due at least partly to thiamine deficiency, but there may be other factors involved.

Axonal degeneration, with flattened membrane-bound sacs and a reduction in the density of neurofilaments and microtubules in the distal parts of axons, occurs in nerves from cases of beriberi and has been produced experimentally in rats.

Pellagra

The neuropathy in pellagra is part of a syndrome with cutaneous lesions, gastrointestinal disturbances and involvement of the CNS and PNS. Little work has been done on the PNS disturbances but the pathological changes indicate an axonal degeneration. Although pellagra is considered to be due to a deficiency of nicotinic acid, or its precursor tryptophan, the relationship of this to the neuropathy has not been established.

Alcoholic neuropathy

The clinical symptoms are somewhat similar to beriberi, as this is also a distal symmetrical sensorimotor neuropathy. The onset is often insidious. There may be vagal involvement and autonomic symptoms, painful hyperaesthesia of the soles of the feet and tenderness of the calf muscles. The predominant pathological finding in the nerves is a distal axonal degeneration, but there is also segmental demyelination. The close similarities to beriberi suggest that the cause is nutritional deficiency, but a contribution from a direct toxic effect of ethanol has not been excluded.

Vitamin E deficiency

Chronic intestinal fat malabsorption, such as that seen in children with chronic biliary atresia and fibrocystic disease, is the most frequent cause of vitamin E deficiency. This may produce a spinocerebellar degeneration and peripheral neuropathy. The neurological effects are probably the result of free radical damage, and have been shown experimentally to be exacerbated by the ingestion of polyunsaturated fatty acids. A biopsy of a sensory neuropathy associated with intestinal malabsorption showed axonal degeneration; in another case, numerous acid-phosphatase-positive membrane-bound structures were seen in the Schwann cells. Similar inclusions have been reported in cases of abetalipoproteinaemia. The neurological syndrome in this condition responds to vitamin E supplementation, raising the possibility of a similar causation. In experimental animals, abnormal axonal inclusions are found in the distal parts of axon, particularly affecting dorsal column axons in the gracile nuclei.

Toxic neuropathies

Industrial toxins

Most of these substances produce a sensorimotor neuropathy with a distal axonopathy, but the details are nearly as varied as the substances involved. Motor symptoms predominate in some instances, such as organophosphate poisoning, and sensory manifestations in others, such as acrylamide toxicity. The symptoms of acrylamide poisoning also include excessive sweating and exfoliative dermatitis, loss of tendon reflexes even in mild cases, and truncal ataxia in more severe ones. Initially there are distal accumulations of neurofilaments in the large fibres in the PNS, followed by axonal degeneration. Recovery is slow and depends on the length of exposure.

In the neuropathy associated with triorthocresyl phosphate (TOCP) and some other organophosphates, there is a dying-back axonal degeneration manifesting as muscle weakness and wasting following a latent period. The initial damage seems particularly to affect the intramuscular nerve endings, but is unrelated to the inhibition of acetylcholinesterase that can cause an acute cholinergic crisis. The dying-back neuropathy produced by 2,5-hexanedione, the toxic metabolite of a range of solvents used in glues and the printing industry, is quite different. 2,5-HD neuropathy is characterized by focal axonal en-largements and complicated by the demyelination produced as a result. Frequently a phenomenon known as 'coasting' occurs. In this, the neuropathy worsens for several weeks after withdrawal of the toxin. Similar morphological changes are seen in carbon disulphide poisoning, suggesting a similar metabolic cause. The metabolic changes may result from interference with glycolysis by the inhibition of glyceraldehyde-3-phosphate dehydrogenase, or may alternatively be due to abnormal neurofilament cross-linking.

Acute exposure to trichloroethylene may result in damage to the facial, trigeminal or optic nerves, whilst chronic intoxication leads to a moderate distal, symmetrical, sensorimotor polyneuropathy and a neuronopathy. Dimethylproprionitrile also produces a dying-back neuropathy affecting the larger fibres first, as do ethylene oxide, chloro-biphenyl, and BHMH (2-t-butylazo-2-hydroxy-5-methylhexane).

Among the metals or metal-like elements, mercury (atomic number 80), thallium (81), lead (82) and arsenic (33), are all highly toxic and all produce a distal axonopathy. This is predominantly sensory in the case of mercury poisoning, which also affects the CNS. Studies of patients with Minamata disease suggested that both myelin and axons are affected, with the initial lesion occurring at the node of Ranvier. There have been no reports of onion bulb formation. Unmyelinated axons are also affected. Lead poisoning, on the other hand, produces a predominantly motor neuropathy, and arsenic and thallium both result in sensorimotor dying-back axonal neuropathies. Mitochondrial abnormalities are particularly prominent in thallium poisoning. Regeneration is frequently poor after withdrawal of either an organic or inorganic toxin.

Drugs

Isoniazid, nitrofurantoin, chloroquine, vincristine, pyridoxine and several other drugs, including gold, are neurotoxic, mostly producing chronic progressive sensorimotor polyneuropathies. Isoniazid causes the degeneration of myelinated and unmyelinated axons, followed by extensive sprouting. Thalidomide, pyridoxine and metronidazole lead to predominantly sensory neuropathies; dapsone and, possibly, cimetidine, lead to motor involvement. Perhexilene maleate affects the Schwann cells, resulting in primary demyelination in addition to severe axonal loss. There may be onion bulb formation. Small, dense membrane-bound inclusions with a variable para-crystalloid structure are just visible by light microscopy, and are found predominantly in the Schwann cells. Lamellar inclusions may be found in amiodarone and chloroquine toxicity. They are more widely distributed than the inclusions associated with perhexilene maleate, and are found in Schwann cells, fibroblasts, capillary endothelial cells and pericytes. Demyelination seems likely to be secondary to the axonal changes, and onion bulb formation is rare. The crystalline bodies found non-specifically in Remak fibres of many axonal neuropathies are a potential source of confusion (Fig. 18.17). There is some evidence that these result from disturbances in cholesterol metabolism, as they can be produced experimentally by treating rats with inhibitors of cholesterol biosynthesis.

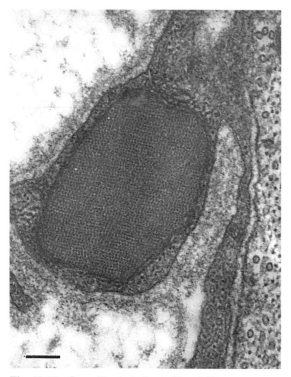

Fig. 18.17 Crystalline inclusion in Remak fibre. (Bar = 0.1 μm.)

Inflammatory demyelinating disorders

Acute inflammatory demyelinating polyradiculoneuropathy (AIDP) (Guillain–Barré syndrome)

This is the commonest acute neuropathy in the UK, particularly in males aged between 20 and 50 years. The majority of patients have an antecedent infection about 1–4 weeks before developing neurological symptoms. Although the causation is still not definitely established, an autoimmune mechanism seems likely. Both cell-mediated immune processes and humoral factors have been implicated. There is a characteristic increase in cerebrospinal fluid protein, without a pleocytosis. Symptoms vary but are predominantly motor and usually symmetrical; distal sensory symptoms and autonomic abnormalities may also occur. Electrodiagnostic studies show reduced nerve conduction velocity, conduction block and signs of denervation. Recovery takes 3–6 months, or longer if there has been extensive axonal loss. Factors associated with a poor outcome are the age at onset, rapid progression, the need for assisted ventilation and small distal evoked muscle action potentials. It is thought that the experimental disease *experimental allergic neuritis* (EAN) is a model. This develops in animals 2 weeks after injection with peripheral nerve antigens plus Freund's adjuvant. However, although P_2 myelin protein has been identified as the causative antigen in EAN, the antigen responsible for AIDP has not yet been identified. There are, however, increases in the levels of acute-phase proteins, and frequently, antineural antibodies, in addition to the presence of immune complexes. Plasma exchange is of benefit in severe cases if performed before deterioration has ceased.

Nerve biopsies reveal inflammatory infiltrates throughout the PNS. These initially appear as perivascular cuffing, but may be difficult to find in a biopsy specimen either because of the patchy distribution of the lesions – which are more numerous in spinal nerve roots – because the invading cells rapidly disperse into the endoneurium, or because only a small number of cells is actually necessary to produce demyelination. The invading cells are mainly lymphocytes and macrophages, and immunolabelling may be useful for characterizing them. Macrophages strip the myelin sheath from its axon by inserting processes between the lamellae and then removing them. Demyelination produces large, temporarily unmyelinated axons. Multiplication of Schwann cells follows and new myelinated segments of varying lengths are formed. Axonal degeneration in differing degrees – sometimes extensive – often occurs, and might represent a bystander effect. The histological changes produced by EAN in animals are quite similar, and the development of the lesions has been extensively studied (see Figs 18.8, 18.9 and 18.10).

Chronic inflammatory demyelinating polyradiculoneuropathy (CIDP)

Closely related to AIDP are chronic progressive and chronic relapsing forms (CIDP) that probably have a different immunological basis. It is not uncommon to find hypertrophic onion bulbs in the chronic forms (see Fig. 18.11a). Occasionally, active cell-mediated demyelination may be identified. The cellular invasion in these chronic cases is often quite limited and difficult to find. Immunocytochemical staining for T_4 and T_8 lymphocytes can be helpful, especially when only occasional cells are present (Fig. 18.18), but occasional cells can also be found in HMSN I (see p. 396), so the clinical history is very important. Intramyelinic oedema is sometimes associated with demyelinating processes. This produces 'bubbles' in the myelin sheaths (see Fig. 18.10).

Rarely, there may be accompanying multifocal demyelinating lesions in the CNS.

Infections

Leprosy

Leprosy, or Hansen's disease, is caused by *Mycobacterium leprae* and is very variable, depending on the individual's reaction to the bacterium. There is a continuous spectrum from lepromatous or pluribacillary leprosy with little reaction to the bacillus through dimorphous leprosy to tuberculoid or paucibacillary leprosy, where

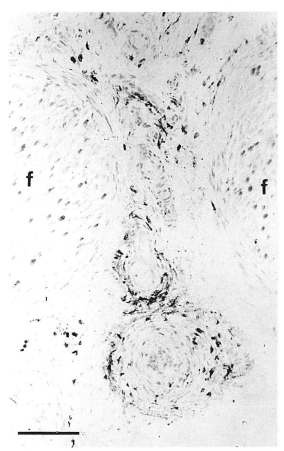

Fig. 18.18 CIDP. Immunochemical staining for T8 lymphocytes. Positive cells are around epineurial blood vessels and fascicles (f). (Frozen sections. Bar = 20 μm.)

there is a vigorous immunological response and severe tissue damage.

In lepromatous leprosy there is a diffuse neuropathy, the changes being maximal in the colder areas of the body, such as the distal extremities. Leprosy bacilli proliferate preferentially at lower temperatures. Sensory loss leads to mutilating lesions, and nerve thickening can produce an entrapment neuropathy. There is loss of myelinated and unmyelinated axons as well as changes in the perineurium. Large numbers of bacteria are present in Schwann cells and in the pale-staining foamy macrophages. They may be demonstrated with Ziehl–Nielsen or Wade-Fite stains, but are more easily seen by electron microscopy. They are present in greater numbers in the Schwann cells associated with unmy-

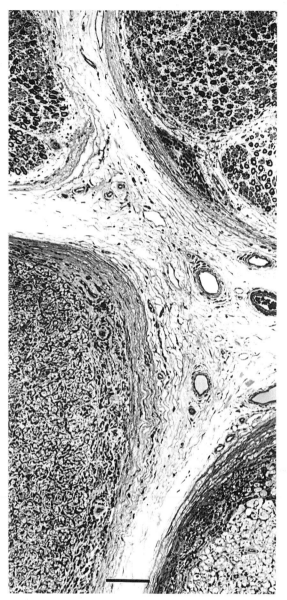

Fig. 18.19 Pleuribacillary (borderline lepromatous) leprosy. There is great variability between fascicles. (Bar = 20 μm.)

In tuberculoid leprosy the disease causes a focal or multifocal neuropathy accompanied by local skin lesions. Damage to cutaneous nerves may lead to the development of focal intraneural 'cold abscesses'. There is an intense immunological response and few bacilli are seen. The typical lesion in skin and nerves is a focal granuloma with giant cells, macrophages and lymphocytes. Severe tissue damage and extensive fibrosis occur. The normal architecture of the nerve can be completely destroyed, so that ultimately no neural elements are left. In this situation the perineurium reverts to disconnected fibroblasts that do not form a complete sheath or possess a basal lamina, and thus have no barrier function (Fig. 18.20).

In borderline cases there are some features of lepromatous and some of tuberculoid leprosy; these may be subdivided into borderline lepromatous and borderline tuberculoid, depending on which predominates. So-called 'reversal reactions' in these cases are sudden exacerbations of the disease. There may be extensive cellular invasion, manifested by perivascular cuffing and invasion of the endoneurium by small lymphocytes, macrophages and other cells.

The traditional theory of the mode of travel of the leprosy bacilli was that they moved up axons from the skin. Although, occasionally, groups of bacilli can be found in axons (Fig. 18.21), this is probably of limited importance and haematogenous spread is of greater significance.

Diphtheria

Although the causative agent, *Corynebacterium diphtheriae*, produces a localized infection of the pharynx or skin, it also produces an exotoxin that damages the myocardium and peripheral nerves. Local injection of this toxin produces focal demyelination. The neuropathy develops after a latent period of some weeks, and complete recovery is possible probably because the axons are not affected. The demyelination is not accompanied by cellular infiltration and particularly affects the spinal ventral and dorsal roots and ganglia, possibly due to a less effective blood–nerve barrier in these regions. The exotoxin has a specific attraction to Schwann cells, and interferes with myelin protein synthesis.

elinated than with myelinated axons. The actual mechanism by which they cause demyelination and axonal loss is unclear. Small myelinated and unmyelinated axons are preferentially affected. Invasion and destruction of the perineurium may hinder identification of individual fascicles in a biopsy specimen. The degree of damage may vary widely between fascicles (Fig. 18.19).

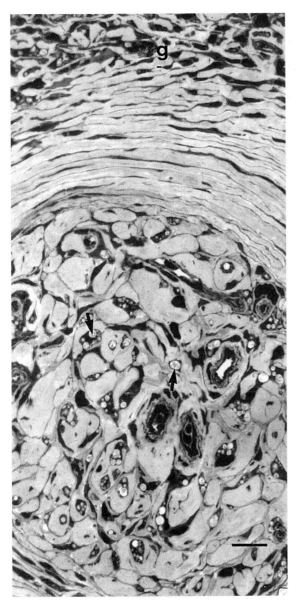

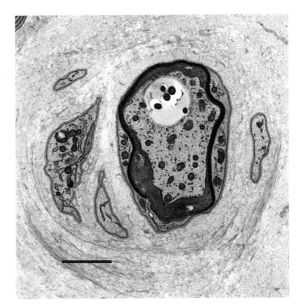

Fig. 18.21 Leprosy bacilli in small myelinated axon. (Bar = 2 μm.)

Fig. 18.20 Severe borderline lepromatous leprosy. The perineurium has reverted to fibroblasts and there is extensive collagen deposition. The epineurium is infiltrated by granulomatous cells (g). Some bacilli are present in the clear spaces (arrows) but are not resolvable at this magnification. (Bar = 20 μm.)

Lyme disease (borreliosis)

This condition, also called tick-bite neuropathy, was first recognized in Europe in the early 1920s. It is caused by the spirochaete *Borrelia burgdorferi* and is transmitted by *Ixodes damnini* or related ticks occurring in deer. The first sign of infection is a typical rash (erythema migrans), starting at the bite. A meningoradiculitis with carditis and arthritis then develop. The peripheral nerve involvement at this stage varies, and may be multifocal or involve the cranial nerves or nerve plexuses or, rarely, produces a syndrome closely resembling the Guillain–Barré syndrome. The third stage is a mild sensorimotor neuropathy, often with a carpal tunnel syndrome due to compression of the median nerve by the transverse carpal segment. Examination of infected nerves and ganglia shows perivascular cuffing by plasma cells and lymphocytes around capillaries. Damage to the nerve is mainly axonal, and affects both myelinated and unmyelinated axons. The mechanism causing the neuropathy is not clear, but may be related to vascular damage or have an allergic origin.

Rabies

Occasionally patients with rabies present with a paralytic rather than an encephalitic syndrome. This can mimic AIDP and show active macrophage-mediated segmental demyelination and remyelination, together with axonal loss.

Human immunodeficiency virus (HIV)

Peripheral neuropathy is common in HIV infection, including the later stage of the acquired immunodeficiency syndrome (AIDS). A variety of diseases may occur, the commonest of which is a sensory neuropathy, which is often painful. Sometimes there is an acute inflammatory demyelinating neuropathy with spontaneous recovery resembling acute inflammatory demyelinating polyradiculoneuropathy (AIDP). CIDP may be encountered more frequently. These inflammatory neuropathies are stated to be most common in the earlier, asymptomatic stages of HIV infection. In the AIDS-related CIDP there is a considerably greater inflammatory reaction. As well as axonal degeneration and variable degrees of demyelination, there may be a necrotizing vasculitis.

More rarely, multiple mononeuropathies giving an asymmetrical picture may occur, with axonal degeneration, perivascular infiltration and vasculitis predominating. Cytomegalovirus infection can cause a rapidly progressive inflammatory lumbosacral polyradiculopathy.

Infectious mononucleosis

Peripheral nervous system complications of infections with the Epstein–Barr virus are varied, and include involvement of the brachial or lumbosacral plexus or facial nerves and AIDP.

Systemic disorders

Diabetes mellitus

This is among the commonest causes of neuropathy, which can be separated into two main groups. One group of disorders, probably metabolic in origin, is predominantly sensory and autonomic symmetrical polyneuropathies, and the other is focal or multifocal neuropathies that may have a vasculitic basis.

In the first type, lesions may be found in dorsal roots and ganglia as well as in nerve trunks, and the symptoms are predominantly distal. In acute painful cases there may be selective involvement of small myelinated and unmyelinated axons, but loss of all fibre calibres may be found and the total myelinated fibre density may be greatly reduced. In some instances the axonal degeneration may be of the dying-back type. Regenerative activity is sometimes prominent, leading to the formation of large clusters of small axon sprouts. Electron microscopy reveals that these are frequently surrounded by an abnormally stiff and persistent basal laminal tube that is often circular in cross-section (Fig. 18.22). In non-diabetic nerves this disappears quite rapidly as the sprouts develop. There may also be segmental demyelination and remyelination, with abnormally thin myelin sheaths and even, occasionally, small onion-bulb formations.

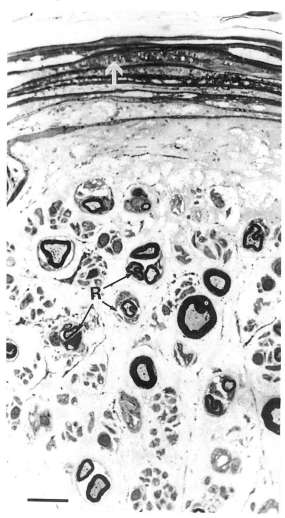

Fig. 18.22 Diabetic neuropathy. There are calcium deposits in the perineurium (arrow) and circular regenerative clusters (R). (Bar = 10 μm.)

The focal and multifocal nerve lesions found in the other main group of diabetic neuropathies may have an ischaemic component, or may even occasionally indicate an abnormal susceptibility to external pressure. The focal lesions are variable: they may be either demyelinating or axonal in nature, and adjacent fascicles are typically differentially affected.

A thickening of the basal laminal sheath around the endoneurial blood vessels, often seen in chronic neuropathies, is particularly common and well developed in diabetic neuropathy (Fig. 18.23).

Uraemia

Chronic renal failure causes a slowly progressive,

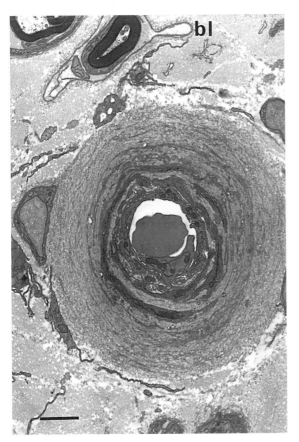

Fig. 18.23 Diabetic neuropathy. There is extensive basal laminal reduplication about an endoneurial blood vessel and a persistent basal laminal tube (bl). (Bar = 2 μm.)

predominantly sensory neuropathy, often with unpleasant dysaesthesias and paraesthesias that may result in a 'restless legs syndrome'. There may also be compression neuropathies of the ulnar or peroneal nerves in bedridden patients. In sural nerve biopsies there is loss of large myelinated fibres and segmental demyelination, probably secondary to axonal atrophy. Deposition of β-2-microglobulin as a form of amyloid has been found to be a cause of the carpal tunnel syndrome in patients on long-term haemodialysis.

Liver disease

A variety of neuropathies have been associated with both acute and chronic liver disease. Acute viral hepatitis may be followed by the Guillain–Barré syndrome, and a subclinical demyelinating neuropathy is sometimes found in patients with chronic cirrhosis. A painful sensory neuropathy is very occasionally associated with primary biliary cirrhosis.

Vasculitis

Neuropathies caused by systemic necrotizing vasculitis are characterized by axonal damage. It is usually possible to find collections of inflammatory cells around epineurial blood vessels (Fig. 18.24). If these are no longer present, staining with MSB for fibrin or immunostaining for fibrinogen will identify the leakage of fibrin that marks the site of previous inflammation. Electron microscopy of the fibrin deposits shows a dense extracellular precipitate with a very fine periodicity. An acute short-lived episode can produce simultaneous degeneration of all fibres. These will then recover together, resulting in replacement of the myelinated fibres with regenerative clusters of the same size and stage of development.

Less commonly, cases with restricted non-systemic vasculitis causing neuropathy are encountered. The histological changes in peripheral nerves are similar.

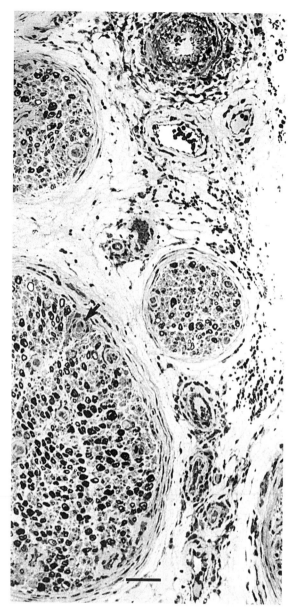

Fig. 18.24 Acute vasculitis. There are inflammatory cells in the epineurium and smaller collections around endoneurial capillaries (arrow). There is also extensive recent axonal degeneration. (Bar = 50 μm.)

Neuropathy associated with paraproteinaemia and dysproteinaemia

Malignant plasma cell dyscrasias: myeloma. Clinically, myeloma is the commonest malignancy with which there may occur an as-

sociated neuropathy. The details are very variable and include the carpal tunnel syndrome due to compression by amyloid deposits, or compression of the spinal roots or cranial nerves due to plasmacytomas. There may rarely be a generalized amyloid neuropathy or, more commonly, a sensorimotor neuropathy similar to that sometimes seen as a non-metastatic complication of carcinoma. This latter is probably a type of dying-back axonal neuropathy. With osteosclerotic myeloma there can also be a chronic demyelinating motor neuropathy, accompanied by widespread oedema, cutaneous changes, endocrine dysfunction and papilloedema (Crow–Fukase syndrome).

Waldenström's macroglobulinaemia. In this condition, a lymphoma is associated with a chronic lymphoreticular proliferation and a monoclonal IgM plasma paraprotein. The neuropathy is chronic, distal and sensorimotor; in biopsies there is either axonal degeneration or segmental demyelination. Extensive basal laminal thickening around the endoneurial capillaries is often prominent in this and in the benign monoclonal paraproteinaemias. In some cases, lymphocytic infiltration is found in the endoneurium. Electron microscopy of myelin sheaths may demonstrate an abnormal periodicity similar to that seen in benign paraproteinaemias (see below). Sometimes extracellular deposits of finely fibrillar material have been recorded in the endoneurium. These are usually granular and close to the Schwann-cell basal lamina, and may be confused with small amyloid deposits. The presumption that these are immunoglobulins has yet to be confirmed, as mucopolysaccharides may be found in this location in many conditions.

Benign monoclonal paraproteinaemia. It is now possible to link some neuropathies whose cause was previously unknown to the presence of benign monoclonal paraproteins, most commonly IgM. With immunocytological techniques, IgM can be found on the myelin sheaths of the nerve (Fig. 18.25), and experimental studies suggest that it may act as an autoantibody. Most patients are older males. As well as a distal sensorimotor neuropathy, patients frequently also suffer from tremor and ataxia.

In nerve biopsies there is often demyelination, but there may also be considerable loss of myseen often, but not exclusively, in remyelinated axons. Close examination is necessary to differentiate this from uncompacted myelin lamellae in which neither major dense nor less dense lines are formed. Although common in paraproteinaemic neuropathy, this latter abnormality may be found in a variety of other diseases, including AIDP, CIDP and paraneoplastic neuropathy. It usually affects either the inner or outer lamellae, but not scattered lamellae within the sheath, as does widely-spaced myelin (Fig. 18.26). It is extremely unusual to find alterations in myelin periodicity other than a threefold increase or complete non-compaction.

Experimentally, it can be shown that applying hyper- or hypo-osmolar solutions to the endoneurium also alters the periodicity, as does irradiation and the intraneural injection of serum from patients or animals with autoimmune diseases.

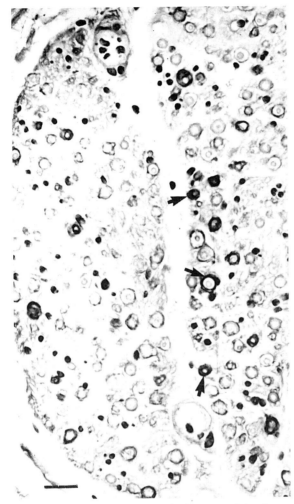

Fig. 18.25 IgM$_k$ paraproteinaemia; immunostaining for IgM on myelin sheaths (arrows). (Bar = 20 μm.)

elinated fibres. There may also be hypertrophic changes due to repeated episodes of demyelination. Intramyelinic oedema may also be found. In about half the cases, the myelin periodicity is about three times that of normal myelin. It seems possible that this is due to the incorporation of the abnormal protein into the Schwann-cell plasma membrane, thus altering its properties and preventing the normal compaction of the outer surfaces to form the less dense line. The two components of this are visible by electron microscopy, but are separated by a much larger gap than normal. The inner surfaces form a normal major dense line. This abnormality is

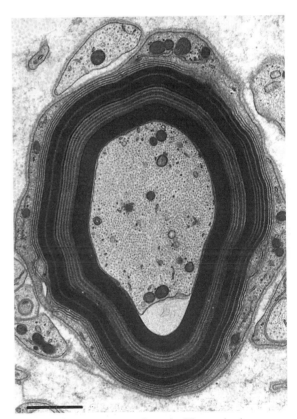

Fig. 18.26 IgM$_k$ paraproteinaemia. The spacing between many of the myelin lamellae is much wider than normal. (Bar = 1 μm.)

Cryoglobulinaemia. The neuropathy that may accompany both essential and secondary cryoglobulinaemia affects the lower limbs. This is related to cryoglobulin deposition, but various mechanisms have been suggested. A vasculitis affecting the vasa nervorum may be due to cryoglobulin deposition and activation of the complement system, but there is also evidence of ischaemic damage to the nerves due to intravascular deposits of cryoglobulin. On electron microscopy of this abnormal protein there are closely packed tubular structures forming electro-dense fingerprint-like arrays in the lumina and capillary walls and, extracellularly, in the endoneurium.

Sarcoidosis

This multisystem disorder affects the PNS in about 5 per cent of cases. The presenting symptoms are very variable and include facial nerve palsies, multiple mononeuropathies, subacute polyradiculoneuritis and a symmetrical sensorimotor polyneuropathy. In nerve biopsies there is axonal loss and segmental demyelination, and there may be sarcoid granulomas. The neuropathy may at times be due to granulomatous angiitis of the vasa nervorum.

Malignancy

A variety of neuropathies may occur as a non-metastatic complication. Sensory neuropathy associated with small-cell carcinoma of the lung is associated with anti-Hu antibodies. Sensorimotor neuropathy may be associated with bronchial and other carcinomas. In some patients the neuropathy resembles AIDP (Guillain–Barré syndrome) or CIDP with segmental demyelination, probably due to an immunological disturbance. No consistent correlation with tumour resection has been found. These patients may respond to plasmapheresis, unlike those with the sensory neuropathy due to lymphocytic infiltration of the dorsal root ganglia and destruction of the sensory neurons. In biopsies of the sural nerve from these cases there is loss of larger myelinated axons.

Very rarely, cases of multiple mononeuropathies occur due to vasculitis associated with malignancy. Morphologically these are the same as other vasculitic neuropathies.

HEREDITARY NEUROPATHIES

Hereditary motor and sensory neuropathy, type I (HMSN I)

Genetic studies have resulted in the identification of a common basis for several diseases previously thought to be distinct, and they are now combined under the heading of HMSN I. These include peroneal muscular atrophy (the hypertrophic form of Charcot–Marie–Tooth disease), and the Roussy–Lévy syndrome. Most commonly the inheritance is autosomal dominant, but a rare autosomal recessive form may also be encountered. Symptoms develop during childhood. Morphologically, the typical change is the presence of extensive circular arrangements of Schwann-cell processes around a central myelinated fibre, due to repeated demyelination and remyelination. There may be loss of the central axon or its replacement by several axon sprouts. The population of myelinated fibres may also be reduced (Fig. 18.27). The development of the excess cell processes and collagen results in an enlarged and thickened nerve trunk.

HMSN II

This is a progressive axonal disorder originally referred to as the neuronal form of Charcot–Marie–Tooth disease. The inheritance is usually autosomal dominant. Symptoms develop slightly later, and may not appear until middle age. Pathologically, mainly the larger myelinated fibres are lost. Collections of axonal sprouts may be seen, indicating attempted regeneration.

X-linked dominant HMSN

In this disorder the clinical picture is similar to HMSN I, with onset in early childhood, pes cavus, atrophy and weakness of the peroneal muscles and intrinsic hand muscles and sensory loss in the hands and feet. The pathological and physiological abnormalities, however, are of an axonal neuropathy that resembles HMSN II,

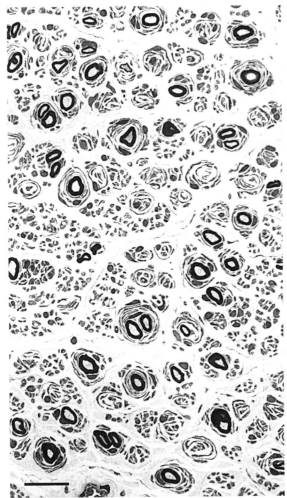

Fig. 18.27 HMSN I. There are hypertrophic whorls of Schwann cells around central myelinated axons. (Bar = 20 μm.)

although the axonal sprouting reported may be more extensive.

HMSN III

Also called Dejerine–Sottas disease, this rare condition is recessively inherited, with an onset in childhood and a progressive clinical course. Severe disability results from delayed motor development, with limb weakness and ataxia. The peripheral nerves are grossly thickened due to the development of extensive hypertrophic whorls. The central axons have either a very thin myelin

sheath (hypomyelination) or none at all, and there is also extensive axonal loss (Fig. 18.28).

Hereditary sensory and autonomic neuropathies (HSAN) type 1

HSAN type 1 is dominantly inherited, with an onset in the second decade or later. The sensory symptoms are due to primary degeneration of the lumbosacral dorsal root ganglion cells and, later, those supplying the upper limbs. The initial symptoms are disturbances of pain and temperature discrimination in the feet and legs. These lead to stress fractures and recurrent plantar ulcers. There may be mild associated motor involvement. Sural nerve biopsies show a loss of unmyelinated and small myelinated axons,

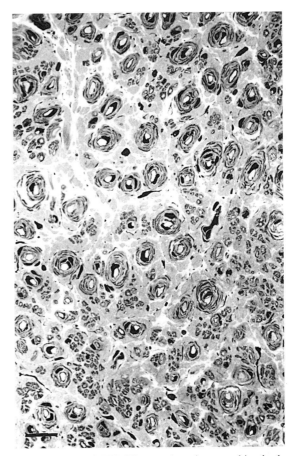

Fig. 18.28 HMSN III. There are large hypertrophic whorls around very thinly myelinated fibres. (Bar = 20 μm.)

with a less marked reduction in the large myelinated fibre population.

HSAN type II

Type II differs from type I in its recessive inheritance and earlier onset, usually in infancy. The sensory loss, which affects all sensory modalities, is more widespread and predominantly involves the distal extremities of the upper and lower limbs. The lips and tongue may be mutilated as a result of the sensory loss, as well as the hands and feet. Autonomic involvement is usually minor. Myelinated fibre loss in the sural nerve may be almost total; the numbers of unmyelinated axons are usually less extensively depleted.

HSAN type III (Riley–Day syndrome)

HSAN type III, or the Riley–Day syndrome, is a recessively inherited disorder most commonly affecting Jewish children. There are prominent autonomic as well as sensory symptoms from birth. In the sural nerve the numbers of unmyelinated axons are greatly reduced and there is a less marked reduction in the densities of small and the largest myelinated fibres. There is a loss of neurons in the dorsal roots, and in sympathetic and parasympathetic ganglia, probably due to developmental aplasia.

HSAN type IV

HSAN type IV is a rare, recessively inherited disorder, with congenital insensitivity to pain, anhidrosis, mild mental retardation and failure to thrive. Sural nerve biopsies show predominantly a loss of unmyelinated axons and a lesser reduction in the small myelinated fibre population.

HSAN type V

This disorder is characterized by congenital insensitivity to pain and a mutilating acropathy. In biopsies of the sural nerve there is a selective loss of small myelinated fibres only.

Friedreich's ataxia

In the early stages of this spinocerebellar degeneration there is areflexia and impaired joint position and vibration sense. This is predominantly a sensory neuropathy, with selective atrophy of large myelinated fibres resulting in secondary demyelination. There is a loss of larger dorsal root ganglion cells. Electrophysiological investigations show normal motor nerve conduction and absent or reduced sensory action potentials. Peripheral nerve involvement may also be found in some other spinocerebellar degenerations.

Hereditary liability to pressure palsies

This autosomal dominant disorder is manifested as a mild generalized neuropathy, superimposed on which there is an excessive liability to the occurrence of pressure palsies. It is possible that the genetic defect results in myelin that is abnormally sensitive to mechanical damage. Both motor and sensory nerves may be affected. The characteristic changes are best seen in fibres teased individually, and take the form of sausage-like thickenings of the myelin sheath called *tomaculi*, from the Latin for a sausage. These often occur preferentially in the paranodal region. There may also be transnodal demyelination and segmental demyelination. Electron microscopy shows that the tomaculi are formed by redundant folds of myelin lamellae.

Familial amyloid polyneuropathies

Amyloids are a heterogeneous group of proteins that vary considerably but have in common a β-pleated sheet configuration. In the amyloidoses that affect the peripheral nerves the deposits occur extracellularly, often around blood vessels. The best-characterized form is type I, or Portuguese hereditary amyloidosis. This is a 'small fibre neuropathy' that initially affects unmyelinated and small myelinated fibres and works its way up the spectrum, so that the last surviving fibres are the largest myelinated ones.

Several different types of hereditary amyloidosis have been identified so far. All except two are due to a single base substitution of the trans-thyretin (TTR) molecule. This abnormal protein is then deposited in many organs, but particularly in peripheral nerves. Specific antibody staining on paraffin sections can be used to distinguish this amyloid from amyloidosis associated with myeloma consisting of κ or λ light chains (Fig. 18.29). The exceptions are the type III or Iowa form, in which the amyloid consists of a variant apolipoprotein A-1 with an arginine for glycine substitution at position 26, and the type IV or Finnish variety, in which the amyloid is derived from plasma gelsoline.

The β-pleated sheet configuration of the amyloid molecules makes them optically active, so that when the section is viewed through crossed polaroid filters, the areas stained red with alkaline Congo red exhibit a bright lime-green birefringence. Alternatively they fluoresce pale blue when stained with thioflavin T and illuminated with UV light and the appropriate filters. This is a very quick, sensitive method of identifying small deposits. They may be closely apposed to Schwann cells or to collagen fibrils. In some cases the deposits are exclusively perivascular (Fig. 18.30a), thus bearing a superficial resemblance to the thickened basal lamina seen around blood vessels in diabetes mellitus and IgM paraproteinaemia. The occurrence of fibrous long-spacing collagen in the adjacent perineurium is very unusual (Fig. 18.30b). In severely affected fascicles the amyloid may replace most of the endoneurial contents, but in milder cases the deposits may be very patchy and difficult to find in a small biopsy.

Neurofibromatosis

This is a relatively common, dominantly inherited disease with very variable expression (see Ch. 13). In the mildest cases of the peripheral form of the disease (von Recklinghausen's disease, NF1) there are only *café au lait* spots on the skin and cutaneous neurofibromas. These consist of proliferated Schwann cells, fibroblasts and collagen through which the nerve fibres course. In more severe cases, the neurofibroma may cause nerve compression or undergo sarcomatous change. In cases with predominantly central involvement (NF2) there are often minimal cutaneous abnormalities. The peripheral nerve tumours are due to proliferation of Schwann cells and may be found on any nerves and roots, including the cranial nerves and the acoustic nerve in particular. There is severe axonal loss. Biopsy of the neurinomas shows masses of Schwann cells and collagen, including widely spaced collagen; axons are very difficult to identify in this region, but unaffected fascicles may pass close by.

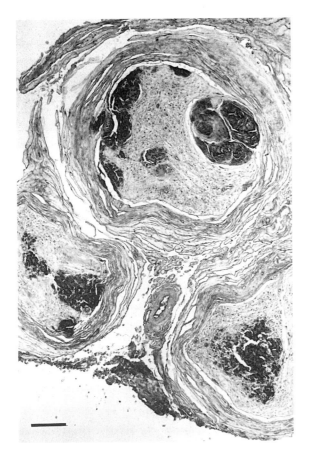

Fig. 18.29 Hereditary (Portuguese type) amyloid neuropathy. (Immunostaining for TTR, frozen section. Bar = 100 μm.)

Lipidoses

Metachromatic leukodystrophy (MLD)

There are late infantile, juvenile and adult variants with onset at 6 months–2 years, 3–16

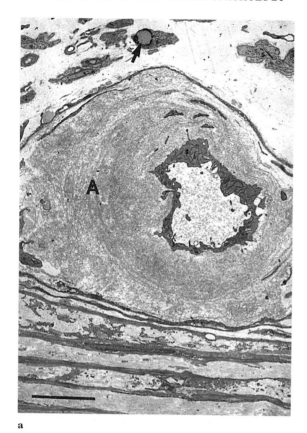

a

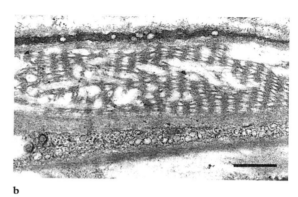

b

Fig. 18.30 Amyloid neuropathy. (a) Perivascular deposits (A) and lipofuscin granule (arrow). (Bar = 5 μm.) (b) Fibrous long-spacing collagen in the adjacent perineurium. (Bar = 0.5 μm.)

years and in adult life respectively. MLD is an autosomal recessive disease caused by a deficiency of arylsulphatase A, leading to an accumulation of cerebroside sulphate in the CNS and ganglia, Schwann cells and kidneys. The late infantile form has the most rapid progression, with onset at 6 months to 2 years of age, and leads to death within about 2 years. Very occasionally the disorder begins with a peripheral neuropathy, with gait disorder, hypotonia and lower limb areflexia preceding CNS signs. More usually it is dominated by CNS disease. Sulphatide is excreted in the urine and the enzyme deficiency can be shown in leucocytes or serum.

MLD is primarily a demyelinating disorder, and biopsies show segmental demyelination and a general thinning of the myelin sheaths. The deposits of cerebroside sulphate in Schwann cells and macrophages give a golden-brown metachromasia with acidified cresyl violet on fresh frozen

sections. Toluidine blue staining of formalin-fixed frozen sections gives a pink metachromasia. The largest deposits are in endoneurial macrophages, and high-power electron microscopy of these shows inclusions with a characteristic periodicity of 6 μm. The smaller amounts in Schwann cells are known as tuffstone bodies, as they are electron-dense with small round holes, giving them some resemblance to tufa (volcanic limestone).

Krabbe's disease (globoid-cell leukodystrophy)

This is an autosomal recessive disease caused by a deficiency of galactocerebroside-β-galactosidase, leading to the accumulation of galactocerebroside in the brain to form large round (globoid) cells. Myelination in both the CNS and PNS is affected. The presenting signs in early infancy are

CNS in origin, but peripheral nerve involvement is soon also demonstrable. There are also very rare cases with very slow progression that do not present until adulthood.

Although the largest deposits of lipid are in the CNS, there are also lesser accumulations in the Schwann cells of the PNS. This lipid is very soluble and is only preserved in frozen sections, but the shape of the crystals may still be seen in epoxy sections for electron microscopy. There are similar inclusions in the macrophages. The myelin sheaths are all thinner than normal, and are often curved around the pale inclusions in the Schwann cells (Fig. 18.31).

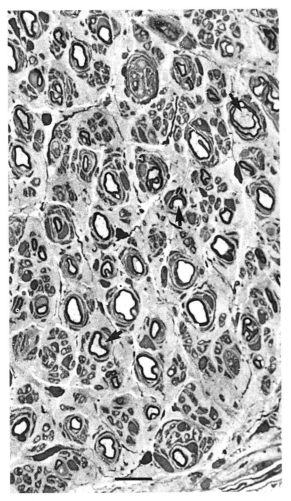

Fig. 18.31 Krabbe's disease; inappropriately thin myelin sheaths and lipid inclusions in Schwann cells (arrows). (Bar = 10 μm.)

Fabry's disease (angiokeratoma corporis diffusum)

This is an X-linked recessive disorder caused by a deficiency of the lysosomal enzyme ceramide-trihexoside-α-galactosidase. Ceramide trihexoside therefore cannot be metabolized, and is deposited in the endothelial and smooth muscle cells of arteries, leading to vascular disease of kidney, heart and brain. Skin involvement leads to the development of dark-red telangiectases (angiokeratomas), especially over the lower trunk. Peripheral nerve symptoms of a painful small fibre neuropathy present in early childhood. Female carriers are often clinically mildly involved as well, although without the renal failure seen in males.

In nerve biopsies there is loss of unmyelinated and small myelinated fibres, probably due to deposition of the glycolipid in ganglion cells. The most striking abnormality is the deposition of ceramide trihexoside in the perineurium and in the walls of the small endoneurial blood vessels. The cytoplasm of the perineurial cells may be almost entirely replaced by lipid deposits (Fig. 18.32). When examined by high-power electron microscopy, the inclusions have a periodicity of 4 nm. The inclusions in the capillary endothelial cells coalesce into large patches, and may be partly dissolved during processing.

Niemann–Pick disease

There are two major groups and various subtypes, all with an autosomal recessive inheritance. The defect in group I is sphingomyelinase deficiency. As well as extensive changes in the CNS there are also deposits of lamellar bodies containing sphingomyelin in Schwann cells, macrophages and endothelial cells. Apart from these deposits the PNS is normal. The defect is not known in group II, but sphingomyelin activity is normal. The PNS is not affected.

Gaucher's disease

Again there are several types, all with an autosomal recessive mode of inheritance. Although the defect in all types is in the enzyme glucocerebroside-β-glucosidase, not all affect the nervous

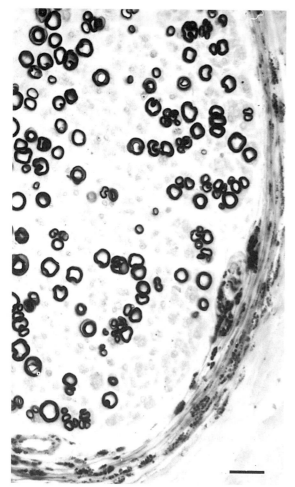

Fig. 18.32 Fabry's disease. Dark-stained lipid inclusions in the perineurium and capillary endothelium. Reduction in myelinated fibre density. (Paraffin section, Flemings fixative, Kultschitsky stain. Bar = 20 μm.)

system. The storage bodies found in type 2 in Schwann cells and macrophages are amorphous and not tubular, as in the Gaucher's cells in the spleen. Axons and myelin are not affected.

Gangliosidoses

There are several types, all with autosomal recessive inheritance with similar clinical presentations but different enzyme abnormalities. The commonest is Tay–Sachs disease. Hexosaminidase A and/or B, or proteins associated with them, are deficient or non-functional. Sandhoff's disease (type 2) has a deficiency of both hexosaminidase A and B, leading to deposits of globoside. There may be some axonal degeneration in peripheral nerves, and lamellar bodies may be found in the axons. The childhood forms are dominated by CNS features. Rare late-onset multisystem degenerations may include a spinal muscular atrophy or neuropathy. Biopsy of the rectal mucosa allows the examination of neuronal cell bodies and axons for deposits of the ganglioside GM_2.

Lipoprotein deficiencies

Tangier disease (α-lipoprotein deficiency)

This is an exceedingly rare autosomal recessive disorder involving α-lipoprotein deficiency. The resultant deposition of cholesterol esters involves many tissues, including nerves. A lipid stain such as Sudan III shows numerous small deposits of stained material in Schwann cells. Both neutral lipid and cholesterol esters are present. Electron microscopy shows these as clear patches in the Schwann cells, as processing largely removes the lipid deposits. The neutral lipid is probably derived from the breakdown of nerve fibres that, for reasons not yet established, are retained in the Schwann cells.

Abetalipoproteinaemia (Bassen–Kornzweig disease)

This rare defect of lipoprotein metabolism is due to the absence of lipoprotein B. The resultant congenital fat malabsorption leads to a deficiency of vitamins A, E and K. Pigmentary retinopathy, peripheral neuropathy and a spinocerebellar degeneration develop during the the first two decades of life. In biopsies of the sural nerve there is a pattern of selective large myelinated fibre loss similar to that seen in vitamin E deficiency. Large doses of vitamin E can prevent or arrest progression of the disease.

Leukodystrophies

Adrenoleukodystrophy

This is an X-linked peroxisomal disorder occurring most commonly in children but also having an adult variant (adrenomyeloneuropathy). There is an accumulation of very long-chain fatty acids (VLFA) in serum, oligodendrocytes and Schwann cells, and cholesterol esters are demonstrable in adrenal and Leydig cells. Motor nerve conduction velocity is reduced and morphologically there is a demyelinating process, with occasional onion bulb formation and some axonal loss. There may be pale, highly curved inclusions in the Schwann cells.

Cockayne's syndrome

The metabolic defect in Cockayne's syndrome is not yet known, but it is a leukodystrophy that may have peripheral nerve involvement, reduced nerve conduction velocity, muscle wasting and areflexia. The peripheral nerves show hypomyelination and occasional onion bulb formations. There may be variable Schwann-cell inclusions.

Miscellaneous

Refsums's disease (phytanic acid storage disease)

Another name for this disease is heredopathia atactica polyneuritiformis. It is a rare autosomal recessive disorder in which a deficiency of α-hydroxyl acid oxidase causes an accumulation of phytanic acid in the serum and tissues. The onset varies between childhood and the third decade. Clinically there is pigmentary retinal degeneration, peripheral neuropathy (often hypertrophic), ataxia and raised CSF protein. Pathologically there is a segmental demyelination, hypertrophic whorls and sometimes crystalline mitochondrial inclusions in the Schwann cells.

Giant axonal neuropathy

This is an autosomal recessive disorder characterized by accumulations of neurofilaments that form tangled masses, distorting and swelling the axons focally to many times their normal diameter (Fig. 18.33). Electron microscopy shows that the unmyelinated axons are also involved. The myelin becomes thinned on the larger giant axons, and may be lost altogether. The swellings are often quite short, and may be found paranodally or internodally. Very high-power magnification shows that the swellings are composed of masses of neurofilaments, often tangled together and sometimes containing denser patches.

Neurofilaments are composed of three proteins described by their molecular weights: 68, 160 and 200 kDa. However, there is no detectable difference in immunocytochemical staining for all three, so there must be some more subtle alteration allowing them to pack together abnormally.

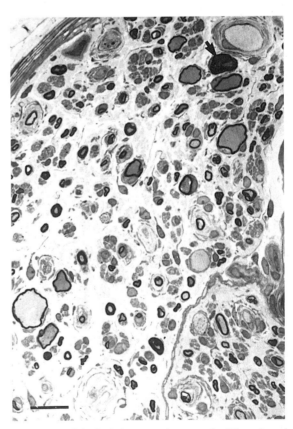

Fig. 18.33 Inherited giant axonal neuropathy. The enlarged axons are thinly myelinated or demyelinated. One axon is atrophic (arrow). (Bar = 20 μm.)

FURTHER READING

Asbury A K & Johnson P C (1978) *Pathology of peripheral nerve*. Philadelphia: W B Saunders.

Babel J, Bischoff A & Spoendlin H (1970) In: *Ultrastructure of the Peripheral Nervous System and Sense Organs*. Edited by A Bischoff. Stuttgart: Georg Thieme Verlag.

Bradley W G, Daroff R B, Fenichel G M & Marsden C D (eds) (1991) *Neurology in Clinical Practice*, Vol. II, Boston: Butterworth-Heinemann.

Thomas P K, Landon D N & King R H M (1991) Diseases of the peripheral nerves. In: *Greenfield's Neuropathology*, 5th edn. Edited by J H Adams, and L W Duchen London: Arnold 1116–1245.

Vital C & Vallet J-M (1987) *Ultrastructural Study of the Human Diseased Peripheral Nerve*, 2nd edn. New York: Elsevier.

Weller R O & Cervos-Navarro, J (1977) *Pathology of Peripheral Nerves*. London: Butterworth.

Index

Abetalipoproteinaemia, 196, 402
Acalculia, 16
Acceleration/deceleration, and brain damage, 133, 140
Acetylcholine, 20
Acid maltase deficiency, 28, 357–358
Acoustic neuromas, 288, 306
Acqueduct, disorders, 235
Acquired immunodeficiency syndrome (AIDS), 1, 122–124, 392
  dementia, 267
  encephalopathy, 122, 123–124
  myelopathy, 123
  myopathy, 362
  opportunistic infections, 123–124
  pathogenesis, 122–123
  see also AIDS-related complex
Actinomycosis, 126
Adamkiewicz artery, 25, 66
Addison's disease, 182
Adenine arabinoside, 201
Adenocarcinoma, lacrimal gland, 331
Adenoid cystic carcinoma, 304, 331–332
Adenomas, pituitary, 19, 270, 299–302
Adenomas, pleomorphic, lacrimal gland, 330–331
Adenosine triphosphate (ATP), 67
Adrenal medulla
  autografts, 151
  fetal, transplantation, 42
Adrenoleukodystrophy, 176, 177–178, 402–403
Adrenomyeloneuropathy, 178
Aesthesioneuroblastomas, 323
Aflatoxin, 186
African trypanosomiasis, 129–130, 206
Ageing, brain, 251–256
  atrophy, 251
  granulovacuolar degeneration, 43
  lacunae, 73–74, 255
  and neurofibrillary tangles, 43
  vascular changes, 255–256
  see also Dementia
Agnosia, visual, 18
Agranular (pyramidal) cortex, 14
Agyria, 231–232
AIDS-related complex (ARC), 122
Alcohol, intoxication, 198–199

neuropathy, 386
nutritional disease, 191, 193–194, 198, 386
Wernicke's encephalopathy, 191, 193–194, 199
see also Fetal alcohol syndrome
Alexander's disease, 176, 178–179, 236
Alpers' disease, 247
Aluminium
  and dialysis dementia, 186–187, 205–206
  neurotoxicity, 186–187, 205–206
Alzheimer type 1 astrocytes, 186
  Wilson's disease, 181–182
Alzheimer type 2 astrocytes, 45, 47, 179
  hepatic encephalopathy, 185
  Wilson's disease, 181, 182
Alzheimer-type dementia, 85, 206
Alzheimer's disease, 9, 43, 44, 213, 257–260
  and βA4-amyloid plaques, 258, 259–260
  cholinergic hypothesis, 260
  head injury, 259
Alzheimer's neurofibrillary degeneration, 42–43, 253–254
Amaurotic familial idiocy, 174
Amblyopia, tobacco, 195, 196
Amino acids
  excitotoxicity, and hypoxia, 68
  metabolic disorders, 179–180
δ-aminobutyric acid, 207
δ-aminolaevulinic acid, 207
Ammon's horn sclerosis, 81, 82
Amoebiasis, 128–129
Amphetamine-related compounds, toxicity, 200
Amphotericin B, 202
Amyloid angiopathy, cerebral, 85
βA4-Amyloid plaques, 252–253, 253, 259–260, 266
Amyloidosis
  familial polyneuropathies, 398–399, 400
  orbital, 315–316
Amyotrophic lateral sclerosis (ALS), 27, 187, 188, 218

Guam variant, 214, 220
Anaesthesia, dissociated, 236–237
Anaesthesia dolorosa, 19
Anencephaly, 228–229
Aneurysms
  congenital, 86
  dissecting, 89
  saccular, 83, 84–88
Angiokeratoma corporis diffusum, 174, 401, 402
Angiomatosis, encephalofacial, 240
Angiopathy
  amyloid, 256, 259
  congophilic, 256, 259
Angiotensin-converting enzyme, 10
Annulus fibrosus, 149
Anterior horn cell loss, 368–369, 370
Antibiotics, intoxication, 201
Antineoplastic agents
  CNS complications, 154
  intoxication, 202
Antiviral agents, intoxication, 201
Anton's syndrome, 17–18
Aortic arch syndrome, 75
Aphasia, conduction, 18
Aponeuroses, orbital, 310
Apoplectic cysts, 84
Apoprotein B, 196
Apraxia, 16, 18
Arachnoid cysts, 231, 298–299
Arachnoidal granulations, and CSF absorption, 60, 238
Arachnoiditis
  chemical, 202
  chronic, 101
Arbovirus infections, 113
Arhinencephaly, 231
Arnold–Chiari malformation, 233–234
  and obstructive hydrocephalus, 60, 238
Arsenic, poisoning, 206, 387
Arsphenamines, complications, 206
Arteries, intracranial/extracranial, irradiation effects, 153
Arteriosclerosis, hyaline, 73, 255
Arteritis see Cerebral arteritis
Artery (ies)
  cerebral hemispheres, 64–65
  hindbrain, 65

Artery (ies) (*contd*)
  spinal, 66
  see also individual arteries
Arthrogryposis multiplex congenita,
  221
Arysulphatase A deficiency, 176
Ascaris strongyloides, 314
Aspartylglycosaminuria, 179
Aspergillosis, 74, 126–127
  orbital, 313–314
Aspergillus flavus, 186
Aspergillus fumigatus, 126
Astrocytes, 31–32
  abnormal, in PML, 116, 117
  Alzheimer type 2, 45, 47
  Bergmann, 199
  cloudy swelling, 45
  fibrillary, 31, 45
  functions, 32
  gemistocytic, 45, 46, 57
  giant, 45
  histological techniques, 8, 9, 10
  immunohistochemistry, 9–10
  protoplasmic, 31–32
  reactive, 48, 105–106, 199
Astrocytomas, 270, 276–281
  anaplastic, 154, 276, 280
  fibrillary, 277–279
  gemistocytic, 279, 280
  histological appearances, 277–281
  pilocytic, 277, 280–281, 284
    intraorbital, 328–329
  pontine, 277
  prognosis. 271
  protoplasmic, 279–280
  subependymal giant-cell, 277, 281
  tectal plate, 306
Astrocytosis, 45–47
  ageing brain, 256
  Creutzfeldt–Jakob disease, 199, 120
Ataxia, 23
  Friedreich's 215, 216, 398
  posterior column, hereditary
    (Biemond), 218
Ataxia-telangiectasia, 217
Atheroma (atherosclerosis)
  ageing brain, 255
  cerebral, and coronary atheroma, 71
  and cerebral infarction, 71–73, 80
  see also Ateriosclerosis
Athetosis, 20
Auditory cortex, 17
Autolysis, post-mortem brain, 36
Autonomic nervous system, diseases,
  221
Autopsy, neonatal, 226
Axolemma, 374
Axonal bulbs, 40, 138, 139
Axonal degeneration, 379–381
Axonal injury, diffuse
  haemorrhagic lesions, 137
  in non-missile injuries, 124, 136–140
Axonal neuropathy, giant, 403
Axonal regeneration, 380, 381–382
Axonotmesis, 384

Axons, 27–28
  histological techniques, 7
  myelination, 374–376
  sodium channels, 376
  transport, 374
  unmyelinated
    degeneration, 380–381 *see*
      Wallerian degeneration
    regeneration, 382
    and Schwann cells, 377
AZT, 360

B virus infection, 111
Babes' nodules, 114
Bacteraemia, reactive microglia, 48
Bacterial infections, 91–101
Balo's disease, 166
Barbiturates, intoxication, 201
Basal ganglia, 18, 20
  calcification, 215
  diseases, 211–212
  status marmoratus (état marbré),
    245
Basilar artery, occlusion, 73
Basilar invagination, 150
Basilary artery, ectasia/tortuosity, and
    hydrocephalus, 60
Basket brain, 238
Bassen–Kornzweig disease, 196, 402
Batten's disease, 171, 174
Becker muscular dystrophy (BMD),
    343–347, 348
Behçet's disease, 75
Bell's palsy, 111
Benedikt's syndrome, 21
Bergmann astrocytes, 32, 199
Beriberi, 191, 194
  neuropathic, 386
BHMH, dying-back neuropathy
    induction, 387
Biemond's ataxia, 218
Bilirubin encephalopathy, 246
Binswanger's disease, 74, 265
Birth injuries, mechanical, 241–242
Blastomyces dermatidis, 125
Blastomycosis, 125
Blepharoplasts, 34, 284
Blood pressure/ICP, Cushing response,
    49, 54
Blood-brain barrier, 36
  dysfunction, 67
Blood-CSF barrier, 36
Bone cysts, aneurysmal, orbital, 325
Bone-forming tumours, orbital, 325,
    326
Borreliosis, 362, 391
Botulism, 205
Bournville's disease, 239–240
Boutons terminaux, 29
  degenerating, 41
Bovine spongiform encephalopathy
    (BSE), 121
Brachiocephalic (innominate) artery, 4
  occlusion, 72

Brain
  ageing *see* Ageing, brain
  biopsy, 8, 271–273
    smear technique, 272, 273
    stains, 273
  blood supply, 35–36
  chemotherapy effects, 154
  coagulation necrosis, 70
  congenital malformations, 225–226
  cysts, post-mortem formation, 36
  development, 223–226
  dissection, 5–6
  fixation, 4–5
  herniae, 50, 52–56
  histological artefacts, 36–37
  hypoxia, selective vulnerability,
    67–68
  and intracranial expanding lesions,
    50, 51–56
  post-mortem autolysis, 36
  purpuric conditions, 90
  removal, 1–3
    newborn, 226
  respirator, Swiss cheese change, 36
  stones, 183, 215
  weight, 251
Brain abscess, 92, 95–97
  amoebic, 129
  in missile head injuries, 146
  in non-missile head injuries, 134,
    145
Brain shift, 24
  and raised ICP, 51–56, 76
Brain stem
  astrocytomas, 277
  blood supply, 65
  compression, 22–23
  damage, and cardiac arrest, 77
  death, and brain autolysis, 36
  neuromelanin, 42
  primary damage, in head injuries,
    137
  reticular formation, 22
  topography, 21
Brain swelling
  congestive, 56, 58
  in non-missile injury, 134, 143
Broca's area
  cerebral cortex, 13, 15
  disease effects, 15
Brodmann areas, cerebral cortex, 14
Brown tumour, orbital, 325
Brown–Séquard syndrome, 148
Brucellosis, 92
Bulbar palsy, progressive, 218
Büngner bands, 380, 381, 382
Bunina bodies, 220
Burning, extradural haematoma,
    141
Burst lobe, 134, 143
Butyrophenones, intoxication, 201

Cachexia, muscular atrophy, 370
Caeruloplasmin deficiency, 181

Calcification, 183, 215
  ageing brain, 256
Calcium, in epileptic neuronal damage, 82
Calcium metabolism, disorders, 183
Canavan–van Bogaert–Bertrand spongy degeneration, 179
Canavan's disease, 179, 236
Candida albicans, 126
Candidosis, 126–127
Capsular haemorrhage, 83
Carbohydrate metabolism, disorders, 180–181
Carbon disulphide, intoxication, 203–204
Carbon monoxide, myelinopathy, 167–168
Carbon monoxide poisoning, 196–197
  brain damage, 80–81, 197
Carbon tetrachloride, 204
Carbonic anhydrase C, 10
Carboxyhaemoglobin, 197
Carcinoid syndrome, 188
Carcinoma
  adenoid cystic, 304, 331–332
  embryonal, 297
  meningeal. 304–305
  metastatic, 304–306
  non-metastatic (remote) effects, 188–190
Cardiac arrest, 68, 76–79
Carnitine deficiency, 360
Caroticocavernous fistula, 88, 140
Carotid arteries, 4
  dissecting aneurysms, 89
  stenosis/occlusion, 71–72
Carpal tunnel syndrome, 394
Caudate nucleus, in Huntington's chorea, 262–263
Central core disease, muscular, 355–356
Central European encephalitis, 113
Cephalohaematomas, 241
Ceramidase deficiency, 174
Cerebellar cortex, microglial shrubwork, 78
Cerebellar degeneration, subacute, 189
Cerebellar hemisphere syndrome, 23
Cerebellar hemispheres, hypoplasia, 234
Cerebello-olivary degeneration (Holmes), 215–216
Cerebello-ocular dysplastic syndrome, 232
Cerebellopontine angle tumours, 306
Cerebellum, 23–24
  blood supply, 65
  irradiation effects, 152–153
  malformations, 233–235
  pan-cerebellar syndrome, 23
  posterior vermis syndrome, 23
Cerebral arteries
  ectasia, 88, 89
  examination, 3–4
Cerebral arteritis

and collagen diseases, 74–75
  giant-cell (temporal), 74–75
  and infarction, 74–75
  micro-organism-associated, 74
  X-irradiation-related, 76
Cerebral atrophy, 251
  alcoholism, 198–199
  hydrocephalus, 58
  Pick's disease, 261
  see also Dementia
Cerebral blood flow (CBF), 66–67
  autoregulation, 66–67
  and hypotension, 76, 79–80
Cerebral contusions
  contrecoup, 136
  coup, 136
  gliding, 134, 136
Cerebral cortex
  damage, and cardiac arrest, 78
  foliation, 224–225
  functional anatomy, 13
  lamination, 224
  layers, 14
Cerebral hemispheres
  arterial supply, 64–65
  dominance, 14
  lobes, 13–14
  venous drainage, 65
Cerebral infarction, 255–256
  anaemic, 69
  and atheroma, 71–73
  developmental stages, 69–70
  haemorrhagic, 69–70
  and hypotension, 76, 79–80
  and hypoxia, 69–70
  and intracranial expanding lesions, 52, 53–54
  partial, 68
  pathogenesis, 70–76
  and ruptured aneurysm, 88
  and strokes, 63, 70–76
Cerebral oedema, 56, 57–58
  definition, 56
  diffuse, 55
  effects and resolution, 58
  hepatic encephalopathy, 185
  hypoglycaemia, 187
  in non-missile injury, 134, 143
Cerebral perfusion pressure (CPP), 49, 66
  failure, cerebral infarction, 76
Cerebral vasomotor paralysis, 49
Cerebrosidosis, 170, 171, 173, 177
Cerebrospinal fluid (CSF)
  in bacterial infections, 92
  cytology, 8
  decreased absorption, 60, 238
  formation/circulation, 34, 58, 59
  gamma-globulin/albumin, multiple sclerosis, 163
  hypersecretion, 60, 238
  otorrhoea/rhinorrhoea, skull fracture, 135
  in virus infections, 104
  volume, 58

Cerebrovascular accidents *see* Strokes
Cerebrovascular disease, 16, 17
Ceroid, in Batten's disease, 174
Cervical myelopathy, 150
Cervical spondylosis, 150
Cervical vertebral arteries, stenosis/occlusion, 71–72
Chagas' disease, 129, 130–131
Charcot–Marie–Tooth disease, 369, 396, 397
Chemotherapy, CNS complications, 154
Chiari malformations, 233–234
Chickenpox, 109–110
Chloramphenicol, 201
Cholesterol metabolism, and Remak fibres, 388
Choline acetyltransferase deficiency, Alzheimer's disease, 260
Chondromas, 304
Chondrosarcomas, 304
Chordomas, 303–304
  sacral, 304
Chorea, 20
  see also Huntington's disease; Sydenham's chorea
Choriocarcinoma, 297
Chorionic gonadotrophin, human, 10, 275
Choristomas, 299
Choroid plexus, 34, 35
  papillomas, 270, 284–285, 286
Chromatolysis, central
  axons, 39, 40
  pellagra, 194
  viral encephalitis, 106
Chromosomal abnormalities, 225, 226–228
Circle of Willis, 64–65
Clioquinol, intoxication, 201
Clostridium botulinum, 205
Clostridium tetani, 205
Coagulation necrosis, 70
Coagulopathy, 90
Coccidioides immitis, 124–125
Coccidioidomycosis, 124–125
Cockayne's syndrome, 176, 179, 403
Coeliac disease, 196
Cold injury, peripheral nerves, 386
Collagen diseases, and cerebral arteritis, 74–75
Coma, diabetic ketoacidotic, 137
Commissural tracts, 224
Computed tomography (CT), 1, 13
  single photon emission (SPECT), 1, 13
  tumour diagnosis, 271, 272
Congenital malformations
  aetiology, 225, 226
  see also named malformations
Coning, cerebellar, 50, 54–55, 56
Connective tissue disorders, inherited, 76
Constructional apraxia, 16
Contusions *see* Cerebral contusions

Convulsions, febrile, 82
Cordotomy, 150–151
Cornea, copper deposition, 181
Corpora amylacea, 32
Corpus callosum
    disease effects, 16
    haemorrhagic lesions, non-missile
        injuries, 137, 140
Corynebacterium diphtheriae, 205, 390
Cot death, 250
Coxsackie viruses, 111
Cranial nerves, tumours, 270, 288–290
Craniopharyngiomas, 303
Craniorrhachischis, 228, 229
Creutzfeldt–Jakob disease, 1, 119–120,
    266
    pathology, 119–120, 121
    safety precautions, 122
    status spongiosus, 258
Cri du chat syndrome, 227
Crow–Fukase syndrome, 394
Cryoglobulinaemia, 396
Cryptococcosis, 74, 124, 125
Cryptococcus neoformans, 124
Cuprizone, toxicity, 167
Cushing response, blood pressure/ICP,
    49, 54
Cushing's syndrome, 188
Cyanide poisoning, 195, 198
Cyanocobalamin deficiency, 195–196
Cyclophosphamide, 202
Cysticercosis, 131
Cysts, 270, 297–299
    arachnoid, 298–299
    colloid, 298
    dermoid, 297–298
        orbital, 315
    enterogenous, 298
    epidermoid, 297–298
    haematic, orbital, 314, 315
    Rathke's cleft, 297
    see also Hydatid cysts
Cytokeratin, 10, 275
Cytomegalovirus (CMV) infection,
    110–111, 392
    fetal, 111, 249
Cytoplasmic bodies, membranous
    Krabbe's disease, 178
    Tay–Sachs' disease, 45, 172, 173
Cytoplasmic inclusions, Pick's disease,
    44
Cytosine arabinoside, 202
Cytosomes, 44

Dacroliths, 332–333
Dacryocystectomy, 332
Dacryocystitis, 332
Dacryocystorhinotomy, 332
Dandy–Walker syndrome, 233, 234
    and obstructive hydrocephalus, 60,
        238
Dapsone, 201
Deafness
    cortical, 17

pure word, 18
Deer/elk, scrapie-like disease, 121
Déjérine–Sottas disease, 397
Déjérine–Thomas cerebellar atrophy,
    217
Delirium tremens, 198
Dementia, 256–267
    AIDS-related, 267
    alcoholic, 198, 266
    Alzheimer type, 85, 206
    definition, 251, 256
    dialysis, 186–187, 205–206
    frontal lobe type, 264
    and malignant disease, 266
    multi-infarct, 74, 255–256, 264–266
    in multiple sclerosis, 266
    and Parkinson's disease, 43, 213,
        214, 220, 264
        cortical Lewy bodies, 264
    post-traumatic, 146
    presenile, 257
    pugilistica, 146, 253, 259, 266
    thalamic, 264
    thiamine, 198
    see also Alzheimer's disease
Demyelination, 24
    autoimmune, 378
    axonal loss, 378
    diabetes mellitus, 187
    and inflammatory disorders,
        388–389
    periaxial, 157, 167
    peripheral nerves, 377–378
    perivenular, 158
    plaques, in multiple sclerosis,
        161–162, 163
    in PML, 116, 117
    primary, 157–166, 377–378
    secondary, 166–168, 378
    tigroid, 179
    toxic, 167
Dendrites, neuronal, 29
Dendritic plaques, 252–253
Denervation atrophy
    anterior horn cell loss, 368–369, 370
    histology, 367–368
    muscle fibres, 366, 367
    and reinnervation, 366–367
Dermatomyositis, 28, 188, 361–364
    age at onset, 361
Desmin, 10
Developmental abnormalities, 223–241
Devic's disease, 166
Di-isopropylfluorophosphonate (DFP),
    intoxication, 205
Diabetes mellitus
    cerebrovascular disease, 187–188
    demyelination, 187
    ketoacidotic coma, 137
    mucor (rhizopus) infections, 188
    peripheral neuropathy, 187, 392–393
Dialysis
    and disequilibrium syndrome, 186
    encephalopathy, 186–187, 205–206
Diastematomyelia, 230, 237

Diencephalon, 224
Dimethylproprionitrile, 387
Diphenylhydantoin, toxicity, 200
Diphtheria, 205, 390
Diplopia, 21
Disconnection syndromes, 13, 18
Disequilibrium syndrome, and dialysis,
    186
Dopamine, 20
    deficiency, fetal tissue
        transplantation, 42
    and Parkinson's disease, 213
Down's syndrome (trisomy 21),
    227–228
    and dementia, 260
    neurofibrillary tangles, 43
Dressing apraxia, 16
Drug abuse
    and cerebral infarction, 76
    and myopathy, 371
Drugs
    allergic sensitivity, 90
    myopathy induction, 371
    peripheral neuropathy induction,
        387–388
Duchenne muscular dystrophy
    (DMD), 343–347
Dura, in brain removal, 1–3
Dysarthria, 23
Dysgraphia, 16
Dyskinesia, reactive, 201
Dyslexia, 16
Dysmyelination, 157, 175–179
Dysphasia, 13
    expressive, 15
        and dementia, 264
    fluent, 16, 17
    receptive, 16, 17
Dysraphic malformations, 223,
    228–231
Dystonia, 20
    musculorum deformans, 20
Dystrophin deficiency
    Duchenne muscular deficiency,
        345–346
    in females, 347

Eaton–Lambert syndrome, 188, 370
Echinococcosis, 131
Echinococcus granulosa, 131
Echoviruses, 111
Ecstasy, myopathy induction, 371
Ectasia, cerebral arteries, 88, 89
Ectoderm, 223
Edwards' syndrome (trisomy 17–18),
    228
Elzholz granules, Schwann cell
    cytoplasm, 377, 380, 385
Embolism
    aorta, 71
    cardiac causes, 71
    and cerebral infarction, 70–71
    fat, 90, 145
    paradoxical, 71

Embolism (contd)
  and strokes, 70–71
Embryonal tumours, 270, 286–288
Emery–Dreifuss muscular dystrophy,
  348–349
Empyema, subdural, pachymeningitis,
  92
Encephalitis, 91
  arbovirus, 113
  herpes simplex virus, 17
  HSV-1 infection, 108
  lethargica, 114, 213–214
  limbic, 189
  viral, acute, 17, 104–107, 158
Encephalocele, 228, 230–231
Encephalomyelitis
  acute disseminated (perivenous), 24,
    157–159
    aetiology, 158–159
    pathology, 157–158
  and carcinoma, 188–189
  experimental autoallergic (EAE),
    and multiple sclerosis, 165
  necrotizing, subacute (Leigh),
    183–184
  viral, 104
Encephalomyopathy, mitochondrial,
  358–360
Encephalopathy
  diabetes mellitus, 187–188
  dialysis, 186–187, 205–206
  hepatic, 184–186, 199
  HIV, 123
  hypertensive, 67, 74
  hypoxic-ischaemic, perinatal,
    243–245
  metabolic, 80–82, 184–188
  pancreatic, 188
  spongiform, 117–122
  subcortical arteriosclerotic, 74
  transmissible, 266
  tuberculous, acute, 98
  uraemic, 186, 188
  see also Wernicke's encephalopathy
Endarteritis, obliterative, tuberculous
  meningitis, 98
Endocarditis, infective
  and brain abscess, 97
  and mycotic aneurysms, 89
Endocrine metabolism disorders,
  182–183
Enolase, neuron-specific, 9, 274
Entamoeba histolytica, 129
Enterovirus infections, 111–113
Eosinophilia-myalgia syndrome,
  364
Eosinophilic granuloma, orbital, 320
Ependyma, 31, 33–34, 35
  reactive, 48
Ependymomas, 270, 282–284, 285
  anaplastic, 282, 284
  myxopapillary, 283, 284, 285
  subependymal, 283, 284, 285
Epilepsy, 17, 81–82
  and calcium influx, 82

idiopathic (primary cryptogenic), 81
post-traumatic, 146–147
symptomatic (secondary), 81–52
temporal lobe (psychomotor), 82
see also Convulsions: Status
  epilepticus
Epithelial membrane antigen, 10
Epstein–Barr virus (EBV), 111
  and AIDS, 122–123
Erdheim–Chester disease, 327–328
Erethism, 208
Erythema migrans, 391
État criblé, 74, 255
État lacunaire, 74, 255
Etat marbré, basal ganglia, 245
Ethanol, intoxication, 198–199
Ethylene glycol, intoxication, 199–200
Exophthalmos, endocrine, 311–312
Experimental autoallergic
  encephalomyelitis (EAE), and
  multiple sclerosis, 165
Eyelids, 310
  capillary haemangiomas, 321

Fabry's disease, 174, 401, 402
Factor VIII/von Willebrand-related
  antigen, 10, 275
Falx cerebri, 49
Farber's lipogranulomatosis, 174
Fascicles, muscle fibres, 339–340
Fasciitis
  eosinophilic, 364
  nodular, 327
Fascioscapulohumeral dystrophy
  (FSHD), 347
Fat embolism, 90
  in non-missile head injuries, 145
Fatty acids, in Krabbe's disease, 178
Fc receptor, 10
Ferrugination, neuronal, 42, 43
Fetal alcohol syndrome, 199, 225, 235
Fetal tissue transplantation, 151
  in dopamine deficiency, 42
  in Parkinson's disease, 42
α-Fetoprotein, 10, 275
Fibres, corticobulbar, 25
Fibronectin, 10
Fibrosarcomas
  meningeal, irradiation-induced, 153
  orbital, 325
Filum terminale, spinal cord, 24
Finnish hereditary amyloidosis, 399
Flexures
  mesencephalic, 224
  spinomedullary, 224
5-fluoruracil, 202
Foix-Alajouanine disease, 89–90
Folch-Lees phospholipid, 33
Foliation, cerebral cortex, 224–225
Follicle-stimulating hormone, 20
Fornix, 14
Fragile X syndrome, 227, 228
Friedreich's ataxia, 215, 216, 398
Frontal lobe, 13, 14

disease symptoms, 15–16
paracentral lobule damage, 'frontal
  incontinence', 15
Fructose metabolism, disorders, 181
Fucosidosis, 179
Fungal infections, 124–128
  orbit, 313–314
  see also named infections

Gait apraxia, 16
Galactocerebroside, 10
Galactocerebroside-β-galactosidase
  deficiency, 177
Galactosaemia, 180
Galactosidases, deficiency, 172, 174
Gangliocytomas, 270, 285
Gangliogliomas, 270, 285–286
Gangliosidosis, 170, 171, 172–173,
  402
  GM1, 171, 172–173
  GM2, 171, 172–173
Gardner's syndrome, 325
Gargoylism, 174
  zebra bodies, 45
Gases, toxic, 196–198
Gaucher's disease, 170, 171, 173, 401
General paralysis of the insane, 100
Gentamicin, 201
Germ-cell tumours, 297
Germinomas, 297
Gerstmann–Strässler–Scheinker
  disease, 120–121
Giant axonal neuropathy, 403
Ginger Jake paralysis, 204
Glia, interfascicular, 32
Glial-axonal junction, 33, 34
Glial fibrillary acidic protein (GFAP),
  9–10, 33, 178, 274
  astrocytosis, 45–47
Glioblastomas, 276, 280, 281
  giant-cell, 280, 282
Gliomas, 270, 275–288
  choroid plexus, 270, 284–285, 286
  definition, 275
  ependymal, 270, 282–284, 285
  grading, 276–281
  mixed, 270, 282, 284
  nasal, 299
  oligodendroglial, 270, 281–282
  optic nerve, 277, 328–329
  Rosenthal fibres, 45
  see also Astrocytomas
Gliomatosis
  cerebri, 277, 281
  meningeal, 275
Gliomesodermal reaction, 45
Gliosarcomas, 280, 282
Gliosis, 45–47
  aqueductal, hydrocephalus, 60
  isomorphic, 45
  subcortical, progressive, 264
  white matter, 245
γ-globulin/albumin, CSF, multiple
  sclerosis, 163

Globus pallidus
  in acquired hepatocerebral
    degeneration, 185–186
  carbon monoxide poisoning, 197
Glomus jugulare tumours, 303
Glucose, blood/CSF levels, 92
Glue-sniffing, 204
Glutamate, excitatory properties, and
    neuronal damage, 69
Glycogen, metabolism disorders,
    muscular, 357–358
Glycogen storage disorders, 180–181
Glycoprotein, myelin-associated, 10
Glycosaminoglycan metabolism,
    disorders, 171, 174–175
Gold, intoxication, 206
Granular cortex, 14
Granulovacuolar degeneration, 254,
    258
  neuronal, 43
Grasp reflex, 15–16
Growth hormone, 20
Growth retardation, intrauterine, 235
Guillain–Barré syndrome, 111,
    388–389
  and acute viral hepatitis, 393
Gummas, neurosyphilis, 100
Gyri, malformations, 231–233

Haemangioblastomas, 240–241, 270,
    294–295
Haemangioendotheliomas, orbital, 322
Haemangiomas
  capillary, eyelids, 321
  cavernous, orbital, 321
Haemangiopericytomas
  meningeal, 269, 270, 293–284
  orbital, 322
Haematomas
  extradural, non-missile injuries, 134,
    141–142
  hypertensive, 84, 85
  intracerebral, 137
    delayed, 141
    non-missile injuries, 134, 143
    and sacular aneurysms, 87–88
  intracranial, 83–84
    non-missile injuries, 134, 135,
      141–143
    raised ICP, 51
    skull fracture, 135
  intradural, non-missile injuries, 134,
    142–143
  subdural, 55, 88
    and dialysis, 187
    non-missile injuries, 134, 142–143
Haematomyelia, 85, 147
Haematopoietic neoplasms, 270,
    295–297
Haemoglobin, carbon monoxide
    affinity for, 80
Haemoglobinopathy, 76
Haemolytic disease, of newborn, 246
Haemorrhage

ball and ring, acute haemorrhagic
    leukoencephalitis, 159, 160
  into spinal cord, 85
  and intracranial expanding lesions,
    52, 53–54
  perinatal, 241–243
  see also various types and regions
Haemosiderosis
  and ruptured aneurysm, 88
  subpial, 88
Hallervordan–Spatz disease, 184,
    211–212
Hallucinations, visual, 18
Hamartomas
  hypothalamic neuronal, 299
  lipomatous, orbit, 325
  retinal, 239
  vascular, 321–322
Hansen's disease, 389–390, 391
Hartnup disease, 180
HBsAg, 1
Head injuries, 133–147
  Alzheimer's disease, 259
  autopsy, 145–146
  incidence, 134
  missile, 133–134, 146–147
    depressed, 146
    penetrating, 146, 147
    perforating, 146
  non-missile, 133, 134–146
    primary damage, 134–141
    secondary damage, 141–145
  petechial haemorrhages, 90
  types, 134
Hemianopia, bitemporal, 20
Hemiballismus, 19, 20
Hemiplegia, 15
  spastic, 21, 22
Hensen's node, 223
Hepatic encephalopathy, 184–186, 199
Hepatic myelopathy, 186
Hepatitis viruses
  and AIDS, 123
  and Guillain-Barré syndrome, 393
Hepatocerebral degeneration, 199
  acquired (non-Wilsonian), 185–186,
    188
Hepatolenticular degeneration
    (Wilson), 20, 181–182
Herniation
  external, 56
  internal, 52
  and intracranial expanding lesions,
    50, 52–56
  reversed tentorial, 56
  supracallosal, 50, 52, 57
  tentorial, 24, 50, 52–54
  tonsillar, 24, 50, 54–55, 56
  transtentorial, 24
Heroin, myopathy induction, 371
Herpes simplex virus (HSV)
  encephalitis, 17, 45, 90
  latency, 108, 109
  RNA transcript, latency-associated,
    109

types, 107
  see also HSV
Herpes zoster, 109–110
Herpesvirus infections, 107–111
  and AIDS, 123
  see also various types
Herpesvirus simiae (B virus) infection,
    111
Heschl's gyrus, 14
Heterotopia, 232, 233, 234
  glial, nasal, 299
  neuron migration failure, 224
Hexacarbons, neuropathies, 204
Hexachlorophane, toxicity, 167, 247
n-Hexane, 204
Hexokinase inhibition, 202
Hexosaminidase deficiency, 172, 402
Hindbrain, blood supply, 65
von Hippel–Landau syndrome,
    240–241, 294–295
Hippocampal formation, 14
Hippocampus, in epilepsy, 81
Hirano bodies, 44, 254–255, 258
Histiocytomas, fibrous
  malignant, 328
  meningeal, 270, 293
  orbital, 327–328
Histiocytosis X, 320
Histological techniques, 6–8
Histoplasma capsulatum, 125
Histoplasmosis, 125
HLA, multiple sclerosis association,
    164
HMSN see Motor/sensory
    neuropathies, hereditary
Hodgkin's disease, 296
  orbital, 317
Holmes' cerebello-olivary
    degeneration, 215–216
Holoprosencephaly, 231, 238
Homocystinuria, 180
Hortega's fountains, 35
HSAN see Sensory/autonomic
    neuropathies, hereditary
HSV-1 infection, 107–109
HSV-2 infection, 107
Human immunodeficiency virus
    (HIV), 1, 122–124
  peripheral neuropathy, 392
Hunter's disease, 171, 174–175, 236
Huntington's disease, 20, 151, 211,
    262–264
Hurler's disease, 171, 174, 175, 236
Hyaline arteriosclerosis, ageing brain,
    255
Hyaline fibres, muscular dystrophies,
    344–345
Hydatid cysts, 131
  and proptosis, 314
Hydranencephaly, 238
Hydrocephalus, 56, 58–61, 233
  active, 58
  acute, 58, 59
  arrested, 58, 59
  choroid plexus papilloma, 285

Hydrocephalus (contd)
  clinical features, 60–61
  communicating, 58, 238
  compensatory (ex vacuo), 58, 78
  definition, 58
  developmental, 238
  external, 58
  hypersecretory, 60, 238
  intermittent, 61
  internal, 58
  and meningitis, 94
  non-communicating, 58
  normal pressure, 61
    dementia, 267
  obstructive, 58, 59–60, 238
  pathogenesis, 58–60, 238
  posthaemorrhagic, 88, 242–243
  and ruptured aneurysm, 88
Hydromyelia, 230
Hygroma, subdural, non-missile injury,
    143
Hypercalcaemia, 188
Hypercapnia, 67
Hypergraphia, 17
Hypermyelination, 379
Hyperpyrexia, malignant, 197–198,
    371–372
Hypertension
  benign intracranial, 61
  and cerebral infarction, 73–74
  microaneuryms, 83
  and multi-infarct dementia, 74
Hypoglycaemia, 188
  brain damage, 81, 82
  cerebral oedema, 187
  perinatal, 246–247
Hyponatraemia, 188
  central pontine myelinolysis, 167
Hypotension
  cerebral infarction, 76, 79–80
  orthostatic, 221
Hypothalamopituitary dysfunction,
    irradiation-induced, 153
Hypothalamus, 19
Hypothyroidism, congenital, 182–183
Hypoxia
  delayed neuronal death, 69
  neuronal damage, 37–39, 68–70
    dendrosomatotoxic/axon-sparing,
      68
    excitatory amino acid-induced,
      68–69
    selective necrosis, 68, 76–77
  perinatal, 20
  selective vulnerability, 67–68
  theories, 68
  structural change, 37–39, 68–70

Idiopathic midline destructive disease
    (IMDD), orbital, 316–317
α-L-iduronidase deficiency, 174
Immunoglobulins, 275
Immunohistochemistry
  techniques, 8–10

tumour diagnosis, 273–275
Inclusion bodies
  in subacute sclerosing
    panencephalitis, 115, 116
  in viral encephalitis, 106, 107, 109
  see also various types
Inclusion body myositis (IBM),
    364–365
  cytoplasmic vacuoles, 364–365
  muscle cell autophagy, 364, 365
Industrial toxins, 203–209, 387
Infantile paralysis, 112
Inflammatory bowel disease, 76
Infratentorial expanding lesions, 56
Iniencephaly, 228
Innominate artery see Brachiocephalic
    (innominate) artery
Insula, cerebral cortex, 14
Intervertebral disc, prolapsed, 148, 149
Intoxications, 196–209
  see also various agents
Intracerebral haemorrhage, amyloid
    angiopathy, 85
Intracranial arteries, occlusion, 72–73
  see also Cerebral arteries
Intracranial expanding lesions, 49–56
  brain herniation, 50, 52–56
  infratentorial, 56
  supratentorial, 52–56
  see also Tumours
Intracranial haemorrhage
  brain tumours, 84–85
  spontaneous, 83–90
    and hypertension, 74, 87
    risk factors, 63
    and strokes, 63
  see also Haematomas
Intracranial pressure (ICP), raised, 24,
    269
  bone erosion, 56
  and intracranial expanding lesions,
    49–56
  pressure-volume curve, 51, 58
  previous episodes, signs, 55–56
  spatial compensation, 49, 51
  stages, 49
  subendocardial haemorrhage, 56
Intraventricular haemorrhage (IVH),
    242, 243
Intraventricular tumours, 306
Iowa hereditary amyloidosis, 399
Irradiation
  brain tumour induction, 153–154
  CNS effects, 151–154
  peripheral nerve damage, 386
Ischaemic cell process, 36, 37–39, 68
Isoniazid, 201

JC virus, and PML, 116
Juvenile xanthogranuloma, orbital, 320

Kainate, 68
Kayser–Fleischer rings, 181

Keratitis, exposure, 328
Kernicterus, 20, 246
Kernohan lesion, 52, 53
Kidneys
  copper deposition, 181
  transplantation, complications, 187
Kimura's disease, 318, 319
Kinky hair disease (Menke), 182
Klebsiella rhinoscleromatosis, 313
Klinefelter's syndrome, 227
Korsakoff's psychosis, 194
Krabbe's disease, 175, 176, 177,
    400–401
Kugelberg–Welander disease, 221, 369
Kuru, 118–119, 266
Kwashiorkor, 191

Lacrimal gland
  lymphomas, 332
  normal structure, 330
  pleomorphic adenoma, 330–331
  tumours, 330–332
Lacrimal sac
  functional anatomy, 332
  inflammatory disease, 332
  tumours, 333
Lacunae, 73–74, 255
Lamina terminalis, 224
Lateral medullary syndrome, 22
Lathyrism, 205
Lead
  inorganic, poisoning, 207
  organic, poisoning, 207–208
  poisoning, 206–208, 387
Leigh's disease, 183–184
Leprosy, 389–390, 391
Leptomeningitis, 91, 92–95
Lesch–Nyhan syndrome, 182
Leucocyte common antigen, 10
Leucotomy, prefrontal, 150
Leukaemia, meningeal, 296
Leukoaraiosis, 256, 266
Leukodystrophy, 169, 175–179,
    402–403
  adreno-, 176, 177–178, 402–403
  Alexander's, 176, 178–179
  globoid-cell (Krabbe), 175, 176,
    177, 400–401
  metachromatic (MLD), 169,
    175–177, 399–400
  Rosenthal fibres, 45
  spongiform, 176, 179
  sudanophilic, 178, 179
Leukoencephalitis, haemorrhagic
  acute, 159–160
  immunological aspects, 159–160
Leukoencephalopathy
  disseminated necrotizing, 202, 203
  irradiation-induced, 152, 153
  progressive multifocal (PML),
    116–117, 123, 168
Leukomalacia
  periventricular, 244
  subcortical, neonatal, 245

Lewy bodies, 44, 211, 212–213, 221
cortical, 264
Lhermitte–Duclos disease, 234–235
Limb girdle dystrophy, 347–348
Limbic structures, 17
Lipid storage diseases
enzyme deficiencies/lipid
interrelations, 171, 172, 173
skeletal muscle, 360
Lipidoses, 399–402
Lipids, metabolic disorders, 170–174
Lipofuscin, 30, 31
Lipofuscinosis, ceroid, neuronal, 171,
174
in Batten's disease, 174
Lipomas, 299
meningeal, 270, 293
orbital, 325
Lipoprotein deficiencies, 402
Liposarcomas, pleomorphic, orbital,
325–326
Lissencephaly, 231–232
Liver, copper deposition, 181
Liver disease, neuropathies, 393
Locked-in syndrome, 22, 73
Lockjaw, 205
Louis–Bar syndrome, 217
Louping-ill encephalitis, 113
Lumbar stenosis, 150
Lupus erythematosus, systemic, 362,
364
Luteinizing hormone, 20
Lyme disease, 362, 391
Lymphadenopathy syndrome (LAS),
122
Lymphocytic proliferations, benign,
orbital, 318–319
Lymphohistioproliferative disorders,
orbital, 317–320
Lymphoid hyperplasia, atypical,
318–319
Lymphoid tissues, mucosa-associated
(MALT), 317
Lymphomas
B-cell, CNS, and AIDS, 124
benign, orbital, 318–319
cerebral, 295–296, 297
grey zone, 318–319
lacrimal gland, 332
malignant
and infections, 190
orbital, 319–320
and renal transplantation, 187
Lymphorrhages, extraocular muscle,
311–312
Lysosomal enzyme disorders, 44–45
Lysosomes, 29, 30
enzyme deficiencies, 169
storage disorders, 169–179, 357–358

McArdle's disease, 28, 357
Macroglobulinaemia, 76
Magnetic resonance imaging (MRI),
13

tumour diagnosis, 271, 272
Malaria, 90, 129
Mamillary bodies, Wernicke's
encephalopathy, 192, 193
Manganese
intoxication, 208
madness, 208
Mannosidosis, 179
Maple syrup urine disease, 180
Marasmus, 83
Marchiafava–Bignami disease, 167, 199
Marie's hereditary cebellar ataxia, 215
Mastoiditis, 92
and brain abscess, 95, 96, 97
Measles virus
inclusion body encephalitis, 116
subacute sclerosing panencephalitis,
114–116
Meckel–Gruber syndrome, 228, 231
Medulla, blood supply, 65
Medulla oblongata, 22–23
Medulloblastomas, 270, 286–288
desmoplastic, 270, 287–288
Megalencephaly, 235–236
Meisserian bodies, 323
Melanin, 42
Melanomas, meningeal, 294
Melanosis, neurocutaneous, 241, 294
MELAS, 358
Membrane attack complex (MAC),
polymyositis, 362
Memory loss, causes, 267
Meninges
carcinomatosis, 304–306
melanocytic lesions, 294
sarcomatosis, 270, 294
tumours, 270, 290–294
Meningiomas, 149, 270, 290–293
anaplastic, 293
angiomatous, 292–293
en-plaque, 291
fibrous, 292
irradiation-induced, 153
meningotheliomatous, 291–292
optic nerve, 329–330
psammomatous, 292, 293
transitional, 292
Meningitis, 35, 91
acute purulent, CSF, 92
aseptic, 104
Epstein–Barr virus, 111
and HSV-1, 108
bacterial subacute, CSF, 92
and cerebral arteritis, 74
exudate, 94
granulomatous, 125
and hydrocephalus, 60, 238
meningococcal, septicaemia, 93
in non-missile head injuries, 134,
145
posterior basal, 94
tuberculous, 74, 92, 97–99
see also Leptomeningitis:
Pachymeningitis
Meningoencephalitis, 91

amoebic, 128–129
and HSV-1, 109
viral, 90, 104
Meningothelial cells, tumours, 270,
290–293
Menke's disease, 182
Menzel cerebellar atrophy, 217
Mercury, poisoning, 208–209, 387
MERRF, 358
Metabolic diseases
and carcinoma, 188
inherited, 169–184
investigations, 169–170
neonatal, 246–247
Metachromatic leukodystrophy
(MLD), 169, 175–177,
399–400
Metals, neurotoxic, 205–209
Metastases, 304–306
Metencephalon, 224
Methanol, intoxication, 199
Methionine synthetase inactivation,
197
Methyl mercury, intoxication, 208–209
N-Methyl-D-aspartate, 68
Methyl-n-ketone, 204
Metronidazole, 202
MHC class II antigens, 10
Microaneurysms, hypertensive, ageing
brain, 255
Microcephaly, 235
Microglia, 34, 35
histological techniques, 8
hyperplasia/proliferation, virus
encephalitis, 105
reactive, 47–48
shrubwork, 78
Microvilli, nodal, Schwann cell, 376
Midbrain, 21
Mikulicz's disease, 332
Mikulicz's syndrome, 332
Millard–Gubler syndrome, 22
Minicore disease, muscular, 356
Mink encephalopathy, 121, 266
Mitochondria
disorders, skeletal muscle, 28
metabolic disorders, 388–360
Mononuclear phagocyte system, CNS,
immunohistochemistry, 10
Mononucleosis, infectious, 392
Morquio syndrome, 171, 175
Morular cells, 130
Mosquito-borne arbovirus encephalitis,
113
Motor cortex damage, and hemiplegia,
15
Motor end plate (MEP) disorders, 366
Motor neuron disease (MND), 188,
218–221, 264, 365, 366, 368
familial forms, 220–221
Guam type, 214, 220
Motor/sensory neuropathies,
hereditary, 369, 378, 379,
396–397
Movement apraxia, 19

Moya Moya disease, 75
MPTP, and parkinsonism, 214
Mucocoele
  lacrimal sac, 332
  orbital, 314, 315
Mucocytes, 37
Mucopolysaccharidoses, 171,
  174–175
Mucormycosis, 74, 127–128, 188
  orbital, 314
Mucosa-associated lymphoid tissue
  (MALT), 317
Multi-infarct dementia, 255–256,
  264–266
  and hypertension, 74
Multiple (disseminated) sclerosis, 24,
  160–166
  acute, 161, 162
  aetiology, 164–165
  Balo's disease, 166
  chronic, 161–162, 163
  diagnosis, 162–164
  and experimental autoallergic
    encephalomyelitis, 165
  genetic aspects, 164, 165
  HLA association, 164
  immunology, 165
  incidence, 160
  neuromyelitis optica (Devic), 166
  pathology, 161–162, 163
  sudanophilic diffuse, 165–166
  variants, 165–166
Multiple system atrophies, 211
Muscles
  biopsy site, 338
  biopsy technique, 337–338
  central core disease, 355–356
  diseases, 337–372
  extraocular, 310, 339
    inflammation, 311–313
  fibre type disproportion, congenital,
    356–357
  fibres, types and staining reactions,
    338–339
  minicore disease, 356
  motor end-point biopsy, 338
  see also Skeletal muscle
Muscular atrophy, progressive, 218
Muscular dystrophies, 28, 343–352
  autosomal recessive, 347
  congenital, 349–350
  see also named types
Mutism, akinetic, 15
Myasthenia
  Eaton–Lambert syndrome, 188, 370
  gravis, 369–370
  neonatal, 370
Mycobacterium leprae, 389
Mycobacterium tuberculosis, 97
Mycosis fungoides, orbital, 317
Mycotic aneurysms, 84, 85–89
Myelin
  basic protein, 164
    antibodies, 10
  degeneration, 41

formation and maintenance, 33
  histological techniques, 7
Myelination, peripheral nerves,
  374–376
Myelinolysis, central pontine, 166–167,
  187, 199
Myelinopathy, carbon dioxide,
  167–168
Myelitis
  necrotic, subacute, 89–90
  transverse, 26, 27, 111, 149
Myelocoele, 229–230
Myeloma, 394
  orbital, 317, 318
Myelomeningocoele, 229, 230, 233,
  238
Myeloneuropathy, nitrous oxide
  poisoning, 197
Myelopathy
  cervical, 150
  hepatic, 186
  HIV-associated, 123
  irradiation-induced, 152
  subacute necrotizing, 189
Myoglobinuria, 357
Myopathies, 188
  AIDS-related, 362
  centronuclear, 353–354
  congenital, 352–353
  drug-induced, 371
  inflammatory, 360–365
    infectious agents, 360–361
  metabolic, 28, 357–360
  myotubular, 353
  nemaline, 354–355
  and systemic disease, 370
Myophosphorylase deficiency, 357
Myosin, 10
Myosin ATPase reaction, 339, 340
Myositis
  inclusion body (IBM), 364–365
  orbital, 312–313
Myotonia, 350–352
  congenita, 351–352
Myotonic dystrophy, 350–351
  congenital, 351, 353
Myxoliposarcomas, orbital, 326–327

Naegleri fowleri, 128
Nageotte residual nodules, 190
Nageotte spiny bracelets, 376
Negri bodies, 106, 114
Nerve biopsy, 28
Nerve sheath tumours, pigmented,
  orbital, 323
Neural crest, 223
Neural folds, 223
Neural plate, 223
Neural tube defects, 223, 228–231
Neural tumours, orbital, 322–323
Neuralgia, post-herpetic, 110
Neurapraxia, 383–384
Neurilemmomas, 270, 288–289, 290

Neuritis, experimental allergic (EAN),
  388–389
Neuroaxonal dystrophies, 184
  Hallervorden-Spatz disease, 184,
    211–212
  infantile, 184
Neuroblastomas, olfactory, 304
Neuroectodermal tumours, primitive
  (PNETs), 288
Neuroepithelial tissue tumours, 270,
  275–288
  see also Gliomas
Neurofibrillary degeneration
  (Alzheimer), 42–43
Neurofibrillary tangles, 206, 211,
  253–254
  Alzheimer's disease, 258
  Down's syndrome, 228
  formation, 254
  and neuritic senile plaques, 260
  supranuclear palsy, 215
Neurofibrils, neuronal, 29
Neurofibromas, 270, 289–290, 291
  orbital, 322
  plexiform, 289
Neurofibromatosis, 238–239, 399
  central, 239
  von Recklinghausen, 238–239, 290,
    322, 399
Neurofilaments (NF), 274
  antibodies, 9
Neurogenesis, 224
Neurogenic disease, skeletal muscle,
  365–369, 370
Neuroglia, 31–34
Neuroleptics, intoxication, 201
Neuromas
  acoustic, 288, 306
  traumatic, 382, 385–386
Neuromelanin, 31, 42
  and ageing, 252
Neuromuscular disease, and
  carcinoma, 188
Neuromyelitis optica (Devic's disease),
  166
Neuronal storage diseases, 169–175
Neuronophagia, 39, 48, 220
  viral encephalitis, 106
Neurons
  abiotrophy, 211
  abnormalities, virus encephalitis, 106
  axonal transection, reaction, 39–41
  ballooned, 45
  central chromatolysis, 39, 40, 182
  cytology, 29–31
  dark cell change, 36, 68
  deafferentation, 39
  dying-back, 196, 205
  ferrugination, 42, 43
  fetal, transplantation, 151
  granulovacuolar degeneration, 43
  histological techniques, 8
  hydropic cell change, 36, 68
  hypoxic damage, 37–39, 68–70
    ghost cell change, 37
Neurinomas, acoustic, 306

Neurons (contd)
  homogenizing cell change, 37, 39
  incrustations, 37, 38
  ischaemic cell change, 36, 37, 38,
    68
  microvacuolation, 37, 38
ischaemic cell process, 36, 37–39, 68
loss, Alzheimer's disease, 258–259
lysosomal enzyme disorders, 44–45
migration/differentiation, 224
necrosis, virus encephalitis, 106, 107
pigments, 42
reactions to disease, 37–45
regeneration, and function recovery,
    40, 41–42
spiny, in Huntington's chorea,
    263–264
transneuronal degeneration, 37
tumours, 285–286
viral inclusions, 45
Neuropathology, techniques, 1–10
  histological, 6–8
  immunohistochemistry, 8–10
Neuropathy
  dying-back, 380, 387
  giant axonal, 403
  peripheral see Peripheral neuropathy
Neuropeptide Y, 264
Neuropeptides, 9
Neuropil, 35
Neuroradiology agents, intoxication,
    202
Neuroradiotherapy agents,
    intoxication, 202
Neurosyphilis, 74
  parenchymatous, 100
  tertiary, 100
Neurotmesis, 384–385
Neurotoxins, 196–209
  environmental, motor neuron
    disease, 368
Neurotransmitters, 9, 20, 29–30
  and Alzheimer's disease, 260
Neurulation, 223
Newborn, autopsy, 226
Nicotinic acid (niacin) deficiency, 194,
    386
Niemann–Pick disease, 170, 171, 173,
    401
Nissl substance, 29, 30
Nitrofurantoin, 201
Nitrogen mustard, 202
Nitroimidazoles, 202
Nitrosoureas, 202
Nitrous oxide, intoxication, 197–198
Nocardia asteroides, 126
Nocardiosis, 126, 127
Non-Hodgkin's lymphomas, 296
Nucleus pulposus, 149
Nutritional deficiencies
  and neuropathy, 386–387
  see also various vitamins

Occipital lobe, 14

diseases, 17–18
Oculomotor nerves, 2
Oculopharyngeal muscular dystrophy,
    349
Oligoastrocyomas, 270, 282
Oligoclonal bands, multiple sclerosis,
    163–164
Oligodendrocytes, 32–33
  abnormal, in PML, 116, 117
  histological techniques, 8
  immunohistochemistry, 10
  reactive, 47
Oligodendrogliomas, 270, 281–282
  anaplastic 270, 282
Olivopontocerebellar degeneration,
    217
Onion bulbs, 378, 379, 388
Opalski cells, 182, 186
Ophthalmoplegia
  progressive external, chronic
    (CPEO), 356–359
  supranuclear, 215
Opiates, intoxication, 201
Opportunistic infections
  AIDS, 123–124
  and renal transplantation, 187
  see also various infections
Optic atrophy, 201
Optic nerve
  gliomas, 277
  tumours, 328–330
Optic neuritis, apraxic, 160
Optic neuropathy, 198
Optic radiation, 16, 17
Oral contraceptives, and cerebral
    infarction, 76
Orbit
  anatomy, 309–310
  apical syndrome, 313
  aponeuroses, 310
  bone-forming tissue-derived tissue
    tumours, 325, 326
  bony, 309–310
  cellulitis, 313
  exenteration specimen, 334
  fibrocyte-derived tumours, 327–328
  fibrosclerosis, multifocal, 309, 310,
    311, 312
  fungal infections, 313–314
  idiopathic inflammation, 310–311
  lipocyte-derived tumours, 325–327
  lymphocytic infiltrates, 310–311
  lymphohistioproliferative disorders,
    317–320
  malignant lymphomas, 319–320
  metastatic tumours, 333
  myositis, acute, 312–313
  parasitic infections, 314
  post-mortem removal, 333–334
  ruptured cysts, 314–315
  sclerosing pseudotumours, 309, 310,
    311, 312
  soft tissue tumours, 322, 323–325
  vascular malformations, 321–322
  vascular neoplasms, 322

Orbital diseases, 309, 334
  clinicopathology, 309
  inflammatory, 310–317
Orbital tumours, 306, 317–328
Orbitofrontal cortex, 15
Organophosphorus compounds,
    intoxication, 204
Osteitis
  and brain abscess, 95–96
  chronic, 92, 93
Osteoarthritis, cervical spine, and
    vertebral artery occlusion, 72
Osteoblastomas, benign, orbital, 325
Osteomas, orbital, 325, 326
Osteosarcomas, orbital, 325, 326
Otitis media, 92
  and brain abscess, 95, 96, 97
Otorrhoea, CSF, 135

Pachygyria, 233
Pachymeningitis, 91, 92
  cervicalis hypertrophica, 100
Pacinian corpuscles, 374
Paget's disease, 150
Pain
  congenital, insensitivity to (HSAN
    type V), 398
  thalamic, 19
Pallidotomy, 150
Palsy, supranuclear, progressive,
    214–215, 264
Panencephalitis
  and congenital rubella, 116
  sclerosing subacute (SSPE), 45,
    114–116, 168
Paralysis, periodic, 351–352
Paramyotonia congenita, 351–352
Paraplegia
  apraxic, in multiple sclerosis, 160
  hareditary spastic (Strümpl),
    217–218
  traumatic, 147, 148
Paraproteinaemia, benign nonoclonal,
    394–395
Paraquat, 214
Parastriate (association visual) cortex,
    17
Parietal lobe, 14
  disease symptoms, 16
Parinaud's syndrome, 21, 24
Parkinsonism, 9, 21
  dementia complex of Guam, 43,
    214, 220
  drug/toxin-induced, 214
  Lewy bodies, 44
  postencephalitic, 43, 114, 213–214
Parkinson's disease, 21, 150, 151,
    212–213
  cortical Lewy bodies, 264
  and dementia, 213, 214, 220, 264
  fetal tissue transplantation, 42
Parkinson's syndrome see Parkinsonism
Patau's syndrome (trisomy 13–15),
    228

Pelizaeus–Merzbacher disease, 176, 179
Pellagra, 167, 194, 196, 386
Perimysium, 339
Perinatal neuropathology, 241–250
Perineuronal satellite cells, 32
Peripheral nerves
  biopsy, 382–383
  cold injury, 386
  demyelination, 377–378
  disorders, 27–28
  epineurium, 374
  fixation problems/handling artefacts, 382–383
  mechanical injury, 383–386
  perineurium, 373
  pressure palsies, 393–395
    hereditary liability to, 398
  radiation damage, 386
  structure, 373–382
    abnormal, 377–382
    normal 373–377
  trunks, 373
Peripheral neuropathy, 28, 383–403
  acquired, 386–396
  in AIDS, 124
  alcoholic, 198, 199
  antibacterial agent-associated, 201
  and coeliac disease, 196
  hereditary, 369
  and infections, 389–392
  and malignant disease, 188
  nutritional, 386–387
  post-gastrectomy, 196
  and systemic disorders, 392–396
Petechial haemorrhages
  acute haemorrhagic leukoencephalitis, 159
  encephalopathy, hypertensive, 90
  non-missile head injury, 140
  Wernicke's encephalopathy, 192, 193
Phakomatoses, 217, 238–241
Phenothiazines, intoxication, 201
Phenylketonuria, 180, 235
4-Phenylpyridine, 214
Phenytoin, toxicity, 200
Phosphorus, intoxication, 209
Phosphorylase deficiency (McArdle), 28, 357
Phytanic acid storage disease, 378, 403
Pick bodies, 44, 261–262
Pick's disease, 260–262
  cytoplasmic inclusions, 44
Pigment metabolism, disorders, 182
Pineal cell tumours, 306
Pinealoblastomas, 325
Pink disease, 208
Pituitary gland, 19–20
  adenomas, 270, 299–302
  anterior, normal, 299, 300
  apoplexy, 302
  carcinoma, 270, 302
  hormones, 19–20
  removal, 4

Pituitary hormones, localization, 10
Placodes, ectodermal, 223
Plaques, neuritic senile, 252–253
  Alzheimer's disease, 258
  Creutzfeldt–Jakob disease, 120
  kuru, 119
  and neurofibrillary tangles, 260
Plasma cell dyscrasias, malignant, 394
Plasmacytomas, orbital, 318
Plasmodium falciparum, 129
Platybasia, 238
Plumbism, 206–208, 387
PML *see* Leukoencephalopathy, progressive multifocal (PML)
Polioencephalitis, 104
Poliomyelitis, 27, 111–113
Polyarteritis nodosa, 74
  arterial fibrinoid necrosis, 364
Polycythaemia rubra vera, 76
Polydystrophy, cerebral progressive (Alpers), 247
Polymicrogyria, 232, 233
Polymyositis, 28, 188, 361–364
Polyneuropathy, amyloid, familial, 398–399, 400
Polyradiculoneuropathy
  acute inflammatory, demyelinating (AIDP), 388–389
  chronic inflammatory, demyelinating (CIDP), 378, 380, 389
Polyribosomes, 29, 30
Pompe's disease, 180, 181, 357
Pons, 21–22
  dorsolateral infarction, 21–22
  paramedian infarction, 22
Pontine myelinolysis, central, 166–167, 187, 199
Porencephaly, 237–238
Porphyria, 182
Portuguese hereditary amyloidosis, 398, 399
Positron emission tomography (PET), 1, 13
Posterior root ganglia, and carcinoma, 190
Potassium, and periodic paralysis, 352
Prealbumin, 275
Prefrontal leucotomy, 150
Pregnancy/puerperium
  and cerebral infarction, 76
  venous/venous sinus thrombosis, 83
Primitive neuroectodermal tumours (PNETs), 288
Prion diseases, 117–124
Prion proteins, 121–122
Prolactin, 20
Proptosis, and hydatid cysts, 314
Prosencephalon, 224
Prosopagnosia, 18
Protein-calorie deficiency, 191, 196
Protozoal infections, 128–131
Protozoal infections, 128–131
Psammoma bodies, orbital astrocytomas, 330
Pseudotabes, 187

Pulseless disease, 75
Punch-drunk syndrome, 146, 253, 259, 266
Purine metabolism, disorders, 182
Purkinje cells, 32
Pyramidal tracts, degeneration, 220
Pyridoxal deficiency, 194–195
Pyridoxamine deficiency, 194–195
Pyridoxine deficiency, 194–195
Pyrimidine metabolism, disorders, 182

Quisqualate, 68

Rabies, 113–114, 391
Radionecrosis, cerebral, 152, 153
Radiotherapy, CNS complications, 151–154
Ragged red fibres, 359–360
Ranvier's node, 33, 376
Rathke's cleft cyst, 297
von Recklinghausen's disease, 238–239, 290, 322, 399
Reflexes, primitive, and frontal lobe damage, 15–16
Refsum's disease, 378, 403
Reich granules, Schwann cell cytoplasm, 377
Reinnervation, and denervation atrophy, 366–367
Remak fibres, 377, 380
  and cholesterol metabolism, 388
Remyelination, 378
Renaut bodies, 384
Respirator brain, 36
Respiratory distress syndrome, 242
Restless legs syndrome, 393
Retinoblastomas, 325
Retroviruses, and multiple sclerosis, 164
Reye's syndrome, 186
Rhabdoid tumours, malignant, orbital, 324
Rhabdomyomas, 239, 240
Rhabdomyosarcomas
  alveolar, 324
  orbital, 322, 323–324
Rheumatic fever, 75
Rheumatoid arthritis, 364
Rhinencephalon, 14
Rhinorrhoea, CSF, 135
Rhombencephalon, 224, 225
Ricin agglutinin, 10
Riley–Day syndrome, 398
Risus sardonicus, 205
Rod cells, 47, 48
Root pain, 25
Rosenthal fibres, 45, 178
Roussy–Lévy syndrome, 396, 397
Rubella, congenital, 249–250
Rubella encephalitis, progressive, 116
Russian (Far Eastern) spring-summer encephalitis, 113

S-100 protein, 9, 274
Saccular aneurysms, 83, 84–88
Sandhoff disease, 171, 172, 402
Sanfilippo syndrome, 171, 175
Sarcoidosis, 396
  meningeal, 101
  orbital, 315, 316
Sarcomas, alveolar soft tissue, 324, 325
Sarcomatosis, meningeal, 270, 294
Satellite cells, perineuronal, 32
Satellitosis, 47
Saturday night palsy, 383
Scalp
  irradiation effects, 151–152
  non-missile injury, 134
Schilder's disease, 178
Schistosoma spp, 131
Schistosomiasis, 131
Schizophrenia, 267
Schmidt–Lanterman incisures, 376,
    377, 379
  fixation artefact, 383
Schwann cells, 33, 374–376
  onion bulbs, 378, 379
  plasma membrane, 376
  and unmyelinated axons, 377
Schwannomas, 149, 270, 288–289,
    290
  acoustic, 288, 306
  orbital, 322–323
  spinal, 289
Sclerosis
  amyotrophic lateral *see* Amyotrophic
    lateral sclerosis (ALS)
  cerebral diffuse, 175
  concentric (Balo's disease), 166
  sudanophilic, diffuse, 165–166
Scrapie, 121, 266
Sellar region, tumours, 270, 299–303
Sensory cortex, 15, 16
Sensory/autonomic neuropathies,
    hereditary, 397–398
Septicaemia, 90
Shock, endotoxic, 90
Shy–Drager syndrome, 221
Sickle-cell disease, 76
Siderophages, 48
Sinusitis, frontal, 92
Sjøgren's syndrome, 332
Skeletal muscle
  diseases, 28
  fibres
    atrophy, 340–341
    hypertrophy, 341
  hypercontraction, 342
  interfibrillary network, 339, 341
  mitochondrial disorders, 28
  necrosis/regeneration, 342
  normal parameters, 339
Skull
  base
    abnormalities, and hydrocephalus,
      60
    examination, 4
  irradiation effects, 151–152
  penetrating injury, epilepsy, 82

Skull fractures, non-missile injury,
    134–135
Sleeping sickness, 129–130, 206
Slow virus infections, 117–124
SMON syndrome, 201
Snout reflex, 16
Soft tissue tumours, orbital, 322,
    323–325
Solvents, industrial, toxicity, 204, 387
Somatostatin, 264
Somites, mesodermal, 223
Spheroids, 220
  in neuroaxonal dystrophy, 184, 211
Sphingolipidoses, 170–174
Sphingomyelinosis, 170, 171, 173, 401
Spina bifida
  cystica, 228, 229–230
  occulta, 228, 230
Spinal arteries, 25
  occlusion, 73
Spinal cord
  anterior horn lesions, 27
  blood supply, 65–66
  central syndrome, 27
  complete transection, 26–27
  compression, 148–150
  disorders, 25–27
  duplication, 230
  examination, 6
  haemorrhage into, 85
  hemisection, 148
  injuries, 147–150
  malformations, 229–231, 236–237
  posterolateral degeneration, 27
  removal, 3
  subacute combined degeneration,
    27, 195
  'toothpaste effect', 3
  topography, 24–25
  tumours, 306
  vascular malformations, 89–90
  vascular syndromes, 27
Spinal injuries, 147–150
Spinal muscular atrophy (SMA),
    347–348, 369, 370, 371, 372
  familial, 221
  reinnervation/compensatory
    hypertrophy, 367
Spinal nerves, tumours, 270, 288–290
Spine, fractures, 147
Spinocerebellar degeneration, 215–221
Spinothalamic tracts, 25
Spondylosis, cervical, 150
Spongiform encephalopathies
  animal-transmissible, 121
  human-transmissible, 118–121
SSPE *see* Panencephalitis, sclerosing
    subacute (SSPE)
Staggers, 194
Status epilepticus, 82
Status marmoratus, basal ganglia, 245
Status spongiosus
  Creutzfeldt–Jakob disease, 119, 258
  kuru, 119
  Leigh's disease, 183
Steatorrhoea, 196

Steroid myopathy, 371
Striatonigral degeneration, 214
Strokes
  and cerebral infarction, 63, 70–76
  incidence, 63
  and ischaemic heart disease, 71
  risk factors, 63
  and spontaneous intracranial
    haemorrhage, 63
  spontaneous intracranial
    haemorrhage, 83
Strümpl hereditary spastic paraplegia,
    217–218
Sturge–Weber syndrome, 240
Subacute necrotizing
    encephalomyelopathy (Leigh),
    183–184
Subarachnoid haemorrhage, 4, 83, 85
  and hydrocephalus, 60, 238
  perinatal, 241–242
  and saccular aneurysms, 87
Subclavian artery, 4
  occlusion, 72
Subclavian steal syndrome, 72
Subdural haemorrhage, birth injury,
    241
Subendocardial haemorrhage, and
    raised ICP, 56
Subependymal haemorrhage, 242
Subependymomas, 283, 284, 285
Substantia nigra
  diseases, 212–215
  fetal, transplantation, 42
Sudanophilic diffuse sclerosis, 165–166
Sudden infant death syndrome, 250
Sulci
  central, development, 225
  malformations, 231–233
Sulphoiduronate sulphatase deficiency,
    175
Superior saggital sinus, 2
Supracallosal hernia, 50, 52, 57
Supranuclear palsy, progressive,
    214–215
  and dementia, 264
Suprasellar tumours, 306
Supratentorial intracranial expanding
    lesions, 52–56
Sydenham's chorea, 20
Sylvian fissures, development, 225
Synapses, 29–30
Synaptic vesicles, 29–30
Synaptophysin, antibodies, 9
Syphilis, 100
  congenital, 247
  meningovascular, 74
Syringomyelia, 27, 230, 236–237
  gliotic tissue, 45
  post-traumatic, 148
Systemic disease
  CNS manifestations, 188–190
  and myopathy, 370

Tabes dorsalis, 27, 100, 101
Taboparesis, 100

Taenia echinococcus, 314
Taenia solium, 131
Takayasu's arteritis, 75
Tangier disease, 402
Tardive dyskinesia, 201
Tay–Sachs' disease, 170, 171, 172–173, 235, 402
    membranous cytoplasmic bodies, 45
Telencephalon, 224
Temporal lobe, 14
    disease symptoms, 16–17
    epilepsy (psychomotor), 82
Tenon's capsule, 310
Tentorial hernia, 50, 52–54
    reversed, 56
Tentorial incisura, 49
Tentorium cerebelli, 49
Teratomas, 297
    orbital, 320, 321
Tetanus, 205
Thalamotomy, 150, 151
Thalamus
    efferent/afferent connections, 18–19
    functional anatomy, 18–19
    haemorrhagic infarction, 54
Thallium, intoxication, 209, 387
Thiamine deficiency, 386
Thiamine dementia, 198
Thrombotic thrombocytopenic purpura, 75, 90
Thyrotoxicosis, 188
Thyrotropin, 20
Tick-bite neuropathy, 362, 391
Tick-borne arbovirus encephalitis, 113
Tin, toxicity, 167, 209
Tobacco amblyopia, 195, 196
Tolosa-Hunt syndrome, 313
Toluene, 204
Tomaculi, 398
Tonsillar hernia, 50, 54–55, 56
Tourniquet paralysis, 383
Toxic encephalopathy, 201
Toxic neuropathies, 387
    see also Intoxications
Toxic oil syndrome, 204
Toxocariasis, 131
Toxoplasma gondii, 128, 247
Toxoplasmosis, 128
    congenital, 248–249
    tissue cysts, 249
Trace metal metabolism, disorders, 181–182
Transient ischaemic attacks (TIAs), 63–64
Transneuronal degeneration, 39
Tremor, 20–21
Trench foot, 386
Treponema pallidum, 100, 247
Trichinosis, 131
Trichloroethylene, 204, 387
Triethyltin, intoxication, 209
Trimethyltin, intoxication, 209
Triorthocresyl phosphate (TOCP), neuropathy, 204–205, 387
Trisomies, 227–228

Triton tumour, 322
Trypanosomiasis, 129–131
    African, 129–130, 206
    South American, 129, 130–131
Tryptophan deficiency, 194
Tuberculomas, 97, 99–100
Tuberculosis, 97–100
    encephalopathy, 98
    meningitis, 92, 97–99
    spinal, 150
Tuberous sclerosis, 239–240
Tuffstone bodies, 400
Tumours, 269–307
    anatomical sites, 305–306
    biopsy, 271–273
    brain stem compression, 22–23
    classification, 269–270
    cranial nerves, 270, 288–290
    diagnosis, 271–275
    embryonal, 270, 286–288
    germ-cell, 297
    haematopoietic, 270, 295–297
    imaging, 271–272
    immunohistochemistry, 273–275
    incidence/prevalence, 270–271
    irradiation, 151
    irradiation-induced, 153–154
    lacrimal sac, 333
    malignant, neuropathy, 396
    meningeal, 270, 290–294
    mesenchymal non-meningothelial, 270, 293–294
    metastatic, 304–306
    neuroectodermal primitive (PNETs), 288
    neuroepithelial tissue, 270, 275–288
    optic nerve, 328–330
    orbital, 306, 317–328
    regional, local extension, 303–304
    sellar region, 270, 299–303
    spinal, cord compression, 148, 149
    spinal nerves, 270, 288–290
    uncertain histogenesis, 294–295
    see also various types and regions
Turner's syndrome, 227

Ulegyria, 245
Uraemia
    encephalopathy, 186, 188
    sensory neuropathy, 393

Varicella zoster (VZ) virus infection, 109–110
Vascular diseases
    and dementia, 264–266
    and malignancy, 190
Vascular malformations
    brain/spinal cord, 84, 86, 89–90
    orbital, 321–322
Vasculitis
    intracranial haemorrhage, 84
    and muscle infarcts, 364
    and neuropathies, 393–394
Vasospasm, in subarachnoid

    haemorrhage, 76
Veins
    cerebral hemispheres, 65
    hindbrain, 65
Venous sinuses, thrombosis, 83
Venous thrombosis, 83
Vermis, agenesis, 234
Vertebrobasilar arteries, 64, 65
Vimentin, 10, 274–275
Vinca alkaloids, 202
Viral inclusions, neuronal, 45
Virchow–Robin space, 35
Virus encephalitis, 104–107
Virus infections, 103–124
    acute encephalitis, 104–107
    aseptic meningitis, 104
    CSF abnormalities, 104
    demyelination, 168
    infection routes, 103–104
    persistent, 114–117
    slow viruses, 117–124
    types, 104
Visual cortex, 17
Vitamin B group deficiencies, 193–196, 386
Vitamin E deficiency, 184, 196, 386–387

Waldenström's macroglobulinaemia, 394
Wallenberg's syndrome, 22
Wallerian degeneration, 39, 40–41, 47, 157
    in diffuse axonal injury, 138, 139
    spinal cord, 147, 148
    staining changes, 41
    tabes dorsalis, 100, 101
Water intoxication, 188
Waterhouse–Friderichsen syndrome, 93
Weber's syndrome, 21
Wegener's granulomatosis, 311
    orbital, 316, 317
Werdnig–Hoffmann disease, 221, 369
Wernicke–Korsakoff syndrome, 194, 196, 266, 267
Wernicke's area, 16
Wernicke's encephalopathy, 17, 167, 191–194, 199
Whipple's disease, 196
White matter, hypoxic-ischaemic lesions, perinatal, 244–245
Wilson's disease, 20, 181–182
Wohlfart–Kugelberg–Welander disease, 221, 369

Xanthogranulomas, juvenile, orbital, 320

Zebra bodies
    gargoylism, 45
    in Hurler's disease, 174, 175
Zidovudine (AZT), and mitochondrial myopathy, 360
Zonula occludens, 36